Pharmacological Management of Neurological Diseases

Pharmacological Management of Neurological Diseases

Editor: Jessie Miller

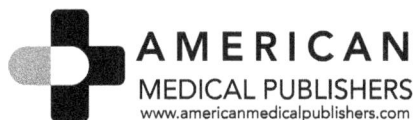

AMERICAN
MEDICAL PUBLISHERS
www.americanmedicalpublishers.com

AMERICAN
MEDICAL PUBLISHERS
www.americanmedicalpublishers.com

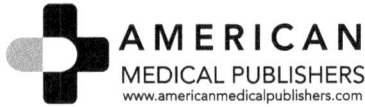

Cataloging-in-Publication Data

Pharmacological management of neurological diseases / edited by Jessie Miller.
  p. cm.
Includes bibliographical references and index.
ISBN 978-1-63927-555-7
1. Neuropharmacology. 2. Nervous system--Diseases. 3. Nervous system--Diseases--Treatment.
4. Neurosciences. 5. Pharmacology. I. Miller, Jessie.
RM315 .P43 2022
615.78--dc23

American Medical Publishers,
41 Flatbush Avenue,
1st Floor, New York,
NY 11217, USA

ISBN 978-1-63927-555-7 (Hardback)

Contents

Preface

I am honored to present to you this unique book which encompasses the most up-to-date data in the field. I was extremely pleased to get this opportunity of editing the work of experts from across the globe. I have also written papers in this field and researched the various aspects revolving around the progress of the discipline. I have tried to unify my knowledge along with that of stalwarts from every corner of the world, to produce a text which not only benefits the readers but also facilitates the growth of the field.

The nervous system transmits signals through the body and coordinates actions and sensory information. Any disorder of the nervous system is known as a neurological disorder. A variety of symptoms can be caused by structural, biochemical, or electrical abnormalities in the brain, spinal cord or other nerves. Paralysis, muscle weakness, poor coordination, loss of sensation, seizures, confusion, pain and altered levels of consciousness are a few such symptoms. There are many known neurological disorders such as Alzheimer's disease, ataxia, cerebral aneurysm, epilepsy, etc. which are studied and treated within the fields of neurology and clinical neuropsychology. Lifestyle changes, physiotherapy, neurorehabilitation, pain management, medication and surgery are some of the treatments for neurological disorders. This book is compiled in such a manner, that it will provide in-depth knowledge about the pharmacological management of neurological diseases. It includes some of the vital pieces of work being conducted across the world, on various topics related to the pharmacological management of neurological diseases. Those in search of information to further their knowledge will be greatly assisted by this book.

Finally, I would like to thank all the contributing authors for their valuable time and contributions. This book would not have been possible without their efforts. I would also like to thank my friends and family for their constant support.

Editor

ASS234, As a New Multi-Target Directed Propargylamine for Alzheimer's Disease Therapy

José Marco-Contelles[1]*, Mercedes Unzeta[2], Irene Bolea[2], Gerard Esteban[2],
Rona R. Ramsay[3], Alejandro Romero[4], Ricard Martínez-Murillo[5], M. Carmo Carreiras[6]
and Lhassane Ismaili[7]

[1] Laboratory of Medicinal Chemistry, Institute of General Organic Chemistry, Cajal Institute (CSIC), Madrid, Spain,
[2] Departament de Bioquímica i Biologia Molecular, Facultat de Medicina, Institut de Neurociències, Universitat Autònoma de
Barcelona, Barcelona, Spain, [3] Biomedical Sciences Research Complex, University of St Andrews, St Andrews, UK,
[4] Department of Toxicology and Pharmacology, Faculty of Veterinary Medicine, Complutense University of Madrid, Madrid,
Spain, [5] Neurovascular Research Group, Department of Molecular, Cellular and Developmental Neurobiology, Cajal Institute
(CSIC), Madrid, Spain, [6] Research Institute for Medicines and Pharmaceutical Sciences (iMed.ULisboa), Faculty of Pharmacy,
University of Lisbon, Lisbon, Portugal, [7] Laboratoire de Chimie Organique et Thérapeutique, Neurosciences Intégratives et
Cliniques EA 481, Université Franche-Comté, Université Bourgogne Franche-Comté, UFR SMP, Besançon, France

Edited by:
Andrew C. McCreary,
Janssen Prevention Center,
Netherlands

Reviewed by:
Alfredo Meneses,
Center for Research and Advanced
Studies of the National Polytechnic
Institute (CINVESTAV), Mexico
Christopher Graham Parsons,
Merz Pharmaceuticals, Germany

*Correspondence:
José Marco-Contelles
iqoc21@iqog.csic.es

Highlights:

- **ASS2324** is a hybrid compound resulting from the juxtaposition of donepezil and the propargylamine **PF9601N**
- **ASS2324** is a multi-target directed propargylamine able to bind to all the AChE/BuChE and MAO A/B enzymes
- **ASS2324** shows antioxidant, neuroprotective and suitable permeability properties
- **ASS2324** restores the scopolamine-induced cognitive impairment to the same extent as donepezil, and is less toxic
- **ASS2324** prevents β-amyloid induced aggregation in the cortex of double transgenic mice
- **ASS2324** is the most advanced anti-Alzheimer agent for pre-clinical studies that we have identified in our laboratories

The complex nature of Alzheimer's disease (AD) has prompted the design of Multi-Target-Directed Ligands (MTDL) able to bind to diverse biochemical targets involved in the progress and development of the disease. In this context, we have designed a number of MTD propargylamines (MTDP) showing antioxidant, anti-beta-amyloid, anti-inflammatory, as well as cholinesterase and monoamine oxidase (MAO) inhibition capacities. Here, we describe these properties in the MTDL **ASS234**, our lead-compound ready to enter in pre-clinical studies for AD, as a new multipotent, permeable cholinesterase/monoamine oxidase inhibitor, able to inhibit Aβ-aggregation, and possessing antioxidant and neuroprotective properties.

Keywords: multi-target directed ligands, Alzheimer's disease, monoamine oxidases, cholinesterases, drugs

INTRODUCTION

Alzheimer's disease (AD) is the most common neurodegenerative disease in the elderly (Karlawish, 2011). AD is characterized by progressive neuronal death resulting in severe cognitive impairment. Two distinctive hallmarks of AD are the presence of accumulated beta-amyloid (Aβ) plaques (Hamley, 2012) and hyperphosphorylated tau protein in the form of intracellular neurofibrillary tangles (NFT) (Wang et al., 2013). Although the precise etiology of AD is not yet known, there is a large consensus in describing it as a complex disorder caused by many factors, including loss of cholinergic transmission, protein misfolding and Aβ aggregation, oxidative stress, free radical formation (Rosini et al., 2014), and metal dyshomeostasis (Huang et al., 2004). AD pathology also involves dysfunctional neurotransmitters and synapse loss (Aisa et al., 2010; Villemagne and Chételat, 2016).

In the following sections we describe the currently accepted AD hypotheses, and our recent contribution to the development of new multipotent propargylamines for AD therapy.

ALZHEIMER'S DISEASE HYPOTHESES

Cholinergic Hypothesis

Cholinergic neurotransmission modulates both cognitive function and cortical plasticity (Arendt and Bigl, 1986) and plays a significant role in the control of cerebral blood flow (Biesold et al., 1989), cortical activity (Détári et al., 1999), learning and memory (Deutsch, 1971). The first physiological evidence of the involvement of the cholinergic system in AD pathology was a reduction of the neurotransmitter acetylcholine (ACh), which constitutes the basis of the cholinergic hypothesis of AD (Deutsch, 1971), used to discover the first anti-AD agents. Acetylcholinesterase (AChE) is expressed in cholinergic neurons, its primary function being the rapid breakdown of ACh during the cholinergic neurotransmission. In addition to rapid breakdown by AChE, ACh can also be metabolized by butyrylcholinesterase (BuChE) (Mesulam et al., 2002) but with different kinetic behavior. Whereas AChE pre-dominates in neurons and exhibits high affinity for ACh, BuChE is present in endothelia, glia and neuronal cells with low affinity for ACh and high K_M values (Soreq and Seidman, 2001).

β-Amyloid Cascade Hypothesis

The amyloid hypothesis postulates that neurodegeneration in AD is caused by abnormal accumulation of Aβ plaques in various areas of the brain (Evin and Weidemann, 2002). The Aβ senile plaques contain Aβ peptides with 39–43 amino acid residues, proteolytically derived from the sequential enzymatic action of β- and γ-secretases of transmembrane APP (Coulson et al., 2000). Within plaques, Aβ peptides in β-sheet conformation assemble and polymerise into fibrillar, protofibers and polymorphic oligomers (Selkoe, 1994). *In vitro*, the Aβ aggregation process is highly susceptible to pH, ionic strength of the solvent,

purification process and temperature. Distinct oligomerization and assembly processes between $A\beta_{1-40}$ and $A\beta_{1-42}$ have been described (Bitan et al., 2003). While dimers and trimers are the most toxic forms of $A\beta_{1-42}$, $A\beta_{1-40}$ reaches equilibrium from monomers to tetramers. Recent findings have shown that soluble oligomeric species were able to disrupt synaptic function (Lambert et al., 1998) and support the belief that soluble dimeric species are highly toxic (Jin et al., 2011). However, direct Aβ-peptide neurotoxicity has been difficult to prove in animal models (Serrano-Pozo et al., 2013). Since the postulation of the amyloid hypothesis, a number, but a number of unsuccessful efforts have been undertaken in clinical research in order to develop novel drugs based on this concept.

Oxidative Stress

Increased production of Reactive Oxygen Species (ROS) have been observed in AD (Praticò, 2008) and, consequently, elevated levels of oxidative markers including damage to proteins, lipids, carbohydrates, and nucleic acids. Antioxidant enzymes were also found to be increased in specific AD brain regions (Sultana et al., 2011). Not surprisingly, the oxidative stress (OS) hypothesis of AD has emerged as a key event in the progress of the disease. In addition, evidence suggests that secretion and deposition of Aβ within the neurons are compensatory measures taken by cells in effort to protect themselves against damage triggered by OS (Hayashi et al., 2007).

Cellular oxidative damage has also been linked to tau hyperphosphorylation and formation of NFTs (Lee et al., 2004). As a consequence, cells succumb to neurodegeneration exhibiting the distinctive cognitive impairment observed in AD patients (Zhu et al., 2007). Altogether, the primary role of OS in AD has been overwhelmingly confirmed, offering the chance to develop specific disease-modifying antioxidant approaches to cure or prevent the development of the disease.

Biometal Hypothesis

The increased levels of ROS are reflected in a deregulated content of biometals such as iron, copper and zinc in the brain of AD patients. Recent findings point to brain OS as one of the earliest changes in AD pathogenesis that might play a central role in the disease progression (Lee et al., 2010). Redox-active metals are capable of stimulating free radical formation *via* the Fenton reaction. Biometals have also been shown to mediate Aβ toxicity in AD (Duce et al., 2010). It has been shown that Aβ peptide itself is a strong redox-active metalloprotein able to directly produce hydrogen peroxide and OH^- in the presence of copper or iron, which, in turn, are enriched in the amyloid cores of senile plaques (Huang et al., 1999). Also, biometals can interact directly with Aβ peptide enhancing its self-aggregation and oligomerization at low physiological concentrations or at mildly acidic conditions (Huang et al., 1999). Moreover, metals can promote tau hyperphosphorylation and subsequent formation of NFTs inducing its aggregation upon interaction with Aβ (Yamamoto et al., 2002).

Abbreviations: AD, Alzheimer's Disease; AChE, acetylcholinesterase; MAO, monoamine oxidase; MTDL, multi-target directed ligand.

DRUGS FOR AD THERAPY

To date, only five drugs have ever been approved for AD therapy. Tacrine, rivastigmine, galantamine and donepezil are AChEI, whereas memantine is a NMDA receptor antagonist.

Tacrine, a competitive AChEI and the first drug to be approved for use in AD by the FDA in 1993, was withdrawn from the market in 2013 due to the high incidence of side effects, mostly derived from hepatotoxicity (Qizilbash et al., 1998). Rivastigmine, a non-selective pseudoreversible ChE inhibitor (Bullock and Lane, 2007), has been reported to have less side effects as well as positive benefit after administration to mild-to-moderate AD patients (Birks and Grimley Evans, 2015). Galantamine, a weak competitive reversible AChEI (Greenblatt et al., 1999) is also a potent allosteric modulator of nicotinic acetylcholine receptors—$\alpha_4\beta_2$, $\alpha_7/5$-HT_3, $\alpha_3\beta_4$, and $\alpha_6\beta_4$—in certain areas of the brain, and potentiates the effects of orthoesteric agonists (Dajas-Bailador et al., 2003; Akk and Steinbach, 2005). Donepezil is a brain-permeable reversible non-competitive ChE inhibitor approved for use in AD (Birks and Harvey, 2006) and currently the most widely prescribed drug for the treatment of this disease. Donepezil is highly selective for AChE over BuChE activity (405:1) (Nochi et al., 1995). Compared to other approved AChEI, donepezil is similarly effective in ameliorating cognitive and functional decline in AD with comparable safety and tolerability (Doody et al., 2014).

Memantine is a glutamatergic agent, the first and only NMDA receptor antagonist approved by FDA in 2003 for the treatment of moderate-to-severe AD and dementia. Memantine binds to NMDA receptors with a low-micromolar IC_{50} value, exhibits neuroprotective activities against Aβ toxicity (Hu et al., 2007), tau phosphorylation (Song et al., 2008), neuroinflammation (Willard et al., 2000), and oxidative stress (Figueiredo et al., 2013).

In the face of general neuronal loss, monoamine oxidase (MAO) inhibitors are used to preserve remaining levels of catecholamine neurotransmitters by inhibiting MAO A in neurons or MAO B in serotonergic neurons, glia and astrocytes. Since MAO B activity is increased in AD, MAO B inhibitors may be of potential therapeutic interest both to maintain neurotransmitter levels and to decrease hydrogen peroxide production (Mandel et al., 2005). For example, rasagiline and selegiline are propargylamines that irreversibly inhibit brain MAO B, but also show neuroprotective activities mainly due to their propargyl moiety (Zindo et al., 2015).

The lack of therapeutic effectiveness of the current drugs based on the single-target paradigm (León et al., 2013) for the treatment of AD prompted the search of MTDL, designed by molecular hybridization of different pharmacophoric moieties from well-known bioactive molecules, able to bind to multiple targets associated with AD. As a result, a number of standard natural or synthetic compounds, including donepezil, tacrine or rivastigmine (Samadi et al., 2011), curcumin (Malar and Devi, 2014), berberine (Jiang et al., 2011) or 8-hydroxyquinoline (Gomes et al., 2014) have been used for this purpose.

Based on this background, we have designed several MTD propargylamines (MTDP) for the potential treatment of AD. All these compounds bear the N-benzylpiperidine group present in donepezil and the N-propargylamine motif present in L-deprenyl (used in Parkinson's disease) and in **PF9601N** (**Figure 1**), a potent and selective MAO B inhibitor with neuroprotective effect demonstrated *in vitro* and *in vivo* using different experimental models (Pérez et al., 1999). The donepezil motif gives inhibition

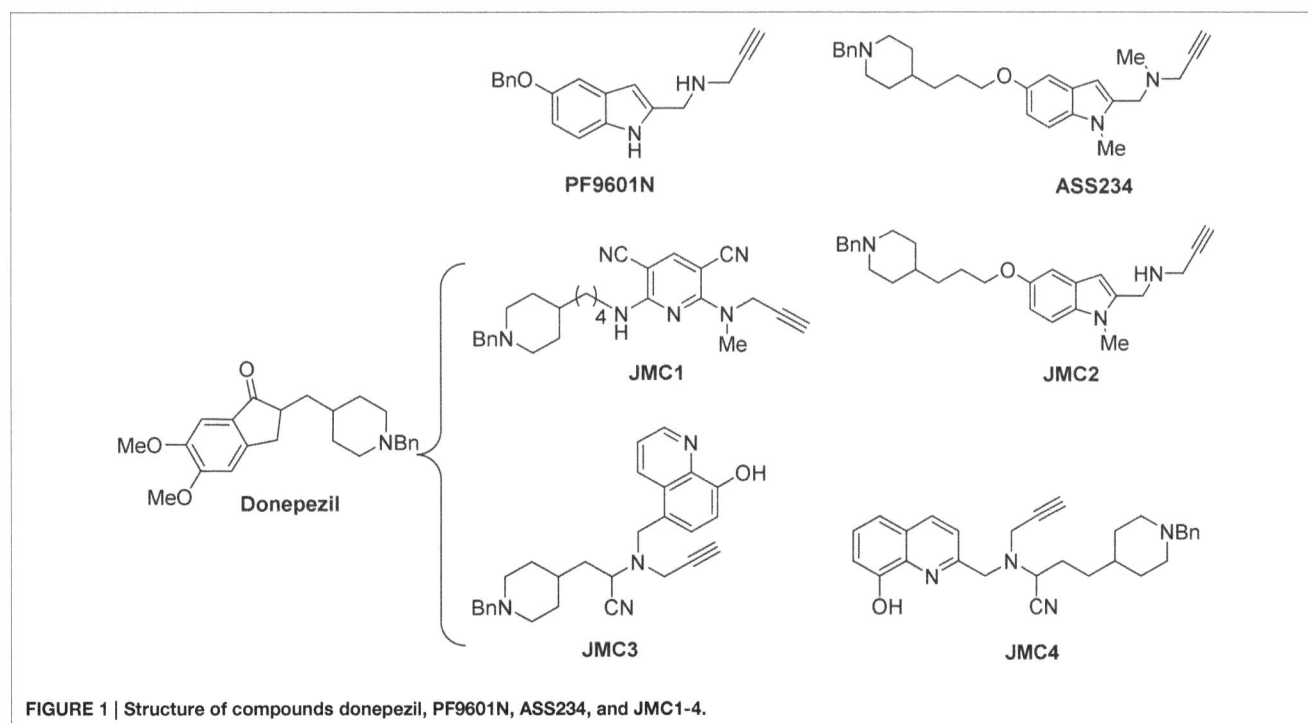

FIGURE 1 | Structure of compounds donepezil, PF9601N, ASS234, and JMC1-4.

of the cholinesterases as well as the ability to inhibit the aggregation of Aβ via the acetylcholinesterase peripheral site, whereas the propargylamine inhibits MAO enzymes and also gives neuroprotection. Both scaffolds were linked by different heterocyclic ring systems, such as pyridine, indole or 8-hydroxyquinoline, affording diverse MTDP as promising drugs to be used in AD therapy (**Figure 1**). This strategy led to **ASS234** (**Figure 1**) with the anti-cholinergic activity of donepezil, selective MAO A inhibition and neuroprotective properties (Bolea et al., 2011).

Next, with the aim of searching for improved MTDLs, two series of novel structurally derived compounds from **ASS234** as multipotent donepezil-pyridyl and donepezil-indolyl hybrids were designed and pharmacologically assessed. Thus, the donepezil-pyridyl compound **JMC1** (**Figure 1**) was identified as a very potent hAChE inhibitor (IC_{50} = 1.1 nM) and a moderate hBuChE inhibitor (IC_{50} = 0.6 µM) with total selectivity toward human MAO B (hMAO B) (Bautista-Aguilera et al., 2014b). The donepezil-indole **JMC2** (**Figure 1**) exhibited the most interesting profile as a potent MAO A inhibitor (IC_{50} = 5.5 nM) moderately able to inhibit MAO B (IC_{50} = 150 nM), AChE (IC_{50} = 190 nM), and BuChE (IC_{50} = 830 nM) (Bautista-Aguilera et al., 2014a). Moreover, the kinetic analysis showed that **JMC2** is a mixed-type AChE inhibitor able to span both the catalytic and peripheral sites (CAS and PAS) of this enzyme, a fact further confirmed by molecular modeling studies. Propargylamines **JMC3** (Wang et al., 2014) and **JMC4** (Wu et al., 2015) bear a N-benzylpiperidine moiety from donepezil and a 8-hydroxyquinoline group (**Figure 1**). **JMC3** (**Figure 1**) was further characterized as an irreversible MAO and mixed-type ChE inhibitor in low micromolar range, and, in addition, it strongly complexed Cu (II), Zn (II), and Fe (III) (Wang et al., 2014). From theoretical ADMET analyses, **JMC3** exhibited proper drug-likeness properties and good brain penetration suitable for CNS activity. **JMC4** (**Figure 1**) showed similar inhibitory behavior as dual ChE/MAO inhibitor (Wu et al., 2015).

The propargylamine **ASS234** (**Figure 1**), deserves further discussion. **ASS234** is a very potent human MAO A and MAO B inhibitor with a IC_{50} values of 5.44 ± 1.74 and 177 ± 25 nM, respectively, inhibiting also both ChEs (IC_{50} (human AChE) = 0.81 ± 0.06 µM; IC_{50} (human BuChE) = 1.82 ± 0.14 µM) (Esteban et al., 2014) (**Figure 2**). In contrast, the reference compounds had only their single expected activity: donepezil was ineffective at inhibiting MAO activities, and **PF9601N**, while potently and selectively inhibiting MAO B displayed no

interaction with the ChEs (Bolea et al., 2011). To sum up, **ASS234** combines the best properties of donepezil and **PF9601N**, simultaneously inhibiting ChE to boost cholinergic transmission and MAO to raise catecholamine levels (Bolea et al., 2013).

Although **ASS234** is a reversible inhibitor of both ChEs with micromolar affinity, it is a highly potent irreversible MAO A inhibitor, similar to clorgyline. Although the initial reversible binding parameter (K_i value of 0.4 µM) indicated that **ASS234** has a lower affinity for MAO A than clorgyline (K_i value of 0.02 µM), and this was also reflected in the higher K_I for the irreversible reaction, the full inactivation of MAO A was rapid. The crystal structure of hMAO B after inactivation by **ASS234** highlighted the formation of a covalent adduct with the flavin N5 atom which, based on the spectral changes, occurs also with the MAO A cofactor (Esteban et al., 2014). Although the N-benzylpiperidine moiety is not fully visible in the electron density in the crystal structure at 1.8 Å resolution, the mass determinations demonstrate that **ASS234** binds as the intact molecule to the MAO B active site, which rules out the possibility that the inhibitor may undergo degradation in the cellular context (Esteban et al., 2014).

Next, the presumed therapeutic potential of **ASS234** was evaluated following its administration to a rat model of vascular dementia based on the permanent bilateral occlusion of the common carotid arteries with experimental vascular dementia to determine its impact on brain neurotransmitter systems. In this rat model, the administration of **ASS234** for 5 days resulted in a potent and selective inhibition of MAO A activity in brain as well as a concurrent increase in concentrations of serotonin and the catecholamines, dopamine and noradrenaline (Stasiak et al., 2014). All these findings allow us to conclude that **ASS234** is able to bind to multiple targets identifying it as an interesting MTDL molecule to be considered for therapeutic development against AD.

The mechanism by which **ASS234** plays a neuroprotective role in AD pathology remains unclear. Recent evidence suggests that the Wingless-Type MMTV Integration Site (Wnt) signaling pathway is important in neuroprotection (Toledo et al., 2008), so we investigated whether **ASS234** activated the Wnt signaling pathway (del Pino et al., 2014). Total RNA was extracted from SH-SY5Y cells incubated with **ASS234** (5 µM) for 24 h and gene expression evaluated for some members of the Wnt1 class signal (Wnt1, Wnt2b, Wnt3a) which represent the "canonical" Wnt/β-catenin pathway, and for some members of the Wnt5a class signal (Wnt6, Wnt5a) which represent

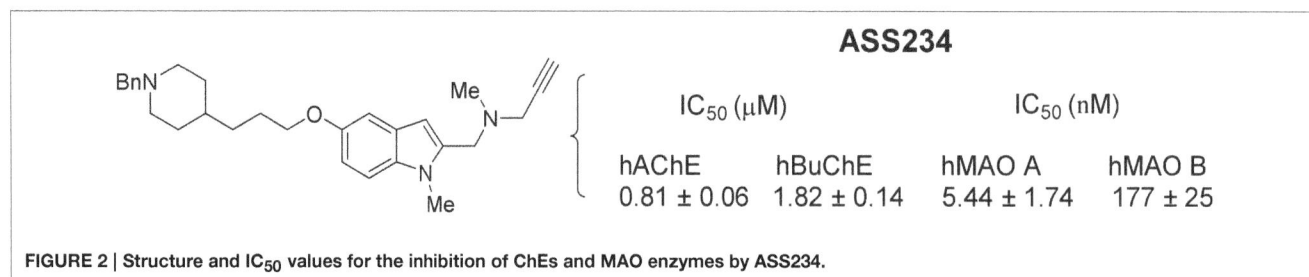

ASS234

	IC_{50} (µM)		IC_{50} (nM)	
hAChE	hBuChE	hMAO A	hMAO B
0.81 ± 0.06	1.82 ± 0.14	5.44 ± 1.74	177 ± 25

FIGURE 2 | Structure and IC_{50} values for the inhibition of ChEs and MAO enzymes by ASS234.

the "non-canonical" Wnt/PCP and Wnt/Ca^{2+} pathways. In ASS234-treated cells, gene expression of Wnt2b, Wnt5a, and Wnt6 was significantly increased. Ingenuity pathways analysis (IPA) identified a number of downstream genes regulated by the Wnt canonical pathways. One of these genes, PPARδ, a key gene related to neuroprotective effects against AD, was significantly increased by ASS234 treatment. From these results, we concluded that ASS234 induced canonical and non-canonical Wnt pathways, which presents another possible mechanism through which this compound can mediate its protective action. Knowing that the activation of Wnt signaling rescues memory loss and improves synaptic dysfunction in transgenic mice model of AD amyloid pathology, these findings indicate that ASS234 could be a novel promising drug for AD therapy.

In order to ascertain the suitability of MTDL ASS234 for pre-clinical studies, the obvious, preliminary and necessary "proof of concept" was assessed. First of all, we investigated the effect of a single-dose of ASS234 (0.62 mg/Kg) on cognition using the scopolamine test. Not surprisingly, scopolamine significantly decreased the exploratory preference for a novel object in the retention trial. Scopolamine-induced cognitive deficit is assessed as a decreased recognition index (RI) in comparison with non-treated and vehicle control groups. After a single dose of ASS234, a significant increase of the RI was observed, indicating reversal of memory impairment induced by scopolamine. Thus, the scopolamine-induced amnesia was reversed by concomitant administration of ASS234 (0.12 mM/kg) which in fact significantly improved the cognitive performance about 13.1%, suggesting that ASS234 exerts its therapeutic effect by enhancing natural memory processes.

Some preliminary studies have been carried out to assess the amyloid plaque burden and gliosis in the cortex of the ASS234 treated group of the transgenic AD model, APPswe/PS1ΔE9 tg mice. Daily administration of ASS234 for 16 weeks at a dose of (0.62 mg/Kg) resulted in apparent reduction in the number of neuritic plaques in the cerebral cortex and hippocampus in comparison to vehicle treated mice. Cortical plaque deposition was significantly decreased in tg mice given the ASS234 treatment compared to tg controls. As in the cortex, the Aβ plaque load in tg mice treated with ASS234 also decreased in the hippocampus, although statistical significance was not reached. These findings indicate that ASS234 has a greater effect upon plaque load in the cerebral cortex than in the hippocampus of APPswe/PS1ΔE9 tg mice.

Next, since microgliosis and astrocytosis, indicative of neuroinflammation, are prominent aspects of this AD mouse model, we proceed to identify the effect of ASS234 on neuroinflammation through the evaluation of the immunohistochemical distribution of the astrocyte marker protein GFAP and of the microglia/macrophage-specific protein iba-1. Significantly decreased GFAP and iba-1 immunostainings were observed in the cortex of the ASS234 treated tg mice compared with that of controls, suggesting a beneficial effect of ASS234 on neuroinflammation. All procedures with animals were carried out in accordance with European Communities Council Directive (2010/63/UE) on animal experiments under a protocol approved by the Animal Welfare Committee of the Cajal Institute (CSIC, Madrid, Spain) and by the Institutional Animal Ethics Committee of the Spain Council for Scientific Research (CSIC), adhering to the recommendations of the European Council and Spanish Department of Health for Laboratory Animals (R.D. 53/2013). A special effort was made to reduce the number of animals used in the study, and the number of animals assigned to each group was to be kept to a minimum necessary to achieve enough significance.

The promising results described above led us to assess the hepatotoxicity and metabolism of compound ASS234. Preliminary toxicity studies of ASS234 along with donepezil and tacrine were performed in parallel in the human cell line HepG2. The results showed that all three compounds reduced cell viability in a concentration-dependent manner, but at very high concentrations (100 and 300 μM) ASS234 exhibited lesser toxicity than the reference compounds, donepezil and tacrine.

CONCLUDING REMARKS

The results presented in this review strongly reinforce the suitability of MTDLs as an appropriate pharmacological approach to be used in AD therapy. Amongst all the compounds tested, MTDL ASS234 particularly has emerged as an interesting lead compound for the design of novel MTDL with a good MAO/AChE inhibitory potency, a significant activity against amyloid aggregation, neuroprotective and anti-apoptotic properties, as well as potent antioxidant capacities, so may have a potential disease-modifying role in the treatment of AD. Given the strong correlation of neuroinflammation with amyloid burden, our results showing that ASS234 considerably reduces both amyloid burden and inflammation in the cerebral cortex of treated tg mice underline the beneficial action of ASS234 in slowing the progression of AD.

From the safety point of view, the affinity of compound ASS234 for MAO A is of concern due to well known "cheese effect," which occurs when tyramine enters the circulation and potentiates sympathetic cardiovascular activity by releasing noradrenaline, and should be considered in future developments of the molecule by analyzing tyramine potentiation and the ASS234 MAO selectivity in the brain. In sum, ASS234 has clearly overcome the "proof of concept," and remains our most advanced anti-Alzheimer agent for pre-clinical studies targeted to find a new therapy for this devastating disease.

AUTHOR CONTRIBUTIONS

JM and MU wrote the manuscript. GE, IB, RR, AR, RM, MC, and LI corrected the manuscript.

ACKNOWLEDGMENTS

MU and JM thank MINECO (Spain) for support (Grant SAF2012-33304; SAF2015-65586-R). RR, MU, GE, and JM thank EU (COST Action 1103) for support.

REFERENCES

Aisa, B., Gil-Bea, F. J., Solas, M., García-Alloza, M., Chen, C. P., Lai, M. K., et al. (2010). Altered NCAM expression associated with the cholinergic system in Alzheimer's disease. *J. Alzheimer's Dis.* 20, 659–668. doi: 10.3233/JAD-2010-1398

Akk, G., and Steinbach, J. H. (2005). Galantamine activates muscle-type nicotinic acetylcholine receptors without binding to the acetylcholine-binding site. *J. Neurosci.* 25, 1992–2001. doi: 10.1523/JNEUROSCI.4985-04.2005

Arendt, T., and Bigl, V. (1986). Alzheimer plaques and cortical cholinergic innervation. *Neuroscience* 17, 277–279. doi: 10.1016/0306-4522(86)90243-5

Bautista-Aguilera, O. M., Esteban, G., Bolea, I., Nikolic, K., Agbaba, D., Moraleda, I., et al. (2014a). Design, synthesis, pharmacological evaluation, QSAR analysis, molecular modeling and ADMET of novel donepezil-indolyl hybrids as multipotent cholinesterase/monoamine oxidase inhibitors for the potential treatment of Alzheimer's disease. *Eur. J. Med. Chem.* 75, 82–95. doi: 10.1016/j.ejmech.2013.12.028

Bautista-Aguilera, O. M., Esteban, G., Chioua, M., Nikolic, K., Agbaba, D., Moraleda, I., et al. (2014b). Multipotent cholinesterase/monoamine oxidase inhibitors for the treatment of Alzheimer's disease: design, synthesis, biochemical evaluation, ADMET, molecular modeling, and QSAR analysis of novel donepezil-pyridyl hybrids. *Drug Des. Devel. Ther.* 8, 1893–1910. doi: 10.2147/DDDT.S69258

Biesold, D., Inanami, O., Sato, A., and Sato, Y. (1989). Stimulation of the nucleus basalis of Meynert increases cerebral cortical blood flow in rats. *Neurosci. Lett.* 98, 39–44. doi: 10.1016/0304-3940(89)90370-4

Birks, J., and Harvey, R. J. (2006). Donepezil for dementia due to Alzheimer's disease. *Cochrane Database Syst. Rev.* CD001190. doi: 10.1002/14651858.CD001190.pub2

Birks, J. S., and Grimley Evans, J. (2015). Rivastigmine for Alzheimer's disease. *Cochrane Database Syst. Rev.* 4:CD001191. doi: 10.1002/14651858.CD001191.pub3

Bitan, G., Kirkitadze, M. D., Lomakin, A., Vollers, S. S., Benedek, G. B., and Teplow, D. B. (2003). Amyloid beta -protein (Abeta) assembly: abeta 40 and Abeta 42 oligomerize through distinct pathways. *Proc. Natl. Acad. Sci. U.S.A.* 100, 330–335. doi: 10.1073/pnas.222681699

Bolea, I., Gella, A., Monjas, L., Pérez, C., Rodríguez-Franco, M. I., Marco-Contelles, J., et al. (2013). Multipotent, permeable drug ASS234 inhibits Abeta aggregation, possesses antioxidant properties and protects from Abeta-induced apoptosis *in vitro. Curr. Alzheimer Res.* 10, 797–808. doi: 10.2174/15672050113109990151

Bolea, I., Juárez-Jimenez, J., de los Ríos, C., Chioua, M., Pouplana, R., Luque, F. J., et al. (2011). Synthesis, biological evaluation, and molecular modeling of donepezil and N-[(5-(benzyloxy)-1-methyl-1H-indol-2-yl)methyl]-N-methylprop-2-yn-1-amine hybrids as new multipotent cholinesterase/monoamine oxidase inhibitors for the treatment of Alzheimer's disease. *J. Med. Chem.* 54, 8251–8270. doi: 10.1021/jm200853t

Bullock, R., and Lane, R. (2007). Executive dyscontrol in dementia, with emphasis on subcortical pathology and the role of butyrylcholinesterase. *Curr. Alzheimer Res.* 4, 277–293. doi: 10.2174/156720507781077313

Coulson, E. J., Paliga, K., Beyreuther, K., and Masters, C. L. (2000). What the evolution of the amyloid protein precursor supergene family tells us about its function. *Neurochem. Int.* 36, 175–184. doi: 10.1016/S0197-0186(99)00125-4

Dajas-Bailador, F. A., Heimala, K., and Wonnacott, S. (2003). The allosteric potentiation of nicotinic acetylcholine receptors by galantamine is transduced into cellular responses in neurons: Ca^{2+} signals and neurotransmitter release. *Mol. Pharmacol.* 64, 1217–1226. doi: 10.1124/mol.64.5.1217

del Pino, J., Ramos, E., Aguilera, O. M., Marco-Contelles, J., and Romero, A. (2014). Wnt signaling pathway, a potential target for Alzheimer's disease treatment, is activated by a novel multitarget compound ASS234. *CNS Neurosci. Ther.* 20, 568–570. doi: 10.1111/cns.12269

Détári, L., Rasmusson, D. D., and Semba, K. (1999). The role of basal forebrain neurons in tonic and phasic activation of the cerebral cortex. *Prog. Neurobiol.* 58, 249–277. doi: 10.1016/S0301-0082(98)00084-7

Deutsch, J. A. (1971). The cholinergic synapse and the site of memory. *Science* 174, 788–794. doi: 10.1126/science.174.4011.788

Doody, R. S., Thomas, R. G., Farlow, M., Iwatsubo, T., Vellas, B., Joffe, S., et al. (2014). Phase 3 trials of solanezumab for mild-to-moderate Alzheimer's disease. *N. Engl. J. Med.* 370, 311–321. doi: 10.1056/NEJMoa1312889

Duce, J. A., Tsatsanis, A., Cater, M. A., James, S. A., Robb, E., Wikhe, K., et al. (2010). Iron-export ferroxidase activity of beta-amyloid precursor protein is inhibited by zinc in Alzheimer's disease. *Cell* 142, 857–867. doi: 10.1016/j.cell.2010.08.014

Esteban, G., Allan, J., Samadi, A., Mattevi, A., Unzeta, M., Marco-Contelles, J., et al. (2014). Kinetic and structural analysis of the irreversible inhibition of human monoamine oxidases by ASS234, a multi-target compound designed for use in Alzheimer's disease. *Biochim. Biophys. Acta* 1844, 1104–1110. doi: 10.1016/j.bbapap.2014.03.006

Evin, G., and Weidemann, A. (2002). Biogenesis and metabolism of Alzheimer's disease Abeta amyloid peptides. *Peptides* 23, 1285–1297. doi: 10.1016/S0196-9781(02)00063-3

Figueiredo, C. P., Clarke, J. R., Ledo, J. H., Ribeiro, F. C., Costa, C. V., Melo, H. M., et al. (2013). Memantine rescues transient cognitive impairment caused by high-molecular-weight abeta oligomers but not the persistent impairment induced by low-molecular-weight oligomers. *J. Neurosci.* 33, 9626–9634. doi: 10.1523/JNEUROSCI.0482-13.2013

Gomes, L. M., Vieira, R. P., Jones, M. R., Wang, M. C., Dyrager, C., Souza-Fagundes, E. M., et al. (2014). 8-Hydroxyquinoline Schiff-base compounds as antioxidants and modulators of copper-mediated Abeta peptide aggregation. *J. Inorg. Biochem.* 139, 106–116. doi: 10.1016/j.jinorgbio.2014.04.011

Greenblatt, H. M., Kryger, G., Lewis, T., Silman, I., and Sussman, J. L. (1999). Structure of acetylcholinesterase complexed with (-)-galanthamine at 2.3 A resolution. *FEBS Lett.* 463, 321–326. doi: 10.1016/S0014-5793(99)01637-3

Hamley, I. W. (2012). The Amyloid beta peptide: a chemist's perspective. *Role in Alzheimer's and fibrillization. Chem. Rev.* 112, 5147–5192. doi: 10.1021/cr3000994

Hayashi, T., Shishido, N., Nakayama, K., Nunomura, A., Smith, M. A., Perry, G., et al. (2007). Lipid peroxidation and 4-hydroxy-2-nonenal formation by copper ion bound to amyloid-beta peptide. *Free Radic. Biol. Med.* 43, 1552–1559. doi: 10.1016/j.freeradbiomed.2007.08.013

Hu, M., Schurdak, M. E., Puttfarcken, P. S., El Kouhen, R., Gopalakrishnan, M., and Li, J. (2007). High content screen microscopy analysis of A beta 1-42-induced neurite outgrowth reduction in rat primary cortical neurons: neuroprotective effects of alpha 7 neuronal nicotinic acetylcholine receptor ligands. *Brain Res.* 1151, 227–235. doi: 10.1016/j.brainres.2007.03.051

Huang, X., Cuajungco, M. P., Atwood, C. S., Hartshorn, M. A., Tyndall, J. D., Hanson, G. R., et al. (1999). Cu(II) potentiation of alzheimer abeta neurotoxicity. *Correlation with cell-free hydrogen peroxide production and metal reduction. J. Biol. Chem.* 274, 37111–37116. doi: 10.1074/jbc.274.52.37111

Huang, X., Moir, R. D., Tanzi, R. E., Bush, A. I., and Rogers, J. T. (2004). Redox-active metals, oxidative stress, and Alzheimer's disease pathology. *Ann. N.Y. Acad. Sci.* 1012, 153–163. doi: 10.1196/annals.1306.012

Jiang, H., Wang, X., Huang, L., Luo, Z., Su, T., Ding, K., et al. (2011). Benzenediol-berberine hybrids: multifunctional agents for Alzheimer's disease. *Bioorg. Med. Chem.* 19, 7228–7235. doi: 10.1016/j.bmc.2011.09.040

Jin, M., Shepardson, N., Yang, T., Chen, G., Walsh, D., and Selkoe, D. J. (2011). Soluble amyloid beta-protein dimers isolated from Alzheimer cortex directly induce Tau hyperphosphorylation and neuritic degeneration. *Proc. Natl. Acad. Sci. U.S.A.* 108, 5819–5824. doi: 10.1073/pnas.1017033108

Karlawish, J. (2011). Addressing the ethical, policy, and social challenges of preclinical Alzheimer disease. *Neurology* 77, 1487–1493. doi: 10.1212/WNL.0b013e318232ac1a

Lambert, M. P., Barlow, A. K., Chromy, B. A., Edwards, C., Freed, R., Liosatos, M., et al. (1998). Diffusible, nonfibrillar ligands derived from Abeta1-42 are potent central nervous system neurotoxins. *Proc. Natl. Acad. Sci. U.S.A.* 95, 6448–6453. doi: 10.1073/pnas.95.11.6448

Lee, H. P., Zhu, X., Casadesus, G., Castellani, R. J., Nunomura, A., Smith, M. A., et al. (2010). Antioxidant approaches for the treatment of Alzheimer's disease. *Expert Rev. Neurother.* 10, 1201–1208. doi: 10.1586/ern.10.74

Lee, Y. J., Jeong, S. Y., Karbowski, M., Smith, C. L., and Youle, R. J. (2004). Roles of the mammalian mitochondrial fission and fusion mediators Fis1, Drp1, and Opa1 in apoptosis. *Mol. Biol. Cell* 15, 5001–5011. doi: 10.1091/mbc.E04-04-0294

León, R., García, A. G., and Marco-Contelles, J. (2013). Recent advances in the multitarget-directed ligands approach for the treatment of Alzheimer's disease. *Med. Res. Rev.* 33, 139–189. doi: 10.1002/med. 20248

Malar, D. S., and Devi, K. P. (2014). Dietary polyphenols for treatment of Alzheimer's disease-future research and development. *Curr. Pharm. Biotechnol.* 15, 330–342. doi: 10.2174/1389201015666140813122703

Mandel, S., Weinreb, O., Amit, T., and Youdim, M. B. H. (2005). Mechanism of neuroprotective action of the anti-Parkinson drug rasagiline and its derivatives. *Brain Res. Rev.* 48, 379–387. doi: 10.1016/j.brainresrev.2004.12.027

Mesulam, M., Guillozet, A., Shaw, P., and Quinn, B. (2002). Widely spread butyrylcholinesterase can hydrolyze acetylcholine in the normal and Alzheimer brain. *Neurobiol. Dis.* 9, 88–93. doi: 10.1006/nbdi.2001.0462

Nochi, S., Asakawa, N., and Sato, T. (1995). Kinetic study on the inhibition of acetylcholinesterase by 1-benzyl-4-[(5,6-dimethoxy-1-indanon)-2-yl]methylpiperidine hydrochloride (E2020). *Biol. Pharm. Bull.* 18, 1145–1147. doi: 10.1248/bpb.18.1145

Pérez, V., Marco, J. L., Fernández-Álvarez, E., and Unzeta, M. (1999). Relevance of benzyloxy group in 2-indolyl methylamines in the selective MAO-B inhibition. *Br. J. Pharmacol.* 127, 869–876. doi: 10.1038/sj.bjp.0702600

Praticò, D. (2008). Evidence of oxidative stress in Alzheimer's disease brain and antioxidant therapy: lights and shadows. *Ann. N.Y. Acad. Sci.* 1147, 70–78. doi: 10.1196/annals.1427.010

Qizilbash, N., Whitehead, A., Higgins, J., Wilcock, G., Schneider, L., and Farlow, M. (1998). Cholinesterase inhibition for Alzheimer disease: a meta-analysis of the tacrine trials. *Dementia Trialists' Collaboration. JAMA* 280, 1777–1782. doi: 10.1001/jama.280.20.1777

Rosini, M., Simoni, E., Milelli, A., Minarini, A., and Melchiorre, C. (2014). Oxidative stress in Alzheimer's disease: are we connecting the dots? *J. Med. Chem.* 57, 2821–2831. doi: 10.1021/jm400970m

Samadi, A., Valderas, C., de los Ríos, C., Bastida, A., Chioua, M., González-Lafuente, L., et al. (2011). Cholinergic and neuroprotective drugs for the treatment of Alzheimer and neuronal vascular diseases. ISynthesis, I., biological assessment, and molecular modelling of new tacrine analogues from highly substituted 2-aminopyridine-3-carbonitriles. *Bioorg. Med. Chem.* 19, 122–133. doi: 10.1016/j.bmc.2010.11.040

Selkoe, D. J. (1994). Alzheimer's disease: a central role for amyloid. *J. Neuropathol. Exp. Neurol.* 53, 438–447. doi: 10.1097/00005072-199409000-00003

Serrano-Pozo, A., Qian, J., Monsell, S. E., Frosch, M. P., Betensky, R. A., and Hyman, B. T. (2013). Examination of the clinicopathologic continuum of Alzheimer disease in the autopsy cohort of the National Alzheimer Coordinating Center. *J. Neuropathol. Exp. Neurol.* 72, 1182–1192. doi: 10.1097/NEN.0000000000000016

Song, M. S., Rauw, G., Baker, G. B., and Kar, S. (2008). Memantine protects rat cortical cultured neurons against beta-amyloid-induced toxicity by attenuating tau phosphorylation. *Eur. J. Neurosci.* 28, 1989–2002. doi: 10.1111/j.1460-9568.2008.06498.x

Soreq, H., and Seidman, S. (2001). Acetylcholinesterase–new roles for an old actor. *Nat. Rev. Neurosci.* 2, 294–302. doi: 10.1038/35067589

Stasiak, A., Mussur, M., Unzeta, M., Samadi, A., Marco-Contelles, J. L., and Fogel, W. A. (2014). Effects of novel monoamine oxidases and cholinesterases targeting compounds on brain neurotransmitters and behavior in rat model of vascular dementia. *Curr. Pharm. Des.* 20, 161–171. doi: 10.2174/13816128113199990026

Sultana, R., Mecocci, P., Mangialasche, F., Cecchetti, R., Baglioni, M., and Butterfield, D. A. (2011). Increased protein and lipid oxidative damage in mitochondria isolated from lymphocytes from patients with Alzheimer's disease: insights into the role of oxidative stress in Alzheimer's disease and initial investigations into a potential biomarker for this dementing disorder. *J. Alzheimers Dis.* 24, 77–84. doi: 10.3233/JAD-2011-101425

Toledo, E. M., Colombres, M., and Inestrosa, N. C. (2008). Wnt signaling in neuroprotection and stem cell differentiation. *Prog. Neurobiol.* 86, 281–296. doi: 10.1016/j.pneurobio.2008.08.001

Villemagne, V. L., and Chételat, G. (2016). Neuroimaging biomarkers in Alzheimer's disease and other dementias. *Ageing Res. Rev.* doi: 10.1016/j.arr.2016.01.004. [Epub ahead of print].

Wang, J.-Z., Xia, Y.-Y., Grundke-Iqbal, I., and Iqbal, K. (2013). Abnormal hyperphosphorylation of tau: sites, regulation, and molecular mechanism of neurofibrillary degeneration. *J. Alzheimer's Dis.* 33, 123–139. doi: 10.3233/JAD-2012-129031

Wang, L., Esteban, G., Ojima, M., Bautista-Aguilera, O. M., Inokuchi, T., Moraleda, I., et al. (2014). Donepezil + propargylamine + 8-hydroxyquinoline hybrids as new multifunctional metal-chelators, ChE and MAO inhibitors for the potential treatment of Alzheimer's disease. *Eur. J. Med. Chem.* 80, 543–561. doi: 10.1016/j.ejmech.2014.04.078

Willard, L. B., Hauss-Wegrzyniak, B., Danysz, W., and Wenk, G. L. (2000). The cytotoxicity of chronic neuroinflammation upon basal forebrain cholinergic neurons of rats can be attenuated by glutamatergic antagonism or cyclooxygenase-2 inhibition. *Exp. Brain Res.* 134, 58–65. doi: 10.1007/s002210000446

Wu, M. Y., Esteban, G., Brogi, S., Shionoya, M., Wang, L., Campiani, G., et al. (2015). Donepezil-like multifunctional agents: design, synthesis, molecular modeling and biological evaluation. *Eur. J. Med. Chem.* doi: 10.1016/j.ejmech.2015.10.001. [Epub ahead of print].

Yamamoto, A., Shin, R. W., Hasegawa, K., Naiki, H., Sato, H., Yoshimasu, F., et al. (2002). Iron (III) induces aggregation of hyperphosphorylated tau and its reduction to iron (II) reverses the aggregation: implications in the formation of neurofibrillary tangles of Alzheimer's disease. *J. Neurochem.* 82, 1137–1147. doi: 10.1046/j.1471-4159.2002.t01-1-01061.x

Zhu, X., Lee, H. G., Perry, G., and Smith, M. A. (2007). Alzheimer disease, the two-hit hypothesis: an update. *Biochim. Biophys. Acta* 1772, 494–502. doi: 10.1016/j.bbadis.2006.10.014

Zindo, F. T., Joubert, J., and Malan, S. F. (2015). Propargylamine as functional moiety in the design of multifunctional drugs for neurodegenerative disorders: MAO inhibition and beyond. *Future Med. Chem.* 7, 609–629. doi: 10.4155/fmc.15.12

Conflict of Interest Statement: The authors declare that the research was conducted in the absence of any commercial or financial relationships that could be construed as a potential conflict of interest.

2

One for All? Hitting Multiple Alzheimer's Disease Targets with One Drug

Rebecca E. Hughes[1], Katarina Nikolic[2] and Rona R. Ramsay[1]*

[1] *School of Biology, BMS Building, University of St Andrews, St Andrews, UK,* [2] *Department of Pharmaceutical Chemistry, Faculty of Pharmacy, University of Belgrade, Belgrade, Serbia*

HIGHLIGHTS

- Many AD target combinations are being explored for multi-target drug design.
- New databases and models increase the potential of computational drug design
- Liraglutide and other antidiabetics are strong candidates for repurposing to AD.
- Donecopride a dual 5-HT/AChE inhibitor shows promise in pre-clinical studies

Edited by:
Eero Vasar,
University of Tartu, Estonia

Reviewed by:
John J. Wagner,
University of Georgia, USA
Min-Yu Sun,
Washington University in St. Louis,
USA
Elizabeth Yuriev,
Monash University, Australia

*Correspondence:
Rona R. Ramsay
rrr@st-andrews.ac.uk

Alzheimer's Disease is a complex and multifactorial disease for which the mechanism is still not fully understood. As new insights into disease progression are discovered, new drugs must be designed to target those aspects of the disease that cause neuronal damage rather than just the symptoms currently addressed by single target drugs. It is becoming possible to target several aspects of the disease pathology at once using multi-target drugs (MTDs). Intended as an introduction for non-experts, this review describes the key MTD design approaches, namely structure-based, *in silico*, and data-mining, to evaluate what is preventing compounds progressing through the clinic to the market. Repurposing current drugs using their off-target effects reduces the cost of development, time to launch, and the uncertainty associated with safety and pharmacokinetics. The most promising drugs currently being investigated for repurposing to Alzheimer's Disease are rasagiline, originally developed for the treatment of Parkinson's Disease, and liraglutide, an antidiabetic. Rational drug design can combine pharmacophores of multiple drugs, systematically change functional groups, and rank them by virtual screening. Hits confirmed experimentally are rationally modified to generate an effective multi-potent lead compound. Examples from this approach are ASS234 with properties similar to rasagiline, and donecopride, a hybrid of an acetylcholinesterase inhibitor and a 5-HT$_4$ receptor agonist with pro-cognitive effects. Exploiting these interdisciplinary approaches, public-private collaborative lead factories promise faster delivery of new drugs to the clinic.

Keywords: **multi-target drugs, Alzheimer's Disease,** *in silico*, **datamining, rational drug design, repurposing**

Abbreviations: AD, Alzheimer's Disease; AChE, acetylcholinesterase; Aβ, amyloid beta; MAO, monoamine oxidase; MTD, multi-target drug; N-methyl-D-aspartate (NMDA receptor; GABA, gamma-aminobutyric acid; 5-HT$_4$R, serotonin (5-HT) receptor type 4; Glucagon-like peptide 1 (GLP-1); BBB, blood brain barrier.

INTRODUCTION

Current therapies available for the treatment of Alzheimer's Disease (AD) show limited ability to modify the disease. To date the focus for AD has been on the depletion of acetylcholine, but AD is a complex multifactorial disease with diverse clinical symptoms. AD causes the gradual onset of multiple cognitive deficits, affecting language, episodic memory and attention (Karran et al., 2011). The disease pathology includes extracellular amyloid beta (Aβ) plaques, intracellular neurofibrillary tangles, inflammation, oxidative stress, iron dysregulation and ultimately neuronal cell death (Carreiras et al., 2013). It is accepted that multifactorial diseases require the simultaneous modulation of multiple targets to manage the course of disease progression (Cavalli et al., 2008), leading to growth in multi-target drug (MTD) design (Hopkins, 2008). This review focuses on possible targets, their combinations, and the three main approaches to designing MTDs: structure-based design, data mining/repurposing, and *in silico* screening. The application of rational drug design to MTDs is difficult but with the recent advances in experimental and computational approaches, a combined approach harnessing the best attributes of each method should ultimately deliver success in the future.

TARGETS AND CURRENT THERAPIES; LIMITATIONS IN ALZHEIMER'S DISEASE

The multifactorial nature of AD means there are many possible therapeutic targets. Current monotherapeutic treatments focus mainly on acetylcholinesterase (AChE) inhibition due to the early cholinergic hypothesis that cognitive dysfunctions of AD may be attributed to decreased neurotransmission at cholinergic synapses as a result of neuronal cell death (Bartus et al., 1982). AChE therapies provide symptomatic relief, but fail to reverse disease progression (Wilkinson et al., 2004; Deardorff et al., 2015), although recent work suggests that donepezil (**Table 1**) may enhance Aβ clearance (Mohamed et al., 2015). The amyloid hypothesis that the generation of toxic Aβ from amyloid precursor protein (APP) and Aβ aggregation result in the pathophysiological changes associated with AD (**Figure 1**) led to compounds targeting Aβ (Karran et al., 2011; Eisele et al., 2015). Although small molecules can target Aβ aggregation (see **Table 1**), the main strategy is immunotherapy, still in clinical trials (Palmer, 2011; Wisniewski and Goñi, 2014). Better understanding of protein aggregation is now available to guide therapeutic intervention on both Aβ and tau aggregation (Eisele et al., 2015).

Following on from direct targeting of Aβ, a relatively new target in AD is the β-secretase (BACE-1) enzyme. Inhibition of this protease BACE-1 should reduce the levels of Aβ in the brain (Vassar, 2014). BACE-1 inhibitors in clinical trials include AZD3293 in phase II/III (NCT02245737) and MK8931 (verubecestat) in phase III (NCT01953601). While these drugs show promise, there are potential complications from a possible role in synaptic function (Kandalepas and Vassar, 2014) and

increased memory impairment and seizures in BACE-1 −/− mice (Hu et al., 2016).

Another major enzyme target, monoamine oxidase (MAO) is inhibited in Parkinson's Disease (PD) to spare the neurotransmitters depleted by neuronal death. The PD drug, rasagiline (see below), is a MAO-B inhibitor in clinical trials for AD (Weinreb et al., 2010).

N-methyl-D-aspartate (NMDA) is a glutamate receptor and is the only other target besides AChE for which a therapy has been approved (Anand et al., 2014). NMDA receptors are over-stimulated in AD brains due to excessive release of glutamate from neurons. This causes high levels of calcium ion influx and activation of enzymes that can cause neuronal cell death (Zheng et al., 2014). NMDA receptors have also been linked to tau hyper-phosphorylation and Aβ toxicity (Couratier et al., 1996). Memantine is the only approved NMDA receptor antagonist for the treatment of moderate to severe AD (Lipton, 2006).

Other receptors being explored are the 5-hydroxytryptamine (5-HT) serotonin receptors, in particular subtype 4 (5-HT$_4$R) that is involved in mood, memory, and learning. 5-HT$_4$R has been linked to memory deficits such as those seen in AD (Cho and Hu, 2007; Lezoualc'h, 2007; Russo et al., 2009). Stimulation causes release of ACh and increases other neurotransmitters (Licht et al., 2010).

Inhibition of these targets individually with current drugs (**Table 1**) has been ineffective at reversing the progression of the disease. A possible answer lies in a polypharmacological approach to modify activities of several of these targets simultaneously, particularly those associated with the progression of the disease. MTDs developed for AD have modified two or more of known targets (cholinesterases, MAOs, acetylcholine receptors, serotonin receptors) or have properties thought to retard disease progression, such as metal chelation, antioxidant or anti-inflammatory activity, or prevention of Aβ or tau aggregation. Ligands for combinations of drug targets should be evaluated against disease progression to define optimal target combinations.

DATAMINING AND REPURPOSING

Repurposing is the development of existing or abandoned drugs for new indications (Boguski et al., 2009), related to the original purpose or after off-target effects are identified by datamining. Repurposing reduces the time to launch, cost of development, and the uncertainty associated with safety and pharmacokinetics (Kim, 2015).

Datamining is a way of using pre-existing knowledge about molecules and applying it to develop new drugs (Sirota et al., 2011; Corbett et al., 2012, 2013). For example, clinical data can be used to identify unanticipated benefits in side effects seen in clinical trials, allowing the early repurposing of therapies (Loging et al., 2011). The most promising drug currently being investigated for repurposing is rasagiline, a selective, irreversible MAO-B inhibitor for the treatment of PD (Youdim et al., 1995, 2001). The repurposing to AD stems from the ability of rasagiline to regulate the non-amyloidogenic processing of

TABLE 1 | Targets, drugs, and new multi-target ligands to combat Alzheimer's Disease (AD).

Targets	Drug name	Structure	Comment
(A) APPROVED DRUGS			
Acetylcholinesterase	Donepezil		Approved drug
	Rivastigmine		Approved drug
	Galantamine		Approved drug
	Tacrine		Withdrawn
Monoamine oxidase	Rasagiline		Approved for PD Phase II for AD

Targets	Parent compounds	Compound	References
(B) MULTI-TARGET DESIGNED LIGANDS			
Cholinesterase Aβ aggregation	Oxoisoaporphine Tacrine		Tang et al., 2011
Cholinesterase Aβ aggregation	Donepezil		Ozer et al., 2013
AChE BACE-1	Huprine Tacrine		Galdeano et al., 2012

(Continued)

TABLE 1 | Continued

Targets	Parent compounds	Compound	References
Cholinesterase MAO Aβ aggregation	Donepezil Compound 28 (Pérez et al., 1999)		Samadi et al., 2012
Cholinesterase MAO	Donepezil Compound 28	Compound 2	Bolea et al., 2011
MAO Cholinesterase	Donepezil PF9601N		Bautista-Aguilera et al., 2014b
MAO Cholinesterase	Tacrine Selegiline (deprenyl)	selegiline	Lu et al., 2013b
Cholinesterase Reactive oxygen species	Memoquin Lipoic acid	lipoic acid	Rosini et al., 2011
MAO Metal chelator Aβ aggregation Cholinesterase	Resveratrol		Lu et al., 2013a
Metal chelator Aβ aggregation	Resveratrol Clioquinol		Li et al., 2014

APP (Yogev-Falach et al., 2003; Bar-Am et al., 2004). Rasagiline also shows neuroprotective activity due to the propargylamine moiety that activates Bcl-2 and down-regulates the Bax proteins (Youdim et al., 2005). It is now in Phase II trial for the treatment of AD (www.clinicaltrials.gov/ct2/show/NCT02359552).

Natural products provide another potential source of MTDs (Ji et al., 2009; Prati et al., 2014). Datamining could harness their potential and then synthetic analogs and derivatives created to enhance their activity (Agis-Torres et al., 2014). Huperzine A, a dietary supplement in China, is an AChE inhibitor (Xing et al., 2014) seemingly with beneficial effects on cognitive function and daily living in AD patients, but the clinical trials to date have poor methodological approaches and so results are inconclusive (Xu et al., 1995; Rafii et al., 2011). Synthetic derivatives like huprine X and huprine-tacrine hybrids have been developed to improve on the potency and efficacy of huperzine A (Galdeano et al., 2012).

One promising repurposing area is from diabetes to AD, first considered because type 2 diabetes is a risk factor for AD (Schrijvers et al., 2010). Insulin signaling is impaired in the brains of Alzheimer's patients (Moloney et al., 2010) so several aspects of insulin signaling and regulation have been targeted. For example, Phase II clinical trials of intranasal insulin administration showed improved biomarkers for early AD including amyloid and tau indicators in cerebrospinal

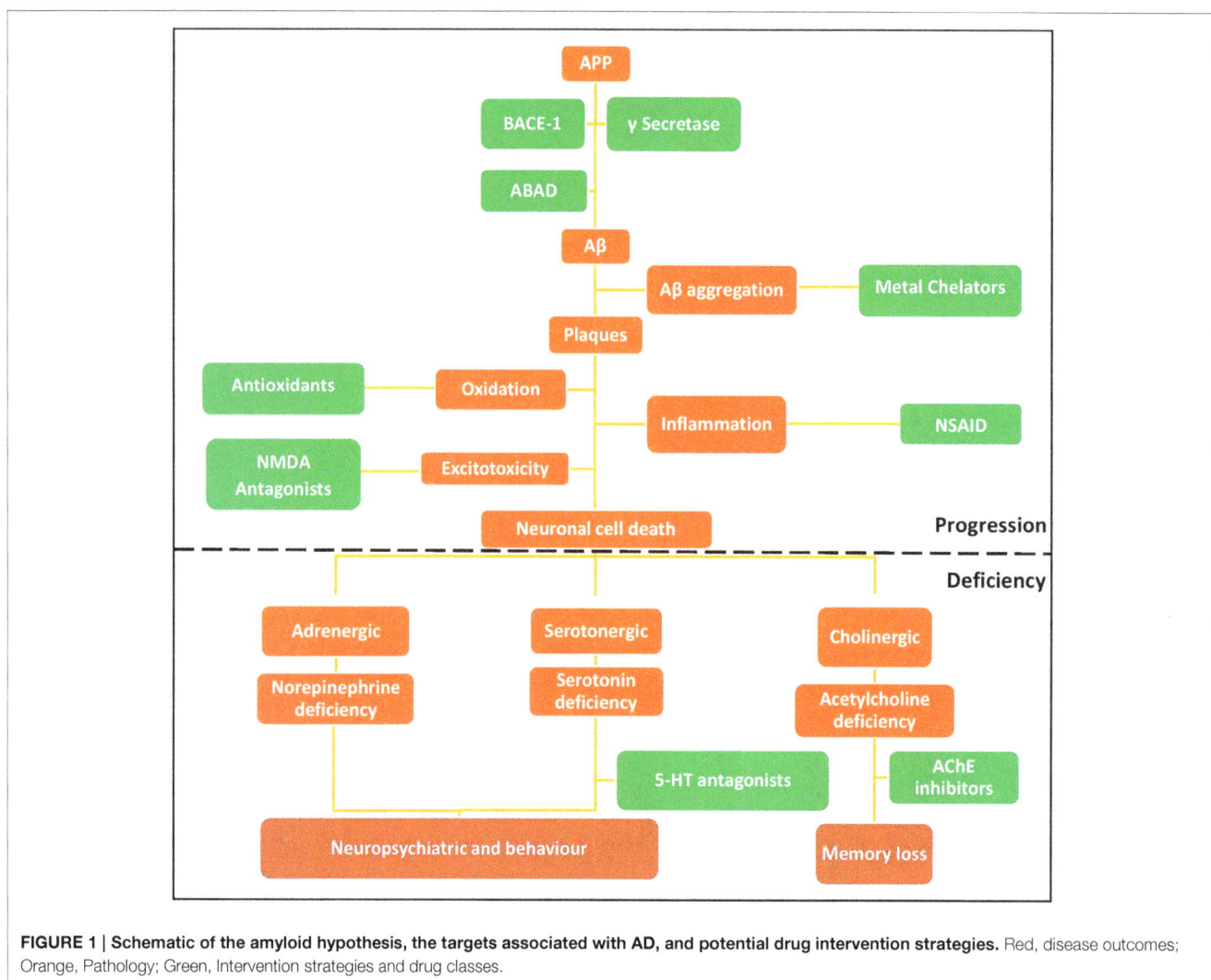

FIGURE 1 | Schematic of the amyloid hypothesis, the targets associated with AD, and potential drug intervention strategies. Red, disease outcomes; Orange, Pathology; Green, Intervention strategies and drug classes.

fluid (CSF) (Craft et al., 2012). Long-lasting glucagon-like peptide 1 (GLP-1) analogs that promote the secretion of insulin are also in clinical trials. Three GLP-1 analogs with potential therapeutic value in AD (Corbett et al., 2012; Hölscher, 2014), have shown *in vivo* benefits in mouse AD models (Gengler et al., 2012). Two of these are Exendin-4 in Phase II clinical trial (See www.clinicaltrials.gov/ct/show/NCT01255163) and Liraglutide, a GLP-1 receptor agonist. Liraglutide crosses the blood brain barrier (BBB) in animal models (Hunter and Hölscher, 2012). It decreases intracellular APP, $A\beta$, and Fe^{2+}-related neurodegeneration, but also improves synaptic plasticity and cognitive function, reducing AD pathology (McClean et al., 2011; McClean and Hölscher, 2014).

DATABASES AND OPEN-ACCESS MINING

The construction of AD knowledge bases will facilitate the repurposing of drugs and our understanding of the neurosignaling pathways involved. One such example

is AlzPlatform, an AD domain-specific chemogenomics database allowing the identification of off-target effects and the repurposing of compounds (Liu et al., 2014). AlzPlatform contains the established computational algorithm TargetHunter, which is an *in silico* target identification tool for small molecules (Wang et al., 2013).

While there is a wealth of open access chemical information available to aid repurposing of FDA approved drugs, compound libraries held by pharmaceutical companies are, for the most part, unavailable. Datamining to find possible targets for these compounds could prove fruitful. An open-innovation drug-repositioning project between AstraZeneca and the Medical Research Council (http://www.labtalk.astrazeneca.com/hot-topics/open-innovation-in-drug-repositioning/) has started and the National Center for Advancing Translational Sciences (NCATS) has created a similar collaboration with 8 pharmaceutical companies. One of the compounds from this program is the Src tyrosine kinase inhibitor, AZD0530 (Saracatinib), being repurposed for the treatment of AD (Larson et al., 2012; Nygaard et al., 2014). The European Lead

Factory (www.europeanleadfactory.eu) is another initiative set up to allow sharing of commercial compound libraries via collaborative public-private partnerships. The compound library, a pool of 30 partner libraries, provides a collection of over 500,000 compounds available for academic groups and pharmaceutical companies to screen experimentally against their chosen targets with great potential to generate new therapeutics.

RATIONAL DRUG DESIGN

Rational drug design is a traditional method for drug development based on structure-function analysis. Successful rational drug design requires the logical and systematic changing of substituents to modify the properties of a compound to reach the desired effect. When applied to MTD design, it means combining pharmacophores of multiple drugs to give complex combinations, then compensating for any disadvantage to the individual targets.

M30, a brain-permeable iron chelator and brain selective MAO inhibitor, was designed on the rationale that MAO and iron are elevated in the brains of AD patients, and this leads to oxidative stress and neurodegeneration (Youdim, 2006). The MAO inhibition is due to the propargylamine of the FDA-approved anti-PD drug rasagiline (Youdim, 2013). The iron chelating activity comes from the prototype iron chelator VK28 (Zheng et al., 2014). M30 irreversibly inhibits both MAO-A and -B with IC_{50} values of 37 ± 2 nM and 57 ± 1 nM respectively, less selective than rasagiline (412 nM and 4.4 nM, respectively) (Zheng et al., 2005). It also regulates APP via its iron chelating ability since APP is a metalloprotein with an iron responsive element in the $5'$ untranslated region (UTR) (Youdim, 2013). Therefore, it has a direct effect on Aβ levels.

To reduce the possibility of adverse effects of metal chelation in the periphery, a second-generation molecule and prodrug, M30D, was designed from tacrine, rivastigmine, and rasagiline (Zheng et al., 2010a,b, 2014). It was 3-fold more potent against MAO-A (IC_{50} of 7.7 nM) than the parental molecule, retaining the same MAO-B inhibition (Zheng et al., 2014). It is metabolized to the active chelator form M30 by AChE and inhibits AChE with an IC_{50} of 500 nM in rat brain homogenates. With these characteristics, M30D is the first site-directed metal chelator with the potential to treat AD.

A similar MTD is ASS234 composed from donepezil and the propargylamine PF9601N. It binds to all the AChE/BuChE and MAO A/B enzymes, shows antioxidant, neuroprotective and suitable permeability properties. *In vivo*, ASS234 restores scopolamine-induced cognitive impairment to the same extent as donepezil, is less toxic, and prevents β-amyloid aggregation in the cortex of AD transgenic mice (Bolea et al., 2013; del Pino et al., 2014).

Another promising structure-based MTD is donecopride. Donecopride is a structural hybrid of donepezil, an AChE inhibitor, and RS67333, a 5-HT$_4$R agonist. RS67333 is a partial 5-HT$_4$R agonist that exerts a procognitive effect via its ability to promote cleavage of APP. RS67333 is structurally similar to donepezil, so it was postulated that it might inhibit AChE. It was indeed a submicromolar AChE inhibitor (Lecoutey et al., 2014; Rochais et al., 2015). Derivatives of RS67333 were then synthesized to improve the AChE activity, from which MR31147 (donecopride) was selected for its remarkable multi-target activity *in vitro*, including an IC50 for AChE of 16 nM (Lecoutey et al., 2014). Donecopride crosses BBB, has a nontoxic profile, and exerts a procognitive effect *in vivo* (Lecoutey et al., 2014). It will be interesting to see how this promising molecule progresses since 5-HT$_4$ targeted therapies have been less commonly explored for AD.

These examples show how methodical rational drug design and experimental screening can be used to generate promising MTD candidates for the treatment of AD.

IN SILICO SCREENING

Rational drug design is currently the approach of choice for MTD design but it is labor intensive, so there is a need for more *in silico* screening to reduce costs and accelerate progress. New computer-based approaches for *in silico* screening (Ekins et al., 2007a; Wang et al., 2013), such as quantitative structure-activity relationships, molecular modeling approaches, machine learning, data mining, and data analysis tools, use *in vitro* data to generate predictive models. Such models are very useful in the discovery and optimization of novel ligands with enhanced affinity to a drug target, as well as for optimization of physicochemical and pharmacokinetic properties of the drug candidates. Several of these *in silico* methods will be evaluated here in the context of selected MTD examples.

Virtual ligand screening is an alternative to experimental high throughput screening (Ekins et al., 2007a). It can be used to screen whole databases of molecules and rank them based on their probability of binding to a drug target. The highest-ranking molecules can then be taken through to an experimental stage to confirm the hits and determine the most promising leads. Virtual screening can be either ligand based, where a diverse set of ligands are analyzed to build up a pharmacophore to score the screen against, or it can be structure-based, where molecules are docked onto the target and scored based on their likely affinity for the target. Quantitative structure-activity relationships (QSAR) is a form of ligand-based virtual screening but it uses a series of logic-based rules describing the chemical properties and substructures linked to activity to screen a database of molecules (Ekins et al., 2007b).

Recently a virtual ligand screen (Bautista-Aguilera et al., 2014a) was used for lead optimization of two donepezil hybrid compounds shown previously to inhibit MAO-A, MAO-B, AChE, and BuChE (Bolea et al., 2011). The 3D-QSAR analysis was carried out both to explain the binding of these compounds to the active sites of the enzymes and to predict substitutions that would increase binding. The QSAR model was used to generate 19 new molecules with substitutions predicted to increase the activity against MAOs and ChEs. The predicted IC50 values suggested that N-[(5-benzyloxy-1-methyl-1-H-indol-2-yl)methyl]-N-methylprop-2-yn-1-amine (compound 2) would be the most potent inhibitor of all four enzymes with values in the nanomolar range for MAO-A, MAO-B, and AChE, while BuChE was predicted at 1.3 µM. The experimental results showed that only 7 of the 19 compounds were active against all four enzymes, which demonstrates how difficult it can be to get activity against four enzymes in one molecule. However, as predicted, compound 2 was the most potent against all four enzymes, confirming the quality of the 3D-pharmacophores. Thus, *in silico* screening can be used to modify a lead compound and generate effective multi-potent inhibitors (Bautista-Aguilera et al., 2014a).

Another option, rather than start from a lead molecule, is to use pharmacophore models to screen existing compound databases with the aim of generating hits against multiple targets. This approach has been used to identify dual inhibitors of BACE-1 and AChE using a combination of virtual screening and molecular docking of compounds from three compound databases. The strategy adopted follows a sequential screening model where the databases were screened in parallel against the two targets sequentially before filters were applied to select for compounds with desirable properties. Finally, docking of the chosen compounds led to 8 compounds from the original 501,799 that fit all the given criteria (Tyagi et al., 2010).

Importantly, *in silico* screening allows the early filtering of compounds based on properties, such as BBB permeability, which can reduce late stage attrition. However, screening sequentially means that compounds that fall below the cut-off criteria in the first round are not screened against the second target. To avoid loss of potential candidates, screening against the targets in parallel is essential (Steindl et al., 2006).

CONCLUDING REMARKS

Over the past decade, there has been a substantial research effort to design MTDs for the treatment of AD. This focus on MTDs is aided by the understanding that AD is a complex and multifactorial disease affecting many interlinked pathological pathways. The lack of efficacy seen with the single target approach is compelling evidence that we needed to rethink the paradigm of drug design to treat these multifactorial diseases. MTD design offers a promising avenue for the progression of AD therapeutic intervention and could ultimately lead to a drug with the ability to reverse disease progression.

While there are many targets for disease-modifying drugs, it remains to be seen which combinations will prove efficacious. It seems logical that in order to reverse disease progression, we must target those aspects of the disease that cause neuronal damage, such as Aβ and oxidative damage, rather than just targeting the breakdown enzymes to alleviate the deficiencies caused by cell death. Of course, targeting a combination of both would relieve symptoms and prevent further neuronal loss.

In terms of the approach to MTD design, an integrated approach using a combination of *in silico* and rational drug design should reduce the cost of high throughput screening and progress discovery more rapidly. The MTD approach is also being used to combat the development of resistance to antimicrobials. MBX-500 has been designed as a hybrid of two classes of antibiotics, fluoroquinolone and anilinouracil, for the treatment of *Clostridium difficile* infections (Butler et al., 2012). TD-1792, a cephalosporin-vancomycin hybrid, has passed a phase II clinical trial for gram-positive skin infections (Stryjewski et al., 2012). While MTD design is in its infancy in the world of antibiotics, there is evidence that it could prove promising here too (East and Silver, 2013; Oldfield and Feng, 2014).

Overall, MTD design is a promising approach to modern medicines for complex diseases. Whether drugs will come from repurposing, rational drug design, *in silico* screening, or a combination approach we cannot predict, but the race is on to develop the first approved MTD capable of reversing AD pathology.

AUTHOR CONTRIBUTIONS

REH reviewed the literature and wrote the draft. All authors contributed to the conception, interpretation, and critical revision of the work. All authors have approved the final version of this review of current literature.

FUNDING

The authors thank COST Action CM1103 for the productive collaborations that inspired this work and for open access funding.

ACKNOWLEDGMENTS

The authors thank the participants in COST Action CM1103 "Structure-based drug design for diagnosis and treatment of neurological diseases: dissecting and modulating complex function in the monoaminergic systems of the brain" for productive collaborations and COST for funding open access publication.

REFERENCES

Agis-Torres, A., Sölhuber, M., Fernandez, M., and Sanchez-Montero, J. M. (2014). Multi-target-directed ligands and other therapeutic strategies in the search of a real solution for alzheimer's disease. *Curr. Neuropharmacol.* 12, 2–36. doi: 10.2174/1570159X113116660047

Anand, R., Gill, K. D., and Mahdi, A. A. (2014). Therapeutics of Alzheimer's disease: past, present and future. *Neuropharmacology* 76, 27–50. doi: 10.1016/j.neuropharm.2013.07.004

Bar-Am, O., Yogev-Falach, M., Amit, T., Sagi, Y., and Youdim, M. B. H. (2004). Regulation of protein kinase C by the anti-parkinson drug, MAO-B inhibitor, rasagiline and its derivatives, *in vivo. J. Neurochem.* 89, 1119–1125. doi: 10.1111/j.1471-4159.2004.02425.x

Bartus, R. T., Dean, R. L. III, Beer, B., and Lippa, A. S. (1982). The cholinergic hypothesis of geriatric memory dysfunction. *Science* 217, 408–417. doi: 10.1126/science.7046051

Bautista-Aguilera, O. M., Esteban, G., Bolea, I., Nikolic, K., Agbaba, D., Moraleda, I., et al. (2014a). Design, synthesis, pharmacological evaluation,

QSAR analysis, molecular modeling and ADMET of novel donepezil-indolyl hybrids as multipotent cholinesterase/monoamine oxidase inhibitors for the potential treatment of Alzheimer's disease. *Eur. J. Med. Chem.* 75, 82–95. doi: 10.1016/j.ejmech.2013.12.028

Bautista-Aguilera, O. M., Samadi, A., Chioua, M., Nikolic, K., Filipic, S., Agbaba, D., et al. (2014b). N-Methyl-N-((1-methyl-5-(3-(1-(2-methylbenzyl)piperidin-4yl)propoxy)-1H- indol-2-yl)methyl)prop-2-yn-1-amine, a new cholinesterase and monoamine oxidase dual. *J. Med. Chem.* 57, 10455–10463. doi: 10.1021/jm501501a

Boguski, M. S., Mandl, K. D., and Sukhatme, V. P. (2009). Repurposing with a difference. *Science* 324, 1394–1395. doi: 10.1126/science.1169920

Bolea, I., Gella, A., Monjas, L., Perez, C., Rodriguez-Franco, M. I., Marco-Contelles, J., et al. (2013). Multipotent, permeable drug ASS234 inhibits A beta aggregation, possesses antioxidant properties and protects from A beta-induced apoptosis *in vitro*. *Curr. Alzheimer Res.* 10, 797–808. doi: 10.2174/15672050113109990151

Bolea, I., Juarez-Jimenez, J., de los Rios, C., Chioua, M., Pouplana, R., Javier Luque, F., et al. (2011). Synthesis, biological evaluation, and molecular modeling of donepezil and N- (5-(Benzyloxy)-1-methyl-1H-indol-2-yl)methyl -N-methylprop-2-yn-1-ami ne hybrids as new multipotent cholinesterase/monoamine oxidase inhibitors for the treatment of Alzheimer's disease. *J. Med. Chem.* 54, 8251–8270. doi: 10.1021/jm200853t

Butler, M. M., Shinabarger, D. L., Citron, D. M., Kelly, C. P., Dvoskin, S., Wright, G. E., et al. (2012). MBX-500, a hybrid antibiotic with *in vitro* and *in vivo* efficacy against toxigenic clostridium difficile. *Antimicrob. Agents Chemother.* 56, 4786–4792. doi: 10.1128/AAC.00508-12

Carreiras, M. C., Mendes, E., Jesus Perry, M. J., Francisco, A. P., and Marco-Contelles, J. (2013). The multifactorial nature of Alzheimer's disease for developing potential therapeutics. *Curr. Top. Med. Chem.* 13, 1745–1770. doi: 10.2174/15680266113139990135

Cavalli, A., Bolognesi, M. L., Minarini, A., Rosini, M., Tumiatti, V., Recanatini, M., et al. (2008). Multi-target-directed ligands to combat neurodegenerative diseases. *J. Med. Chem.* 51, 347–372. doi: 10.1021/jm7009364

Cho, S., and Hu, Y. (2007). Activation of 5-HT4 receptors inhibits secretion of beta-amyloid peptides and increases neuronal survival. *Exp. Neurol.* 203, 274–278. doi: 10.1016/j.expneurol.2006.07.021

Corbett, A., Pickett, J., Burns, A., Corcoran, J., Dunnett, S. B., Edison, P., et al. (2012). Drug repositioning for Alzheimer's disease. *Nat. Rev. Drug Discov.* 11, 833–846. doi: 10.1038/nrd3869

Corbett, A., Williams, G., and Ballard, C. (2013). Drug repositioning: an opportunity to develop novel treatments for Alzheimer's disease. *Pharmaceuticals* 6, 1304–1321. doi: 10.3390/ph6101304

Couratier, P., Lesort, M., Sindou, P., Esclaire, F., Yardin, C., and Hugon, J. (1996). Modifications of neuronal phosphorylated tau immunoreactivity induced by NMDA toxicity. *Mol. Chem. Neuropathol.* 27, 259–273. doi: 10.1007/BF02815108

Craft, S., Baker, L. D., Montine, T. J., Minoshima, S., Watson, G. S., Claxton, A., et al. (2012). Intranasal insulin therapy for Alzheimer disease and amnestic mild cognitive impairment a pilot clinical trial. *Arch. Neurol.* 69, 29–38. doi: 10.1001/archneurol.2011.233

Deardorff, W. J., Feen, E., and Grossberg, G. T. (2015). The use of cholinesterase inhibitors across all stages of Alzheimer's disease. *Drugs Aging* 32, 537–547. doi: 10.1007/s40266-015-0273-x

del Pino, J., Ramos, E., Bautista-Aguilera, O. M., Marco-Contelles, J., and Romero, A. (2014). Wnt signaling pathway, a potential target for Alzheimer's disease treatment, is activated by a novel multitarget compound ASS234. *CNS Neurosci. Ther.* 20, 568–570. doi: 10.1111/cns.12269

East, S. P., and Silver, L. L. (2013). Multitarget ligands in antibacterial research: progress and opportunities. *Expert Opin. Drug Discov.* 8, 143–156. doi: 10.1517/17460441.2013.743991

Eisele, Y. S., Monteiro, C., Fearns, C., Encalada, S. E., Wiseman, R. L., Powers, E. T., et al. (2015). Targeting protein aggregation for the treatment of degenerative diseases. *Nat. Rev. Drug Discov.* 14, 759–780. doi: 10.1038/nrd4593

Ekins, S., Mestres, J., and Testa, B. (2007a). *In silico* pharmacology for drug discovery: methods for virtual ligand screening and profiling. *Br. J. Pharmacol.* 152, 9–20. doi: 10.1038/sj.bjp.0707305

Ekins, S., Mestres, J., and Testa, B. (2007b). *In silico* pharmacology for drug discovery: applications to targets and beyond. *Br. J. Pharmacol.* 152, 21–37. doi: 10.1038/sj.bjp.0707306

Galdeano, C., Viayna, E., Sola, I., Formosa, X., Camps, P., Badia, A., et al. (2012). Huprine-tacrine heterodimers as anti-amyloidogenic compounds of potential interest against Alzheimer's and Prion diseases. *J. Med. Chem.* 55, 661–669. doi: 10.1021/jm200840c

Gengler, S., McClean, P. L., McCurtin, R., Gault, V. A., and Hoelscher, C. (2012). Val(8)GLP-1 rescues synaptic plasticity and reduces dense core plaques in APP/PS1 mice. *Neurobiol. Aging* 33, 265–276. doi: 10.1016/j.neurobiolaging.2010.02.014

Hölscher, C. (2014). Central effects of GLP-1: new opportunities for treatments of neurodegenerative diseases. *J. Endocrinol.* 221, T31–T41. doi: 10.1530/JOE-13-0221

Hopkins, A. L. (2008). Network pharmacology: the next paradigm in drug discovery. *Nat. Chem. Biol.* 4, 682–690. doi: 10.1038/nchembio.118

Hu, X., Fan, Q., Hou, H., and Yan, R. (2016). Neurological dysfunctions associated with altered BACE1-dependent neuregulin-1 signaling. *J. Neurochem.* 136, 234–249. doi: 10.1111/jnc.13395

Hunter, K., and Hölscher, C. (2012). Drugs developed to treat diabetes, liraglutide and lixisenatide, cross the blood brain barrier and enhance neurogenesis. *BMC Neurosci.* 13:33. doi: 10.1186/1471-2202-13-33

Ji, H.-F., Li, X.-J., and Zhang, H.-Y. (2009). Natural products and drug discovery can thousands of years of ancient medical knowledge lead us to new and powerful drug combinations in the fight against cancer and dementia? *EMBO Rep.* 10, 194–200. doi: 10.1038/embor.2009.12

Kandalepas, P. C., and Vassar, R. (2014). The normal and pathologic roles of the Alzheimer's beta-secretase, BACE1. *Curr. Alzheimer Res.* 11, 441–449. doi: 10.2174/1567205011666140604122059

Karran, E., Mercken, M., and De Strooper, B. (2011). The amyloid cascade hypothesis for Alzheimer's disease: an appraisal for the development of therapeutics. *Nat. Rev. Drug Discov.* 10, 698–U1600. doi: 10.1038/nrd3505

Kim, T.-W. (2015). Drug repositioning approaches for the discovery of new therapeutics for Alzheimer's disease. *Neurotherapeutics* 12, 132–142. doi: 10.1007/s13311-014-0325-7

Larson, M., Sherman, M. A., Amar, F., Nuvolone, M., Schneider, J. A., Bennett, D. A., et al. (2012). The complex PrPc-Fyn couples human oligomeric A beta with pathological tau changes in Alzheimer's disease. *J. Neurosci.* 32, 16857. doi: 10.1523/JNEUROSCI.1858-12.2012

Lecoutey, C., Hedou, D., Freret, T., Giannoni, P., Gaven, F., Since, M., et al. (2014). Design of donecopride, a dual serotonin subtype 4 receptor agonist/acetylcholinesterase inhibitor with potential interest for Alzheimer's disease treatment. *Proc. Natl. Acad. Sci. U.S.A.* 111, E3825–E3830. doi: 10.1073/pnas.1410315111

Lezoualc'h, F. (2007). 5-HT4 receptor and Alzheimer's disease: the amyloid connection. *Exp. Neurol.* 205, 325–329. doi: 10.1016/j.expneurol.2007.02.001

Li, S.-Y., Wang, X.-B., and Kong, L.-Y. (2014). Design, synthesis and biological evaluation of imine resveratrol derivatives as multi-targeted agents against Alzheimer's disease. *Eur. J. Med. Chem.* 71, 36–45. doi: 10.1016/j.ejmech.2013.10.068

Licht, C. L., Knudsen, G. M., and Sharp, T. (2010). Effects of the 5-HT4 receptor agonist RS67333 and paroxetine on hippocampal extracellular 5-HT levels. *Neurosci. Lett.* 476, 58–61. doi: 10.1016/j.neulet.2010.04.002

Lipton, S. A. (2006). Paradigm shift in neuroprotection by NMDA receptor blockade: memantine and beyond. *Nat. Rev. Drug Discov.* 5, 160–170. doi: 10.1038/nrd1958

Liu, H., Wang, L., Lv, M., Pei, R., Li, P., Pei, Z., et al. (2014). AlzPlatform: an Alzheimer's disease domain-specific chemogenornics knowledgebase for polypharmacology and target identification research. *J. Chem. Inf. Model.* 54, 1050–1060. doi: 10.1021/ci500004h

Loging, W., Rodriguez-Esteban, R., Hill, J., Freeman, T. B., and Miglietta, J. (2011). Cheminformatic/bioinformatic analysis of large corporate databases: application to drug repurposing. *Drug Discov. Today Ther. Strateg.* 8, 109–116. doi: 10.1016/j.ddstr.2011.06.004

Lu, C., Guo, Y., Yan, J., Luo, Z., Luo, H.-B., Yan, M., et al. (2013a). Design, synthesis, and evaluation of multitarget-directed resveratrol derivatives for the treatment of Alzheimer's disease. *J. Med. Chem.* 56, 5843–5859. doi: 10.1021/jm400567s

Lu, C., Zhou, Q., Yan, J., Du, Z., Huang, L., and Li, X. (2013b). A novel series of tacrine-selegiline hybrids with cholinesterase and monoamine oxidase inhibition activities for the treatment of Alzheimer's disease. *Eur. J. Med. Chem.* 62, 745–753. doi: 10.1016/j.ejmech.2013.01.039

McClean, P. L., and Hölscher, C. (2014). Liraglutide can reverse memory impairment, synaptic loss and reduce plaque load in aged APP/PS1 mice, a model of Alzheimer's disease. *Neuropharmacology* 76, 57–67. doi: 10.1016/j.neuropharm.2013.08.005

McClean, P. L., Parthsarathy, V., Faivre, E., and Hölscher, C. (2011). The diabetes drug liraglutide prevents degenerative processes in a mouse model of Alzheimer's disease. *J. Neurosci.* 31, 6587–6594. doi: 10.1523/JNEUROSCI.0529-11.2011

Mohamed, L. A., Qosa, H., and Kaddoumi, A. (2015). Age-related decline in brain and hepatic clearance of amyloid-beta is rectified by the cholinesterase inhibitors donepezil and rivastignnine in rats. *ACS Chem. Neurosci.* 6, 725–736. doi: 10.1021/acschemneuro.5b00040

Moloney, A. M., Griffin, R. J., Timmons, S., O'Connor, R., Ravid, R., and O'Neill, C. (2010). Defects in IGF-1 receptor, insulin receptor and IRS-1/2 in Alzheimer's disease indicate possible resistance to IGF-1 and insulin signalling. *Neurobiol. Aging* 31, 224–243. doi: 10.1016/j.neurobiolaging.2008.04.002

Nygaard, H. B., van Dyck, C. H., and Strittmatter, S. M. (2014). Fyn kinase inhibition as a novel therapy for Alzheimer's disease. *Alzheimers Res. Ther.* 6:8 doi: 10.1186/alzrt238

Oldfield, E., and Feng, X. (2014). Resistance-resistant antibiotics. *Trends Pharmacol. Sci.* 35, 664–674. doi: 10.1016/j.tips.2014.10.007

Ozer, E. O., Tan, O. U., Ozadali, K., Kucukkilinc, T., Balkan, A., and Ucar, G. (2013). Synthesis, molecular modeling and evaluation of novel N '-2-(4-benzylpiperidin-/piperazin-1-yl)acylhydrazone derivatives as dual inhibitors for cholinesterases and A beta aggregation. *Bioorg. Med. Chem. Lett.* 23, 440–443. doi: 10.1016/j.bmcl.2012.11.064

Palmer, A. M. (2011). Neuroprotective therapeutics for Alzheimer's disease: progress and prospects. *Trends Pharmacol. Sci.* 32, 141–147. doi: 10.1016/j.tips.2010.12.007

Pérez, V., Marco, J. L., Férnandez-Alvarez, E., and Unzeta, M. (1999). Relevance of benzyloxy group in 2-indolyl methylamines in the selective MAO-B inhibition. *Br. J. Pharmacol.* 127, 869–876. doi: 10.1038/sj.bjp.0702600

Prati, F., Uliassi, E., and Bolognesi, M. L. (2014). Two diseases, one approach: multitarget drug discovery in Alzheimer's and neglected tropical diseases. *MedChemComm* 5, 853–861. doi: 10.1039/c4md00069b

Rafii, M. S., Walsh, S., Little, J. T., Behan, K., Reynolds, B., Ward, C., et al. (2011). A phase II trial of huperzine A in mild to moderate Alzheimer disease. *Neurology* 76, 1389–1394. doi: 10.1212/WNL.0b013e318216eb7b

Rochais, C., Lecoutey, C., Gaven, F., Giannoni, P., Hamidouche, K., Hedou, D., et al. (2015). Novel multitarget-directed ligands (MTDLs) with acetylcholinesterase (AChE) inhibitory and serotonergic subtype 4 receptor (5-HT4R) agonist activities as potential agents against Alzheimer's disease: the design of donecopride. *J. Med. Chem.* 58, 3172–3187. doi: 10.1021/acs.jmedchem.5b00115

Rosini, M., Simoni, E., Bartolini, M., Tarozzi, A., Matera, R., Milelli, A., et al. (2011). Exploiting the lipoic acid structure in the search for novel multitarget ligands against Alzheimer's disease. *Eur. J. Med. Chem.* 46, 5435–5442. doi: 10.1016/j.ejmech.2011.09.001

Russo, O., Cachard-Chastel, M., Riviere, C., Giner, M., Soulier, J.-L., Berthouze, M., et al. (2009). Design, synthesis, and biological evaluation of new 5-HT(4) receptor agonists: application as amyloid cascade modulators and potential therapeutic utility in Alzheimer's disease. *J. Med. Chem.* 52, 2214–2225. doi: 10.1021/jm801327q

Samadi, A., de los Ríos, C., Bolea, I., Chioua, M., Iriepa, I., Moraleda, I., et al. (2012). Multipotent MAO and cholinesterase inhibitors for the treatment of Alzheimer's disease: synthesis, pharmacological analysis and molecular modeling of heterocyclic substituted alkyl and cycloalkyl propargyl amine. *Eur. J. Med. Chem.* 52, 251–262. doi: 10.1016/j.ejmech.2012.03.022

Schrijvers, E. M. C., Witteman, J. C. M., Sijbrands, E. J. G., Hofman, A., Koudstaal, P. J., and Breteler, M. M. B. (2010). Insulin metabolism and the risk of Alzheimer disease the rotterdam study. *Neurology* 75, 1982–1987. doi: 10.1212/WNL.0b013e3181ffe4f6

Sirota, M., Dudley, J. T., Kim, J., Chiang, A. P., Morgan, A. A., Sweet-Cordero, A., et al. (2011). Discovery and preclinical validation of drug indications using

compendia of public gene expression data. *Sci. Transl. Med.* 3:96ra77. doi: 10.1126/scitranslmed.3001318

Steindl, T. M., Schuster, D., Laggner, C., and Langer, T. (2006). Parallel screening: A novel concept in pharmacophore modeling and virtual screening. *J. Chem. Inf. Model.* 46, 2146–2157. doi: 10.1021/ci6002043

Stryjewski, M. E., Potgieter, P. D., Li, Y.-P., Barriere, S. L., Churukian, A., Kingsley, J., et al. (2012). TD-1792 versus vancomycin for treatment of complicated skin and skin structure infections. *Antimicrob. Agents Chemother.* 56, 5476–5483. doi: 10.1128/AAC.00712-12

Tang, H., Zhao, L.-Z., Zhao, H.-T., Huang, S.-L., Zhong, S.-M., Qin, J.-K., et al. (2011). Hybrids of oxoisoaporphine-tacrine congeners: novel acetylcholinesterase and acetylcholinesterase-induced beta-amyloid aggregation inhibitors. *Eur. J. Med. Chem.* 46, 4970–4979. doi: 10.1016/j.ejmech.2011.08.002

Tyagi, A., Gupta, S., Pandey, A., and Mohan, C. G. (2010). Alzheimer's disease multi-target directed inhibitor design using sequential virtual screening techniques. *Curr. Res. Inf. Pharm. Sci.* 11, 29–32. Available online at: http://www.niper.ac.in/29_crips.pdf

Vassar, R. (2014). BACE1 inhibitor drugs in clinical trials for Alzheimer's disease. *Alzheimer's Res. Ther.* 6, 89–89. doi: 10.1186/s13195-014-0089-7

Wang, L., Ma, C., Wipf, P., Liu, H., Su, W., and Xie, X.-Q. (2013). Target hunter: an *in silico* target identification tool for predicting therapeutic potential of small organic molecules based on chemogenomic database. *Aaps J.* 15, 395–406. doi: 10.1208/s12248-012-9449-z

Weinreb, O., Amit, T., Bar-Am, O., and Youdim, M. B. H. (2010). Rasagiline: a novel anti-parkinsonian monoamine oxidase-B inhibitor with neuroprotective activity. *Prog. Neurobiol.* 92, 330–344. doi: 10.1016/j.pneurobio.2010.06.008

Wilkinson, D. G., Francis, P. T., Schwam, E., and Payne-Parrish, J. (2004). Cholinesterase inhibitors used in the treatment of Alzheimer's disease the relationship between pharmacological effects and clinical efficacy. *Drugs Aging* 21, 453–478. doi: 10.2165/00002512-200421070-00004

Wisniewski, T., and Goñi, F. (2014). Immunotherapy for Alzheimer's disease. *Biochem. Pharmacol.* 88, 499–507. doi: 10.1016/j.bcp.2013.12.020

Xing, S.-H., Zhu, C.-X., Zhang, R., and An, L. (2014). Huperzine a in the treatment of Alzheimer's disease and vascular dementia: a meta-analysis. *Evid. Based Complement. Alternat. Med.* 2014, 363985–363985. doi: 10.1155/2014/363985

Xu, S. S., Gao, Z. X., Zheng, W., Du, Z. M., Xu, W. A., Yang, J. S., et al. (1995). Efficacy of tablet huperzine-a on memory, cognition, and behavior in Alzheimers-disease. *Acta Pharmacol. Sin.* 16, 391–395.

Yogev-Falach, M., Amit, T., Bar-Am, O., and Youdim, M. B. H. (2003). The importance of propargylamine moiety in the anti-Parkinson drug rasagiline and its derivatives for MAPK-dependent amyloid precursor protein processing. *FASEB J.* 17, 2325. doi: 10.1096/fj.03-0078fje

Youdim, M. B. H. (2006). The path from anti Parkinson drug selegiline and rasagiline to multi-functional neuroprotective anti Alzheimer drugs ladostigil and M30. *Curr. Alzheimer Res.* 3, 541–550. doi: 10.2174/156720506779025288

Youdim, M. B. H. (2013). Multi target neuroprotective and neurorestorative anti-Parkinson and anti-Alzheimer drugs ladostigil and m30 derived from rasagiline. *Exp. Neurobiol.* 22, 1–10. doi: 10.5607/en.2013.22.1.1

Youdim, M. B. H., Finberg, J. P. M., Levy, R., Sterling, J., Lerner, D., Berger-Paskin, T., et al. (1995). *R-Enantiomers of N-Propargyl-Aminoindan Compounds, their Preparation and Pharmaceutical Compositions Containing Them.* U.S. Patent No: US5457133 A

Youdim, M. B. H., Gross, A., and Finberg, J. P. M. (2001). Rasagiline N-propargyl-1R(+)-aminoindan, a selective and potent inhibitor of mitochondrial monoamine oxidase B. *Br. J. Pharmacol.* 132, 500–506. doi: 10.1038/sj.bjp.0703826

Youdim, M. B. H., Maruyama, W., and Naoi, M. (2005). Neuropharmacological, neuroprotective and amyloid precursor processing properties of selective MAO-B inhibitor antiparkinsonian drug, rasagiline. *Drugs Today* 41, 369–391. doi: 10.1358/dot.2005.41.6.893613

Zheng, H., Fridkin, M., and Youdim, M. (2014). From single target to multitarget/network therapeutics in Alzheimer's therapy. *Pharmaceuticals* 7, 113–135. doi: 10.3390/ph7020113

Zheng, H., Fridkin, M., and Youdim, M. B. H. (2010a). Site-activated chelators derived from anti-parkinson drug rasagiline as a potential safer and more effective approach to the treatment of Alzheimer's disease. *Neurochem. Res.* 35, 2117–2123. doi: 10.1007/s11064-010-0293-1

Zheng, H., Gal, S., Weiner, L. M., Bar-Am, O., Warshawsky, A., Fridkin, M., et al. (2005). Novel multifunctional neuroprotective iron chelator-monoamine oxidase inhibitor drugs for neurodegenerative diseases: *in vitro* studies on antioxidant activity, prevention of lipid peroxide formation and monoamine oxidase inhibition. *J. Neurochem.* 95, 68–78. doi: 10.1111/j.1471-4159.2005.03340.x

Zheng, H., Youdim, M. B. H., and Fridkin, M. (2010b). Site-activated chelators targeting acetylcholinesterase and monoamine oxidase for Alzheimer's therapy. *ACS Chem. Biol.* 5, 603–610. doi: 10.1021/cb900264w

Conflict of Interest Statement: The authors declare that the research was conducted in the absence of any commercial or financial relationships that could be construed as a potential conflict of interest.

3

Monoaminergic Mechanisms in Epilepsy may Offer Innovative Therapeutic Opportunity for Monoaminergic Multi-Target Drugs

Dubravka Svob Strac[1], Nela Pivac[1], Ilse J. Smolders[2], Wieslawa A. Fogel[3], Philippe De Deurwaerdere[4] and Giuseppe Di Giovanni[5]*

[1] *Division of Molecular Medicine, Rudjer Boskovic Institute, Zagreb, Croatia,* [2] *Department of Pharmaceutical Chemistry and Drug Analysis, Vrije Universiteit Brussel, Brussels, Belgium,* [3] *Department of Hormone Biochemistry, Medical University of Lodz, Lodz, Poland,* [4] *Centre National de la Recherche Scientifique (Unité Mixte de Recherche 5293), Bordeaux, France,* [5] *Laboratory of Neurophysiology, Department of Physiology and Biochemistry, University of Malta, Msida, Malta*

Edited by:
Alfredo Meneses,
CINVESTAV, Mexico

Reviewed by:
Hiram Luna-Munguia,
University of Michigan, USA
Władysław Lasoń,
Institute of Pharmacology, Polish
Academy of Sciences, Poland
Javad Mirnajafi-Zadeh,
Tarbiat Modares University, Iran

*Correspondence:
Giuseppe Di Giovanni
giuseppe.digiovanni@um.edu.mt

A large body of experimental and clinical evidence has strongly suggested that monoamines play an important role in regulating epileptogenesis, seizure susceptibility, convulsions, and comorbid psychiatric disorders commonly seen in people with epilepsy (PWE). However, neither the relative significance of individual monoamines nor their interaction has yet been fully clarified due to the complexity of these neurotransmitter systems. In addition, epilepsy is diverse, with many different seizure types and epilepsy syndromes, and the role played by monoamines may vary from one condition to another. In this review, we will focus on the role of serotonin, dopamine, noradrenaline, histamine, and melatonin in epilepsy. Recent experimental, clinical, and genetic evidence will be reviewed in consideration of the mutual relationship of monoamines with the other putative neurotransmitters. The complexity of epileptic pathogenesis may explain why the currently available drugs, developed according to the classic drug discovery paradigm of "one-molecule-one-target," have turned out to be effective only in a percentage of PWE. Although, no antiepileptic drugs currently target specifically monoaminergic systems, multi-target directed ligands acting on different monoaminergic proteins, present on both neurons and glia cells, may represent a new approach in the management of seizures, and their generation as well as comorbid neuropsychiatric disorders.

Keywords: monoamine receptors, multi-target direct ligands, epilepsy, epileptogenesis, antiepileptic drugs, quad-partite synapse, astrocytes, microglia

INTRODUCTION

Epilepsy is a complex chronic group of neurological disorders that affects ~60 million people worldwide, with 6 million in Europe alone (Baulac et al., 2015).

Epilepsy is characterized by spontaneous and recurrent unprovoked seizures (bursts of neuronal hyperactivity) arising in the brain that can be "focal" or "partial" if they remain confined to their area of origin, or "generalized" if they spread to the entire cerebral hemispheres. Recently, seizures have been classified in focal and generalized convulsive and non-convulsive epilepsies according to their different electrophysiological and clinical characteristics (Berg et al., 2010). Epilepsy can be symptomatic, for example, due to stroke, infections, brain tumors, prolonged febrile seizures, and other occurrences of status epilepticus (SE). Additionally, about 40% of all epilepsies, especially during childhood, and adolescence (Guerrini, 2006), are idiopathic epilepsies. Several defects in ion channel or neurotransmitter genes or proteins that control brain excitability have been recently identified in some idiopathic epilepsies (Scharfman, 2007). In addition, various epidemiological and family studies have suggested a genetic basis of epilepsy (Myers and Mefford, 2015). A number of genes have been associated with epilepsy disorders in a Mendelian manner (Harden, 2002). However, it has been suggested that most epilepsies have a polygenic basis, with multiple genetic susceptibility factors which have only partial effects, but act in concert, and interact with various environmental factors (Ferraro and Buono, 2006; Tan and Berkovic, 2010). The genes associated with epilepsy are involved in different molecular pathways, including the regulation of development and function of the nervous system (Holmes and Noebels, 2016). Although, the majority of genes associated with epilepsies are coding for different voltage and ligand-gated ion channels or regulating the action of excitatory or inhibitory neurotransmission (i.e., CHRNA4, CHRNA2, CHRNB2, GABRG2, GABRA1, KCNQ2, KCNQ3, SCN1B, SCN1A, SCN2A), the potential role of several other genes (i.e., ARX, CDKL5, LGI1, PCDH19, SLC2A1, SPTAN1, STXBP1) in the epilepsy has also been also suggested (Rees, 2010; Hildebrand et al., 2013).

Genetics therefore plays a role, although a complex one, in almost all acquired epilepsies.

The lifetime prevalence of epilepsy is 1–2%, and it affects individuals of all ages regardless of gender or socio-economic status. Epilepsy is a significant health concern for the human population and people with epilepsy (PWE) carry a risk of

---

Abbreviations: SERT, 5-HT transporter; 5-HTTLPR, 5-HT-transporter-linked polymorphic region; 6-OHDA, 6-hydroxydopamine; AC, adenylyl cyclase; AR, adrenoceptor; AT1, angiotensin; AEDs, antiepileptic drugs; DBH, beta-hydroxylase; SNDRIs, block the synaptic reuptake of 5-HT, NA and DA; BDNF, brain-derived neurotrophic factor; beta-alanyl-L-histidine, carnosine; COMT, catechol-O-methyltransferase; CNS, Central Nervous System; CSF, cerebrospinal fluid; ChE, cholinesterase; cAMP, cyclic adenosine monophosphate; DAT, DA transporter; DBA, Dilute Brown Non-Agouti; DA, dopamine; FDA, Food and Drug Administration; GAT-1, GABA transporter-1; GAERS, Genetic Absence Epilepsy Rats from Strasbourg; GEPR, genetic epilepsy-prone rat; GLU, glutamate; HRs, histamine receptors; IAE, idiopathic absence epilepsy; JME, juvenile myoclonic epilepsy; KA, kainic acid; KO, knock out; L-DOPA, L-3,4-dihydroxyphenylalanine; L, long; MAO-I, MAO inhibitors; MAO-BIs, MAO-B inhibitors; MES, maximal electroshock seizure; mTOR, mechanistic target of rapamycin; MT, melatonin; MTE-HS, mesial TLE with hippocampal sclerosis; mCPP, meta-chlorophenylpiperazine; MAO-A and MAO-B, monoamine oxidase A and B; MATs, monoamine transporters; MTDL, multi-target-directed ligands; DSP4, N-(2-chloroethyl)-N-ethyl-2-bromobenzylamine; NAT, NA transporter; NMDA, N-methyl-d-aspartate; PTZ, pentylenetretrazole; PWE, people with epilepsy; PLC, phospholipase C; PET, positron emission tomography; SSRIs, selective serotonin reuptake inhibitors; 5-HT, Serotonin; SNRIs, serotonin-noradrenaline reuptake inhibitors; S, short; SCN1A, sodium voltage gated channel alpha subunit 1; SCN2A, sodium voltage-gated channel alpha subunit 2; SRSs, spontaneous recur rent seizures; SE, status epilepticus; TLE, temporal lobe epilepsy; SUDEP, unexpected death in epilepsy; VNS, vagus nerve stimulation; WAG/Rij, Wistar Albino Glaxo rats from Rijswijk.

---

premature mortality, with a life expectancy 10 years less than the general population (Gaitatzis et al., 2004).

There is currently no cure or prevention for epilepsy. Most, if not all of the approved antiepileptic drugs (AEDs) are not truly "antiepileptic" but merely "anti-seizures" (Van Liefferinge et al., 2013). Indeed, the AEDs do not stop epileptogenesis, the process of converting a normal brain to a brain with epilepsy, but at the most they reach complete seizure control. Unfortunately, not all PWE respond to the therapies, with 30–40% of them possessing pharmacoresistant epilepsy (Kobau et al., 2008). Although, the efforts in antiepileptic drug development have not solved the issue, they have encouraged experimental and clinical research to focus on different mechanisms involved in the neurological disorder. Indeed, many candidate processes and molecular targets are currently under intense scrutiny and hopefully will improve treatment and quality of life of PWE.

Monoamines are major neuromodulator systems in the central nervous system (CNS) and compelling evidence accumulated in the last 30 years has also established their pivotal role in epilepsy (Kobayashi and Mori, 1977; Kurian et al., 2011). Serotonin (5-HT; Bagdy et al., 2007; Guiard and Di Giovanni, 2015), dopamine (DA; Bozzi and Borrelli, 2013), noradrenaline (NA; Giorgi et al., 2004), histamine (Bhowmik et al., 2012), and melatonin (MT; Tchekalarova et al., 2015b; Brigo and Igwe, 2016) are all known to halt seizure activity.

Further proof of monoaminergic involvement in the pathogenesis of epilepsy is the evidence that depression, bipolar disorders, and other neuropsychiatric disorders classically related to monoamine dysfunctions, may augment the risk of seizures and/or vice versa. As matter of fact, PWE with longer duration of active epilepsy show higher comorbidity of depressive disorders, bipolar disorder and anxiety (Rocha et al., 2014), and in depressed patients there is a higher rate of epilepsy compared to general population (Garcia, 2012). It has been suggested that epilepsy and mood disorders may be different manifestations of the same disturbances in transmission and/or signal transduction mediated by monoamines, hyperactivity of the hypothalamic-pituitary-adrenal axis, and CNS inflammation (Rocha et al., 2014). As both epilepsy and monoamine-based neuropsychiatric disorders are complex diseases that imply changes in multiple neurotransmitters and both neuronal and glial cells activity, a comprehensive understanding of the underlying mechanisms is still in its infancy. Nevertheless, this evidence of dual link between these two disorders suggest that drugs targeting monoamines may be useful for both epilepsy and its neuropsychiatric comorbidities (Guiard and Di Giovanni, 2015; Venzi et al., 2016).

Although, the role of monoamines in epilepsy was reviewed for the first time by Kobayashi and Mori (1977), followed by intensive exploration in pre-clinical and clinical research over the last 40 years, this has not led to new treatments. Indeed, the questions asked by Kobayashi and Mori (1977) "Is there an abnormal metabolism of monoamines in the brain of epileptic patients? If so, how is it related to the elaboration or maintenance of epileptic seizures?" do not yet have definitive answers.

Compelling evidence shows that monoaminergic systems appear dysregulated in animal (Szabo et al., 2015) and human epileptic brain and increased monoamines and metabolite levels in the cerebrospinal fluid (CSF) of PWE have been consistently observed (Pintor et al., 1990; Naffah-Mazzacoratti et al., 1996).

Nevertheless, the elevated levels of 5-HT and DA metabolites during epilepsy may represent an epiphenomenon, rather than a concerted strategy of local or distal neurons to contain an epileptogenic focus (Lowy and Meltzer, 1988). Indeed, the rate of monoaminergic metabolism (i.e., synthesis, uptake, and clearance) does not significantly correlate with the epileptic condition in baboon (Szabo et al., 2015). Moreover, it has recently been shown that receptor antagonism completely prevented all kainic acid-induced increases in extracellular hippocampal 5-HT levels in rats without affecting seizure development *per se*. This result suggested a lack of a direct relationship between seizure susceptibility and alterations in hippocampal 5-HT levels, at least in this rat model (Tchekalarova et al., 2015b).

These findings, however, do not necessarily exclude the monoaminergic system as a potential source of pathogenesis in epilepsy and sudden unexpected death in epilepsy (SUDEP; Richerson and Buchanan, 2011).

As a further complication, monoamines seem to have a dual effect being proconvulsant when in high concentration in the epileptic foci. Indeed, within a certain concentration range, intrahippocampally applied 5-HT contributed to the prevention of hippocampally evoked limbic seizures. On the other hand, excessive 5-HT increases worsened seizure outcome (Clinckers et al., 2004) and elevated, endogenous noradrenergic transmission is for example an etiological factor in some cases of epilepsy (Fitzgerald, 2010).

In the following sections of this review, we will focus on the role of different monoamines in seizure onset and spread, discussing anatomical, pharmacological, and genetic evidence obtained in animal and human studies. We will provide the rationale for the use of drugs targeting monoamines or their related molecules in epilepsy, some already representing good examples of multi-target directed drugs. We finish by exploring the interesting possibility that the monoaminergic treatment may cure the dysfunction of the quad-partite synapse acting at the level of their different components, i.e., (pre- and postsynaptic) neurons, astrocytes, and microglia cells.

MONOAMINES IN EPILEPSY: PRECLINICAL AND CLINICAL EVIDENCE

Serotonergic System in Epilepsy

It goes without saying that 5-HT is involved in epilepsy mechanisms. According to a variety of recent findings, neurodevelopmental alterations of serotonergic circuits in mice are crucial in controlling seizure susceptibility to the well-established chemoconvulsant kainic acid (KA; i.e., a glutamatergic kainate receptor agonist) in later life (Tripathi and Bozzi, 2015). Clinical presentations of human epilepsy have often been attributed to deficiencies of cerebral monoamines, including

5-HT (Kurian et al., 2011). Serotonin (but also DA) enhancement may even be involved to a certain extent in the mechanisms of action of several clinically used antiepileptic drugs (Yan et al., 1992; Ahmad et al., 2005; Biton, 2007).

Nevertheless, the picture is not always that clear-cut. The classical view is that the monoamine enhancing antidepressant drugs are contraindicated in PWE, or should at least be used with caution. Against this assumption, more and more reports provided evidence that several 5-HT enhancing antidepressants were not proconvulsant but rather displayed anticonvulsant properties (Hamid and Kanner, 2013). Dailey and Naritoku (1996) deducted that non-monoaminergic off-target effects of antidepressants are most likely responsible for the increased risk of seizures.

The most straightforward answer to the question—why 5-HT seems to exert such a complex role in the modulation of enhanced brain excitability and epilepsy phenomena—is of course the fact that 5-HT interacts with a variety of different receptor subtypes linked to divergent signal transduction cascades, thereby often exerting opposing control on cell membrane potentials (De Deurwaerdere and Di Giovanni, 2016). Moreover, these 5-HTR subtypes are differently distributed in distinct brain areas and diverse brain circuitries involved in various types of epilepsy. Moreover, as will be illustrated in following sections, the same holds true for the other monoamines described within this review.

For the remainder of this 5-HT section, we will focus merely on 5-HTR subtype-specific seizure-modulating actions. Most evidence can be found on the roles of $5\text{-}HT_1R$ and $5\text{-}HT_2R$ subtypes and the $5\text{-}HT_3R$, while—to the best of our knowledge—less literature is available with regard to the possible involvement of $5\text{-}HT_4$ and $5\text{-}HT_6Rs$ in epilepsy mechanisms. No data has been published on $5\text{-}HT_5Rs$ in epilepsy. Finally, the involvement of the $5\text{-}HT_7R$ in mechanisms of epilepsy is still ambiguous (Ciranna and Catania, 2014; Nikiforuk, 2015).

Within the scope of the current manuscript, it will be impossible to review all the available data to date, but we will focus on the most prominent and/or recent findings. We also refer to the review paper by Panczyk et al. (2015) who listed the evidence for the involvement of $5\text{-}HT_{1A}$, $5\text{-}HT_{2C}$, $5\text{-}HT_3$, $5\text{-}HT_4$, and $5\text{-}HT_7Rs$ as well as the 5-HT transporter (SERT) in epilepsy (Panczyk et al., 2015).

With regard to the $5\text{-}HT_{2A}R$ and its seizure modulating effects, literature is abundant but also very complex. For a complete and recent overview on the role of the $5\text{-}HT_{2A}R$ in rodent epilepsy models, we refer to the detailed review by Guiard and Di Giovanni (2015). They summarized the evidence for $5\text{-}HT_{2A}R$ modulation in both generalized and focal epilepsies, and concluded that both proconvulsant and anticonvulsant roles have been established for this $5\text{-}HT_{2A}R$ subtype, depending on the dose of the ligands used, the experimental rodent model investigated and the different populations of the receptors. At high doses of the $5\text{-}HT_{2A}R$ ligands, proconvulsant effects were often noted which may be attributed—at least partly—to other non-selective off-target effects (Guiard and Di Giovanni, 2015). Because of this complexity, we refer the readers to this in deep review.

Focal Seizures

Human data

In PWE suffering from TLE, hippocampal 5-HT depletion (da Fonseca et al., 2015) and reduced 5-HT$_{1A}$R availability have been observed. The latter somatodendritic 5-HT$_{1A}$ autoreceptor is one of the best characterized subtypes of the 14 known 5-HTRs and is clearly implicated in seizure modulation. A large body of evidence on this receptor subtype in epilepsy has arisen from many positron emission tomography (PET) studies in PWE, and reduced 5-HT$_{1A}$R binding in the epileptic focus has been repeatedly and consistently found in these temporal lobe epilepsy (TLE) patients (Hasler et al., 2007; Lothe et al., 2008; Giovacchini et al., 2009; Assem-Hilger et al., 2010). All of these studies point to the fact that diminished 5-HT$_{1A}$R expression and subsequent less activation by endogenous 5-HT may lead to the epileptic phenotype. PET imaging of brain 5-HT$_{1A}$Rs has also helped in the correct identification of the epileptogenic zone during the preoperative evaluation of temporal lobe of PWE subjected to epilepsy surgery (Didelot et al., 2008; Theodore et al., 2012).

More recently, it has been shown that both 5-HT$_6$Rs (Wang et al., 2015) and 5-HT$_7$Rs (Yang et al., 2012) were upregulated in the human neocortex of PWE with refractory TLE. These interesting findings call for more studies with 5-HT$_6$R and 5-HT$_7$R ligands.

Animal data

Acute seizure evocation with KA led to increases in hippocampal 5-HT tissue content and extracellular 5-HT levels (Alfaro-Rodriguez et al., 2011; Tchekalarova et al., 2015a) while during the spontaneous recurrent limbic seizures in the KA model decreases in 5-HT content were found (Tchekalarova et al., 2011). In another well-established post-SE rat model for focal epilepsy using pilocarpine (i.e., a muscarinergic receptor agonist) as the chemoconvulsant, 5-HT hippocampal content (Cavalheiro et al., 1994) and hippocampal 5-HT levels (Meurs et al., 2008) were increased during the acute seizure phase but not during the following spontaneous recurrent seizure phase (Cavalheiro et al., 1994; Szyndler et al., 2005). Comparing three acute limbic seizure models, which differed only in the chemoconvulsant used to evoke the seizures in rats, no straightforward correlation between the seizure activity and increased hippocampal extracellular 5-HT concentrations could be found (Meurs et al., 2008).

Concerning the role of the somatodendritic 5-HT$_{1A}$ autoreceptor in focal epilepsy, the majority of pharmacological studies clearly highlight the anticonvulsant effects of 5-HT$_{1A}$R agonists against limbic seizures evoked in various rat models, e.g., against pilocarpine-induced seizures (Clinckers et al., 2004; Lopez-Meraz et al., 2005; Pericic et al., 2005; Orban et al., 2013), as well as against status epilepticus evoked by lithium pilocarpine (Yang et al., 2014).

Activation of the 5-HT$_{2C}$Rs do not appear to play a pivotal role in focal epilepsy or on the contrary is proepileptic (Di Giovanni and De Deurwaerdere, 2016). Indeed, 5-HT$_{2C}$R agonists with different pharmacological profiles such as meta-chlorophenylpiperazine (mCPP) and lorcaserin, but not RO60-0175, were able to stop the elongation of the electrically triggered hippocampal maximal dentate gyrus activation in a limbic seizure model in anesthetized rats, an effect that was not blocked but rather potentiated by pre-treatment of SB 242084 (Orban et al., 2014), a selective 5-HT$_{2C}$R antagonist. In addition, 5-HT$_3$Rs display also no importance in focal hippocampal seizures (Watanabe et al., 1998).

A selective 5-HT$_6$R antagonist was able to attenuate spontaneous recurrent seizures in the post-SE pilocarpine rat model, and diminished hippocampal mechanistic target of rapamycin (mTOR) activity, suggesting that 5-HT$_6$Rs may mediate limbic seizures via mTOR signaling (Wang et al., 2015). Moreover, 5-HT$_6$R expression was upregulated in the hippocampus and neocortex of the pilocarpine-treated rats (Wang et al., 2015), confirming the finding in PWE as described above. There is one study showing that 5-HT$_7$R antagonism also diminished the number of limbic seizures in pilocarpine-treated rats (Yang et al., 2012). More confirmatory results with 5-HT$_6$R and 5-HT$_7$R antagonists in focal epilepsy models might be interesting to obtain.

In vitro data

Serotonin inhibited bicuculline (i.e., a GABA$_A$ receptor antagonist)- and KA-evoked epileptiform activity in brain slices via membrane hyperpolarization (Salgado and Alkadhi, 1995). The use of a 5-HT$_3$R agonist showed no effect on cortical epileptiform activity (Bobula et al., 2001). In rat hippocampal brain slices, 5-HT$_4$R agonism aggravated population spikes, evoked by electrical stimulation and spontaneous epileptiform activity (Tokarski et al., 2002). The influence of many other 5-HT receptor subtypes on epileptiform activity remains elusive.

Generalized Convulsive Seizures

Animal data

Hippocampal 5-HT$_{1A}$ and 5-HT$_{1B}$R immunoreactivities were decreased in the rat unilateral hypoxic-induced epilepsy model (An and Kim, 2011). Anticonvulsant effects of 5-HT$_{1A}$R agonists have also been repeatedly reported in models for generalized seizures, such as the pentylenetretrazole (PTZ, a prototypic antagonist of GABA$_A$ receptors) model (Lopez-Meraz et al., 2005), tonic-clonic seizures evoked by amygdala kindling (Lopez-Meraz et al., 2005), and the picrotoxin (another typically used antagonist of GABA$_A$ receptors) model (Peričić et al., 2005). The seizure modulating roles of specific 5-HT$_{1B}$, 5-HT$_{1D}$, and 5-HT$_{1E}$Rs are less studied, but anticonvulsant properties upon 5-HT$_{1B}$ activation in the PTZ model were described (Wesolowska et al., 2006).

Strong evidence for decreased excitability upon 5-HT$_{2C}$R activation was obtained from the 5-HT$_{2C}$R knock out (KO) mice that displayed a clear generalized epileptic phenotype and exhibited an increased sensitivity to chemoconvulsant PTZ (Tecott et al., 1995; Heisler et al., 1998).

The first report using a 5-HT$_3$R ligand in relation to epilepsy was described by Cutler and Piper (Cutler, 1990) who showed that 5-HT$_3$R antagonism had no effects upon seizure susceptibility or severity in Mongolian gerbils. Unclear effects of 5-HT$_3$R antagonists were noted on audiogenic seizures in Dilute Brown Non-Agouti (DBA)/2 mice (Semenova and Ticku, 1992) and on alcohol withdrawal seizures (Kostowski et al., 1993; Grant et al., 1994). A 5-HT$_3$R agonist facilitated generalized seizure development in the well-characterized rat amygdala kindling model (Wada et al., 1997). Despite all these initial negative results, recent interest in the 5-HT$_3$R subtype emerged in the PTZ model for generalized seizures and in PTZ kindling. Indeed, 5-HT$_3$R agonism exhibited dose-dependent anticonvulsant effects in the PTZ model (Li et al., 2014). Moreover, the 5-HT$_3$R subtype seems to play a prominent role in mediating the anticonvulsant effects of various selective 5-HT reuptake inhibitors in this classical PTZ model for generalized epilepsy (Payandemehr et al., 2012; Alhaj et al., 2015).

PTZ-induced convulsive responses were aggravated in 5-HT$_4$R KO mice (Compan et al., 2004). Potent and selective 5-HT$_6$R antagonists displayed clear anticonvulsant effects in the maximal electroshock test in rats (Routledge et al., 2000; Stean et al., 2002; Hirst et al., 2006).

Some pharmacological studies with 5-HT$_7$R antagonists pointed to anticonvulsant effects in various rodent models. For instance, antagonism of 5-HT$_7$Rs protected DBA/2J mice against audiogenic seizures (Bourson et al., 1997). Anticonvulsant effects of 5-HT$_7$R agonists were also described against picrotoxin-evoked seizures in mice (Pericic and Svob Strac, 2007). In line with these findings, constitutive deletion of the 5-HT$_7$R resulted in proconvulsant effects as the KO mice exhibited decreased thresholds for electroshock-induced seizures and decreased seizure thresholds for PTZ- and cocaine-induced seizures (Witkin et al., 2007). More investigations are therefore needed to clarify the exact role of the 5-HT$_7$R in generalized epilepsy.

Generalized Non-convulsive Seizures and Epilepsy Syndromes
Human data
Insufficient human evidence on generalized non-convulsive seizures and epilepsy syndromes exists so far. Treatment of a male patient suffering from drug-resistant epilepsy, resulting from a deleterious de novo sodium voltage-gated channel alpha subunit 2 (SCN2A), gene splice-site mutation, with the 5-HT precursor 5-hydroxytryptophan, led to mild clinical improvement (Horvath et al., 2016).

Animal data
Some typical 5-HT$_{2C}$R agonists dose-dependently suppressed absence seizures in the Genetic Absence Epilepsy Rats from Strasbourg (GAERS), a well-established polygenic rat model of absence epilepsy and non-convulsive seizures; these effects were prevented when administering a selective 5-HT$_{2C}$R antagonist, indicating the potential of selective 5-HT$_{2C}$R agonists as novel anti-absence drugs (Venzi et al., 2016). Experiments on Wistar Albino Glaxo rats from Rijswijk (WAG/Rij) rats, another polygenic rat model of absence epilepsy, have found that mCPP decreased spike-wave discharges (SWDs) cumulative duration via the activation of 5-HT$_{2C}$Rs (Jakus et al., 2003). Strikingly, while SB 242084 had no effect on SWDs when administered on its own in WAG/Rij rats, (Jakus et al., 2003; Jakus and Bagdy, 2011) it showed some anti-absence effects in GAERS. The 5-HT$_{2B}$R is less characterized and/or without effect on

the threshold for generalized seizures (Upton et al., 1998; Di Giovanni and De Deurwaerdere, 2016). Antagonism of 5-HT$_7$Rs reduced spontaneous spike-wave discharges in the WAG/Rij rats (Graf et al., 2004).

In vitro data
Sourbron et al. (2016) were able to demonstrate that selective 5-HT$_{1D}$-, 5-HT$_{1E}$-, 5-HT$_{2A}$-, 5-HT$_{2C}$-, and 5-HT$_7$-R agonists significantly decreased epileptiform activity in a homozygous sodium voltage gated channel alpha subunit 1 (SCN1A) mutant zebrafish model for Dravet syndrome (Sourbron et al., 2016).

Dopaminergic System in Epilepsy
The seizure modulating effects of DA have received a lot of attention since the 1960s, so it is almost an impossible task to review the abundant evidence to date. This section will therefore summarize the most obvious findings and highlight a few recent studies. For a more expanded review, we recommend the fine manuscript by Bozzi and Borrelli (2013) who reviewed the intracellular signaling pathways triggered by activation of different DA receptors (DARs) in relation to their role in limbic seizures and epileptogenesis (Bozzi and Borrelli, 2013).

For years, it has been known that innate deficiencies in DA contributed to the seizure-prone states of some genetic rodent models and therefore may be a predisposing factor for human epilepsy (Starr, 1996). Generally, excitability is affected in a biphasic fashion via DAergic actions: D$_1$-like receptor activation merely increases excitation while D$_2$-like receptor activation largely leads to anticonvulsant actions. The important role of D$_2$-like receptors in regulating brain excitability is clinically supported by the well-known decrease in the seizure thresholds in PWE treated with antipsychotic D$_2$R antagonists. However, information on selective D$_3$R, D$_4$R, and D$_5$R modulating effects on seizures are scarce.

Focal Seizures
Human data
In PWE suffering from TLE, alterations in the neocortical DA content, D1-like and D2-like receptor expression, and DA transporter (DAT) binding have been reported (Rocha et al., 2012). Reduced D$_2$R/D$_3$R binding, sustained impairment of the DAergic system, was demonstrated in extrastriatal and/or striatal brain regions of PWE, specifically with TLE (Bernedo Paredes et al., 2015).

Animal data
Similarly as described above for 5-HT, acute kainic acid-induced seizures increased hippocampal DA tissue content and extracellular DA levels, (Alfaro-Rodriguez et al., 2011; Tchekalarova et al., 2015b) while during the spontaneous recurrent limbic seizures in the kainic acid model, decreases in DA content were found (Tchekalarova et al., 2011). In the pilocarpine rat model, DA hippocampal content (Cavalheiro et al., 1994) and hippocampal DA levels (Meurs et al., 2008) were increased during the acute seizure phase. During the chronic recurrent seizure phase in the pilocarpine model, hippocampal DA content was elevated in one study (Cavalheiro et al., 1994)

while no alterations were described in another study (Szyndler et al., 2005). Interestingly, when comparing three acute limbic seizure models, a direct relationship between the seizure activity and increased hippocampal extracellular concentrations of DA were established (Meurs et al., 2008).

In line with the majority of data described for generalized seizures, D_1-like receptor-activation results in seizure enhancement in the limbic pilocarpine model (Barone et al., 1990). Activation of hippocampal D_2-like receptors, leading to inhibition of adenylyl cyclase (AC) via Gi coupling, consistently protected rodents against limbic motor seizures, supporting seizure facilitation via D_1R-mediated increases in cyclic adenosine monophosphate (cAMP; Bozzi and Borrelli, 2013). Moreover, the D_2-like receptors seem to play a pivotal role in the overall anticonvulsant effect of hippocampal DA since a selective D_2R antagonist abolished DA-mediated anticonvulsant effects in the acute pilocarpine limbic seizure model (Clinckers et al., 2004). Most interestingly, D_2-like receptor signaling in the hippocampus also leads to glycogen synthase kinase 3β inhibition and hippocampal cell survival following kainic acid administration (Dunleavy et al., 2013).

In vitro data
Electrophysiological data demonstrated that DA can affect hippocampal excitability in a biphasic fashion but the predominant DA action was an D_2-like receptor-mediated inhibitory effect via hyperpolarization of the resting membrane potential and a long-lasting increase in after-hyperpolarization (Benardo and Prince, 1982). D_4R KO mice displayed cortical hyperexcitability, as measured with electrophysiological current and voltage-clamp recordings, suggesting that D_4R activation can negatively modulate glutamate (GLU) activity in the frontal cortex (Rubinstein et al., 2001). This is not unexpected from a receptor from the D_2-like receptor family that mainly exhibits decreased excitation upon activation.

Generalized Convulsive Seizures
Human data
Patients with juvenile myoclonic epilepsy showed a reduction in D_2R/D_3R binding restricted to the bilateral posterior putamen, suggesting an alteration of the DAergic system within this region (Landvogt et al., 2010).

Animal data
Repeated D_1-like receptor activation results in generalized seizures, disrupted hippocampal plasticity, and impaired long-term recognition memory (Gangarossa et al., 2014). Initially, the majority of results on D_1-like receptor agonist effects on behavioral seizure thresholds clearly indicated proconvulsant effects (Starr, 1996). Nevertheless, recent reports showed that D_1-like receptor agonists, linked to stimulation of adenylate cyclase (AC; but not phospholipase C, PLC), led to prominent behavioral seizures in rodents, whereas D_1-like receptor agonists, linked to stimulation of phospholipase C (PLC, but not AC), did not (O'sullivan et al., 2008). The D_5R belongs to the D_1-like receptor family and upon its activation mainly increased excitation is

observed, although less prominent in comparison with D_1R activation and subsequent increases in cAMP (O'sullivan et al., 2008).

The role of the D_3R in seizure modulation appears to be more complex. D_3R KOs were less sensitive to picrotoxin-induced clonic seizures and mortality suggesting proconvulsant D_3R-mediated signaling (Micale et al., 2009). On the other hand, D_3R-mediated agonist actions protected against acute and cocaine-kindled seizures in mice and reduced lethal effects of acute cocaine toxicity (Witkin et al., 2008). Most probably, different D_3R downstream signaling cascades in different implicated brain regions may explain the contrasting results (Bozzi and Borrelli, 2013); however more investigations are required.

Generalized Non-convulsive Seizures and Epilepsy Syndromes
Human data
The DA precursor L-3,4-dihydroxyphenylalanine (L-DOPA) improved the clinical outcome of a male patient suffering from intractable epileptic encephalopathy (Horvath et al., 2016), again sustaining an overall anticonvulsant DA-mediated action. Nevertheless, DA concentrations in media collected from neural cultures, derived from induced pluripotent stem cells from a patient with the Dravet syndrome, were higher than those from wild-type neural cultures (Maeda et al., 2016).

Animal data
Activation of both D_1-like and D_2-like receptors showed anti-absence effects (Deransart et al., 2000), probably by decreasing $GABA_A$ receptor-mediated tonic inhibition (Yague et al., 2013) that is altered in animal models of absence seizures (Cope et al., 2009). Up-regulation of D_3 (but not D_1, D_2, or D_5) receptor mRNA seems part of the epileptic phenotype in absence-epilepsy prone rats (Deransart et al., 2001). The role of D_1-like and D_2-like receptors in non-convulsive epilepsy is thus less clear-cut in comparison with the data obtained in focal and generalized seizure and epilepsy models.

Noradrenergic System in Epilepsy
The suggestion that NA may act as an anticonvulsant was posed over 60 years ago (Chen et al., 1954). Subsequent experimental studies provided firm evidence that the noradrenergic system modifies seizure activity. Nowadays, vagus nerve stimulation (VNS) is an adjunctive treatment for resistant epilepsy and depression (Panebianco et al., 2016).

Focal Seizures
Human data
In this context, the receptor-binding assays with prazosin as a ligand, performed on isolated cortical cell membranes from 10 PWE subjected to temporal lobectomy due to intractable partial epilepsy, showed a reduced density of $α_1$ adrenoceptor (AR) in the sites of the epileptic foci with no change in affinity. It was concluded that the lower receptor density may result in noradrenergic hyposensitivity that could contribute to a localized

diminution in inhibitory mechanisms in epileptic foci (Briere et al., 1986).

Animal data

Likewise, VNS is an effective adjunctive treatment for medically refractory epilepsy, and was found to produce its anticonvulsive effect by increasing NA levels in the hippocampus that is critically involved in the generation of limbic seizures (Raedt et al., 2011). The anticonvulsant action of VNS on pilocarpine-induced seizures in rats can be abolished by the blockade of hippocampal α_2-AR, indicating a strong causal link between the seizure-suppressing effect of VNS and hippocampal noradrenergic signaling (Raedt et al., 2011). Interestingly, combined but not separate α_2- and β_2-AR stimulation inhibited limbic seizures induced by pilocarpine infusion in the hippocampus of rats. On the other hand, α_{1A}-AR stimulation and α_{1D}-AR antagonism alone also inhibited seizures associated with respectively significant hippocampal GABA increases and GLU decreases (Clinckers et al., 2010).

In vitro data

NA has demonstrated both proconvulsant and antiepileptic properties; however, the specific pharmacology of these actions has not been clearly established. For instance, under conditions of impaired GABAergic inhibition, the excitatory and inhibitory effects of NA on hippocampal CA3 epileptiform activity are mediated primarily via β- and α_2-ARs respectively. Moreover, the NA antiepileptic effect in CA3 epileptiform in vitro is not dependent on the increase in GABAergic function (Jurgens et al., 2005) but is due to the activation of the α_2-AR on presynaptic glutamatergic terminals of the recurrent axon collaterals of the CA3 pyramidal neurons (Jurgens et al., 2007). While the α_1-AR antagonists prazosin and terazosin had no effect on hippocampal CA3 epileptiform activity in slice with GABA system blocked, (Jurgens et al., 2005) there is in vitro evidence showing that α_1-AR subtype activation was able to release GABA and somatostatin at the single cell level. This suggests that α_1-AR activation may also represent one mechanism by which NA exerts anti-epileptic effects within the hippocampus.

Generalized Convulsive Seizures

Human data

NA may have proconvulsant and anticonvulsant properties under certain conditions; activated noradrenergic transmission could be an etiological factor in some epilepsies. The available clinical data on the subject (NA boosting antidepressants, α_2 AR agonists, pheophromocytoma, etc.) are discussed in detail by Fitzgerald (Fitzgerald, 2010). It has been shown that co-administration of β-ARs ligands with conventional AEDs, i.e., diazepam, phenobarbital, lamotrigine, valproate, enhance the anticonvulsive efficacy of the latter ones (De Sarro et al., 2002; Fischer, 2002; Luchowska et al., 2002).

Animal data

It has been shown that the animals treated with the monoaminergic toxin 6-hydroxydopamine (6-OHDA)

or the noradrenergic toxin N-(2-chloroethyl)-N-ethyl-2-bromobenzylamine (DSP4), as well as DA beta-hydroxylase (DBH) KO mice that lack NA, expressed increased susceptibility to convulsing stimuli (Bortolotto and Cavalheiro, 1986; McIntyre and Edson, 1989) while, on the contrary, the stimulation of the locus coeruleus in the same animals consistently reduced it (Libet et al., 1977; Weiss et al., 1990). Further confirmation of inhibitory effects of NA on epileptogenesis was obtained by studying the genetic epilepsy-prone rat (GEPR) model (Yan et al., 1993, 1998). With regard to a question related to the receptors involved, the studies yielded conflicting results; the same ligands—agonists or antagonists, could have proconvulsant or anticonvulsant effects, depending on the animal species, the strain, the model of epilepsy employed (for refs see Fitzgerald, 2010) and also receptor location, as in case of α_2-AR (Szot et al., 2004). Specifically, in flurothyl model of generalized convulsive seizures, it has been suggested that presynaptic α_2-AR is responsible for the proconvulsant effect of α_2-AR agonists, while the postsynaptic α_2-AR is responsible for the anticonvulsant effect of α_2-AR agonists (Szot et al., 2004). That α_2-ARs mediate anticonvulsive effects is supported also by the observation that D79N mice which carry a point mutation in the locus of α_2-AR develop amygdala kindling very easily (Janumpalli et al., 1998). Fewer studies concerned with α_1-AR have been conducted. In DBH KO mice, pre-treatment with α_1-AR agonist protected these mice against PTZ induced seizures while α_1-AR antagonist exacerbated PTZ induced seizures in the control mice (Weinshenker et al., 2001b). As to β-ARs, the anticonvulsive activity of propranolol, a non-selective antagonist, has been demonstrated in a variety of animal models of generalized tonic-clonic seizures. Propranolol reduced seizures induced in mice by lidocaine, PTZ, strychnine, low frequency, and maximal electroshock (Saelens et al., 1977; Akkan et al., 1989; Fischer, 2002) as well as by sound in DBA/2 mice (Anlezark et al., 1979; De Sarro et al., 2002), and increased the threshold for lidocaine-induced convulsions in awake animals (Nakamura et al., 2008). Other beta blockers that showed some protective effects include metoprolol, for instance against audio seizures (De Sarro et al., 2002). On the other hand, the anticonvulsant effects of higher doses of clenbuterol against generalized tonic-clonic seizures has also been demonstrated in a couple of used tests (Fischer et al., 2001). Pre-treatment with α_1-AR or β_2-AR, but not α_2-AR or β_1-AR agonist significantly protected against PTZ-induced seizures in DBH$^{-/-}$ mice. Therefore, activation of the α_1-AR is primarily responsible for the anticonvulsant activity of endogenous NA in the murine PTZ model of epilepsy. Endogenous NA probably does not activate the β_2-AR under these conditions, but exogenous activation of the β_2-AR produces an anticonvulsant effect (Weinshenker et al., 2001a).

Generalized Non-convulsive Seizures and Epilepsy Syndromes

Animal data

Further confirmation of inhibitory effects of NA on epileptogenesis was obtained in GAERS (Micheletti et al., 1987). It has also been shown that various antiepileptic drugs, i.e., carbamazepine, have a modulatory, activating effect on NA system (Olpe and Jones, 1983; Post, 1988).

Melatonin System in Epilepsy

Melatonin (MT), N-acetyl-5-methoxytryptamine, is a major hormone of the pineal gland chiefly involved in circadian and seasonal rhythm regulations. Beyond that, it exerts a multitude of anti-excitatory and sedating effects that have been reviewed recently (Reiter et al., 2010; Hardeland et al., 2011). The majority of data indicates anticonvulsant properties of MT when applied at pharmacological doses in both pre- and clinical investigations.

Focal Seizures
In vitro data
In an early electrophysiological study, epileptiform field potentials were elicited by omission of Mg^{2+} from the superfusate and recorded from layers II–V of human temporal neocortical slices cut from tissue resected for surgical treatment of epilepsy. The frequency of occurrence of epileptiform field potentials was halved with application of MT (Fauteck et al., 1995).

Generalized Convulsive Seizures
Human data
Clinical studies on a group of 54 children have demonstrated that during a convulsive crisis, the MT concentration in blood, as measured in patient's serum, significantly peaked but normalized within 1 h. The MT production stimulated by the convulsive crisis may be part of the response of the organism counteracting the seizures effects (Molina-Carballo et al., 2007). Nevertheless, in other studies no changes in serum or salivary MT concentrations were found after epileptic seizures (Rao et al., 1989; Motta et al., 2014). Clinical reports have shown the beneficial effect of MT treatment on seizure activity during the day and night (Goldberg and Spealman, 1983; Peled et al., 2001) in patients with intractable epilepsy. Systematic review of all so far published clinical data on MT in relation to epilepsy, including therapeutic use of MT, lead to the conclusion that there is no marked improvement or worsening of seizures with MT (Jain and Besag, 2013) or its use as add-on treatment (Brigo and Igwe, 2016). Only large randomized double blind placebo-controlled trials could give the final answer. In addition, it has been recently suggested that melatonergic drugs may be effective in treating comorbid depression in PWE (Tchekalarova et al., 2015b)

Animal data
The anticonvulsant activity exerted by MT seen in animal models of epilepsy (Golombek et al., 1992, 1996; Cardinali et al., 2008; Solmaz et al., 2009) has been suggested to be executed via increasing the activity of GABAergic system (Golombek et al., 1996). A selective MT_1/MT_2R agonist mimicked the MT effects in rat rapid kindling model and in the spontaneously epileptic mice lacking voltage-gated Kv1.1 channels (Kcna1-null mice; Fenoglio-Simeone et al., 2009). Beneficial actions of MT in epilepsy have also been attributed to its free radical

scavenging properties (Mohanan and Yamamoto, 2002). MT has been reported to have an anticonvulsant action in many models of acute seizures, such as those produced by the administration of PTZ, picrotoxin, bicuculline, pilocarpine, l-cysteine, kainate, 3-mercaptopropionic acid, quinolinate, GLU, strychnine, N-methyl-d-aspartate (NMDA), or penicillin, as well as in the maximal electroshock seizure (MES) test in rats, mice, gerbils, and hamsters (see Banach et al., 2011). MT treatment during epileptogenesis can have beneficial effects against the deleterious consequences of SE in the KA model of TLE. Melatonin chronic treatment increased the seizure-latent period, decreased the frequency of spontaneous recurrent seizures (SRSs), and attenuated the circadian rhythm of seizure activity (Petkova et al., 2014; Tchekalarova et al., 2015b). These findings are in agreement with the earlier evidence that pinealectomy facilitates the epileptogenic process that follows the long-lasting SE. This facilitation can be partially reverted by the simultaneous administration of MT (De Lima et al., 2005). Agomelatine is a novel antidepressant agent, which is structurally homologous to MT. It is a potent MT1 and MT2 MTR agonist as well as a 5-$HT_{2C}R$ receptor antagonist (Millan et al., 2003). It was recently approved as an antidepressant medication with comparable efficacy to classical antidepressant drugs (Sansone and Sansone, 2011). Agomelatine has anticonvulsant activity shown in PTZ- or pilocarpine-induced seizure models due to its combined action at MT1/2 and 5-$HT_{2C}Rs$ (Aguiar et al., 2012).

Generalized Non-convulsive Seizures and Epilepsy Syndromes
Animal data
It has been shown that subchronic and systemic administration of agomelatine and MT displayed considerable antiepileptic effects on absence seizures in WAG/Rij rats (Hatice et al., 2015).

Agomelatine seems to be recommendable as a potential drug for absence epilepsy and many other complications such as depression and sleep disorders associated with epilepsy.

Histaminergic System in Epilepsy

The CNS histaminergic system is involved in variety of physiological and behavioral functions among them sleep-wake cycle, appetite control, cognitive functions, neuroendocrine functions, locomotor activity, emotion, and stress behavior. Histamine is formed locally in the CNS; the synthesizing enzyme histidine decarboxylase operates under subsaturating concentration of L-histidine. An increase in the substrate supply results in enhancement of cerebral histamine pool. Of the four histamine receptors (HRs), in the cerebral tissues H1–H_3Rs are undoubtedly present. While H_1 and H_2Rs are located postsynaptically, the H_3 ones are presynaptic auto- or heteroreceptors, controlling the release and synthesis of histamine, and modulating release of other neurotransmitters, e.g., acetylcholine, DA, NA, 5-HT, glutamate, and GABA (Schwartz et al., 1991; Haas and Panula, 2003). The involvement of cerebral histamine in regulation of seizure susceptibility is sufficiently documented by both clinical and experimental studies, which strongly point to histamine as an anticonvulsant. The antiepileptic activity seems to be mediated by H_1 and H_3Rs.

Focal Seizures
Animal data

In a comprehensive study on amygdala kindled seizures in rats, convincing evidence for the suppressive role of central histamine in epilepsy was provided (Kamei, 2001). In the amygdala of kindled rats, a significant decrease of histamine concentrations was disclosed. Exogenous histamine administered to kindled animals elicited the seizure inhibiting effect that was mimicked by H_1R agonists but not H_2R agonists. Moreover, when administered repeatedly to rats, L-histidine retarded development of amygdala kindling (Kamei et al., 1998). Histidine and metoprine also inhibited seizures, and both treatments were associated with enhanced histamine levels in cerebral cortex, hippocampus, hypothalamus, and amygdala. H_3R antagonists evoked an antiepileptic effect, which was prevented by pretreatment with an H_3R agonist and was sensitive to H_1R antagonists. As shown by others (Jin et al., 2005) amygdala kindled seizure inhibition could also be achieved by administration of dipeptide carnosine (beta-alanyl-L-histidine). The antiepileptic effect was antagonized by H_1R blockers of the first generation (pyrilamine, diphenhydramine), indicating histamine participation.

Generalized Convulsive Seizures

Accordingly, manipulations of the endogenous histamine level that resulted in its increase (stimulation of synthesis, inhibition of degradation) was invariably associated with the inhibition of convulsions or increased threshold for seizure induction, the opposite being true for procedures that caused either decrease of brain histamine concentration or blocked histamine signaling via H_1 or activated H_3Rs. For instance, metoprine, an inhibitor of histamine catabolizing enzyme, histamine N-methyl transferase, inhibited electroshock seizures (Tuomisto and Tacke, 1986).

Animal data

Metoprine inhibited seizures evoked by amygdala kindling in rats (Kamei et al., 1998; Kamei, 2001), as well as reduced audiogenic convulsions in genetically audiogenic seizure sensitive rats (Tuomisto et al., 1987). Likewise, L-histidine inhibited amygdala kindled seizures (Kamei et al., 1998) as well as PTZ-induced seizures in rats (Chen et al., 2002), an effect potentiated by H_3R antagonist, thioperamide, and antagonized by α-fluoromethylhistidine (inhibitor of histidine decarboxylase) as well as by pyrilamine, H_1R antagonist (Chen et al., 2002). In audiogenic epilepsy prone Krushinski–Molodkina rats, as opposed to epilepsy resistant Wistar rats, brain histamine concentrations are significantly lower (Onodera et al., 1992). In different animal models of epilepsy, imidazole and non-imidazole H_3R antagonists facilitating the release of histamine have proven to be beneficial (Yokoyama et al., 1993; Kakinoki et al., 1998; Kamei, 2001). Pitolisant, an H_3R antagonist, showed excellent antiepileptic activity in animal models of seizure, predictive for generalized, MES test in mice (Sadek et al., 2014).

Clinical data

Interestingly, children with febrile seizures showed significantly lower histamine concentrations in cerebrospinal fluid than febrile children without seizures. Based on these findings, the suggestion was made that brain histaminergic system may be involved in inhibiting seizures associated with febrile illnesses in childhood (Kiviranta et al., 1995). The clinical data amply documented proconvulsant effects of H_1R antagonists administered in clinically relevant doses (Churchill and Gammon, 1949; Yokoyama et al., 1993; Takano et al., 2010; Miyata et al., 2011; Zolaly, 2012). Therefore, centrally acting H_1R antagonists which may increase seizure susceptibility in patients with febrile seizures are neither recommended to these patients nor to PWE. Also, they should be avoided in young infants, more sensitive to the drugs that could potentially disturb the anticonvulsive central histaminergic system. The potential antiseizure activity of pitolisant, a non-imidazole H_3R inverse agonist, was examined in 14 photosensitive adults using the photosensitivity standard model and employing 20/40/60 mg dose. Significant suppression of generalized epileptiform discharges was observed in the majority of the PWE (Kasteleijn-Nolst Trenite et al., 2013; Bialer et al., 2015). Unfortunately, a recent multicenter, national, pragmatic, noncomparative, open-label, exploratory phase II trial reported there was no clinical effects of pitolisant in human epilepsy, in spite of the existing promising animal data (Collart Dutilleul et al., 2016).

Generalized Non-convulsive Seizures and Epilepsy Syndromes
Animal data

WAG/Rij strain showed an increase in the density of H_1R binding in the frontal motor cortex and interposed nucleus of cerebellum and a decrease in the substantia nigra compacta compared to the non-epileptic control group (Midzyanovskaya et al., 2016). Taking into account the bidirectional effect of the H_1R antagonist pyrilamine on SWDs in WAG/Rij rats (Midzyanovskaya et al., 2005), it may be speculated that histamine modulates different areas involved in opposite absence seizure modulation.

MONOAMINES IN EPILEPSY: GENETIC EVIDENCE

Genetic Animal Studies
Genetics of Serotonergic System

As shown in **Table 1**, various KO animal studies have investigated the contribution of the serotonergic system in the neurobiology of epilepsy (Theodore, 2003; Bagdy et al., 2007).

Some of the first such studies involved GEPRs, which displayed deficits in serotonergic system (Dailey et al., 1989). Specifically, these rats had lower brain 5-HT concentration, synaptosomal 5-HT uptake, and tryptophan hydroxylase activity in regions of forebrain and brainstem (Statnick et al., 1996). Moreover, various studies demonstrated reduced hippocampal 5-HTR density in the GEPRs (Dailey et al., 1992; Statnick et al., 1996; Salgado-Commissariat and Alkadhi, 1997) suggesting the critical importance of serotonergic activity in seizure regulation (Jobe et al., 1999). In line with these findings, results obtained on GEPRs also suggest that antiepileptic drugs such as carbamazepine and valproate increase 5-HT concentrations as a part of their mechanism of action (Yan

TABLE 1 | Animal studies investigating the involvement of monoamine systems in epilepsy.

Animal model	Findings	References
SEROTONERGIC SYSTEM		
Genetically epilepsy-prone rats	Deficits in serotonergic and noradrenergic systems	Dailey et al., 1989
	Lower brain 5-HT concentration, synaptosomal 5-HT uptake, and tryptophan hydroxylase activity in regions of forebrain and brainstem	Statnick et al., 1996
	Reduced hippocampal 5-HT receptor density	Dailey et al., 1992; Statnick et al., 1996; Salgado-Commissariat and Alkadhi, 1997
	Antiepileptic drugs such as carbamazepine and valproate increase 5-HT concentrations	Yan et al., 1992; Dailey et al., 1997
Genetic mutant mice lacking 5-HT1A receptors	Increased seizure susceptibility	Sarnyai et al., 2000
Genetic mutant mice lacking 5-HT2C receptors	Increased seizure susceptibility	Tecott et al., 1995; Brennan et al., 1997
C57BL/6J (6J) and C57BL/6ByJ (6ByJ) mice	5-HT2 receptors mediate genetic sensitivity to cocaine-induced convulsions	O'dell et al., 2000
DOPAMINERGIC AND NORADRENERGIC SYSTEMS		
Genetic Absence Epilepsy Rats from Strasbourg	Reduced D2 receptor binding sites in the caudate–putamen and CA3 hippocampal region	Jones et al., 2010
Wistar Albino Glaxo rats from Rijswijk	Reduced D2 receptor binding sites in the caudate–putamen and CA3 hippocampal region	Birioukova et al., 2005
D2 receptor knockout (D2R$^{-/-}$) mice	Increased susceptibility to seizures induced by kainic acid	Bozzi et al., 2000; Tripathi et al., 2010
	Increased susceptibility to seizures induced by pilocarpine	Bozzi and Borrelli, 2002, 2006
	CA3 hippocampal apoptotic cell death	Bozzi et al., 2000; Bozzi and Borrelli, 2006; Tripathi et al., 2010
Congenic D4 "knockout" mice	D4 receptors in the interaction with D1 receptors positively regulate D1 receptor-mediated seizures	O'sullivan et al., 2006
D4 receptor knockout (D4R$^{-/-}$) mice	Spontaneous synaptic activity and epileptic discharges induced by 4-aminopyridine or bicuculline increased in cortical slices	Rubinstein et al., 2001
D1 and D5 receptor knockout mice	D1 and D5 receptor-dependent induction of seizures	O'sullivan et al., 2008
DBH (DBH$^{-/-}$ mice) knock-out mice	Mice susceptible to of pentylenetetrazole-induced seizures, activation of the a1AR is responsible for the anticonvulsant activity of endogenous noradrenaline; noradrenergic agonists have protective effects against seizures	Weinshenker et al., 2001a
HISTAMINERGIC SYSTEM		
H1 receptor gene knockout, histidine decarboxylase deficient and mast cell-deficient mice	Faster development of pentylenetetrazole-induced seizures and increased histamine content in diencephalon	Chen et al., 2003
EL mice-genetic model of human temporal lobe epilepsy	Inhibitory actions of the histaminergic neurons on the epileptogenesis; Pretreatment with histidine and metoprine delayed, while H1 blockade speed up the time of seizure onset	Yawata et al., 2004

et al., 1992; Dailey et al., 1997). In addition to rats, genetic mutant mice lacking 5-HT$_{1A}$Rs (Sarnyai et al., 2000) or 5-HT$_{2C}$Rs (Tecott et al., 1995; Brennan et al., 1997) displayed increased seizure susceptibility, suggesting the involvement of these receptors in the regulation of neuronal excitability. In addition, 5-HT$_{2C}$Rs have been suggested to mediate genetic sensitivity to cocaine-induced convulsions (O'dell et al., 2000).

Genetics of Dopaminergic and Noradrenergic Systems

Genetically altered rats and mice were used to provide an insight into the role of the DAergic system in the epileptogenesis (**Table 1**). DA D$_2$R binding sites were found to be reduced in the caudate-putamen and CA3 hippocampal region of GAERS (Jones et al., 2010) and WAG/Rij rats (Birioukova et al., 2005). In mice, inactivation of the D$_2$R gene and consequently impaired D$_2$R-mediated signaling resulted in more severe seizures. Namely, D$_2$R KO mice showed an increased susceptibility to seizures induced by kainic acid (Bozzi et al., 2000) and pilocarpine (Bozzi and Borrelli, 2002, 2006). In these mice, CA3 hippocampal apoptotic cell death was observed (Bozzi et al., 2000; Bozzi and Borrelli, 2006; Tripathi et al., 2010), suggesting that D$_2$R activation may be neuroprotective. Further studies on DAR KO mice investigated the intracellular pathways activated by different DARs in response to seizures (Bozzi et al., 2000; Rubinstein et al., 2001; Bozzi and Borrelli, 2002; O'sullivan et al., 2008; Tripathi et al., 2010; Dunleavy et al.,

2013). These experiments also established the role of D_1 and D_5Rs in the regulation of synaptic activity (O'sullivan et al., 2008). Moreover, spontaneous synaptic activity and epileptic discharges induced by 4-aminopyridine or bicuculline were increased in cortical slices from D_4R KO mice (Rubinstein et al., 2001). It has been suggested that D_4Rs in interaction with D_1Rs positively regulate D_1R-mediated seizures (O'sullivan et al., 2006).

In the evaluation of the contribution of NA to neuronal excitability (**Table 1**), an animal model of DBH KO mice was used (Weinshenker et al., 2001b). These mice lacking NA were susceptible to seizures, and noradrenergic agonists showed protective effects against seizures. Endogenous NA had anticonvulsant effects and was confirmed to represent a potent endogenous inhibitor of neuronal excitability, and these results suggest that future strategies should be focused on noradrenergic drugs to treat epilepsy (Weinshenker et al., 2001b).

Genetics of Histaminergic System

As demonstrated in **Table 1**, histaminergic neurons have also been postulated to have important role in the inhibition of convulsions and seizures (Yawata et al., 2004), since it has been shown that increased H concentrations suppressed seizures and presumably have neuroprotective properties (Bhowmik et al., 2012). In an animal model of epilepsy with PTZ-induced chemical kindling, behavioral, and neurochemical characteristics were examined in various strains of mutant mice (in H_1R KO mice, histidine decarboxylase deficient, and mast cell-deficient mice) compared to their wild type mice (Lai et al., 2003). Mutant mice displayed faster development of seizures and increased histamine content in diencephalon compared to the corresponding wild type mice, suggesting that histamine has protective anticonvulsive effects on seizures achieved via H_1Rs (Lai et al., 2003). In another animal model, in EL mouse (genetic model of human temporal lobe epilepsy), inhibitory actions of the histaminergic neurons on the epileptogenesis were reported (Yawata et al., 2004). In these mice, pretreatment with histidine, a precursor of histamine, and with metoprine, an inhibitor of the histamine N-methyltransferase, delayed the time of onset of the seizures, while H_1R blockade with antagonist speed it up (Yawata et al., 2004).

Genetic Human Studies
Genetics of Serotonergic System

As shown in **Table 2**, the genetic background regarding serotonergic system in epileptogenesis has been most frequently investigated using the association between SERT (or 5-HTT) gene variants and epilepsy. Genetic mutations in the 5-HTT gene influence 5-HTT expression and change extracellular 5-HT levels, therefore increasing susceptibility to seizures (Ottman and Risch, 2012; Salzmann and Malafosse, 2012). One of the most studied polymorphisms in this gene is a variable number of tandem repeats (5-HTTVNTR) polymorphism, located in the second intron, with a repetition unit containing 17 bp. There are three alleles of 5-HTTVNTR that contain 9, 10, or 12 repetitions. Less efficient transcriptional genotypes (10/10) of the 5-HTTVNTR were found more frequently in PWE with juvenile myoclonic epilepsy (JME) compared to control subjects of Egyptian origin (Esmail et al., 2015). The similar result, with the higher frequency of the 10-repeat allele of the 5-HTTVNTR in PWE with TLE in comparison to controls, was observed in Brazilian subjects (Schenkel et al., 2011). In Han Chinese population, one study reported higher frequency of the 10-repeat allele (Li et al., 2012), whereas the other found higher frequencies of transcriptionally more efficient 12/12 genotype and allele 12 (Che et al., 2010), in the PWE with TLE than in normal controls. On the other hand, Italian PWE with TLE showed lower frequencies of the 10 repeat of the 5-HTTVNTR in comparison to control subjects (Manna et al., 2007), whereas results obtained on Croatian subjects demonstrated lack of association of 5-HTTVNTR polymorphism with TLE (Stefulj et al., 2010). In subjects suffering from mesial TLE with hippocampal sclerosis (MTE-HS), the treatment response to antiepileptic drug was evaluated: 12/12 genotype of 5-HTTVNTR polymorphism was found to be associated with significantly increased risk for a nonresponse to medical treatment compared to carriers of the 10-repeat allele (Kauffman et al., 2009). Moreover, PWE with TLE carrying the combination of transcriptionally more efficient 5-HTTVNTR (12/12) genotype and L/L genotype of another common 5-HTT polymorphism, 5-HT-transporter-linked polymorphic region (5-HTTLPR), displayed poorer treatment response to antiepileptic medication therapy (Hecimovic et al., 2010). 5-HTTLPR is a biallelic polymorphism located in the 5′ regulatory region of 5-HTT gene. 5-HTTLPR short (S) allele has been associated with lower transcriptional efficiency of this gene and lower 5-HT uptake activity, in comparison to the long (L) allele (Lesch et al., 1994; Heils et al., 1996). Although the homozygous S genotype was found to significantly increase risk of developing alcohol withdrawal seizures and delirium (Sander et al., 1997), no significant differences were observed in the frequencies of 5-HTTLPR genotypes and alleles in PWE with TLE and normal controls in Chinese Han (Che et al., 2010) and Croatian (Stefulj et al., 2010) populations, as well as in the PWE suffering from IGE (Sander et al., 2000). In addition, a meta-analysis including 5-HTTVNTR and 5-HTTLPR polymorphisms, suggested that 5-HTT gene may not be the primary determinant of epilepsy susceptibility, but in the interaction with other genes involved in different signaling pathways, it might participate in epileptogenesis (Yang et al., 2013).

Studies investigating the role of 5-HTR gene variants in susceptibility to seizure generation demonstrated no association of Cys23Ser polymorphism located in the gene HTR2C with IGE or alcohol withdrawal seizures (Samochowiec et al., 1999; Stefulj et al., 2010). Moreover, genetic variants of the C1019G polymorphism in the HTR1A gene also displayed similar distribution among PWE with TLE and control subjects (Stefulj et al., 2010). However, the 5-HT_{1A}R mRNA expression was found to be higher in hippocampal tissue of PWE with TLE homozygous for the C-allele of rs6295 polymorphism, located in the promoter region of the human HTR1A gene, as compared to

TABLE 2 | Human studies investigating the involvement of monoamine systems in epilepsy.

Human study	Findings	References
SEROTONERGIC SYSTEM		
Juvenile myoclonic epilepsy (JME)	Less efficient transcriptional genotypes (10/10) of the 5-HTTVNTR polymorphism were more frequent in patients with JME	Esmail et al., 2015
Temporal lobe epilepsy (TLE)	Higher frequency of the 10-repeat allele of the 5-HTTVNTR polymorphism in patients with TLE in comparison to controls	Schenkel et al., 2011
	Higher frequency of the 10-repeat allele of the 5-HTTVNTR polymorphism in patients with TLE than in normal controls	Li et al., 2012
	Higher frequencies of transcriptionally more efficient 12/12 genotype and allele 12 of the 5-HTTVNTR polymorphism in patients with TLE than in normal controls	Che et al., 2010
	Lower frequencies of the 10 repeat of the 5-HTTVNTR polymorphism in comparison to control subjects	Manna et al., 2007
	Lack of association of 5-HTTVNTR polymorphism with TLE	Stefulj et al., 2010
	TLE patients carrying the combination of transcriptionally more efficient 5-HTTVNTR (12/12) genotype and L/L genotype of 5-HTTLPR polymorphism had poorer treatment response to antiepileptic therapy	Hecimovic et al., 2010
Mesial temporal lobe epilepsy with hippocampal sclerosis (MTE-HS)	12/12 genotype of 5-HTTVNTR polymorphism associated with increased risk for a nonresponse to medical treatment compared to carriers of the 10-repeat allele	Kauffman et al., 2009
Alcohol withdrawal seizures	Homozygous S genotype of 5-HTTLPR polymorphism significantly increase risk to develop alcohol withdrawal seizures	Sander et al., 1997
Temporal lobe epilepsy (TLE)	Lack of association of 5-HTTLPR polymorphism with TLE	Che et al., 2010; Stefulj et al., 2010
Idiopathic generalized epilepsy	Lack of association of 5-HTTLPR polymorphism with IGE	Sander et al., 2000
Idiopathic generalized epilepsy or alcohol withdrawal seizures	Lack of association of Cys23Ser polymorphism of HTR2C with IGE or alcohol withdrawal seizures	Samochowiec et al., 1999; Stefulj et al., 2010
Temporal lobe epilepsy (TLE)	Lack of association of C1019G polymorphism of HTR1A with TLE	Stefulj et al., 2010
	Higher expression of 5-HT$_{1A}$ receptor mRNA expression in hippocampal tissue of TLE patients homozygous for the C-allele of rs6295 polymorphism in HTR1A, as compared to patients with the GG-genotype	Pernhorst et al., 2013
	Marginally increased frequency of 861G allele of the G861C polymorphism in 5-HT1B receptor gene in the patients with TLE	Stefulj et al., 2010
	T variant of 1354CT polymorphism in HTR2A may influence an earlier age of onset of TLE	Manna et al., 2012
DOPAMINERGIC AND NORADRENERGIC SYSTEMS		
Epilepsy and antiepileptic drug response	Lack of association between DBH C-1021T polymorphism and epilepsy, several epilepsy subtypes, or response to antiepileptic drugs	Depondt et al., 2004
Effects of antiepileptic drug	Patients with genetic variants of DBH rs1611115, COMT rs4680 and dopamine receptor D2 rs1800497 polymorphisms, associated with decreased dopaminergic activity, have higher susceptibility to negative psychotropic effects of levetiracetam	Helmstaedter et al., 2013
Idiopathic generalized epilepsy (Dailey et al.) Idiopathic absence epilepsy (IAE)	Higher frequency of the 9-copy allele of DAT polymorphism was observed in IGE and IAE patients compared to the control group	Sander et al., 2000
ENZYMES INVOLVED IN THE MONOAMINE SYNTHESIS AND METABOLISM		
Neurological syndrome with learning disabilities, epilepsy, and psychiatric symptoms	Mutation-induced deficiency of the 6 pyruvoyl tetrahydropterin synthase, necessary for normal function of tyrosine and tryptophan hydroxylases	Ng et al., 2015
Neurological syndrome with mental retardation and epilepsy	Inherited duplication of Xp11.3, including MAOA and MAOB genes	Tzschach et al., 2008; Klitten et al., 2011
	Inherited deletion of Xp11.3, including MAOA and MAOB genes	Whibley et al., 2010
Idiopathic generalized epilepsies (Dailey et al.)	Lack of association between the MAOA-uVNTR polymorphism and different IGE subtypes	Haug et al., 2000
Temporal lobe epilepsy (TLE)	Lack of association between the MAOA-uVNTR polymorphism and TLE	Stefulj et al., 2010

PWE with the GG-genotype (Pernhorst et al., 2013). On the other hand, the frequency of 861G allele of the G861C polymorphism in the HTR1B gene was found to be marginally increased in the PWE with TLE, implicating this allele in the susceptibility to TLE (Stefulj et al., 2010). The 861G allele has been linked with fewer 5-HT$_{1B}$Rs in the human brain, in comparison to 861C allele (Huang et al., 1999). In addition, Manna et al. (2012) demonstrated that the T variant of 1354CT polymorphism in HTR2A gene may be implicated in an earlier age of onset of TLE (Manna et al., 2012).

Genetics of Dopaminergic and Noradrenergic Systems

DBH, another enzyme involved in conversion of DA to NA, is important for the maintenance of central DA and NA concentrations (**Table 2**). It is presumed that endogenous NA has an antiepileptic effect, especially in limbic regions, and regulates seizure threshold (Giorgi et al., 2004). Plasma DBH was shown to decrease during epileptic seizures (Miras-Portuga et al., 1975). The functional polymorphism in the *DBH* gene, the DBH (rs1611115 or C-970T or DBH C-1021T) polymorphism affects DBH activity and is responsible for almost 50% of the plasma DBH variations. However, there were no significant differences in the frequency of the TT, TC, and CC genotypes in the DBH C-1021T between large numbers of PWE and control subjects (Depondt et al., 2004). Depondt and colleagues detected no significant association between DBH C-1021T polymorphism and epilepsy, several epilepsy subtypes, or response to antiepileptic drugs, implying that this polymorphism does not contribute to epilepsy (Depondt et al., 2004). On the other hand, epileptic PWE carrying genetic variants of rs1611115 polymorphism in *DBH* gene, rs4680 polymorphism located in the gene coding for catechol-O-methyltransferase (COMT) and rs1800497 polymorphism in DA D$_2$R gene, all genetic variants associated with decreased DAergic activity, showed a higher susceptibility to negative psychotropic effects of the antiepileptic drug levetiracetam (Helmstaedter et al., 2013). These findings suggested that decreased DAergic transmission in PWE may worsen the outcome and adverse effects of treatment with specific AEDs.

Genetic studies investigating other components of DAergic system in epilepsy, include polymorphisms in the human DAT gene, which may explain inter-individual differences in the density or affinity of DAT (**Table 2**). The study of Sander et al. (2000) reported the association of the 40 bp repeats polymorphism in the 3′ untranslated region of the *DAT* gene with IGE, and especially with idiopathic absence epilepsy (IAE) (Sander et al., 2000). Significantly higher frequency of the 9-copy allele of this polymorphism was observed in IGE and IAE PWE compared to the control group (Sander et al., 2000). In addition, various studies demonstrated that the A9 allele (9-copy repeat) of the *DAT* gene contributed to the risk of alcohol-withdrawal seizures and delirium (Sander et al., 1997; Gorwood et al., 2003), suggesting that variations of the *DAT* gene may modulate neuronal excitability and contribute to epileptogenesis.

Genetics of Enzymes Involved in the Monoamine Synthesis and Metabolism

Some insights about the involvement of the human monoaminergic genes in epilepsy have come from a neurological syndrome, which includes learning disabilities, epilepsy, and psychiatric symptoms (**Table 2**). This syndrome is probably caused by the mutation-induced deficiency of the 6 pyruvoyl tetrahydropterin synthase, necessary for normal function of tyrosine and tryptophan hydroxylases, enzymes enrolled in the synthesis of monoamines (Ng et al., 2015). Moreover, PWE with mental retardation carry an inherited duplication (Tzschach et al., 2008; Klitten et al., 2011), or deletion (Whibley et al., 2010) of Xp11.3, including genes coding for monoamine oxidase A and B (MAO-A and MAO-B), suggested that these genes are important for normal development of the CNS. This is not surprising, as MAO-A and MAO-B play a role in the degradation of monoamine neurotransmitters such as DA, NA, and 5-HT. In PWE with idiopathic generalized epilepsies, like childhood absence epilepsy, JAE, and juvenile myoclonic epilepsy (Blümcke et al.), the functional polymorphism located in the promoter of *MAOA* gene (MAOA-uVNTR) was evaluated to test whether allelic variation has a role in the etiology of IGE (Haug et al., 2000). Although, it was expected that the higher activity promoter alleles (3a and 4 copy alleles) would be associated with susceptibility to epilepsy, the frequencies of the high and low (3 copy allele) activity allele groups were similar between PWE and controls, and these results did not confirm any association between the MAOA-uVNTR polymorphism and different IGE subtypes (Haug et al., 2000). In line with these results, genetic variants of MAOA-uVNTR polymorphism were also similarly distributed among PWE with TLE and control subjects (Stefulj et al., 2010).

Despite the large body of evidence reviewed here, relatively scanty evidence from both animal and human studies is available to support the direct association between epilepsy and variation of genes involved in different aspects of monoaminergic neurotransmission, including synthesis, metabolism, transport, reuptake, or packaging (Ng et al., 2015).

MONOAMINERGIC STRATEGIES TO TREAT EPILEPSY

As of yet, there are still no fully effective drugs for treating epilepsy. Despite the emergence of new agents, a consistent proportion of PWE remain resistant to drug treatments. It appears clear that Paul Ehrlich's "magic bullets" do not work in complex CNS pathologies such as epilepsy for which "magic shotguns" are instead needed (Roth et al., 2004). Indeed, single-target AED may not always induce the desired effect even if they successfully inhibit or activate a specific target known to be altered in epilepsy (Csermely et al., 2005). One of the expansions is that effectiveness can be affected in compensatory ways. There is a need to develop multi-target anticonvulsants with the ability to prevent or delay the onset of epilepsy and/or the potential for disease modification.

Unfortunately, in contrast to other CNS disorders (i.e., Alzheimer Disorder, AD), a multi-target ligand approach, acting simultaneously on different receptors or enzymatic systems implicated in epilepsy has not yet attracted the attention of medicinal chemists. Specifically, targeting multiple monoamine systems via multi-target-directed ligands (MTDL) may represent a successful approach, since the experimental and clinical evidence reviewed here has demonstrated the pivotal role of different monoaminergic proteins/enzymes in epilepsy. The rational discovery of multi-target drugs this may represent is an emerging area in epilepsy. These drugs may be also useful for the frequent comorbid psychiatric disorders seen in PWE (Bialer and White, 2010; Cardamone et al., 2013).

Some of standard or herbal monoaminergic medicines already show a profile of multi-target drugs acting via modulation of multiple proteins/systems rather than single targets (Di Matteo et al., 2000; Quesseveur et al., 2013), a phenomenon known as polypharmacology (Hopkins, 2008).

Lu et al. (2012) compared the drug targets and the market sales of the new molecular entities approved by the Food and Drug Administration (FDA) using network analysis tools. There are several monoaminergic targets, such as DARs, 5-HTRs, ARs, MAO-B, etc., that are common to the CNS complex diseases, confirming that these targets play crucial roles in the development of complex diseases and in drug discovery (Lu et al., 2012).

MAO Enzymes As Targets to Treat Epilepsy

MAO (EC 1.4.3.4, amine-oxygen oxidoreductase) exists as two isozymes: MAO-A and MAO-B, both showing different substrate specificities, sensitivity to inhibitors, and amino acid sequences. MAO catalyzes the oxidative deamination of a variety of biogenic and xenobiotic amines, with the concomitant production of hydrogen peroxide (Youdim et al., 1988). MAO-A preferentially oxidizes NA and 5-HT and is selectively inhibited by clorgyline, while MAO-B preferentially deaminates β-phenylethylamine and is irreversibly inhibited by l-deprenyl (Ramsay, 2013). MAO activity has been shown to be linked to epilepsy since the 1960s (Plotnikoff et al., 1963; Kohli et al., 1967). For instance, MAO-B activity is elevated in hypometabolic regions of PWE with TLE due to activated astrocytes and gliosis (Kumlien et al., 1992), the most common histopathological abnormality seen in this focal epilepsy (Blümcke et al., 2013). PET studies with ^{11}C-deprenyl (Kumlien et al., 2001) or autoradiographic studies in human brain slices with ^{3}H-deprenyl (Kumlien et al., 1992) have therefore been used for identification of epileptogenic regions in patients with focal epilepsy for surgical resection.

Although, several studies showed that the old MAO inhibitors exhibit anticonvulsant activity (Plotnikoff et al., 1963; Kohen et al., 1996), they have not been used clinically due to their adverse effects. In addition, the magnitude of the anticonvulsant response in animals models vary between MAO inhibitors (MAO-I), while the role of MAO subtypes underscoring the anticonvulsant action of MAO-I is not well understood. More specifically, both selective MAO-A and MAO-B inhibitors (MAO-AIs and MAO-BIs) exert anticonvulsant activity in different preclinical models of seizure (Sparks and Buckholtz,

1985; Mukhopadhyay et al., 1987; Löscher and Lehmann, 1996, 1998; Loscher et al., 1999).

However, the anticonvulsant and the antiepileptogenic effects of l-deprenyl, the most extensively studied drug in this respect, seem to be mediated by MAO-A inhibition instead of the irreversible MAO-B inhibition (Loscher et al., 1999). On the one hand, this interpretation agrees with the lack of anticonvulsant efficacy of the selective MAO-BI LU 53439, but potent anticonvulsant activity of the selective MAO-AI esuprone, in the kindling model of epilepsy (Loscher et al., 1999). These results point strongly to MAO-A but not MAO-B inhibition as an effective means of inducing anticonvulsant effects. On the other hand, other MAO-BIs including safinamide or zonisamide have been shown to be efficacious in some seizure models (Bialer, 2012; Park et al., 2015) and zonisamide was approved for epilepsy recently (Bialer, 2012). Zonisamide has been shown to physically interact with human MAO-B, but not MAO-A enzyme (Binda et al., 2011) highlighting that MAO-B inhibition can be worth targeting to achieve an anticonvulsant effect. The fact that MAO-A could indirectly mediate the anticonvulsant properties of MAO-BIs could be related to the complex relationships between MAO-A and MAO-B. Indeed, despite the existence of preferring substrates for each enzyme, the selective blockade of one enzyme has been shown to alter the activity of the other one, particularly after chronic administration (Youdim et al., 2006; Finberg, 2014). In spite of the complex relationships between MAO-A and MAO-B, these studies stress that MAO inhibition may be an interesting strategy for developing novel anticonvulsant agents in considering also the better tolerability of the newer compounds compared to the early MAO-Is (Löscher and Lehmann, 1996, 1998; Loscher et al., 1999; Youdim et al., 2006; Bialer, 2012).

Aside from monoaminergic mechanisms, l-deprenyl has been shown to affect the polyamine binding site of the NMDA subtype of GLURs, to stimulate neurotrophic factors, and to modulate gene expression and protein synthesis, which again is unrelated to MAO-B inhibition (Magyar, 2011). Moreover, MAO-BIs seem to be effective by acting on different pathways, along with their enhancing effect on monoaminergic transmission. For instance they possess neuroprotective properties (Aluf et al., 2013) by blocking oxidative stress and ROS formation (Riederer et al., 2004). Accordingly, compelling evidence supports the idea that rasagiline-induced neuroprotection is not related to the inhibition of MAO enzymatic activity. This action has been ascribed to the presence of the reactive propargylamino moiety which might interfere with many other cellular processes such as different key steps of the apoptotic cascade (Al-Nuaimi et al., 2012). In view of these various effects, it is impossible to foresee which effect(s) are most likely to explain the anticonvulsant and antiepileptogenic activity of l-deprenyl. Indeed, MAO-BIs show multimodal effects and a MTDL profile (Pisani et al., 2011; Bolea et al., 2013).

To date, the only MTDL strategy targeting monoaminergic systems has focused on MAO inhibition among other targets with cholinesterase (ChE) as a new strategy for AD (Bolea et al., 2013) even if it has not yet led to novel clinical therapeutics (Pisani et al., 2011) with the exception of rasagiline (Youdim, 2003). Interestingly, some drug candidates have emerged from MTDL design showing promising multi-target properties and have been submitted to extensive bio-pharmacological profiling (Cavalli et al., 2008). Members of the Cost ACTION CM1103 (http://www.cost.eu/COST_Actions/cmst/CM1103) have designed, synthetized and evaluated new different MTDL compounds acting on ChE and MAO-I that may elicit better outcomes in the complex nature of AD than the current selective drugs (Benek et al., 2015; Ismaili et al., 2016; Unzeta et al., 2016). Moreover, MAO-Is with additional ion-chelating and/or antioxidant activities, compounds with dual MAO-I and adenosine A2aR antagonist activity have been characterized (Pisani et al., 2011; Guzior et al., 2015). Among these MTDLs based on MAO inhibition, several compounds seem to be promising drug candidates, while others may serve as a valuable inspiration in the search for new effective therapies for epilepsy. Crucial experimental evidence supporting these assumptions is now warranted.

Monoamine Transporters As Targets to Treat Epilepsy

The other important class of monoaminergic drugs that may be useful for treating epilepsy is the monoamine transporters (MATs). MATs (DAT, SERT, and NA transporter or NAT) are transmembrane proteins located in plasma membranes of monoaminergic neurons, while SERT is also expressed in platelets (Amara and Kuhar, 1993). Due to amino acid sequence and proposed structural similarity among the three plasma membrane transporters, many MAT inhibitors have affinity for all three transporters.

Antidepressants are commonly prescribed to PWE to treat comorbid depression and/or anxiety. These include selective serotonin reuptake inhibitors (SSRIs), serotonin-noradrenaline reuptake inhibitors (SNRIs), and related medications (Cardamone et al., 2013). Strikingly, several preclinical and human studies have shown that antidepressants have an anticonvulsant effect and in PWE can improve seizure outcomes, with some patients experiencing dramatic and complete seizure freedom during antidepressant treatment (see Cardamone et al., 2013 for recent review of the literature). Mounting experimental and clinical evidence indicates that antidepressants are anticonvulsants, not proconvulsants as was earlier believed (Jobe and Browning, 2005). Indeed, the proconvulsant effects of antidepressants are mainly reported in cases of overdose, or when therapeutic relevant doses are excessive for slow metabolizers (Preskorn and Fast, 1992). Nevertheless, this erroneous convulsant liability of antidepressants has hindered their use in epilepsy.

SSRIs and SNRIs selectively inhibit monoamine reuptake at the neuronal presynaptic membrane by blocking the 5-HT and 5-HT/NA reuptake transporters, respectively, increasing 5-HT and/or NA levels in the synapse and in the peri-extrasynaptic space. Serotonin and NA may therefore modulate neuronal (i.e., excitability and release of other neurotransmitters) and neuroglial activity. Different lines of enquiries have indicated that SSRIs and SNRIs possess a wealth of potentially therapeutic targets apart from simply increasing monoamine in the CNS, including anti-inflammatory, antioxidant, neuroprotective, and immunomodulatory effects, increase in the brain-derived neurotrophic factor (BDNF), and modulation in the mTOR pathway (Dale et al., 2015).

This list is by no means exhaustive, and other processes, including genetic/genomic and epigenetic mechanisms may be equally important. SSRIs and SNRIs may impact on the different neurobiological alterations occurring in epileptogenesis, and may potentially influence disease course. Alper et al. (2007) reviewed the effects of some SSRIs and SNRIs on seizure incidence in a large cohort of non-epileptic patients in phase II and III of FDA clinical trials of depression treatment between 1985 and 2004. Among the outputs of this study, it appeared that the incidence of seizures occurring in depressed patients treated with antidepressants was significantly lower, compared to those treated with a placebo (Alper et al., 2007). Unfortunately, there have been no double-blind, randomized controlled studies yet; most of the studies have been small and on highly selected patient populations recruited from epilepsy clinics or following epilepsy surgery, and with few longitudinal, follow-up studies.

It is possible that SSRIs and SNRIs, by targeting mechanisms that are both involved in seizure generation and psychiatric comorbidities, may induce both seizure suppression and antidepressant effects. This multi-target profile possessed by SSRIs and SNRIs provides them with the potential to meet some of the criteria for MTDLs. The introduction of drugs such as duloxetine for the treatment of major depression (Carter and McCormack, 2009) indicates the clinical feasibility of designing multifunctional ligands to treat CNS disorders with complex disease pathways, such as epilepsy. Another example is a class of compounds known as triple reuptake inhibitors (i.e., amitifadine) that simultaneously block the synaptic reuptake of 5-HT, NA, and DA (SNDRIs; Skolnick et al., 2006; Weng et al., 2015). Again, as for the MAO-based MTDLs experimental evaluation in animal models of epilepsy and in PWE is needed.

Monoamine Receptors As Targets to Treat Epilepsy

A more successful approach with fewer side effects would be to selectively target some monoaminergic receptors instead of increasing monoamine concentrations with MAO and/or MAT inhibitors treatment. Based on the evidence reviewed here, it might be inferred that the development of MTDLs with optimal polypharmacological profile would exhibit, for example, agonistic activity at $5\text{-HT}_{2C}\text{Rs}/\text{D}_2\text{Rs}/\alpha_2\text{-ARs}$ and antagonistic activity at H_3Rs but also antagonistic effects at $5\text{-HT}_{2C}\text{Rs}/\text{MT}_{1/2}\text{Rs}$ (agomelatine). Polypharmacological approaches are therefore likely to be extensively applied for rational design of ligands with optimal multitarget profile and for the discovery of multipotent drug candidates with improved efficacy and safety in therapy of complex brain diseases (Nikolic et al., 2016).

NEW RESEARCH TRENDS IN MONOAMINERGIC STRATEGIES TO TREAT EPILEPSY

Epilepsy is no longer believed to be strictly a disturbance in the functioning of neurons and specifically of their contact points, the synapses. Instead, it is now seen as an imbalance of the physiological extracellular milieu, due to a plethora of different mechanisms. Therefore, the final imbalance between excitation and inhibition in synaptic transmission that underlies hyperexcitability of the epileptic brain (see van Gelder and Sherwin, 2003 for a review) is far from being a mere direct alteration of the excitatory glutamatergic and the inhibitory GABAergic neurotransmission. Indeed, the pathophysiology underlying ictogenesis and the development of epilepsy is very complex, and clearly does not involve only neuronal cells. Much recent evidence points to a significant contribution made by glial cells to the pathophysiology of epilepsy (Devinsky et al., 2013). This follows the new concept that glial cells interact closely with neurons and play an active role in brain functions. Astrocytes, the major type of glia, make direct contact with neurons via a structure that has been defined as the *tripartite synapse*, in which the astrocytic process is associated with the pre- and post-synapse areas of neurons (Araque et al., 1999). Many normal astrocytic functions are depressed in epilepsy, including K^+ homeostasis and accompanying changes in aquaporin, gap-junction expression and function, local blood flow and the blood-brain barrier (BBB), uptake and metabolism of GLU and glucose in astrocytes, and neurotransmitter supply, particularly in inhibitory neurons (see Devinsky et al., 2013; Coulter and Steinhauser, 2015 for extensive reviews). Moreover, glial GABA transporter-1 (GAT-1) activity in thalamic astrocytes is impaired in absence epilepsy causing the enhanced GABA levels typical of this generalized non convulsive epilepsy (Richards et al., 1995) and leading to an aberrant $GABA_A$ receptor-mediated tonic inhibition (Cope et al., 2009; Pirttimaki et al., 2013).

Emerging evidence suggests that also microglia cells, the CNS resident macrophage cells, play important physiological roles at synapses to such as extent that the concept of a quad-partite synapse has been recently suggested (Schafer et al., 2013).

It is instead well-known that inflammation is due to microglia activation and linked to different CNS diseases. For instance, a large body of evidence indicates that inflammatory changes sustained by uncontrolled glial-mediated immunity contribute to epileptogenesis (Devinsky et al., 2013). Moreover, activated microglia promote astrocytic activation and *vice versa* (Liu et al., 2011), thus sustaining a vicious circle. All these biochemical changes, often linked with gliosis, have significant functional consequences, contributing to epileptogenesis.

Considering the fact that monoamines modulate human behaviors and CNS functions, the antiepileptic, and anticonvulsant action of monoamine ligands may be due to their effect on different targets.

It is well-known that monoamines classically modulate cell excitability by controlling release of GLU, GABA and, other neurotransmitters and ion channels as we have reviewed (for detailed reviews see also Ciranna, 2006; Fink and Goethert, 2007). However, it is a relative new evidence that astrocytes contribute in the cellular action of antidepressants (Schipke et al., 2011; Bernstein et al., 2015; Hertz et al., 2015). Moreover, as further proof of a glial dysfunction in depression, decreased density and number of glia cells has been observed in cortical regions, including the prefrontal and cingulate areas in humans (Rajkowska and Stockmeier, 2013), In addition, selective destruction of frontocortical astrocytes (Banasr and Duman, 2008), NG2-expressing glia (NG2 glia) in the prefrontal cortex (Birey et al., 2015) or pharmacological and genetic inhibition of the activity of the glial glutamate transporter GLT-1 in subcortical areas i.e., the lateral habenula (Cui et al., 2014), were capable of triggering a depressive-like phenotype in rodents.

Astrocytes express virtually all of the receptor systems and ion channels found in neurons (Verkhratsky and Kettenmann, 1996) including transporters critical for synaptic uptake of glutamate (Tanaka et al., 1997) and GABA (De Biasi et al., 1998). Monoamine receptors, (Azmitia et al., 1996), such as $5\text{-HT}_{2A/2B/2C}$ receptors are expressed on astrocytes (Hirst et al., 1998; Sanden et al., 2000; Hwang et al., 2008), but also 5-HT_4, 5-HT_5, and 5-HT_7 receptors (Quesseveur et al., 2013), α-ARs (Bekar et al., 2008) and β_2-ARs (Mantyh et al., 1995), and all the DA receptors (Miyazaki et al., 2004) are detected. The SERT, NAT, DAT, and the catabolic isoenzymes responsible for the degradation of monoamines (i.e., MAO-A and MAO-B; COMT) were clearly identified in this cell type (see Quesseveur et al., 2013 for a recent review and references within). These observations emphasize the fact that astrocytes can regulate the extracellular monoamine levels by modulating the expression and function of MAO-A, MAO-B, and COMT and at the same time are regulated by feedback by monoamines via the glial monoamine receptors.

SSRIs citalopram and fluoxetine can excite astrocytes directly by inducing astrocytic calcium transients that, differently from the glutamate-induced calcium responses in astrocytes, occur time-delayed, asynchronously and sometimes in an oscillatory manner (Schipke et al., 2011).

Monoamines can change expression of various molecules (Shishkina et al., 2012) involved in epileptogenesis acting on microglial cells. The link between monoamines and microglia is bidirectional. Indeed, microglial pro-inflammatory cytokines, levels of which increase during epileptogenesis, can decrease 5-HT, DA, and NA availability by acting on their presynaptic reuptake transporters through activation of mitogen-activated protein kinase pathways (Zhu et al., 2010) and by reducing monoamine synthesis through decreasing enzymatic co-factors such as tetrahydrobiopterin (Neurauter et al., 2008). Moreover, many cytokines activate the enzyme indoleamine 2,3-dioxygenase which converts tryptophan into kynurenine (Maes et al., 2011).

From the analysis of the experimental and clinical evidence reviewed here it is possible to hypothesize that a dysfunction of the monoaminergic quad-partite synapse due to an insult (i.e., neurotrauma, infectious injury, genetic disorders...) may be a common pathophysiological mechanism of epilepsy and mood disorders. Depending on the alterations of the quad-partite synapse functions we might have particular mood disorders, epilepsy, or neuropsychiatric disorders with epilepsy (or *vice versa*?). In the latter scenario, depression may be a biologic marker for more severe epilepsy since it is a predictor of a worse seizure outcome in PWE with TLE (Kanner et al., 2003; **Figure 1**). Some of the antiepileptic/antiepileptogenic effects exerted by monoamines might be due to their ability to act on glia targets. For instance, we have suggested that Ro 60-0175 may normalize the aberrant enhanced $GABA_A$ tonic current of the thalamic neurons of GAERS (Cavaccini et al., 2012) by activating astrocytic $5-HT_{2C}Rs$ that increase activity of glial GAT-1 transporter leading to a reduction of extrasynaptic GABA levels. This hypothesis reinforce the idea of a glial dysfunction in epilepsy and glial cells as new therapeutic targets for this disorder (Crunelli and Carmignoto, 2013; Crunelli et al., 2015). Nevertheless, the role of 5-HT in the function of glial GABA transporters and in general in the modulation of GABA homeostasis, although earlier suggested (Voutsinos et al., 1998), remains to be fully investigated in epilepsy. Interestingly, other early findings showed that 5-HT is capable of modulating the activity of glial Na^+/K^+-ATPase but not in the kindled glial fraction (Hernandez and Condes-Lara,

1989). The failure of this 5-HT control of reactive astrocytes due to repeated seizures may contribute to seizure-like activity and epileptogenesis.

CONCLUSION

In this review, recent evidence from both animal and human studies supporting the role of monoamines in epilepsy was described. The possible therapeutic application of these findings has been long disregarded, mainly due the severe side effects of some monoaminergic drugs or due to interpretative bias on research evidence.

As further reasons of this stall are that the both the pathophysiological mechanisms underlying epileptogenesis and the genetics of epilepsy are still not clear. Therefore, further research on different aspects of monoaminergic neurotransmission using human genetic biomarkers in combination with novel animal genetic models, might elucidate the complex role of monoamines in the pathophysiology of

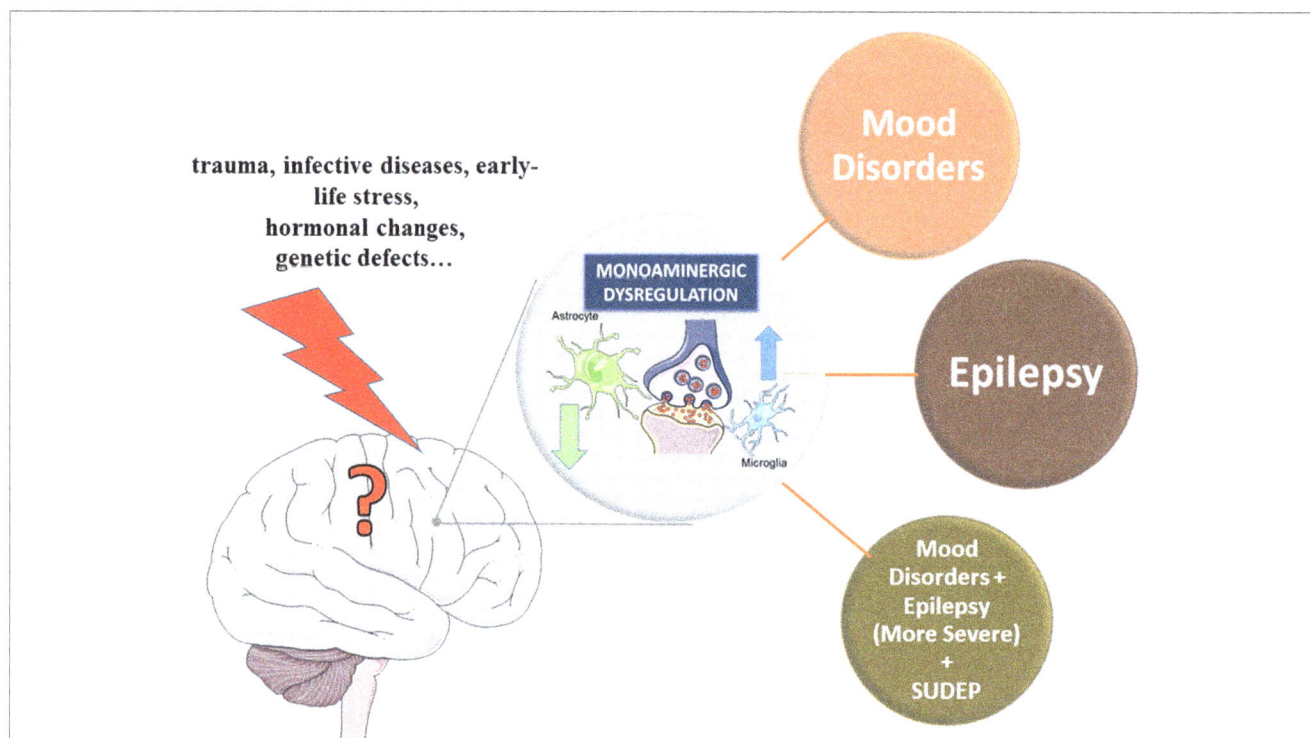

FIGURE 1 | **Hypothetical monoaminergic quad-partite synapse dysfunction as a common pathological mechanism of mood disorders and epilepsy.** The processing of information in synapses is not only defined by neurons, but also by glia cells, namely by astrocytes, which enwrap synapses, and microglia, which dynamically interact with synapses in an activity-dependent manner. This new evidence has brought the development of the quad-partite synapse model, as a further evolution of the tripartite synapse, made up of four elements i.e., presynaptic and postsynaptic neuronal terminals, astrocyte and microglia cells (Schafer et al., 2013). Numerous lines of evidence support the contention that a modification of the quad-partite synapse astrocytes and microglia in different brain regions is associated with depression, and epilepsy (Crunelli and Carmignoto, 2013; Quesseveur et al., 2013). We propose that there may be shared underlying pathology that predisposes patients to depression, epilepsy or both seizures and depression (the latter "seizure/depression phenotype"). For example, traumas, infective disease, early life stress, hormonal changes, genetic and developmental defects, just to cite a few, might induce a dysfunction of the monoaminergic quad-partite synapse and different pathogenic scenarios might cause depression, epilepsy or both conditions. The underlying pathology in the monoaminergic systems of patients with epilepsy (PWE) lowers the threshold for seizures, while also increasing the risk of depression. Moreover, PWE suffering of mood disorders have a higher risk to develop severe and drug-resistant epilepsy (Kanner et al., 2003) and sudden unexpected death in epilepsy (SUDEP; Richerson and Buchanan, 2011). Arrows indicate hypo- or hyperfunction of the glial cells.

epilepsy and might accelerate development of novel therapeutic strategies targeting various components of monoaminergic systems. This is desperately needed, firstly because the number of anti-seizure drugs in clinical development has been decreasing over the years (Bialer et al., 2013) and secondly for the increasing number of PWE with refractory epilepsy. Therefore, the beneficial effects of ligands at D_2R, $5-HT_{2C}R$, MTRs, α-ARs, H_3Rs, MAO-Is, and MTAs inhibitors observed in both animal and human epilepsy would deserve more attention both from preclinical and clinical researchers and above all medicinal chemists.

In our opinion, adequate control of epileptogenesis and convulsions and comorbid psychiatric disorders will likely benefit from MTDLs that target different synergistic monoaminergic pathways and different elements of the quad-partite synapse. Nevertheless, their synthesis and experimental validation needs significant efforts and time. There is a scientific and economic incentive for their synthesis as anti-epileptic and/or anti-epileptogenic drug targets. New monoaminergic drugs with fewer side effects and a multi-target profile are warranted.

AUTHOR CONTRIBUTIONS

All authors contributed to the conception and interpretation of the work and to its critical revision. All authors have approved the final version and may be held accountable for the integrity of this review of current literature.

ACKNOWLEDGMENTS

Support was kindly provided by the EU COST Action CM1103. GDG kindly acknowledges MCST R&I 2013-014.

REFERENCES

Aguiar, C. C., Almeida, A. B., Araújo, P. V., Vasconcelos, G. S., Chaves, E. M., Do Vale, O. C., et al. (2012). Anticonvulsant effects of agomelatine in mice. *Epilepsy Behav.* 24, 324–328. doi: 10.1016/j.yebeh.2012.04.134

Ahmad, S., Fowler, L. J., and Whitton, P. S. (2005). Lamotrigine, carbamazepine and phenytoin differentially alter extracellular levels of 5-hydroxytryptamine, dopamine and amino acids. *Epilepsy Res.* 63, 141–149. doi: 10.1016/j.eplepsyres.2005.02.002

Akkan, A. G., Yillar, D. O., Eskazan, E., Akcasu, A., and Ozüner, Z. (1989). The effect of propranolol on maximal electroshock seizures in mice. *Int. J. Clin. Pharmacol. Ther. Toxicol.* 27, 255–257.

Alfaro-Rodríguez, A., González-Piña, R., Bueno-Nava, A., Arch-Tirado, E., Ávila-Luna, A., Uribe-Escamilla, R., et al. (2011). Effects of oxcarbazepine on monoamines content in hippocampus and head and body shakes and sleep patterns in kainic acid-treated rats. *Metab. Brain Dis.* 26, 213–220. doi: 10.1007/s11011-011-9254-x

Alhaj, M. W., Zaitone, S. A., and Moustafa, Y. M. (2015). Fluvoxamine alleviates seizure activity and downregulates hippocampal GAP-43 expression in pentylenetetrazole-kindled mice: role of 5-HT3 receptors. *Behav. Pharmacol.* 26, 369–382. doi: 10.1097/FBP.0000000000000127

Al-Nuaimi, S. K., MacKenzie, E. M., and Baker, G. B. (2012). Monoamine oxidase inhibitors and neuroprotection: a review. *Am. J. Ther.* 19, 436–448. doi: 10.1097/MJT.0b013e31825b9eb5

Alper, K., Schwartz, K. A., Kolts, R. L., and Khan, A. (2007). Seizure incidence in psychopharmacological clinical trials: an analysis of Food and Drug Administration (FDA) summary basis of approval reports. *Biol. Psychiatry* 62, 345–354. doi: 10.1016/j.biopsych.2006.09.023

Aluf, Y., Vaya, J., Khatib, S., Loboda, Y., and Finberg, J. P. (2013). Selective inhibition of monoamine oxidase A or B reduces striatal oxidative stress in rats with partial depletion of the nigro-striatal dopaminergic pathway. *Neuropharmacology* 65, 48–57. doi: 10.1016/j.neuropharm.2012.08.023

Amara, S. G., and Kuhar, M. J. (1993). Neurotransmitter transporters: recent progress. *Annu. Rev. Neurosci.* 16, 73–93. doi: 10.1146/annurev.ne.16.030193.000445

An, S. J., and Kim, D. S. (2011). Alterations in serotonin receptors and transporter immunoreactivities in the hippocampus in the rat unilateral hypoxic-induced epilepsy model. *Cell. Mol. Neurobiol.* 31, 1245–1255. doi: 10.1007/s10571-011-9726-x

Anlezark, G., Horton, R., and Meldrum, B. (1979). The anticonvulsant action of the (−)- and (+)-enantiomers of propranolol. *J. Pharm. Pharmacol.* 31, 482–483. doi: 10.1111/j.2042-7158.1979.tb13563.x

Araque, A., Parpura, V., Sanzgiri, R. P., and Haydon, P. G. (1999). Tripartite synapses: glia, the unacknowledged partner. *Trends Neurosci.* 22, 208–215. doi: 10.1016/S0166-2236(98)01349-6

Assem-Hilger, E., Lanzenberger, R., Savli, M., Wadsak, W., Mitterhauser, M., Mien, L. K., et al. (2010). Central serotonin 1A receptor binding in temporal lobe epilepsy: a [carbonyl-(11)C]WAY-100635 PET study. *Epilepsy Behav.* 19, 467–473. doi: 10.1016/j.yebeh.2010.07.030

Azmitia, E. C., Gannon, P. J., Kheck, N. M., and Whitaker-Azmitia, P. M. (1996). Cellular localization of the 5-HT1A receptor in primate brain neurons and glial cells. *Neuropsychopharmacology* 14, 35–46. doi: 10.1016/S0893-133X(96)80057-1

Bagdy, G., Kecskemeti, V., Riba, P., and Jakus, R. (2007). Serotonin and epilepsy. *J. Neurochem.* 100, 857–873. doi: 10.1111/j.1471-4159.2006.04277.x

Banach, M., Gurdziel, E., Jedrych, M., and Borowicz, K. K. (2011). Melatonin in experimental seizures and epilepsy. *Pharmacol. Rep.* 63, 1–11. doi: 10.1016/S1734-1140(11)70393-0

Banasr, M., and Duman, R. S. (2008). Glial loss in the prefrontal cortex is sufficient to induce depressive-like behaviors. *Biol. Psychiatry* 64, 863–870. doi: 10.1016/j.biopsych.2008.06.008

Barone, P., Parashos, S. A., Palma, V., Marin, C., Campanella, G., and Chase, T. N. (1990). Dopamine D1 receptor modulation of pilocarpine-induced convulsions. *Neuroscience* 34, 209–217. doi: 10.1016/0306-4522(90)90314-T

Baulac, M., De Boer, H., Elger, C., Glynn, M., Kälviäinen, R., Little, A., et al. (2015). Epilepsy priorities in Europe: a report of the ILAE-IBE Epilepsy Advocacy Europe Task Force. *Epilepsia* 56, 1687–1695. doi: 10.1111/epi.13201

Bekar, L. K., He, W., and Nedergaard, M. (2008). Locus coeruleus alpha-adrenergic-mediated activation of cortical astrocytes in vivo. *Cereb. Cortex* 18, 2789–2795. doi: 10.1093/cercor/bhn040

Benardo, L. S., and Prince, D. A. (1982). Dopamine modulates a Ca2+-activated potassium conductance in mammalian hippocampal pyramidal cells. *Nature* 297, 76–79. doi: 10.1038/297076a0

Benek, O., Soukup, O., Pasdiorova, M., Hroch, L., Sepsova, V., Jost, P., et al. (2015). Design, synthesis and in vitro evaluation of indolotacrine analogues as multitarget-directed ligands for the treatment of Alzheimer's disease. *Chem. Med. Chem.* 11, 1264–1269. doi: 10.1002/cmdc.201500383

Berg, A. T., Berkovic, S. F., Brodie, M. J., Buchhalter, J., Cross, J. H., Van Emde Boas, W., et al. (2010). Revised terminology and concepts for organization of seizures and epilepsies: report of the ILAE Commission on Classification and Terminology, 2005-2009. *Epilepsia* 51, 676–685. doi: 10.1111/j.1528-1167.2010.02522.x

Bernedo Paredes, V. E., Buchholz, H. G., Gartenschlager, M., Breimhorst, M., Schreckenberger, M., and Werhahn, K. J. (2015). Reduced D2/D3 receptor binding of extrastriatal and striatal regions in temporal lobe epilepsy. *PLoS ONE* 10:e0141098. doi: 10.1371/journal.pone.0141098

Bernstein, H. G., Steiner, J., Guest, P. C., Dobrowolny, H., and Bogerts, B. (2015). Glial cells as key players in schizophrenia pathology: recent insights and concepts of therapy. *Schizophr. Res.* 161, 4–18. doi: 10.1016/j.schres.2014.03.035

Bhowmik, M., Khanam, R., and Vohora, D. (2012). Histamine H3 receptor antagonists in relation to epilepsy and neurodegeneration: a systemic consideration of recent progress and perspectives. *Br. J. Pharmacol.* 167, 1398–1414. doi: 10.1111/j.1476-5381.2012.02093.x

Bialer, M. (2012). Chemical properties of antiepileptic drugs (AEDs). *Adv. Drug Deliv. Rev.* 64, 887–895. doi: 10.1016/j.addr.2011.11.006

Bialer, M., and White, H. S. (2010). Key factors in the discovery and development of new antiepileptic drugs. *Nat. Rev. Drug Discov.* 9, 68–82. doi: 10.1038/nrd2997

Bialer, M., Johannessen, S. I., Levy, R. H., Perucca, E., Tomson, T., and White, H. S. (2013). Progress report on new antiepileptic drugs: a summary of the Eleventh Eilat Conference (EILAT XI). *Epilepsy Res.* 103, 2–30. doi: 10.1016/j.eplepsyres.2012.10.001

Bialer, M., Johannessen, S. I., Levy, R. H., Perucca, E., Tomson, T., and White, H. S. (2015). Progress report on new antiepileptic drugs: a summary of the Twelfth Eilat Conference (EILAT XII). *Epilepsy Res.* 111, 85–141. doi: 10.1016/j.eplepsyres.2015.01.001

Binda, C., Aldeco, M., Mattevi, A., and Edmondson, D. E. (2011). Interactions of monoamine oxidases with the antiepileptic drug zonisamide: specificity of inhibition and structure of the human monoamine oxidase B complex. *J. Med. Chem.* 54, 909–912. doi: 10.1021/jm101359c

Birey, F., Kloc, M., Chavali, M., Hussein, I., Wilson, M., Christoffel, D. J., et al. (2015). Genetic and stress-induced loss of NG2 glia triggers emergence of depressive-like behaviors through reduced secretion of FGF2. *Neuron* 88, 941–956. doi: 10.1016/j.neuron.2015.10.046

Birioukova, L. M., Midzyanovskaya, I. S., Lensu, S., Tuomisto, L., and van Luijtelaar, G. (2005). Distribution of D1-like and D2-like dopamine receptors in the brain of genetic epileptic WAG/Rij rats. *Epilepsy Res.* 63, 89–96. doi: 10.1016/j.eplepsyres.2004.12.001

Biton, V. (2007). Clinical pharmacology and mechanism of action of zonisamide. *Clin. Neuropharmacol.* 30, 230–240. doi: 10.1097/wnf.0b013e3180413d7d

Blümcke, I., Thom, M., Aronica, E., Armstrong, D. D., Bartolomei, F., Bernasconi, A., et al. (2013). International consensus classification of hippocampal sclerosis in temporal lobe epilepsy: a Task Force report from the ILAE commission on diagnostic methods. *Epilepsia* 54, 1315–1329. doi: 10.1111/epi.12220

Bobula, B., Zahorodna, A., and Bijak, M. (2001). Different receptor subtypes are involved in the serotonin-induced modulation of epileptiform activity in rat frontal cortex *in vitro. J. Physiol. Pharmacol.* 52, 265–274.

Bolea, I., Gella, A., and Unzeta, M. (2013). Propargylamine-derived multitarget-directed ligands: fighting Alzheimer's disease with monoamine oxidase inhibitors. *J. Neural Transm.* 120, 893–902. doi: 10.1007/s00702-012-0948-y

Bortolotto, Z. A., and Cavalheiro, E. A. (1986). Effect of DSP4 on hippocampal kindling in rats. *Pharmacol. Biochem. Behav.* 24, 777–779. doi: 10.1016/0091-3057(86)90591-5

Bourson, A., Kapps, V., Zwingelstein, C., Rudler, A., Boess, F. G., and Sleight, A. J. (1997). Correlation between 5-HT7 receptor affinity and protection against sound-induced seizures in DBA/2J mice. *Naunyn Schmiedebergs Arch. Pharmacol.* 356, 820–826. doi: 10.1007/PL00005123

Bozzi, Y., and Borrelli, E. (2002). Dopamine D2 receptor signaling controls neuronal cell death induced by muscarinic and glutamatergic drugs. *Mol. Cell. Neurosci.* 19, 263–271. doi: 10.1006/mcne.2001.1064

Bozzi, Y., and Borrelli, E. (2006). Dopamine in neurotoxicity and neuroprotection: what do D2 receptors have to do with it? *Trends Neurosci.* 29, 167–174. doi: 10.1016/j.tins.2006.01.002

Bozzi, Y., and Borrelli, E. (2013). The role of dopamine signaling in epileptogenesis. *Front. Cell. Neurosci.* 7:157. doi: 10.3389/fncel.2013.00157

Bozzi, Y., Vallone, D., and Borrelli, E. (2000). Neuroprotective role of dopamine against hippocampal cell death. *J. Neurosci.* 20, 8643–8649.

Brennan, T. J., Seeley, W. W., Kilgard, M., Schreiner, C. E., and Tecott, L. H. (1997). Sound-induced seizures in serotonin 5-HT2c receptor mutant mice. *Nat. Genet.* 16, 387–390. doi: 10.1038/ng0897-387

Brière, R., Sherwin, A. L., Robitaille, Y., Olivier, A., Quesney, L. F., and Reader, T. A. (1986). Alpha-1 adrenoceptors are decreased in human epileptic foci. *Ann. Neurol.* 19, 26–30. doi: 10.1002/ana.410190106

Brigo, F., and Igwe, S. C. (2016). Melatonin as add-on treatment for epilepsy. *Cochrane Database Syst. Rev.* 3:CD006967. doi: 10.1002/14651858.CD006967.pub3

Cardamone, L., Salzberg, M. R., O'brien, T. J., and Jones, N. C. (2013). Antidepressant therapy in epilepsy: can treating the comorbidities affect the underlying disorder? *Br. J. Pharmacol.* 168, 1531–1554. doi: 10.1111/bph.12052

Cardinali, D. P., Pandi-Perumal, S. R., and Niles, L. P. (2008). "Melatonin and its receptors: biological function in circadian sleep-wake regulation," in *Neurochemistry of Sleep and Wakefulness*, eds J. M. Monti, S. R. Pand-Perumal, and C. M. Sinton (Cambridge: Cambridge University Press), 283–314.

Carter, N. J., and McCormack, P. L. (2009). Duloxetine: a review of its use in the treatment of generalized anxiety disorder. *CNS Drugs* 23, 523–541. doi: 10.2165/00023210-200923060-00006

Cavaccini, A., Yagüe, J. G., Errington, A. C., Crunelli, V., and Di Giovanni, G. (2012). "Opposite effects of thalamic 5-HT2A and 5-HT2C receptor activation on tonic GABA-A inhibition: implications for absence epilepsy," in *Annual Meeting of Neuroscience Society* (New Orleans, LA), 138.103/B157.

Cavalheiro, E. A., Fernandes, M. J., Turski, L., and Naffah-Mazzacoratti, M. G. (1994). Spontaneous recurrent seizures in rats: amino acid and monoamine determination in the hippocampus. *Epilepsia* 35, 1–11. doi: 10.1111/j.1528-1157.1994.tb02905.x

Cavalli, A., Bolognesi, M. L., Minarini, A., Rosini, M., Tumiatti, V., Recanatini, M., et al. (2008). Multi-target-directed ligands to combat neurodegenerative diseases. *J. Med. Chem.* 51, 347–372. doi: 10.1021/jm7009364

Che, F. Y., Wei, Y. Y., Heng, X. Y., Fu, Q. X., and Jiang, J. Z. (2010). Association between serotonin transporter gene polymorphisms and non-lesional temporal lobe epilepsy in a Chinese Han population. *Neural Regen. Res.* 5, 1270–1273.

Chen, G., Ensor, C. R., and Bohner, B. (1954). A facilitation action of reserpine on the central nervous system. *Proc. Soc. Exp. Biol. Med.* 86, 507–510. doi: 10.3181/00379727-86-21149

Chen, Z., Li, W. D., Zhu, L. J., Shen, Y. J., and Wei, E. Q. (2002). Effects of histidine, a precursor of histamine, on pentylenetetrazole-induced seizures in rats. *Acta Pharmacol. Sin.* 23, 361–366.

Chen, Z., Li, Z., Sakurai, E., Mobarakeh, J. I., Ohtsu, H., Watanabe, T., et al. (2003). Chemical kindling induced by pentylenetetrazol in histamine H1 receptor gene knockout mice (H1KO), histidine decarboxylase-deficient mice ($HDC^{-/-}$) and mast cell-deficient W/Wv mice. *Brain Res.* 968, 162–166. doi: 10.1016/S0006-8993(03)02229-7

Churchill, J. A., and Gammon, G. D. (1949). The effect of antihistaminic drugs on convulsive seizures. *J. Am. Med. Assoc.* 141, 18–21. doi: 10.1001/jama.1949.02910010020004

Ciranna, L. (2006). Serotonin as a modulator of glutamate- and GABA-mediated neurotransmission: implications in physiological functions and in pathology. *Curr. Neuropharmacol.* 4, 101–114. doi: 10.2174/157015906776359540

Ciranna, L., and Catania, M. V. (2014). 5-HT7 receptors as modulators of neuronal excitability, synaptic transmission and plasticity: physiological role and possible implications in autism spectrum disorders. *Front. Cell. Neurosci.* 8:250. doi: 10.3389/fncel.2014.00250

Clinckers, R., Smolders, I., Meurs, A., Ebinger, G., and Michotte, Y. (2004). Anticonvulsant action of hippocampal dopamine and serotonin is independently mediated by D2 and 5-HT1A receptors. *J. Neurochem.* 89, 834–843. doi: 10.1111/j.1471-4159.2004.02355.x

Clinckers, R., Zgavc, T., Vermoesen, K., Meurs, A., Michotte, Y., and Smolders, I. (2010). Pharmacological and neurochemical characterization of the involvement of hippocampal adrenoreceptor subtypes in the modulation of acute limbic seizures. *J. Neurochem.* 115, 1595–1607. doi: 10.1111/j.1471-4159.2010.07065.x

Collart Dutilleul, P., Ryvlin, P., Kahane, P., Vercueil, L., Semah, F., Biraben, A., et al. (2016). Exploratory phase II trial to evaluate the safety and the antiepileptic effect of pitolisant (BF2.649) in refractory partial seizures, given as adjunctive treatment during 3 months. *Clin. Neuropharmacol.* 39, 188–193. doi: 10.1097/WNF.0000000000000159

Compan, V., Zhou, M., Grailhe, R., Gazzara, R. A., Martin, R., Gingrich, J., et al. (2004). Attenuated response to stress and novelty and hypersensitivity to seizures in 5-HT4 receptor knock-out mice. *J. Neurosci.* 24, 412–419. doi: 10.1523/JNEUROSCI.2806-03.2004

Cope, D. W., Di Giovanni, G., Fyson, S. J., Orbán, G., Errington, A. C., Lorincz, M. L., et al. (2009). Enhanced tonic GABAA inhibition in typical absence epilepsy. *Nat. Med.* 15, 1392–1398. doi: 10.1038/nm.2058

Coulter, D. A., and Steinhäuser, C. (2015). Role of astrocytes in epilepsy. *Cold Spring Harb. Perspect. Med.* 5:a022434. doi: 10.1101/cshperspect.a022434

Crunelli, V., and Carmignoto, G. (2013). New vistas on astroglia in convulsive and non-convulsive epilepsy highlight novel astrocytic targets for treatment. *J. Physiol.* 591, 775–785. doi: 10.1113/jphysiol.2012.243378

Crunelli, V., Carmignoto, G., and Steinhäuser, C. (2015). Novel astrocyte targets: new avenues for the therapeutic treatment of epilepsy. *Neuroscientist* 21, 62–83. doi: 10.1177/1073858414523320

Csermely, P., Agoston, V., and Pongor, S. (2005). The efficiency of multi-target drugs: the network approach might help drug design. *Trends Pharmacol. Sci.* 26, 178–182. doi: 10.1016/j.tips.2005.02.007

Cui, W., Mizukami, H., Yanagisawa, M., Aida, T., Nomura, M., Isomura, Y., et al. (2014). Glial dysfunction in the mouse habenula causes depressive-like behaviors and sleep disturbance. *J. Neurosci.* 34, 16273–16285. doi: 10.1523/JNEUROSCI.1465-14.2014

Cutler, M. G. (1990). Behavioural effects in gerbils of the 5-HT3 receptor antagonists, BRL 43694 and ICS 205-930, under circumstances of high and low light intensity. *Neuropharmacology* 29, 515–520. doi: 10.1016/0028-3908(90)90062-V

da Fonseca, N. C., Joaquim, H. P., Talib, L. L., de Vincentiis, S., Gattaz, W. F., and Valente, K. D. (2015). Hippocampal serotonin depletion is related to the presence of generalized tonic-clonic seizures, but not to psychiatric disorders in patients with temporal lobe epilepsy. *Epilepsy Res.* 111, 18–25. doi: 10.1016/j.eplepsyres.2014.12.013

Dailey, J. W., Mishra, P. K., Ko, K. H., Penny, J. E., and Jobe, P. C. (1992). Serotonergic abnormalities in the central nervous system of seizure-naive genetically epilepsy-prone rats. *Life Sci.* 50, 319–326. doi: 10.1016/0024-3205(92)90340-U

Dailey, J. W., and Naritoku, D. K. (1996). Antidepressants and seizures: clinical anecdotes overshadow neuroscience. *Biochem. Pharmacol.* 52, 1323–1329. doi: 10.1016/S0006-2952(96)00509-6

Dailey, J. W., Reigel, C. E., Mishra, P. K., and Jobe, P. C. (1989). Neurobiology of seizure predisposition in the genetically epilepsy-prone rat. *Epilepsy Res.* 3, 3–17. doi: 10.1016/0920-1211(89)90063-6

Dailey, J. W., Reith, M. E., Yan, Q. S., Li, M. Y., and Jobe, P. C. (1997). Anticonvulsant doses of carbamazepine increase hippocampal extracellular serotonin in genetically epilepsy-prone rats: dose response relationships. *Neurosci. Lett.* 227, 13–16. doi: 10.1016/S0304-3940(97)00288-7

Dale, E., Bang-Andersen, B., and Sánchez, C. (2015). Emerging mechanisms and treatments for depression beyond SSRIs and SNRIs. *Biochem. Pharmacol.* 95, 81–97. doi: 10.1016/j.bcp.2015.03.011

De Biasi, S., Vitellaro-Zuccarello, L., and Brecha, N. C. (1998). Immunoreactivity for the GABA transporter-1 and GABA transporter-3 is restricted to astrocytes in the rat thalamus. A light and electron-microscopic immunolocalization. *Neuroscience* 83, 815–828. doi: 10.1016/S0306-4522(97)00414-4

De Deurwaerdère, P., and Di Giovanni, G. (2016). Serotonergic modulation of the activity of mesencephalic dopaminergic systems: therapeutic implications. *Prog. Neurobiol.* doi: 10.1016/j.pneurobio.2016.03.004. [Epub ahead of print].

De Lima, E., Soares, J. M. Jr., Del Carmen Sanabria Garrido, Y., Gomes Valente, S., Priel, M. R., Chada Baracat, E., et al. (2005). Effects of pinealectomy and the treatment with melatonin on the temporal lobe epilepsy in rats. *Brain Res.* 1043, 24–31. doi: 10.1016/j.brainres.2005.02.027

De Sarro, G., Di Paola, E. D., Ferreri, G., De Sarro, A., and Fischer, W. (2002). Influence of some beta-adrenoceptor antagonists on the anticonvulsant potency of antiepileptic drugs against audiogenic seizures in DBA/2 mice. *Eur. J. Pharmacol.* 442, 205–213. doi: 10.1016/S0014-2999(02)01536-4

Depondt, C., Cock, H. R., Healy, D. G., Burley, M. W., Weinshenker, D., Wood, N. W., et al. (2004). The -1021C->T DBH gene variant is not associated with epilepsy or antiepileptic drug response. *Neurology* 63, 1497–1499. doi: 10.1212/01.WNL.0000142092.16719.AD

Deransart, C., Landwehrmeyer, G. B., Feuerstein, T. J., and Lücking, C. H. (2001). Up-regulation of D3 dopaminergic receptor mRNA in the core of the nucleus accumbens accompanies the development of seizures in a genetic model of absence-epilepsy in the rat. *Brain Res. Mol. Brain Res.* 94, 166–177. doi: 10.1016/S0169-328X(01)00240-6

Deransart, C., Riban, V., Lê, B. T., Marescaux, C., and Depaulis, A. (2000). Dopamine in the striatum modulates seizures in a genetic model of absence epilepsy in the rat. *Neuroscience* 100, 335–344. doi: 10.1016/S0306-4522(00)00266-9

Devinsky, O., Vezzani, A., Najjar, S., De Lanerolle, N. C., and Rogawski, M. A. (2013). Glia and epilepsy: excitability and inflammation. *Trends Neurosci.* 36, 174–184. doi: 10.1016/j.tins.2012.11.008

Di Giovanni, G., and De Deurwaerdère, P. (2016). New therapeutic opportunities for 5-HT2C receptor ligands in neuropsychiatric disorders. *Pharmacol. Ther.* 157 125–162. doi: 10.1016/j.pharmthera.2015.11.009

Di Matteo, V., Di Giovanni, G., Di Mascio, M., and Esposito, E. (2000). Effect of acute administration of hypericum perforatum-CO2 extract on dopamine and serotonin release in the rat central nervous system. *Pharmacopsychiatry* 33, 14–18. doi: 10.1055/s-2000-8449

Didelot, A., Ryvlin, P., Lothe, A., Merlet, I., Hammers, A., and Mauguière, F. (2008). PET imaging of brain 5-HT1A receptors in the preoperative evaluation of temporal lobe epilepsy. *Brain* 131, 2751–2764. doi: 10.1093/brain/awn220

Dunleavy, M., Provenzano, G., Henshall, D. C., and Bozzi, Y. (2013). Kainic acid-induced seizures modulate Akt (SER473) phosphorylation in the hippocampus of dopamine D2 receptor knockout mice. *J. Mol. Neurosci.* 49, 202–210. doi: 10.1007/s12031-012-9927-x

Esmail, E. H., Labib, D. M., and Rabie, W. A. (2015). Association of serotonin transporter gene (5HTT) polymorphism and juvenile myoclonic epilepsy: a case-control study. *Acta Neurol. Belg.* 115, 247–251. doi: 10.1007/s13760-014-0400-1

Fauteck, J. D., Bockmann, J., Bockers, T. M., Wittkowski, W., Köhling, R., Lücke, A., et al. (1995). Melatonin reduces low-Mg2+ epileptiform activity in human temporal slices. *Exp. Brain Res.* 107, 321–325. doi: 10.1007/BF00230052

Fenoglio-Simeone, K., Mazarati, A., Sefidvash-Hockley, S., Shin, D., Wilke, J., Milligan, H., et al. (2009). Anticonvulsant effects of the selective melatonin receptor agonist ramelteon. *Epilepsy Behav.* 16, 52–57. doi: 10.1016/j.yebeh.2009.07.022

Ferraro, T. N., and Buono, R. J. (2006). Polygenic epilepsy. *Adv. Neurol.* 97, 389–398.

Finberg, J. P. (2014). Update on the pharmacology of selective inhibitors of MAO-A and MAO-B: focus on modulation of CNS monoamine neurotransmitter release. *Pharmacol. Ther.* 143, 133–152. doi: 10.1016/j.pharmthera.2014.02.010

Fink, K. B., and Göethert, M. (2007). 5-HT receptor regulation of neurotransmitter release. *Pharmacol. Rev.* 59, 360–417. doi: 10.1124/pr.59.07103

Fischer, W. (2002). Anticonvulsant profile and mechanism of action of propranolol and its two enantiomers. *Seizure* 11, 285–302. doi: 10.1053/seiz.2001.0644

Fischer, W., Kittner, H., Regenthal, R., Malinowska, B., and Schlicker, E. (2001). Anticonvulsant and sodium channel blocking activity of higher doses of clenbuterol. *Naunyn Schmiedebergs Arch. Pharmacol.* 363, 182–192. doi: 10.1007/s002100000341

Fitzgerald, P. J. (2010). Is elevated norepinephrine an etiological factor in some cases of epilepsy? *Seizure* 19, 311–318. doi: 10.1016/j.seizure.2010.04.011

Gaitatzis, A., Johnson, A. L., Chadwick, D. W., Shorvon, S. D., and Sander, J. W. (2004). Life expectancy in people with newly diagnosed epilepsy. *Brain* 127, 2427–2432. doi: 10.1093/brain/awh267

Gangarossa, G., Ceolin, L., Paucard, A., Lerner-Natoli, M., Perroy, J., Fagni, L., et al. (2014). Repeated stimulation of dopamine D1-like receptor and hyperactivation of mTOR signaling lead to generalized seizures, altered dentate gyrus plasticity, and memory deficits. *Hippocampus* 24, 1466–1481. doi: 10.1002/hipo.22327

Garcia, C. S. (2012). Depression in temporal lobe epilepsy: a review of prevalence, clinical features, and management considerations. *Epilepsy Res. Treat.* 2012, 809843. doi: 10.1155/2012/809843

Giorgi, F. S., Pizzanelli, C., Biagioni, F., Murri, L., and Fornai, F. (2004). The role of norepinephrine in epilepsy: from the bench to the bedside. *Neurosci. Biobehav. Rev.* 28, 507–524. doi: 10.1016/j.neubiorev.2004.06.008

Giovacchini, G., Conant, S., Herscovitch, P., and Theodore, W. H. (2009). Using cerebral white matter for estimation of nondisplaceable binding of 5-HT1A receptors in temporal lobe epilepsy. *J. Nucl. Med.* 50, 1794–1800. doi: 10.2967/jnumed.109.063743

Goldberg, S. R., and Spealman, R. D. (1983). Suppression of behavior by intravenous injections of nicotine or by electric shocks in squirrel monkeys: effects of chlordiazepoxide and mecamylamine. *J. Pharmacol. Exp. Ther.* 224, 334–340.

Golombek, D. A., Fernández Duque, D., De Brito Sánchez, M. G., Burin, L., and Cardinali, D. P. (1992). Time-dependent anticonvulsant activity of melatonin in hamsters. *Eur. J. Pharmacol.* 210, 253–258. doi: 10.1016/0014-2999(92)90412-W

Golombek, D. A., Pévet, P., and Cardinali, D. P. (1996). Melatonin effects on behavior: possible mediation by the central GABAergic system. *Neurosci. Biobehav. Rev.* 20, 403–412. doi: 10.1016/0149-7634(95)00052-6

Gorwood, P., Limosin, F., Batel, P., Hamon, M., Adès, J., and Boni, C. (2003). The A9 allele of the dopamine transporter gene is associated with delirium tremens and alcohol-withdrawal seizure. *Biol. Psychiatry* 53, 85–92. doi: 10.1016/S0006-3223(02)01440-3

Graf, M., Jakus, R., Kantor, S., Levay, G., and Bagdy, G. (2004). Selective 5-HT1A and 5-HT7 antagonists decrease epileptic activity in the WAG/Rij rat model of absence epilepsy. *Neurosci. Lett.* 359, 45–48. doi: 10.1016/j.neulet.2004.01.072

Grant, K. A., Hellevuo, K., and Tabakoff, B. (1994). The 5-HT3 antagonist MDL-72222 exacerbates ethanol withdrawal seizures in mice. *Alcohol. Clin. Exp. Res.* 18, 410–414. doi: 10.1111/j.1530-0277.1994.tb00034.x

Guerrini, R. (2006). Epilepsy in children. *Lancet* 367, 499–524. doi: 10.1016/S0140-6736(06)68182-8

Guiard, B. P., and Di Giovanni, G. (2015). Central serotonin-2A (5-HT2A) receptor dysfunction in depression and epilepsy: the missing link? *Front. Pharmacol.* 6:46. doi: 10.3389/fphar.2015.00046

Guzior, N., Wieckowska, A., Panek, D., and Malawska, B. (2015). Recent development of multifunctional agents as potential drug candidates for the treatment of Alzheimer's disease. *Curr. Med. Chem.* 22, 373–404. doi: 10.2174/0929867321666141106122628

Haas, H., and Panula, P. (2003). The role of histamine and the tuberomamillary nucleus in the nervous system. *Nat. Rev. Neurosci.* 4, 121–130. doi: 10.1038/nrn1034

Hamid, H., and Kanner, A. M. (2013). Should antidepressant drugs of the selective serotonin reuptake inhibitor family be tested as antiepileptic drugs? *Epilepsy Behav.* 26, 261–265. doi: 10.1016/j.yebeh.2012.10.009

Hardeland, R., Cardinali, D. P., Srinivasan, V., Spence, D. W., Brown, G. M., and Pandi-Perumal, S. R. (2011). Melatonin–a pleiotropic, orchestrating regulator molecule. *Prog. Neurobiol.* 93, 350–384. doi: 10.1016/j.pneurobio.2010.12.004

Harden, C. L. (2002). The co-morbidity of depression and epilepsy: epidemiology, etiology, and treatment. *Neurology* 59, S48–S55. doi: 10.1212/wnl.59.6_suppl_4.s48

Hasler, G., Bonwetsch, R., Giovacchini, G., Toczek, M. T., Bagic, A., Luckenbaugh, D. A., et al. (2007). 5-HT1A receptor binding in temporal lobe epilepsy patients with and without major depression. *Biol. Psychiatry* 62, 1258–1264. doi: 10.1016/j.biopsych.2007.02.015

Hatice, A., Duygu, A., Sema, İ., Fatih, E., Mustafa, A., and Erda, L. A. (2015). The effects of agomelatine and melatonin on ECoG activity of absenceepilepsy model in WAG/Rij rats. *Turk. J. Biol.* 39, 904–910. doi: 10.3906/biy-1507-32

Haug, K., Sander, T., Hallmann, K., Lentze, M. J., Propping, P., Elger, C. E., et al. (2000). Association analysis between a regulatory-promoter polymorphism of the human monoamine oxidase A gene and idiopathic generalized epilepsy. *Epilepsy Res.* 39, 127–132. doi: 10.1016/S0920-1211(99)00116-3

Hecimovic, H., Stefulj, J., Cicin-Sain, L., Demarin, V., and Jernej, B. (2010). Association of serotonin transporter promoter (5-HTTLPR) and intron 2 (VNTR-2) polymorphisms with treatment response in temporal lobe epilepsy. *Epilepsy Res.* 91, 35–38. doi: 10.1016/j.eplepsyres.2010.06.008

Heils, A., Teufel, A., Petri, S., Stöber, G., Riederer, P., Bengel, D., et al. (1996). Allelic variation of human serotonin transporter gene expression. *J. Neurochem.* 66, 2621–2624. doi: 10.1046/j.1471-4159.1996.66062621.x

Heisler, L. K., Chu, H. M., and Tecott, L. H. (1998). Epilepsy and obesity in serotonin 5-HT2C receptor mutant mice. *Ann. N.Y. Acad. Sci.* 861, 74–78. doi: 10.1111/j.1749-6632.1998.tb10175.x

Helmstaedter, C., Mihov, Y., Toliat, M. R., Thiele, H., Nuernberg, P., Schoch, S., et al. (2013). Genetic variation in dopaminergic activity is associated with the risk for psychiatric side effects of levetiracetam. *Epilepsia* 54, 36–44. doi: 10.1111/j.1528-1167.2012.03603.x

Hernandez, J., and Condés-Lara, M. (1989). Serotonin-dependent (Na+,K+)ATPase in kindled rats: a study in various brain regions. *Brain Res.* 480, 403–406. doi: 10.1016/0006-8993(89)90743-9

Hertz, L., Rothman, D. L., Li, B., and Peng, L. (2015). Chronic SSRI stimulation of astrocytic 5-HT2B receptors change multiple gene expressions/editings and metabolism of glutamate, glucose and glycogen: a potential paradigm shift. *Front. Behav. Neurosci.* 9:25. doi: 10.3389/fnbeh.2015.00308

Hildebrand, M. S., Dahl, H. H., Damiano, J. A., Smith, R. J., Scheffer, I. E., and Berkovic, S. F. (2013). Recent advances in the molecular genetics of epilepsy. *J. Med. Genet.* 50, 271–279. doi: 10.1136/jmedgenet-2012-101448

Hirst, W. D., Cheung, N. Y., Rattray, M., Price, G. W., and Wilkin, G. P. (1998). Cultured astrocytes express messenger RNA for multiple serotonin receptor subtypes, without functional coupling of 5-HT1 receptor subtypes to adenylyl cyclase. *Brain Res. Mol. Brain Res.* 61, 90–99. doi: 10.1016/S0169-328X(98)00206-X

Hirst, W. D., Stean, T. O., Rogers, D. C., Sunter, D., Pugh, P., Moss, S. F., et al. (2006). SB-399885 is a potent, selective 5-HT6 receptor antagonist with cognitive enhancing properties in aged rat water maze and novel object recognition models. *Eur. J. Pharmacol.* 553, 109–119. doi: 10.1016/j.ejphar.2006.09.049

Holmes, G. L., and Noebels, J. L. (2016). The epilepsy spectrum: targeting future research challenges. *Cold Spring Harb. Perspect. Med.* 6:a028043. doi: 10.1101/cshperspect.a028043

Hopkins, A. L. (2008). Network pharmacology: the next paradigm in drug discovery. *Nat. Chem. Biol.* 4, 682–690. doi: 10.1038/nchembio.118

Horvath, G. A., Demos, M., Shyr, C., Matthews, A., Zhang, L., Race, S., et al. (2016). Secondary neurotransmitter deficiencies in epilepsy caused by voltage-gated sodium channelopathies: a potential treatment target? *Mol. Genet. Metab.* 117, 42–48. doi: 10.1016/j.ymgme.2015.11.008

Huang, Y. Y., Grailhe, R., Arango, V., Hen, R., and Mann, J. J. (1999). Relationship of psychopathology to the human serotonin1B genotype and receptor binding kinetics in postmortem brain tissue. *Neuropsychopharmacology* 21, 238–246. doi: 10.1016/S0893-133X(99)00030-5

Hwang, J., Zheng, L. T., Ock, J., Lee, M. G., and Suk, K. (2008). Anti-inflammatory effects of m-chlorophenylpiperazine in brain glia cells. *Int. Immunopharmacol.* 8, 1686–1694. doi: 10.1016/j.intimp.2008.08.004

Ismaili, L., Refouvelet, B., Benchekroun, M., Brogi, S., Brindisi, M., Gemma, S., et al. (2016). Multitarget compounds bearing tacrine- and donepezil-like structural and functional motifs for the potential treatment of Alzheimer's disease. *Prog. Neurobiol.* doi: 10.1016/j.pneurobio.2015.12.003. [Epub ahead of print].

Jain, S., and Desag, F. M. (2013). Does melatonin affect epileptic seizures? *Drug Saf.* 36, 207–215. doi: 10.1007/s40264-013-0033-y

Jakus, R., and Bagdy, G. (2011). "The role of 5-HT2C receptor in epilepsy," in *5-HT2C Receptors in the Pathophysiology of CNS Disease*, eds G. Di Giovanni, E. Esposito, and V. Di Matteo (Wien: Springer-Verlag), 429–444.

Jakus, R., Graf, M., Juhasz, G., Gerber, K., Levay, G., Halasz, P., et al. (2003). 5-HT2C receptors inhibit and 5-HT1A receptors activate the generation of spike-wave discharges in a genetic rat model of absence epilepsy. *Exp. Neurol.* 184, 964–972. doi: 10.1016/S0014-4886(03)00352-2

Janumpalli, S., Butler, L. S., Macmillan, L. B., Limbird, L. E., and McNamara, J. O. (1998). A point mutation (D79N) of the alpha2A adrenergic receptor abolishes the antiepileptogenic action of endogenous norepinephrine. *J. Neurosci.* 18, 2004–2008.

Jin, C. L., Yang, L. X., Wu, X. H., Li, Q., Ding, M. P., Fan, Y. Y., et al. (2005). Effects of carnosine on amygdaloid-kindled seizures in Sprague-Dawley rats. *Neuroscience* 135, 939–947. doi: 10.1016/j.neuroscience.2005.06.066

Jobe, P. C., and Browning, R. A. (2005). The serotonergic and noradrenergic effects of antidepressant drugs are anticonvulsant, not proconvulsant. *Epilepsy Behav.* 7, 602–619. doi: 10.1016/j.yebeh.2005.07.014

Jobe, P. C., Dailey, J. W., and Wernicke, J. F. (1999). A noradrenergic and serotonergic hypothesis of the linkage between epilepsy and affective disorders. *Crit. Rev. Neurobiol.* 13, 317–356.

Jones, N. C., Martin, S., Megatia, I., Hakami, T., Salzberg, M. R., Pinault, D., et al. (2010). A genetic epilepsy rat model displays endophenotypes of psychosis. *Neurobiol. Dis.* 39, 116–125. doi: 10.1016/j.nbd.2010.02.001

Jurgens, C. W., Boese, S. J., King, J. D., Pyle, S. J., Porter, J. E., and Doze, V. A. (2005). Adrenergic receptor modulation of hippocampal CA3 network activity. *Epilepsy Res.* 66, 117–128. doi: 10.1016/j.eplepsyres.2005.07.007

Jurgens, C. W., Hammad, H. M., Lichter, J. A., Boese, S. J., Nelson, B. W., Goldenstein, B. L., et al. (2007). Alpha2A adrenergic receptor activation inhibits epileptiform activity in the rat hippocampal CA3 region. *Mol. Pharmacol.* 71, 1572–1581. doi: 10.1124/mol.106.031773

Kakinoki, H., Ishizawa, K., Fukunaga, M., Fujii, Y., and Kamei, C. (1998). The effects of histamine H3-receptor antagonists on amygdaloid kindled seizures in rats. Brain Res. Bull. 46, 461–465. doi: 10.1016/S0361-9230(98)00048-3

Kamei, C. (2001). Involvement of central histamine in amygdaloid kindled seizures in rats. Behav. Brain Res. 124, 243–250. doi: 10.1016/S0166-4328(01)00218-2

Kamei, C., Ishizawa, K., Kakinoki, H., and Fukunaga, M. (1998). Histaminergic mechanisms in amygdaloid-kindled seizures in rats. Epilepsy Res. 30, 187–194. doi: 10.1016/S0920-1211(98)00005-9

Kanner, A., Tilwalli, S., Smith, M., Bergen, D., Palac, S., Balabanov, A., et al. (2003). Presurgical history of depression is associated with a worse postsurgical seizure outcome following a temporal lobectomy. Neurology 62 (Suppl. 5), A389.

Kasteleijn-Nolst Trenité, D., Parain, D., Genton, P., Masnou, P., Schwartz, J. C., and Hirsch, E. (2013). Efficacy of the histamine 3 receptor (H3R) antagonist pitolisant (formerly known as tiprolisant; BF2.649) in epilepsy: dose-dependent effects in the human photosensitivity model. Epilepsy Behav. 28, 66–70. doi: 10.1016/j.yebeh.2013.03.018

Kauffman, M. A., Consalvo, D., Gonzalez-Morón, D., Aguirre, F., D'alessio, L., and Kochen, S. (2009). Serotonin transporter gene variation and refractory mesial temporal epilepsy with hippocampal sclerosis. Epilepsy Res. 85, 231–234. doi: 10.1016/j.eplepsyres.2009.03.010

Kiviranta, T., Tuomisto, L., and Airaksinen, E. M. (1995). Histamine in cerebrospinal fluid of children with febrile convulsions. Epilepsia 36, 276–280. doi: 10.1111/j.1528-1157.1995.tb00996.x

Klitten, L. L., Møller, R. S., Ravn, K., Hjalgrim, H., and Tommerup, N. (2011). Duplication of MAOA, MAOB, and NDP in a patient with mental retardation and epilepsy. Eur. J. Hum. Genet. 19, 1–2. doi: 10.1038/ejhg.2010.149

Kobau, R., Zahran, H., Thurman, D. J., Zack, M. M., Henry, T. R., Schachter, S. C., et al. (2008). Epilepsy surveillance among adults–19 States, behavioral risk factor surveillance system, 2005. MMWR. Surveill. Summ. 57, 1–20.

Kobayashi, K., and Mori, A. (1977). Brain monoamines in seizure mechanism (review). Folia Psychiatr. Neurol. Jpn. 31, 483–489. doi: 10.1111/j.1440-1819.1977.tb02637.x

Kohen, R., Metcalf, M. A., Khan, N., Druck, T., Huebner, K., Lachowicz, J. E., et al. (1996). Cloning, characterization, and chromosomal localization of a human 5-HT6 serotonin receptor. J. Neurochem. 66, 47–56. doi: 10.1046/j.1471-4159.1996.66010047.x

Kohli, R. P., Gupta, T. K., Parmar, S. S., and Arora, R. C. (1967). Anticonvulsant properties of some newer monoamine oxidase inhibitors. Jpn. J. Pharmacol. 17, 409–415. doi: 10.1254/jjp.17.409

Kostowski, W., Dyr, W., and Krzascik, P. (1993). The abilities of 5-HT3 receptor antagonist ICS 205-930 to inhibit alcohol preference and withdrawal seizures in rats. Alcohol 10, 369–373. doi: 10.1016/0741-8329(93)90022-G

Kumlien, E., Hilton-Brown, P., Spännare, B., and Gillberg, P.-G. (1992). In vitro quantitative autoradiography of [3H]-L-deprenyl and [3H]-PK 11195 binding sites in human epileptic hippocampus. Epilepsia 33, 610–617. doi: 10.1111/j.1528-1157.1992.tb02336.x

Kumlien, E., Nilsson, A., Hagberg, G., Långström, B., and Bergström, M. (2001). PET with 11C-deuterium-deprenyl and 18F-FDG in focal epilepsy. Acta Neurol. Scand. 103, 360–366. doi: 10.1034/j.1600-0404.2001.103006360.x

Kurian, M. A., Gissen, P., Smith, M., Heales, S. Jr., and Clayton, P. T. (2011). The monoamine neurotransmitter disorders: an expanding range of neurological syndromes. Lancet Neurol. 10, 721–733. doi: 10.1016/S1474-4422(11)70141-7

Lai, M. K., Tsang, S. W., Francis, P. T., Esiri, M. M., Hope, T., Lai, O. F., et al. (2003). [3H]GR113808 binding to serotonin 5-HT(4) receptors in the postmortem neocortex of Alzheimer disease: a clinicopathological study. J. Neural Transm. 110, 779–788. doi: 10.1007/s00702-003-0825-9

Landvogt, C., Buchholz, H. G., Bernedo, V., Schreckenberger, M., and Werhahn, K. J. (2010). Alteration of dopamine D2/D3 receptor binding in patients with juvenile myoclonic epilepsy. Epilepsia 51, 1699–1706. doi: 10.1111/j.1528-1167.2010.02569.x

Lesch, K. P., Balling, U., Gross, J., Strauss, K., Wolozin, B. L., Murphy, D. L., et al. (1994). Organization of the human serotonin transporter gene. J. Neural Transm. Gen. Sect. 95, 157–162. doi: 10.1007/BF01276434

Li, B., Wang, L., Sun, Z., Zhou, Y., Shao, D., Zhao, J., et al. (2014). The anticonvulsant effects of SR 57227 on pentylenetetrazole-induced seizure in mice. PLoS ONE 9:e93158. doi: 10.1371/journal.pone.0093158

Li, J., Lin, H., Zhu, X., Li, L., Wang, X., Sun, W., et al. (2012). Association study of functional polymorphisms in serotonin transporter gene with temporal lobe epilepsy in Han Chinese population. Eur. J. Neurol. 19, 351–353. doi: 10.1111/j.1468-1331.2011.03521.x

Libet, B., Gleason, C. A., Wright, E. W. Jr., and Feinstein, B. (1977). Suppression of an epileptiform type of electrocortical activity in the rat by stimulation in the vicinity of locus coeruleus. Epilepsia 18, 451–462. doi: 10.1111/j.1528-1157.1977.tb04991.x

Liu, W., Tang, Y., and Feng, J. (2011). Cross talk between activation of microglia and astrocytes in pathological conditions in the central nervous system. Life Sci. 89, 141–146. doi: 10.1016/j.lfs.2011.05.011

López-Meraz, M. L., González-Trujano, M. E., Neri-Bazán, L., Hong, E., and Rocha, L. L. (2005). 5-HT1A receptor agonists modify epileptic seizures in three experimental models in rats. Neuropharmacology 49, 367–375. doi: 10.1016/j.neuropharm.2005.03.020

Löscher, W., and Lehmann, H. (1996). L-deprenyl (selegiline) exerts anticonvulsant effects against different seizure types in mice. J. Pharmacol. Exp. Ther. 277, 1410–1417.

Löscher, W., and Lehmann, H. (1998). Anticonvulsant efficacy of L-deprenyl (selegiline) during chronic treatment in mice: continuous versus discontinuous administration. Neuropharmacology 37, 1587–1593. doi: 10.1016/S0028-3908(98)00130-0

Loscher, W., Lehmann, H., Teschendorf, H. J., Traut, M., and Gross, G. (1999). Inhibition of monoamine oxidase type A, but not type B, is an effective means of inducing anticonvulsant activity in the kindling model of epilepsy. J. Pharmacol. Exp. Ther. 288, 984–992.

Lothe, A., Merlet, I., Demarquay, G., Costes, N., Ryvlin, P., and Mauguière, F. (2008). Interictal brain 5-HT1A receptors binding in migraine without aura: a 18F-MPPF-PET study. Cephalalgia 28, 1282–1291. doi: 10.1111/j.1468-2982.2008.01677.x

Lowy, M. T., and Meltzer, H. Y. (1988). Stimulation of serum cortisol and prolactin secretion in humans by MK-212, a centrally active serotonin agonist. Biol. Psychiatry 23, 818–828. doi: 10.1016/0006-3223(88)90070-4

Lu, J. J., Pan, W., Hu, Y. J., and Wang, Y. T. (2012). Multi-target drugs: the trend of drug research and development. PLoS ONE 7:e40262. doi: 10.1371/journal.pone.0040262

Luchowska, E., Luchowski, P., Wielosz, M., Kleinrok, Z., Czuczwar, S. J., and Urbanska, E. M. (2002). Propranolol and metoprolol enhance the anticonvulsant action of valproate and diazepam against maximal electroshock. Pharmacol. Biochem. Behav. 71, 223–231. doi: 10.1016/S0091-3057(01)00654-2

Maeda, H., Chiyonobu, T., Yoshida, M., Yamashita, S., Zuiki, M., Kidowaki, S., et al. (2016). Establishment of isogenic iPSCs from an individual with SCN1A mutation mosaicism as a model for investigating neurocognitive impairment in Dravet syndrome. J. Hum. Genet. 61, 565–569. doi: 10.1038/jhg.2016.5

Maes, M., Leonard, B. E., Myint, A. M., Kubera, M., and Verkerk, R. (2011). The new '5-HT' hypothesis of depression: cell-mediated immune activation induces indoleamine 2,3-dioxygenase, which leads to lower plasma tryptophan and an increased synthesis of detrimental tryptophan catabolites (TRYCATs), both of which contribute to the onset of depression. Prog. Neuropsychopharmacol. Biol. Psychiatry 35, 702–721. doi: 10.1016/j.pnpbp.2010.12.017

Magyar, K. (2011). The pharmacology of selegiline. Int. Rev. Neurobiol. 100, 65–84. doi: 10.1016/B978-0-12-386467-3.00004-2

Manna, I., Labate, A., Gambardella, A., Forabosco, P., La Russa, A., Le Piane, E., et al. (2007). Serotonin transporter gene (5-Htt): association analysis with temporal lobe epilepsy. Neurosci. Lett. 421, 52–56. doi: 10.1016/j.neulet.2007.05.022

Manna, I., Labate, A., Mumoli, L., Palamara, G., Ferlazzo, E., Aguglia, U., et al. (2012). A functional genetic variation of the 5-HTR2A receptor affects age at onset in patients with temporal lobe epilepsy. Ann. Hum. Genet. 76, 277–282. doi: 10.1111/j.1469-1809.2012.00713.x

Mantyh, P. W., Rogers, S. D., Allen, C. J., Catton, M. D., Ghilardi, J. R., Levin, L. A., et al. (1995). Beta 2-adrenergic receptors are expressed by glia in vivo in the normal and injured central nervous system in the rat, rabbit, and human. J. Neurosci. 15, 152–164.

McIntyre, D. C., and Edson, N. (1989). Kindling-based status epilepticus: effect of norepinephrine depletion with 6-hydroxydopamine. Exp. Neurol. 104, 10–14. doi: 10.1016/0014-4886(89)90002-2

Meurs, A., Clinckers, R., Ebinger, G., Michotte, Y., and Smolders, I. (2008). Seizure activity and changes in hippocampal extracellular glutamate, GABA, dopamine and serotonin. *Epilepsy Res.* 78, 50–59. doi: 10.1016/j.eplepsyres.2007. 10.007

Micale, V., Cristino, L., Tamburella, A., Petrosino, S., Leggio, G. M., Drago, F., et al. (2009). Altered responses of dopamine D3 receptor null mice to excitotoxic or anxiogenic stimuli: possible involvement of the endocannabinoid and endovanilloid systems. *Neurobiol. Dis.* 36, 70–80. doi: 10.1016/j.nbd.2009.06.015

Micheletti, G., Warter, J. M., Marescaux, C., Depaulis, A., Tranchant, C., Rumbach, L., et al. (1987). Effects of drugs affecting noradrenergic neurotransmission in rats with spontaneous petit mal-like seizures. *Eur. J. Pharmacol.* 135, 397–402. doi: 10.1016/0014-2999(87)90690-X

Midzyanovskaya, I., Kopilov, M., Fedotova, E., Kuznetsova, G., and Tuomisto, L. (2005). Dual effect of pyrilamine on absence seizures in WAG/Rij rats. *Inflamm. Res.* 54, S40–S41. doi: 10.1007/s00011-004-0418-6

Midzyanovskaya, I. S., Birioukova, L. M., Shatskova, A. B., van Luijtelaar, G., and Tuomisto, L. M. (2016). H1 histamine receptor densities are increased in brain regions of rats with genetically generalized epilepsies. *Epilepsy Res.* 127, 135–140. doi: 10.1016/j.eplepsyres.2016.08.029

Millan, M. J., Gobert, A., Lejeune, F., Dekeyne, A., Newman-Tancredi, A., Pasteau, V., et al. (2003). The novel melatonin agonist agomelatine (S20098) is an antagonist at 5-hydroxytryptamine2C receptors, blockade of which enhances the activity of frontocortical dopaminergic and adrenergic pathways. *J. Pharmacol. Exp. Ther.* 306, 954–964. doi: 10.1124/jpet.103.051797

Miras-Portuga, M. T., Aunis, D., Mandel, P., Warter, J. M., Coquillat, G., and Kurtz, D. (1975). Human circulating dopamine-B-hydroxylase and epilepsy. *Pharmacologia* 41, 5.

Miyata, I., Saegusa, H., and Sakurai, M. (2011). Seizure-modifying potential of histamine H1 antagonists: a clinical observation. *Pediatr. Int.* 53, 706–708. doi: 10.1111/j.1442-200X.2011.03328.x

Miyazaki, I., Asanuma, M., Diaz-Corrales, F. J., Miyoshi, K., and Ogawa, N. (2004). Direct evidence for expression of dopamine receptors in astrocytes from basal ganglia. *Brain Res.* 1029, 120–123. doi: 10.1016/j.brainres.2004.09.014

Mohanan, P. V., and Yamamoto, H. A. (2002). Preventive effect of melatonin against brain mitochondria DNA damage, lipid peroxidation and seizures induced by kainic acid. *Toxicol. Lett.* 129, 99–105. doi: 10.1016/S0378-4274(01)00475-1

Molina-Carballo, A., Muñoz-Hoyos, A., Sánchez-Forte, M., Uberos-Fernández, J., Moreno-Madrid, F., and Acuña-Castroviejo, D. (2007). Melatonin increases following convulsive seizures may be related to its anticonvulsant properties at physiological concentrations. *Neuropediatrics* 38, 122–125. doi: 10.1055/s-2007-985138

Motta, E., Czuczwar, S. J., Ostrowska, Z., Golba, A., Soltyk, J., Norman, R., et al. (2014). Circadian profile of salivary melatonin secretion and its concentration after epileptic seizure in patients with drug-resistant epilepsy–preliminary report. *Pharmacol. Rep.* 66, 492–498. doi: 10.1016/j.pharep.2013.10.006

Mukhopadhyay, M., Upadhyay, S. N., and Bhattacharya, S. K. (1987). Neuropharmacological studies on selective monoamine oxidase A and B inhibitors. *Indian J. Exp. Biol.* 25, 761–770.

Myers, C. T., and Mefford, H. C. (2015). Advancing epilepsy genetics in the genomic era. *Genome Med.* 7, 91. doi: 10.1186/s13073-015-0214-7

Naffah-Mazzacoratti, M. G., Amado, D., Cukiert, A., Gronich, G., Marino, R., Calderazzo, L., et al. (1996). Monoamines and their metabolites in cerebrospinal fluid and temporal cortex of epileptic patients. *Epilepsy Res.* 25, 133–137. doi: 10.1016/0920-1211(96)00030-7

Nakamura, T., Oda, Y., Takahashi, R., Tanaka, K., Hase, I., and Asada, A. (2008). Propranolol increases the threshold for lidocaine-induced convulsions in awake rats: a direct effect on the brain. *Anesth. Analg.* 106, 1450–1455. doi: 10.1213/ane.0b013e31816ba49d

Neurauter, G., Schröcksnadel, K., Scholl-Bürgi, S., Sperner-Unterweger, B., Schubert, C., Ledochowski, M., et al. (2008). Chronic immune stimulation correlates with reduced phenylalanine turnover. *Curr. Drug Metab.* 9, 622–627. doi: 10.2174/138920008785821738

Ng, J., Papandreou, A., Heales, S. J., and Kurian, M. A. (2015). Monoamine neurotransmitter disorders-clinical advances and future perspectives. *Nat. Rev. Neurol.* 11, 567–584. doi: 10.1038/nrneurol.2015.172

Nikiforuk, A. (2015). Targeting the serotonin 5-HT7 receptor in the search for treatments for CNS disorders: rationale and progress to date. *CNS Drugs* 29, 265–275. doi: 10.1007/s40263-015-0236-0

Nikolic, K., Mavridis, L., Djikic, T., Vucicevic, J., Agbaba, D., Yelekci, K., et al. (2016). Drug design for CNS diseases: polypharmacological profiling of compounds using cheminformatic, 3D-QSAR and virtual screening methodologies. *Front. Neurosci.* 10:265. doi: 10.3389/fnins.2016. 00265

O'dell, L. E., Li, R., George, F. R., and Ritz, M. C. (2000). Molecular serotonergic mechanisms appear to mediate genetic sensitivity to cocaine-induced convulsions. *Brain Res.* 863, 213–224. doi: 10.1016/S0006-8993(00)02141-7

Olpe, H. R., and Jones, R. S. (1983). The action of anticonvulsant drugs on the firing of locus coeruleus neurons: selective, activating effect of carbamazepine. *Eur. J. Pharmacol.* 91, 107–110. doi: 10.1016/0014-2999(83)90369-2

Onodera, K., Tuomisto, L., Tacke, U., and Airaksinen, M. (1992). Strain differences in regional brain histamine levels between genetically epilepsy-prone and resistant rats. *Methods Find. Exp. Clin. Pharmacol.* 14, 13–16.

Orban, G., Bombardi, C., Marino Gammazza, A., Colangeli, R., Pierucci, M., Pomara, C., et al. (2014). Role(s) of the 5-HT2C receptor in the development of maximal dentate activation in the hippocampus of anesthetized rats. *CNS Neurosci. Ther.* 20, 651–661. doi: 10.1111/cns.12285

Orban, G., Pierucci, M., Benigno, A., Pessia, M., Galati, S., Valentino, M., et al. (2013). High dose of 8-OH-DPAT decreases maximal dentate gyrus activation and facilitates granular cell plasticity in vivo. *Exp. Brain Res.* 230, 441–451. doi: 10.1007/s00221-013-3594-1

O'sullivan, G. J., Dunleavy, M., Hakansson, K., Clementi, M., Kinsella, A., Croke, D. T., et al. (2008). Dopamine D1 vs D5 receptor-dependent induction of seizures in relation to DARPP-32, ERK1/2 and GluR1-AMPA signalling. *Neuropharmacology* 54, 1051–1061. doi: 10.1016/j.neuropharm.2008.02.011

O'sullivan, G. J., Kinsella, A., Grandy, D. K., Tighe, O., Croke, D. T., and Waddington, J. L. (2006). Ethological resolution of behavioral topography and D2-like vs. D1-like agonist responses in congenic D4 dopamine receptor "knockouts": identification of D4:D1-like interactions. *Synapse* 59, 107–118. doi: 10.1002/syn.20225

Ottman, R., and Risch, N. (2012). "Genetic epidemiology and gene discovery in epilepsy," in *Jasper's Basic Mechanisms of the Epilepsies, 4th Edn,* eds J. L. Noebels, M. Avoli, M. A. Rogawski, R. W. Olsen, and A. V. Delgado-Escueta (Bethesda, MD: National Center for Biotechnology Information).

Panczyk, K., Golda, S., Waszkielewicz, A., Zelaszczyk, D., Gunia-Krzyzak, A., and Marona, H. (2015). Serotonergic system and its role in epilepsy and neuropathic pain treatment: a review based on receptor ligands. *Curr. Pharm. Des.* 21, 1723–1740. doi: 10.2174/1381612821666141121114917

Panebianco, M., Zavanone, C., Dupont, S., Restivo, D. A., and Pavone, A. (2016). Vagus nerve stimulation therapy in partial epilepsy: a review. *Acta Neurol. Belg.* 116, 241–248. doi: 10.1007/s13760-016-0616-3

Park, K. D., Yang, X. F., Dustrude, E. T., Wang, Y., Ripsch, M. S., White, F. A., et al. (2015). Chimeric agents derived from the functionalized amino acid, lacosamide, and the alpha-aminoamide, safinamide: evaluation of their inhibitory actions on voltage-gated sodium channels, and antiseizure and antinociception activities and comparison with lacosamide and safinamide. *ACS Chem. Neurosci.* 6, 316–330. doi: 10.1021/cn5002182

Payandemehr, B., Bahremand, A., Rahimian, R., Ziai, P., Amouzegar, A., Sharifzadeh, M., et al. (2012). 5-HT(3) receptor mediates the dose-dependent effects of citalopram on pentylenetetrazole-induced clonic seizure in mice: involvement of nitric oxide. *Epilepsy Res.* 101, 217–227. doi: 10.1016/j.eplepsyres.2012.04.004

Peled, N., Shorer, Z., Peled, E., and Pillar, G. (2001). Melatonin effect on seizures in children with severe neurologic deficit disorders. *Epilepsia* 42, 1208–1210. doi: 10.1046/j.1528-1157.2001.28100.x

Peričić, D., Lazić, J., Jazvinšćak Jembrek, M., and Švob Štrac, D. (2005). Stimulation of 5-HT1A receptors increases the seizure threshold for picrotoxin in mice. *Eur. J. Pharmacol.* 527, 105–110. doi: 10.1016/j.ejphar.2005.10.021

Pericic, D., Lazic, J., Jazvinscak Jembrek, M., and Svob Strac, D. (2005). Stimulation of 5-HT 1A receptors increases the seizure threshold for picrotoxin in mice. *Eur. J. Pharmacol.* 527, 105–110. doi: 10.1016/j.ejphar.2005.10.021

Pericic, D., and Svob Strac, D. (2007). The role of 5-HT(7) receptors in the control of seizures. *Brain Res.* 1141, 48–55. doi: 10.1016/j.brainres.2007.01.019

Pernhorst, K., Van Loo, K. M., Von Lehe, M., Priebe, L., Cichon, S., Herms, S., et al. (2013). Rs6295 promoter variants of the serotonin type 1A receptor are differentially activated by c-Jun *in vitro* and correlate to transcript levels in human epileptic brain tissue. *Brain Res.* 1499, 136–144. doi: 10.1016/j.brainres.2012.12.045

Petkova, Z., Tchekalarova, J., Pechlivanova, D., Moyanova, S., Kortenska, L., Mitreva, R., et al. (2014). Treatment with melatonin after status epilepticus attenuates seizure activity and neuronal damage but does not prevent the disturbance in diurnal rhythms and behavioral alterations in spontaneously hypertensive rats in kainate model of temporal lobe epilepsy. *Epilepsy Behav.* 31, 198–208. doi: 10.1016/j.yebeh.2013.12.013

Pintor, M., Mefford, I. N., Hutter, I., Pocotte, S. L., Wyler, A. R., and Nadi, N. S. (1990). Levels of biogenic amines, their metabolites, and tyrosine hydroxylase activity in the human epileptic temporal cortex. *Synapse* 5, 152–156. doi: 10.1002/syn.890050210

Pirttimaki, T., Parri, H. R., and Crunelli, V. (2013). Astrocytic GABA transporter GAT-1 dysfunction in experimental absence seizures. *J. Physiol.* 591, 823–833. doi: 10.1113/jphysiol.2012.242016

Pisani, L., Catto, M., Leonetti, F., Nicolotti, O., Stefanachi, A., Campagna, F., et al. (2011). Targeting monoamine oxidases with multipotent ligands: an emerging strategy in the search of new drugs against neurodegenerative diseases. *Curr. Med. Chem.* 18, 4568–4587. doi: 10.2174/092986711797379302

Plotnikoff, N., Huang, J., and Havens, P. (1963). Effect of monoamino oxidase inhibitors on audiogenic seizures. *J. Pharm. Sci.* 52, 172–173. doi: 10.1002/jps.2600520217

Post, R. M. (1988). Time course of clinical effects of carbamazepine: implications for mechanisms of action. *J. Clin. Psychiatry* 49(Suppl.), 35–48.

Preskorn, S. H., and Fast, G. A. (1992). Tricyclic antidepressant-induced seizures and plasma drug concentration. *J. Clin. Psychiatry* 53, 160–162.

Quesseveur, G., Gardier, A. M., and Guiard, B. P. (2013). The monoaminergic tripartite synapse: a putative target for currently available antidepressant drugs. *Curr. Drug Targets* 14, 1277–1294. doi: 10.2174/13894501113149990209

Raedt, R., Clinckers, R., Mollet, L., Vonck, K., El Tahry, R., Wyckhuys, T., et al. (2011). Increased hippocampal noradrenaline is a biomarker for efficacy of vagus nerve stimulation in a limbic seizure model. *J. Neurochem.* 117, 461–469. doi: 10.1111/j.1471-4159.2011.07214.x

Rajkowska, G., and Stockmeier, C. A. (2013). Astrocyte pathology in major depressive disorder: insights from human postmortem brain tissue. *Curr. Drug Targets* 14, 1225–1236. doi: 10.2174/13894501113149990156

Ramsay, R. R. (2013). Inhibitor design for monoamine oxidases. *Curr. Pharm. Des.* 19, 2529–2539. doi: 10.2174/1381612811319140004

Rao, M. L., Stefan, H., and Bauer, J. (1989). Epileptic but not psychogenic seizures are accompanied by simultaneous elevation of serum pituitary hormones and cortisol levels. *Neuroendocrinology* 49, 33–39. doi: 10.1159/000125088

Rees, M. I. (2010). The genetics of epilepsy–the past, the present and future. *Seizure* 19, 680–683. doi: 10.1016/j.seizure.2010.10.029

Reiter, R. J., Tan, D. X., and Fuentes-Broto, L. (2010). Melatonin: a multitasking molecule. *Prog. Brain Res.* 181, 127–151. doi: 10.1016/S0079-6123(08)81008-4

Richards, D. A., Lemos, T., Whitton, P. S., and Bowery, N. G. (1995). Extracellular GABA in the ventrolateral thalamus of rats exhibiting spontaneous absence epilepsy: a microdialysis study. *J. Neurochem.* 65, 1674–1680. doi: 10.1046/j.1471-4159.1995.65041674.x

Richerson, G. B., and Buchanan, G. F. (2011). The serotonin axis: shared mechanisms in seizures, depression, and SUDEP. *Epilepsia* 52(Suppl. 1), 28–38. doi: 10.1111/j.1528-1167.2010.02908.x

Riederer, P., Danielczyk, W., and Grünblatt, E. (2004). Monoamine oxidase-B inhibition in Alzheimer's disease. *Neurotoxicology* 25, 271–277. doi: 10.1016/S0161-813X(03)00106-2

Rocha, L., Alonso-Vanegas, M., Orozco-Suárez, S., Alcantara-González, D., Cruzblanca, H., and Castro, E. (2014). Do certain signal transduction mechanisms explain the comorbidity of epilepsy and mood disorders? *Epilepsy Behav.* 38, 25–31. doi: 10.1016/j.yebeh.2014.01.001

Rocha, L., Alonso-Vanegas, M., Villeda-Hernández, J., Mújica, M., Cisneros-Franco, J. M., López-Gómez, M., et al. (2012). Dopamine abnormalities in the neocortex of patients with temporal lobe epilepsy. *Neurobiol. Dis.* 45, 499–507. doi: 10.1016/j.nbd.2011.09.006

Roth, B. L., Sheffler, D. J., and Kroeze, W. K. (2004). Magic shotguns versus magic bullets: selectively non-selective drugs for mood disorders and schizophrenia. *Nat. Rev. Drug Discov.* 3, 353–359. doi: 10.1038/nrd1346

Routledge, C., Bromidge, S. M., Moss, S. F., Price, G. W., Hirst, W., Newman, H., et al. (2000). Characterization of SB-271046: a potent, selective and orally active 5-HT(6) receptor antagonist. *Br. J. Pharmacol.* 130, 1606–1612. doi: 10.1038/sj.bjp.0703457

Rubinstein, M., Cepeda, C., Hurst, R. S., Flores-Hernandez, J., Ariano, M. A., Falzone, T. L., et al. (2001). Dopamine D4 receptor-deficient mice display cortical hyperexcitability. *J. Neurosci.* 21, 3756–3763.

Sadek, B., Kuder, K., Subramanian, D., Shafiullah, M., Stark, H., Lazewska, D., et al. (2014). Anticonvulsive effect of nonimidazole histamine H3 receptor antagonists. *Behav. Pharmacol.* 25, 245–252. doi: 10.1097/FBP.0000000000000042

Saelens, D. A., Walle, T., Gaffney, T. E., and Privitera, P. J. (1977). Studies on the contribution of active metabolites to the anticonvulsant effects of propranolol. *Eur. J. Pharmacol.* 42, 39–46. doi: 10.1016/0014-2999(77)90188-1

Salgado, D., and Alkadhi, K. A. (1995). Inhibition of epileptiform activity by serotonin in rat CA1 neurons. *Brain Res.* 669, 176–182. doi: 10.1016/0006-8993(94)01235-A

Salgado-Commissariat, D., and Alkadhi, K. A. (1997). Serotonin inhibits epileptiform discharge by activation of 5-HT1A receptors in CA1 pyramidal neurons. *Neuropharmacology* 36, 1705–1712. doi: 10.1016/S0028-3908(97)00134-2

Salzmann, A., and Malafosse, A. (2012). Genetics of temporal lobe epilepsy: a review. *Epilepsy Res. Treat.* 2012:863702. doi: 10.1155/2012/863702

Samochowiec, J., Smolka, M., Winterer, G., Rommelspacher, H., Schmidt, L. G., and Sander, T. (1999). Association analysis between a Cys23Ser substitution polymorphism of the human 5-HT2c receptor gene and neuronal hyperexcitability. *Am. J. Med. Genet.* 88, 126–130. doi: 10.1002/(SICI)1096-8628(19990416)88:2<126::AID-AJMG6>3.0.CO;2-M

Sanden, N., Thorlin, T., Blomstrand, F., Persson, P. A. I., and Hansson, E. (2000). 5-Hydroxytryptamine(2B) receptors stimulate Ca2+ increases in cultured astrocytes from three different brain regions. *Neurochem. Int.* 36, 427–434. doi: 10.1016/S0197-0186(99)00134-5

Sander, T., Berlin, W., Ostapowicz, A., Samochowiec, J., Gscheidel, N., and Hoehe, M. R. (2000). Variation of the genes encoding the human glutamate EAAT2, serotonin and dopamine transporters and susceptibility to idiopathic generalized epilepsy. *Epilepsy Res.* 41, 75–81. doi: 10.1016/S0920-1211(00)00120-0

Sander, T., Harms, H., Podschus, J., Finckh, U., Nickel, B., Rolfs, A., et al. (1997). Allelic association of a dopamine transporter gene polymorphism in alcohol dependence with withdrawal seizures or delirium. *Biol. Psychiatry* 41, 299–304. doi: 10.1016/S0006-3223(96)00044-3

Sansone, R. A., and Sansone, L. A. (2011). Agomelatine: a novel antidepressant. *Innov. Clin. Neurosci.* 8, 10–14.

Sarnyai, Z., Sibille, E. L., Pavlides, C., Fenster, R. J., McEwen, B. S., and Toth, M. (2000). Impaired hippocampal-dependent learning and functional abnormalities in the hippocampus in mice lacking serotonin(1A) receptors. *Proc. Natl. Acad. Sci. U.S.A.* 97, 14731–14736. doi: 10.1073/pnas.97.26.14731

Schafer, D. P., Lehrman, E. K., and Stevens, B. (2013). The "quad-partite" synapse: microglia-synapse interactions in the developing and mature CNS. *Glia* 61, 24–36. doi: 10.1002/glia.22389

Scharfman, H. E. (2007). The neurobiology of epilepsy. *Curr. Neurol. Neurosci. Rep.* 7, 348–354. doi: 10.1007/s11910-007-0053-z

Schenkel, L. C., Bragatti, J. A., Torres, C. M., Martin, K. C., Gus-Manfro, G., Leistner-Segal, S., et al. (2011). Serotonin transporter gene (5HTT) polymorphisms and temporal lobe epilepsy. *Epilepsy Res.* 95, 152–157. doi: 10.1016/j.eplepsyres.2011.03.013

Schipke, C. G., Heuser, I., and Peters, O. (2011). Antidepressants act on glial cells: SSRIs and serotonin elicit astrocyte calcium signaling in the mouse prefrontal cortex. *J. Psychiatr. Res.* 45, 242–248. doi: 10.1016/j.jpsychires.2010.06.005

Schwartz, J. C., Arrang, J. M., Garbarg, M., Pollard, H., and Ruat, M. (1991). Histaminergic transmission in the mammalian brain. *Physiol. Rev.* 71, 1–51.

Semenova, T. P., and Ticku, M. K. (1992). Effects of 5-HT receptor antagonists on seizure susceptibility and locomotor activity in DBA/2 mice. *Brain Res.* 588, 229–236. doi: 10.1016/0006-8993(92)91580-8

Shishkina, G. T., Kalinina, T. S., and Dygalo, N. N. (2012). Effects of swim stress and fluoxetine on 5-HT1A receptor gene expression and monoamine metabolism in the rat brain regions. *Cell. Mol. Neurobiol.* 32, 787–794. doi: 10.1007/s10571-012-9828-0

Skolnick, P., Krieter, P., Tizzano, J., Basile, A., Popik, P., Czobor, P., et al. (2006). Preclinical and clinical pharmacology of DOV 216,303, a "triple" reuptake inhibitor. *CNS Drug Rev.* 12, 123–134. doi: 10.1111/j.1527-3458.2006.00123.x

Solmaz, I., Gürkanlar, D., Gökçil, Z., Göksoy, C., Ozkan, M., and Erdogan, E. (2009). Antiepileptic activity of melatonin in guinea pigs with pentylenetetrazol-induced seizures. *Neurol. Res.* 31, 989–995. doi: 10.1179/174313209X385545

Sourbron, J., Schneider, H., Kecskés, A., Liu, Y., Buening, E. M., Lagae, L., et al. (2016). Serotonergic modulation as effective treatment for dravet syndrome in a zebrafish mutant model. *ACS Chem. Neurosci.* 7, 588–598. doi: 10.1021/acschemneuro.5b00342

Sparks, D. L., and Buckholtz, N. S. (1985). Combined inhibition of serotonin uptake and oxidative deamination attenuates audiogenic seizures in DBA/2J mice. *Pharmacol. Biochem. Behav.* 23, 753–757. doi: 10.1016/0091-3057(85)90067-X

Starr, M. S. (1996). The role of dopamine in epilepsy. *Synapse* 22, 159–194. doi: 10.1002/(SICI)1098-2396(199602)22:2<159::AID-SYN8>3.0.CO;2-C

Statnick, M. A., Dailey, J. W., Jobe, P. C., and Browning, R. A. (1996). Abnormalities in brain serotonin concentration, high-affinity uptake, and tryptophan hydroxylase activity in severe-seizure genetically epilepsy-prone rats. *Epilepsia* 37, 311–321. doi: 10.1111/j.1528-1157.1996.tb00565.x

Stean, T. O., Hirst, W. D., Thomas, D. R., Price, G. W., Rogers, D., Riley, G., et al. (2002). Pharmacological profile of SB-357134: a potent, selective, brain penetrant, and orally active 5-HT(6) receptor antagonist. *Pharmacol. Biochem. Behav.* 71, 645–654. doi: 10.1016/S0091-3057(01)00742-0

Stefulj, J., Bordukalo-Niksic, T., Hecimovic, H., Demarin, V., and Jernej, B. (2010). Epilepsy and serotonin (5HT): variations of 5HT-related genes in temporal lobe epilepsy. *Neurosci. Lett.* 478, 29–31. doi: 10.1016/j.neulet.2010.04.060

Szabó, C. Á., Patel, M., and Uteshev, V. V. (2015). Cerebrospinal fluid levels of monoamine metabolites in the epileptic baboon. *J. Primatol.* 4:129. doi: 10.4172/2167-6801.1000129

Szot, P., Lester, M., Laughlin, M. L., Palmiter, R. D., Liles, L. C., and Weinshenker, D. (2004). The anticonvulsant and proconvulsant effects of alpha2-adrenoreceptor agonists are mediated by distinct populations of alpha2A-adrenoreceptors. *Neuroscience* 126, 795–803. doi: 10.1016/j.neuroscience.2004.04.030

Szyndler, J., Wierzba-Bobrowicz, T., Skórzewska, A., Maciejak, P., Walkowiak, J., Lechowicz, W., et al. (2005). Behavioral, biochemical and histological studies in a model of pilocarpine-induced spontaneous recurrent seizures. *Pharmacol. Biochem. Behav.* 81, 15–23. doi: 10.1016/j.pbb.2005.01.020

Takano, T., Sakaue, Y., Sokoda, T., Sawai, C., Akabori, S., Maruo, Y., et al. (2010). Seizure susceptibility due to antihistamines in febrile seizures. *Pediatr. Neurol.* 42, 277–279. doi: 10.1016/j.pediatrneurol.2009.11.001

Tan, N. C., and Berkovic, S. F. (2010). The Epilepsy Genetic Association Database (epiGAD): analysis of 165 genetic association studies, 1996-2008. *Epilepsia* 51, 686–689. doi: 10.1111/j.1528-1167.2009.02423.x

Tanaka, K., Watase, K., Manabe, T., Yamada, K., Watanabe, M., Takahashi, K., et al. (1997). Epilepsy and exacerbation of brain injury in mice lacking the glutamate transporter GLT-1. *Science* 276, 1699–1702. doi: 10.1126/science.276.5319.1699

Tchekalarova, J., Loyens, E., and Smolders, I. (2015a). Effects of AT1 receptor antagonism on kainate-induced seizures and concomitant changes in hippocampal extracellular noradrenaline, serotonin, and dopamine levels in Wistar-Kyoto and spontaneously hypertensive rats. *Epilepsy Behav.* 46, 66–71. doi: 10.1016/j.yebeh.2015.03.021

Tchekalarova, J., Moyanova, S., Fusco, A. D., and Ngomba, R. T. (2015b). The role of the melatoninergic system in epilepsy and comorbid psychiatric disorders. *Brain Res. Bull.* 119, 80–92. doi: 10.1016/j.brainresbull.2015.08.006

Tchekalarova, J., Pechlivanova, D., Atanasova, T., Markova, P., Lozanov, V., and Stoynev, A. (2011). Diurnal variations in depression-like behavior of Wistar and spontaneously hypertensive rats in the kainate model of temporal lobe epilepsy. *Epilepsy Behav.* 20, 277–285. doi: 10.1016/j.yebeh.2010.12.021

Tecott, L. H., Sun, L. M., Akana, S. F., Strack, A. M., Lowenstein, D. H., Dallman, M. F., et al. (1995). Eating disorder and epilepsy in mice lacking 5-HT2c serotonin receptors. *Nature* 374, 542–546. doi: 10.1038/374542a0

Theodore, W. H. (2003). Does serotonin play a role in epilepsy? *Epilepsy Curr.* 3, 173–177. doi: 10.1046/j.1535-7597.2003.03508.x

Theodore, W. H., Martinez, A. R., Khan, O. I., Liew, C. J., Auh, S., Dustin, I. M., et al. (2012). PET of serotonin 1A receptors and cerebral glucose metabolism for temporal lobectomy. *J. Nucl. Med.* 53, 1375–1382. doi: 10.2967/jnumed.112.103093

Tokarski, K., Zahorodna, A., Bobula, B., and Hess, G. (2002). Comparison of the effects of 5-HT1A and 5-HT4 receptor activation on field potentials and epileptiform activity in rat hippocampus. *Exp. Brain Res.* 147, 505–510. doi: 10.1007/s00221-002-1259-6

Tripathi, P. P., and Bozzi, Y. (2015). The role of dopaminergic and serotonergic systems in neurodevelopmental disorders: a focus on epilepsy and seizure susceptibility. *Bioimpacts* 5, 97–102. doi: 10.15171/bi.2015.07

Tripathi, P. P., Santorufo, G., Brilli, E., Borrelli, E., and Bozzi, Y. (2010). Kainic acid-induced seizures activate GSK-3beta in the hippocampus of D2R−/− mice. *Neuroreport* 21, 846–850. doi: 10.1097/WNR.0b013e32833d5891

Tuomisto, L., and Tacke, U. (1986). Is histamine an anticonvulsive inhibitory transmitter? *Neuropharmacology* 25, 955–958. doi: 10.1016/0028-3908(86)90029-8

Tuomisto, L., Tacke, U., and Willman, A. (1987). Inhibition of sound-induced convulsions by metoprine in the audiogenic seizure susceptible rat. *Agents Actions* 20, 252–254. doi: 10.1007/BF02074683

Tzschach, A., Chen, W., Erdogan, F., Hoeller, A., Ropers, H. H., Castellan, C., et al. (2008). Characterization of interstitial Xp duplications in two families by tiling path array CGH. *Am. J. Med. Genet. A* 146A, 197–203. doi: 10.1002/ajmg.a.32070

Unzeta, M., Esteban, G., Bolea, I., Fogel, W. A., Ramsay, R. R., Youdim, M. B., et al. (2016). Multi-Target Directed Donepezil-Like Ligands for Alzheimer's Disease. *Front. Neurosci.* 10:205. doi: 10.3389/fnins.2016.00205

Upton, N., Stean, T., Middlemiss, D., Blackburn, T., and Kennett, G. (1998). Studies on the role of 5-HT2C and 5-HT2B receptors in regulating generalised seizure threshold in rodents. *Eur. J. Pharmacol.* 359, 33–40. doi: 10.1016/S0014-2999(98)00621-9

van Gelder, N. M., and Sherwin, A. L. (2003). Metabolic parameters of epilepsy: adjuncts to established antiepileptic drug therapy. *Neurochem. Res.* 28, 353–365. doi: 10.1023/A:1022433421761

Van Liefferinge, J., Massie, A., Portelli, J., Di Giovanni, G., and Smolders, I. (2013). Are vesicular neurotransmitter transporters potential treatment targets for temporal lobe epilepsy? *Front. Cell. Neurosci.* 7:139. doi: 10.3389/fncel.2013.00139

Venzi, M., David, F., Bellet, J., Cavaccini, A., Bombardi, C., Crunelli, V., et al. (2016). Role for serotonin2A (5-HT2A) and 2C (5-HT2C) receptors in experimental absence seizures. *Neuropharmacology* 108, 292–304. doi: 10.1016/j.neuropharm.2016.04.016

Verkhratsky, A., and Kettenmann, H. (1996). Calcium signalling in glial cells. *Trends Neurosci.* 19, 346–352. doi: 10.1016/0166-2236(96)10048-5

Voutsinos, B., Dutuit, M., Reboul, A., Fevre-Montange, M., Bernard, A., Trouillas, P., et al. (1998). Serotoninergic control of the activity and expression of glial GABA transporters in the rat cerebellum. *Glia* 23, 45–60. doi: 10.1002/(SICI)1098-1136(199805)23:1<45::AID-GLIA5>3.0.CO;2-3

Wada, Y., Shiraishi, J., Nakamura, M., and Koshino, Y. (1997). Effects of the 5-HT3 receptor agonist 1-(m-chlorophenyl)-biguanide in the rat kindling model of epilepsy. *Brain Res.* 759, 313–316. doi: 10.1016/S0006-8993(97)00366-1

Wang, L., Lv, Y., Deng, W., Peng, X., Xiao, Z., Xi, Z., et al. (2015). 5-HT6 receptor recruitment of mTOR modulates seizure activity in epilepsy. *Mol. Neurobiol.* 51, 1292–1299. doi: 10.1007/s12035-014-8806-6

Watanabe, K., Minabe, Y., Ashby, C. R. Jr., and Katsumori, H. (1998). Effect of acute administration of various 5-HT receptor agonists on focal hippocampal seizures in freely moving rats. *Eur. J. Pharmacol.* 350, 181–188. doi: 10.1016/S0014-2999(98)00255-6

Weinshenker, D., Szot, P., Miller, N. S., and Palmiter, R. D. (2001a). Alpha(1) and beta(2) adrenoreceptor agonists inhibit pentylenetetrazole-induced seizures in mice lacking norepinephrine. *J. Pharmacol. Exp. Ther.* 298, 1042–1048.

Weinshenker, D., Szot, P., Miller, N. S., Rust, N. C., Hohmann, J. G., Pyati, U., et al. (2001b). Genetic comparison of seizure control by norepinephrine and neuropeptide Y. *J. Neurosci.* 21, 7764–7769.

Weiss, G. K., Lewis, J., Jimenez-Rivera, C., Vigil, A., and Corcoran, M. E. (1990). Antikindling effects of locus coeruleus stimulation: mediation by ascending noradrenergic projections. *Exp. Neurol.* 108, 136–140. doi: 10.1016/0014-4886(90)90020-S

Weng, Z., Zheng, Y., and Li, J. (2015). Synthesis, antidepressant activity, and toxicity of the erythro/threo racemates and optical isomers of 2-(4-benzylpiperazin-1-yl)-1-(5-chloro-6-methoxynaphthalen-2-yl)hexan-1-ol. *Chem. Biol. Drug Design* 85, 454–460. doi: 10.1111/cbdd.12438

Wesolowska, A., Nikiforuk, A., and Chojnacka-Wójcik, E. (2006). Anticonvulsant effect of the selective 5-HT1B receptor agonist CP 94253 in mice. *Eur. J. Pharmacol.* 541, 57–63. doi: 10.1016/j.ejphar.2006.04.049

Whibley, A., Urquhart, J., Dore, J., Willatt, L., Parkin, G., Gaunt, L., et al. (2010). Deletion of MAOA and MAOB in a male patient causes severe developmental delay, intermittent hypotonia and stereotypical hand movements. *Eur. J. Hum. Genet.* 18, 1095–1099. doi: 10.1038/ejhg.2010.41

Witkin, J. M., Baez, M., Yu, J., Barton, M. E., and Shannon, H. E. (2007). Constitutive deletion of the serotonin-7 (5-HT(7)) receptor decreases electrical and chemical seizure thresholds. *Epilepsy Res.* 75, 39–45. doi: 10.1016/j.eplepsyres.2007.03.017

Witkin, J. M., Levant, B., Zapata, A., Kaminski, R., and Gasior, M. (2008). The dopamine D3/D2 agonist (+)-PD-128,907 [(R-(+)-trans-3,4a,10b-tetrahydro-4-propyl-2H,5H-[1]benzopyrano[4,3-b]-1,4-oxazin -9-ol)] protects against acute and cocaine-kindled seizures in mice: further evidence for the involvement of D3 receptors. *J. Pharmacol. Exp. Ther.* 326, 930–938. doi: 10.1124/jpet.108.139212

Yagüe, J. G., Cavaccini, A., Errington, A. C., Crunelli, V., and Di Giovanni, G. (2013). Dopaminergic modulation of tonic but not phasic GABA(A)-receptor-mediated current in the ventrobasal thalamus of Wistar and GAERS rats. *Exp. Neurol.* 247, 1–7. doi: 10.1016/j.expneurol.2013.03.023

Yan, Q. S., Dailey, J. W., Steenbergen, J. L., and Jobe, P. C. (1998). Anticonvulsant effect of enhancement of noradrenergic transmission in the superior colliculus in genetically epilepsy-prone rats (GEPRs): a microinjection study. *Brain Res.* 780, 199–209. doi: 10.1016/S0006-8993(97)01139-6

Yan, Q. S., Jobe, P. C., and Dailey, J. W. (1993). Thalamic deficiency in norepinephrine release detected via intracerebral microdialysis: a synaptic determinant of seizure predisposition in the genetically epilepsy-prone rat. *Epilepsy Res.* 14, 229–236. doi: 10.1016/0920-1211(93)90047-B

Yan, Q. S., Mishra, P. K., Burger, R. L., Bettendorf, A. F., Jobe, P. C., and Dailey, J. W. (1992). Evidence that carbamazepine and antiepilepsirine may produce a component of their anticonvulsant effects by activating serotonergic neurons in genetically epilepsy-prone rats. *J. Pharmacol. Exp. Ther.* 261, 652–659.

Yang, K., Su, J., Hu, Z., Lang, R., Sun, X., Li, X., et al. (2013). Serotonin transporter (5-HTT) gene polymorphisms and susceptibility to epilepsy: a meta-analysis and meta-regression. *Genet. Test. Mol. Biomarkers* 17, 890–897. doi: 10.1089/gtmb.2013.0341

Yang, Y., Guo, Y., Kuang, Y., Wang, S., Jiang, Y., Ding, Y., et al. (2014). Serotonin 1A receptor inhibits the status epilepticus induced by lithium-pilocarpine in rats. *Neurosci. Bull.* 30, 401–408. doi: 10.1007/s12264-013-1396-x

Yang, Z., Liu, X., Yin, Y., Sun, S., and Deng, X. (2012). Involvement of 5-HT(7) receptors in the pathogenesis of temporal lobe epilepsy. *Eur. J. Pharmacol.* 685, 52–58. doi: 10.1016/j.ejphar.2012.04.011

Yawata, I., Tanaka, K., Nakagawa, Y., Watanabe, Y., Murashima, Y. L., and Nakano, K. (2004). Role of histaminergic neurons in development of epileptic seizures in EL mice. *Brain Res. Mol. Brain Res.* 132, 13–17. doi: 10.1016/j.molbrainres.2004.08.019

Yokoyama, H., Iinuma, K., Yanai, K., Watanabe, T., Sakurai, E., and Onodera, K. (1993). Proconvulsant effect of ketotifen, a histamine H1 antagonist, confirmed by the use of d-chlorpheniramine with monitoring electroencephalography. *Methods Find. Exp. Clin. Pharmacol.* 15, 183–188.

Youdim, M., Finberg, J., and Tipton, K. (1988). "Monoamine Oxidase," in *Handbook of Experimental Pharmacology*, eds U. Tredelenburg and N. Weiner (Berlin: Springer-Verlag), 119–192.

Youdim, M. B. (2003). Rasagiline: an anti-Parkinson drug with neuroprotective activity. *Expert Rev. Neurother.* 3, 737–749. doi: 10.1586/14737175.3.6.737

Youdim, M. B. H., Edmondson, D., and Tipton, K. F. (2006). The therapeutic potential of monoamine oxidase inhibitors. *Nat. Rev. Neurosci.* 7, 295–309. doi: 10.1038/nrn1883

Zhu, C. B., Lindler, K. M., Owens, A. W., Daws, L. C., Blakely, R. D., and Hewlett, W. A. (2010). Interleukin-1 receptor activation by systemic lipopolysaccharide induces behavioral despair linked to MAPK regulation of CNS serotonin transporters. *Neuropsychopharmacology* 35, 2510–2520. doi: 10.1038/npp.2010.116

Zolaly, M. A. (2012). Histamine H1 antagonists and clinical characteristics of febrile seizures. *Int. J. Gen. Med.* 5, 277–281. doi: 10.2147/IJGM.S29320

Conflict of Interest Statement: The authors declare that the research was conducted in the absence of any commercial or financial relationships that could be construed as a potential conflict of interest.

4

Monoaminergic and Histaminergic Strategies and Treatments in Brain Diseases

Giuseppe Di Giovanni [1], Dubravka Svob Strac [2], Montse Sole [3], Mercedes Unzeta [3], Keith F. Tipton [4], Dorotea Mück-Šeler [2], Irene Bolea [3], Laura Della Corte [5], Matea Nikolac Perkovic [2], Nela Pivac [2], Ilse J. Smolders [6], Anna Stasiak [7], Wieslawa A. Fogel [7] and Philippe De Deurwaerdère [8]*

[1] Department of Physiology and Biochemistry, University of Malta, Msida, Malta, [2] Division of Molecular Medicine, Rudjer Boskovic Institute, Zagreb, Croatia, [3] Departament de Bioquímica i Biologia Molecular, Facultat de Medicina, Institut de Neurociències, Universitat Autònoma de Barcelona, Barcelona, Spain, [4] School of Biochemistry and Immunology, Trinity College Dublin, Dublin, Ireland, [5] Department of Neuroscience, University of Florence, Florence, Italy, [6] Department of Pharmaceutical Chemistry and Drug Analysis, Vrije Universiteit Brussel, Brussels, Belgium, [7] Department of Hormone Biochemistry, Medical University of Lodz, Lodz, Poland, [8] Centre National de la Recherche Scientifique (Unité Mixte de Recherche 5293), Institut of Neurodegenerative Diseases, Bordeaux Cedex, France

Edited by:
Arjan Blokland,
Maastricht University, Netherlands

Reviewed by:
Grzegorz Kreiner,
Polish Academy of Sciences, Poland
John Finberg,
Technion – Israel Institute of Technology, Israel

*Correspondence:
Philippe De Deurwaerdère
deurwaer@u-bordeaux.fr

The monoaminergic systems are the target of several drugs for the treatment of mood, motor and cognitive disorders as well as neurological conditions. In most cases, advances have occurred through serendipity, except for Parkinson's disease where the pathophysiology led almost immediately to the introduction of dopamine restoring agents. Extensive neuropharmacological studies first showed that the primary target of antipsychotics, antidepressants, and anxiolytic drugs were specific components of the monoaminergic systems. Later, some dramatic side effects associated with older medicines were shown to disappear with new chemical compounds targeting the origin of the therapeutic benefit more specifically. The increased knowledge regarding the function and interaction of the monoaminergic systems in the brain resulting from in vivo neurochemical and neurophysiological studies indicated new monoaminergic targets that could achieve the efficacy of the older medicines with fewer side-effects. Yet, this accumulated knowledge regarding monoamines did not produce valuable strategies for diseases where no monoaminergic drug has been shown to be effective. Here, we emphasize the new therapeutic and monoaminergic-based strategies for the treatment of psychiatric diseases. We will consider three main groups of diseases, based on the evidence of monoamines involvement (schizophrenia, depression, obesity), the identification of monoamines in the diseases processes (Parkinson's disease, addiction) and the prospect of the involvement of monoaminergic mechanisms (epilepsy, Alzheimer's disease, stroke). In most cases, the clinically available monoaminergic drugs induce widespread modifications of amine tone or excitability through neurobiological networks and exemplify the overlap between therapeutic approaches to psychiatric and neurological conditions. More recent developments that have resulted in improved drug specificity and responses will be discussed in this review.

Keywords: antipsychotic, antidepressant, monoamine oxidase inhibitor, multi-target pharmacology, neurodegenerative diseases, stroke, antiparkinsonian treatments, drug addiction

INTRODUCTION

Monoaminergic systems are important cellular targets in a variety of neuropsychiatric and neurological conditions. Improved knowledge of these systems, in terms of function and molecular organization, has confirmed their roles in the efficacy of older medications. Medicinal chemistry has detected some newer compounds that affect identified molecular targets and additional monoaminergic targets are still being investigated. Although monoaminergic systems have a pivotal role in the effect of many existing medicines, there is a need for further developments, as additional targets have been identified that could be as interesting as monoamines (Millan et al., 2015b).

Monoaminergic systems, involving dopamine (DA), serotonin (5-HT), noradrenaline (NA) and histamine are involved in virtually all cerebral functions and modification of their activity has been identified in most, if not all, neuropsychiatric and neurological diseases. Some of these diseases, including schizophrenia, depression and Parkinson's disease (PD) benefit from monoaminergic-based treatments, but there is still scope for therapeutic improvement. In spite of clear monoaminergic disturbances in other devastating diseases, including Alzheimer's disease, addiction and epilepsy, no approved monoamine-based treatments are yet available. The discovery of the most pertinent drugs in numerous psychiatric diseases was serendipitous while the causal implication of monoaminergic systems in several diseases is still unclear. In this context, the identification of drug targets as well as more detailed neuropharmacological analysis should allow for the improvement of existing drugs.

The complexity of the organization of monoaminergic systems in the brain limits the likelihood of drugs acting on a single target to correct a disease selectively, although recent examples suggest that this strategy might be worth continuing (Meltzer and Roth, 2013). Moreover, specific targets for a neurotransmitter are often distributed in numerous neurobiological circuits so that a selective compound may produce a plethora of distinct effects, some of which may be undesirable. Such a situation may occur in the treatment of diseases like schizophrenia where the use of DA receptor antagonists is associated with undesirable side effects, as discussed below. The complexity of these circuits may lead to the proposed use of either agonists or antagonists for correcting the same diseases (Di Giovanni and De Deurwaerdère, 2016). There is a growing body of evidence demonstrating that most neuropsychiatric disorders are multifactorial and that an action on a single target is elusive both in terms of

symptomatic and curative treatments (Millan et al., 2015a,b). Increased understanding of the mechanisms involved in such diseases led to the use of combinations of drugs targeting distinct receptors/enzymes or to the development of multi-target drugs. Finally, it is clear that the action on one target of one monoaminergic system will have repercussion on the activity of the other systems, which can affect the efficacy of medicines and may also introduce unwanted side-effects.

Therapeutic approaches that target monoaminergic systems are completely different and depend on the disease. The aim of this review is to present the development of new chemical compounds and therapeutic strategies aimed at modulating monoaminergic function in various brain disorders. We used the angle depicted in **Figure 1** arbitrarily categorizing three groups of diseases. Thus, after briefly presenting the physiology of the four main monoamine systems in the brain, this review will summarize past and current developments in the treatment of neuropsychiatric diseases that have monoaminergic-based medication (schizophrenia, depression, obesity) without a clear pathophysiological picture. Thereafter, we will present therapeutic strategies for brain diseases where the cause of the disease has been identified but with distinct success regarding the treatments and their amelioration (PD, drug addiction). The review will finish by presenting some strategies aimed at ameliorating the symptoms of brain diseases that still do not benefit from monoaminergic-based treatments in spite of the numerous evidence that it could be beneficial (epilepsy, AD, and ischemic stroke). The choice has been also driven by the involvement of the various researchers in the COST action CM1103, which was dedicated to drug design in the field of monoamines. The overall picture should give a clearer indication of the neuropharmacological significance of targeting monoaminergic systems in neuropsychiatric diseases and the need for future research.

MONOAMINERGIC SYSTEMS IN THE BRAIN

Pathways of monoaminergic systems project from the brainstem to different brain areas and the spinal cord, and they include dopaminergic neurons, located in the ventral tegmental area (VTA) and the substantia nigra pars compacta (SNc), noradrenergic neurons, arising from locus coeruleus (LC), serotonergic neurons, originating from median and dorsal raphe nuclei (Hale and Lowry, 2011) and histaminergic neurons arriving from tuberomamillary nucleus of the hypothalamus (Taylor, 1975). **Figure 2** illustrates approximately the, still limited, knowledge of the pharmacological and biochemical identities for each of these systems. DA is a catecholamine synthesized by the enzyme tyrosine hydroxylase (TH), which catalyzes the conversion of the amino acid L-tyrosine to L-3,4-dihydroxyphenylalanine (L-DOPA), and by the aromatic L-amino acid decarboxylase (AADC) which converts L-DOPA into DA (Cooper et al., 2003). DA can be metabolized by dopamine β-hydroxylase (DBH) into NA. DBH is mainly present in vesicles and can be found in the cytosol (Gagnon et al., 1976). 5-HT is

Abbreviations: COMT, catechol-O-methyl transferase; DA, dopamine; 5-HT, serotonin; NA, noradrenaline; MAO, monoamine oxidase; MAO-I, monoamine oxidase inhibitor; SSRI, selective serotonin reuptake inhibitor; SNRI, serotonin noradrenaline reuptake inhibitor; AD, Alzheimer's disease; PD, Parkinson's disease; VTA, ventral tegmental area; SNc, substantia nigra pars compacta; LC, locus coeruleus; L-DOPA, L-3,4-dihydroxyphenylalanine; AADC, aromatic L-amino acid decarboxylase; DBH, dopamine β-hydroxylase; TPH, tryptophan hydroxylase; VMAT2, vesicular monoamine transporter; SERT, 5-HT transporter; DAT, DA transporter; NET, NA transporter; OCT, organic cation transporters; PMAT, plasma membrane monoamine transporter; EPS, extrapyramidal side-effects; TCA, tricyclic antidepressant; AChEI, acetylcholinesterase inhibitor; VAP-1, vascular adhesion protein 1.

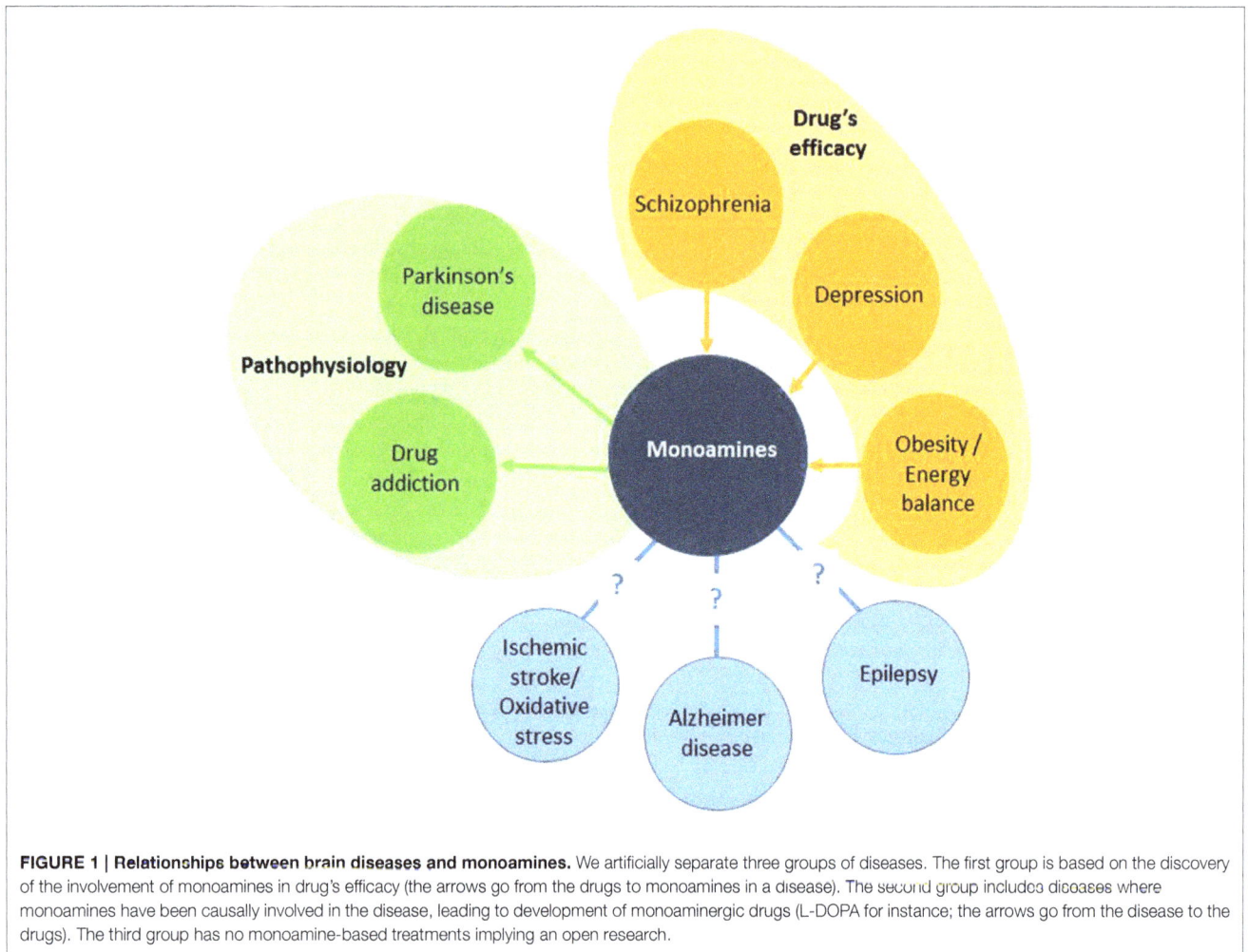

FIGURE 1 | Relationships between brain diseases and monoamines. We artificially separate three groups of diseases. The first group is based on the discovery of the involvement of monoamines in drug's efficacy (the arrows go from the drugs to monoamines in a disease). The second group includes diseases where monoamines have been causally involved in the disease, leading to development of monoaminergic drugs (L-DOPA for instance; the arrows go from the disease to the drugs). The third group has no monoamine-based treatments implying an open research.

produced from L-tryptophan by tryptophan hydroxylase (TPH) and AADC. Unlike in the case of the catecholamines and 5-HT, the decarboxylase involved in the synthesis of histamine is L-histidine decarboxylase (Taylor, 1975).

The degradation of biogenic amines is a complex mechanism that is not fully understood because it involves several enzymes and cell types. The monoamine oxidases (MAO) are a family of flavin adenine dinucleotide (FAD)-containing enzymes that catalyze the oxidative deamination of primary, secondary or tertiary amines. They produce hydrogen peroxide, ammonia and the corresponding aldehyde. There are two isoforms of MAO present in mammals: MAO-A and MAO-B, which share approximately 70% sequence identity and are encoded by separate genes located on the X chromosome (Youdim et al., 2006). The anatomical distribution of MAO isoforms in human brains was confirmed by positron-emission topography (PET) using intravenous ^{11}C-labeled irreversible inhibitors (Fowler et al., 1987). Autoradiographic and *in situ* hybridization studies have revealed that histaminergic and serotonergic neurons as well as astrocytes are rich in MAO-B whereas catecholaminergic neurons mainly contain MAO-A (Saura et al., 1992, 1996). DA, NA and 5-HT can be degraded

by MAO-A (Youdim et al., 2006; Finberg, 2014). The aldehyde derivatives, which are more toxic than the parent compounds, are catabolized by aldehyde dehydrogenase/reductase (Eisenhofer et al., 2004). MAO-B is involved in the glial metabolism of catecholamines and can affect the metabolism of biogenic amines in diverse conditions including PD (Youdim et al., 2006; Riederer and Laux, 2011). It is also involved in the metabolism of other amines, including 2-phenylethylamine and N(tele)-methylhistamine.

Catechol-O-methyltransferase (COMT) can also metabolize DA and NA (Eisenhofer et al., 2004). Two isoforms have been described (soluble COMT, S-COMT; membrane-bound COMT, MB-COMT) having different subcellular compartmentation. In the brain, S-COMT is found in the cytosol of glial cells, whereas MB-COMT is bound to the endoplasmic reticulum and present in neurons. MB-COMT mainly inactivates catecholamines and derivatives originating from DA and NA neurotransmission, whereas S-COMT preferentially transforms exogenous catecholamines (Myohanen et al., 2010; Tammimäki et al., 2010). COMT is not present in DA terminals (Schendzielorz et al., 2013), implying that glial cells or other neurons reuptake extracellular DA in tissues where the clearance

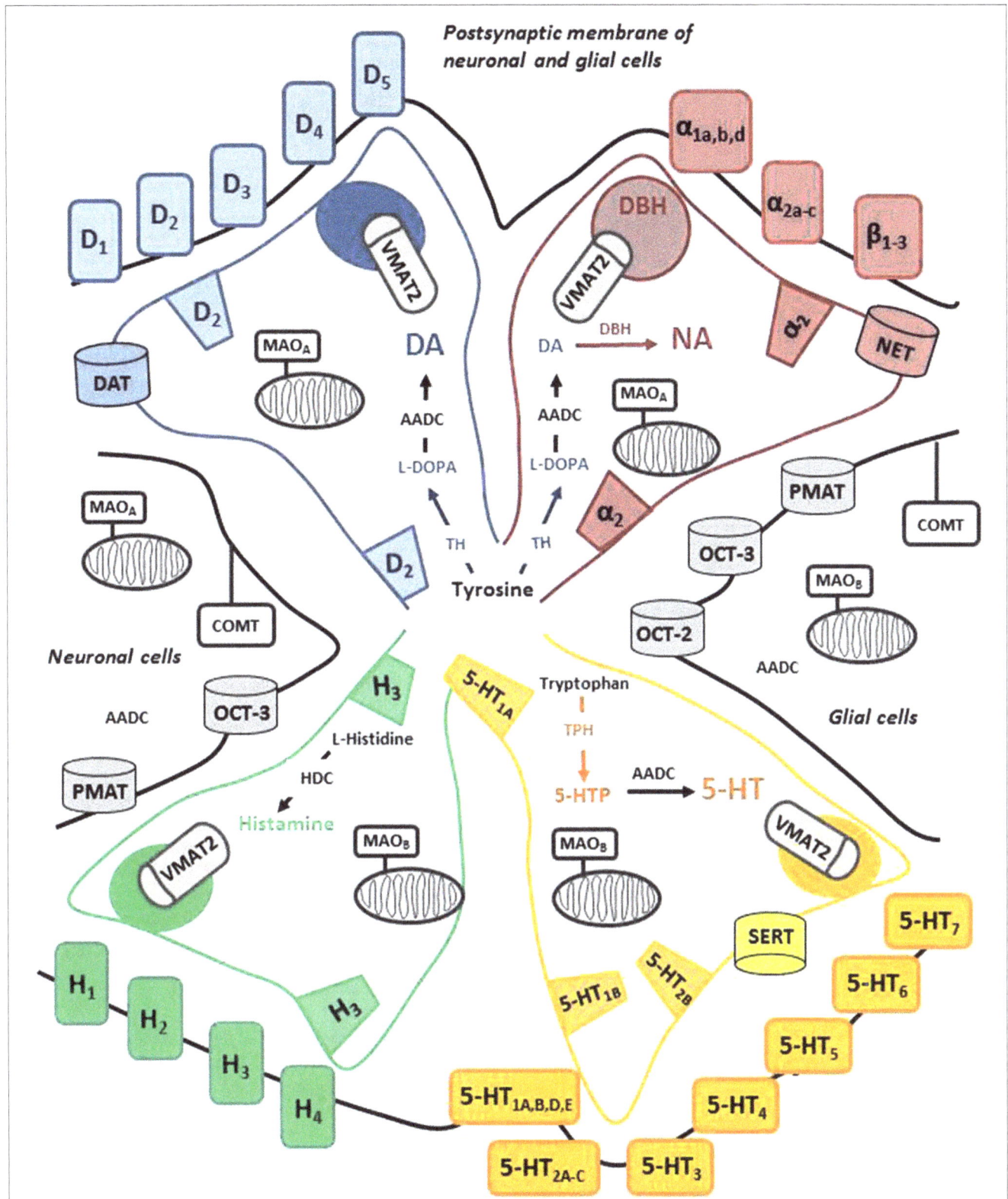

FIGURE 2 | Cellular and molecular organization of central monoaminergic systems. The figure depicts each monoamine system (dopamine, DA; noradrenaline, NA; serotonin, 5-HT; histamine) the biosynthesis, metabolism, the receptors and transporters. The color is used to identify the proteins that are selective for each system while the black color is used for non-specific proteins. The terminals of each monoaminergic neurons contact post-synaptic elements that express a variety of receptors which are more or less specific for each monoamine. Autoreceptors can be located at terminals and cell bodies for most systems. In the

(Continued)

of DA is low. COMT is also involved in the degradation of metabolites generated by MAO activities. The final products from these two distinct catabolic pathways is homovanillic acid for DA metabolism and either vanillylmandelic acid or a conjugated form of 3-methoxy-4-hydroxyphenylglycol for NA metabolism (Eisenhofer et al., 2004). Histamine follows distinct pathways. It is converted in the brain by histamine N-methyltransferase to N(tele)-methylhistamine, which undergoes degradation by MAO-B followed by the aldehyde oxidation to N(tele)-methylimidazole acetic acid, while in periphery histamine is degraded by diamine oxidase (Taylor, 1975; Morisset et al., 2000).

Once synthesized, all monoamines are concentrated in the vesicular compartment by the vesicular monoamine transporter or VMAT2 (Wimalasena, 2011). Regarding the extracellular space, various transporters are involved in the clearance of monoamines. Three major classes of monoamine transporters, 5-HT transporter (SERT), DA transporter (DAT), and NA transporter (NET), are responsible for the reuptake of 5-HT, DA and NA, respectively, from the synaptic cleft back to pre-synaptic neuron (Torres et al., 2003). Of note, the reuptake of DA occurs physiologically through the NET in extrastriatal tissues (Di Chiara et al., 1992). The reuptake of these monoamines is not totally selective and there are also several low affinity/high capacitance transporters including the organic cation transporters (OCT1-3 subtypes) and the plasma membrane monoamine transporter (PMAT) (Daws, 2009; Hensler et al., 2013; De Deurwaerdère et al., 2016). These systems, which are expressed by glial cells and other types of neurons, are involved in the reuptake of histamine (no preferential transporter) and the other monoamines. Thus, while the first step of synthesis can be selective, most of the other steps are overlapping and the catabolism involves cells other than monoaminergic neurons (**Figure 2**). Furthermore, the enzymes of biogenic amine catabolism are involved in several additional processes.

The main selectivity regarding these systems, although limited to some extent, is conferred by the receptors; two families for DA (D$_1$-like including D$_1$ and D$_5$R and D$_2$-like including D$_2$L, D$_2$S, D$_3$, D$_4$ receptor subtypes) (Emilien et al., 1999; Beaulieu and Gainetdinov, 2011), three families also for NA ($\alpha_{1a,b,d}$ or α_{2a-d} receptor subtypes, and β receptor subtypes including β_{1-3}) (Andersson, 1980; Ahles and Engelhardt, 2014; Ghanemi and Hu, 2015), four for histamine (H$_{1-4}$) (Panula et al., 2015) and seven for 5-HT (5-HT$_{1-7}$) (Barnes and Sharp, 1999; Hoyer et al., 2002). They are mostly G-protein-coupled receptors (GPCR), except for the 5-HT$_3$ receptor subtypes which are channel receptors. The cerebral distribution is distinct for each receptor. The differential

distribution in some brain regions for a subtype can be a hint with regards to its participation in some specific functions. Details related to brain expression of monoamine receptors are found in the above-cited authoritative reviews. In any case, most of them are expressed in several neurobiological networks. Moreover, several subtypes may directly, as autoreceptors (see below), or indirectly modify the activity of monoaminergic neurons, thereby altering neurobiological networks beyond their specific distribution.

Each monoaminergic neuronal system has its own autoreceptor(s). Thus, adrenergic cells express the α_{2c} receptor while histaminergic neurons express H$_3$ receptors. Dopaminergic and serotonergic neurons express D$_2$/D$_3$ receptors and 5-HT$_{1A}$, 5-HT$_{1B/1D}$ and 5-HT$_{2B}$ receptors, respectively. The function of these autoreceptors located at both cell bodies and/or neuron terminals is usually to inhibit the electrical activity, excitability, synthesis and/or release. They also regulate the activity of the transporters presumably via intracellular signaling pathways. As illustrated in **Figure 2**, these autoreceptors are also expressed by other cell types (heteroreceptors).

The last point to consider when dealing with neuropharmacology of monoaminergic systems is that, either by acting on non-selective enzymes such as MAO, or by selectively targeting one receptor, the biological responses likely involve all systems due to their interaction throughout the brain (Fitoussi et al., 2013; Hensler et al., 2013). The complex interaction between these systems overwhelms the single target and the integrative views of the newer monoaminergic treatments must clearly include this dimension (De Deurwaerdère and Di Giovanni, 2016).

FROM THE DRUGS TO MONOAMINES

Treatments of Schizophrenia
Historical Perspectives

It is logical to start the overview of the monoaminergic potentials in psychiatry by the discovery of neuroleptic drugs (antipsychotic drugs), which may be considered as the birth of biological psychiatry. Schizophrenia is a complex neuropsychiatric disorder with high prevalence (Owen et al., 2016). In the early 1950s, chlorpromazine was initially used by the French physicians Laborit and Charpentier for its antihistaminic properties, to calm down patients before anesthesia. The effect of chlorpromazine was spectacular and it was transposed successfully to the treatment of schizophrenia by Deniker and Delay (López-Muñoz et al., 2005). Other drugs from different chemical classes were found to mimic the antipsychotic action of chlorpromazine, but it was several years before the understanding that dopaminergic system could be involved (Carlsson and Lindqvist, 1963), and that the DA (D_2) receptor subtype was a common target of all antipsychotic drugs (Seeman et al., 1975, 1976). Nowadays, central D_2 receptors, among other receptor types, remain an essential target in drug design of newer antipsychotic drugs (Butini et al., 2016).

Mechanisms of Action of Antipsychotic Drugs

All antipsychotic drugs block the D_2 receptor subtype and the antipsychotic efficacy depends on the proportion of occupied D_2 receptors, which is directly related to the affinity of the compound at D_2 receptor and the free plasma concentration of the antipsychotic drug. Most of these drugs including chlorpromazine or haloperidol are efficacious against positive symptoms of schizophrenia such as delusion, paranoia or hallucinations. Their therapeutic benefit is assumed to be related to the blockade of D_2 receptors in the ventral striatum (nucleus accumbens). On the other hand, these compounds are not efficacious against the negative symptoms which may even aggravate (Millan et al., 2014; Remington et al., 2016). These drugs also induce several serious side-effects, either due to their off-targets including H_1, α_2, muscarinic2 (M_2) receptor antagonist properties, or to chronic central D_2 receptor blockade. Notably the extrapyramidal side-effects (EPS) include parkinsonism, akathisia, dystonia and tardive dyskinesia (Ebadi and Srinivasan, 1995).

Although clozapine is more efficacious against negative and cognitive symptoms than other antipsychotic drugs and has fewer EPS (Ashby and Wang, 1996), its clinical use was discontinued due to its propensity to induce agranulocytosis. However, it was subsequently reintroduced if carefully monitored (Deutch et al., 1991; Ashby and Wang, 1996). The peculiar clinical responses gave rise to the concept of the typical and atypical antipsychotic drugs, the latter inducing less EPS and vegetative effects (Meltzer, 1993, 1999). Studies of the pharmacological behavior of drugs like clozapine or risperidone led to the proposal that the atypical profile corresponds to a higher affinity of the drug toward 5-HT_2 (i.e., 5-HT_{2A}) vs. D_2 receptor subtypes (Meltzer et al., 1989a,b). This pharmacological constraint has been added to the D_2 receptor target in the selection of drugs possibly exhibiting an atypical antipsychotic profile. Drugs like olanzapine, quetiapine, ziprasidone and more recently brexpiprazole are representatives of this class (**Table 1**). These newer antipsychotic drugs have lower propensity to induce EPS, but another concern emerges regarding the development of metabolic side effects such as weight excess. It is possible that their antagonist/inverse agonist profile at 5-HT_{2C} receptors in addition to the H_1 receptor antagonism participate to the development of increased body weight and obesity side effect (see below) (**Table 1**).

The superiority of clozapine in terms of low incidence of EPS has been also related to its low affinity at D_2 receptors, implying a fast dissociation from the receptor and avoiding unsurmountable D_2 receptor blockade, either acutely or chronically (Kapur and Seeman, 2001). This property has not been verified for all antipsychotics but it introduces the notion that antipsychotic drugs could correct rather than block central DA transmission. Aripiprazole brexpiprazole or cariprazine display partial agonist

activities at some signaling pathways connected to D_2 receptors (Kiss et al., 2010; Citrome, 2013, 2015). In spite of the high occupancy of D_2 receptors *in vivo* presumably overwhelming the 80% threshold occupancy, these partial or biased agonists do not induce catalepsy in rats and induce fewer EPS in humans compared to typical neuroleptics (Citrome, 2015).

Questions and Directions

There are several outstanding questions for neuropharmacology. In spite of the availability of antipsychotic drugs minimizing the occurrence of EPS, abnormal motor responses are still present with some of these medications.

(i) The reason why 5-HT_{2A} receptor antagonism has beneficial effects is still not fully understood with respect to the lower EPS and the involvement of motor part of the basal ganglia. There are reasonable amounts of data showing that the impact of D_2 receptor blockade in the presence of 5-HT_{2A} receptor antagonism would be reinforced in the mesolimbic system and conversely dampened in the mesocortical system (Meltzer and Huang, 2008). Indeed, 5-HT_{2A} receptor antagonists enhance DA release induced by D_2 receptor blockade in the cortex. A similar property has been observed with 5-HT_{1A} receptor agonism (Meltzer and Massey, 2011; Hensler et al., 2013; Schreiber and Newman-Tancredi, 2014). This may explain the fact that antipsychotic drugs like cariprazine, with low affinity for 5-HT_{2A} receptor and moderate to high affinity for 5-HT_{1A} receptors, display atypical antipsychotic drug profiles in the clinic (Kiss et al., 2010; De Deurwaerdère, 2016). The favorable profile regarding motor parts of the basal ganglia is not likely to be related to a putative disinhibitory action of 5-HT_2 receptor blockade on DA neuron activity, as had been previously speculated (Kapur and Remington, 1996; De Deurwaerdère and Di Giovanni, 2016). Rather, their cortical effects could have beneficial effects on cognitive symptoms of the disease that are, in part, independent from D_2 receptor blockade. The categorization in typical vs. atypical antipsychotics is not always clear in considering only the binding profiles (**Table 1**).

(ii) The negative symptoms remain one of the most difficult challenges in the treatment of schizophrenia (Millan et al., 2014; Remington et al., 2016). Interestingly, neuropsychopharmacological analysis tends to dissociate various symptoms of schizophrenia which could have distinct etiology (Buckley et al., 2009). Acting on these distinct dimensions implies a combination of selective drugs or the use of multi-target medicines (Butini et al., 2016), and animal models adapted for the different symptoms (Millan et al., 2014). This implies, in turn, an extensive preclinical evaluation for testing the suitability of any new compound (Millan et al., 2015b; De Deurwaerdère, 2016; Di Giovanni and De Deurwaerdère, 2016). Some of the most advanced treatments focus on the following targets (**Table 1**): D_2 receptor antagonism regarding the positive symptoms, 5-HT_{1A} receptor agonism/5-HT_{2A} receptor antagonism and/or increase in cortical acetylcholine release for the

TABLE 1 | Receptor-binding affinities of typical and atypical antipsychotic drugs.

Antipsychotics	D_2	D_3	$5\text{-}HT_{1A}$	$5\text{-}HT_{2A}$	Other targets*
TYPICAL ANTIPSYCHOTICS					
Haloperidol	8.84	8.56	6.29	7.28	D_4 (8.83); α_{1A} (7.9); σ_1 (8.52)
flupentixol	9.46	8.76	5.1	7.06	D_1 (8.46); H_1 (9.07)
Thioridazine	9.4	8.82	6.84	7.56	α_{1A} (8.5); α_{1B} (8.62); M_1 (7.89); M_5 (7.9); H_1 (7.78)
Pimozide	9.48	9.6	6.19	7.32	$5\text{-}HT_7$ (9.3); D_4 (8.74)
Perphenazine	8.47	9.89	6.38	8.25	$5\text{-}HT_6$ (7.77); $5\text{-}HT_7$ (7.64); D_1 (7.52); D_4 (7.77); α_{1A} (8); H1 (8.1); σ_1 (7.73)
Loxapine	7.96	7.71	5.61	8.18	$5\text{-}HT_{2C}$ (7.88); $5\text{-}HT_6$ (7.51); $5\text{-}HT_7$ (7.06); D_1 (7.27); D_4 (8.08); D_5 (7.12); α_{1A} (7.51); α_{1B} (7.28); α_{2A} (6.82); α_{2B} (6.97); α_{2C} (7.1); M_1 (6.92); H_1 (8.3)
ATYPICAL ANTIPSYCHOTICS					
Clozapine	6.87	6.66	7.06	8.39	$5\text{-}HT_{1B}$ (6.28)b; $5\text{-}HT_{2B}$ (8.79); $5\text{-}HT_{2C}$ (8.56 - IA); $5\text{-}HT_3$ (6.62); $5\text{-}HT_6$ (7.87); $5\text{-}HT_7$ (7.75); D_1 (7.64); D_4 (7.33); D5 (6.63); α_{1A} (8.79); α_{1B} (8.15); α_{2A} (7.43); α_{2B} (7.58); α_{2C} (8.22); M_1 (8.21); M_2 (7.44); M_3 (7.72); M_4 (7.81); M_5 (7.81); H_1(8.95); H_2 (6.82); H_4 (6.18)
Risperidone	8.21	8.16	6.75	9.69	$5\text{-}HT_{1B}$ (7.83); $5\text{-}HT_{1D}$ (7.07); $5\text{-}HT_{2B}$ (7.8); $5\text{-}HT_{2C}$ (8.17); $5\text{-}HT_6$ (8.18); D_4 (8.21); D_5 (7.8); α_{1A} (8.3); α_{1B} (8.04); α_{2A} (7.78); α_{2C} (8.89); H_1 (7.7)
Olanzapine	7.67	7.46	5.82	8.88	$5\text{-}HT_{2B}$ (8.41); $5\text{-}HT_{2C}$ (8.41); $5\text{-}HT_3$ (6.69); $5\text{-}HT_6$ (8.09); $5\text{-}HT_7$ (6.98); D_4 (7.75); D_5 (7.04); α_{1A} (6.95); α_{1B} (6.58); α_{2A} (6.5); α_{2B} (7.09); α_{2C} (7.54); M_1 (7.58); M_2 (7.2); M_3 (7.28); M_4 (7.61); M_5 (8.12); H_1 (8.66); H_2 (7.36)
Ziprasidone	8.09	8.35	9.01	9.51	$5\text{-}HT_{1B}$ (8.4); $5\text{-}HT_{1D}$ (8.64); $5\text{-}HT_{2B}$ (9.08); $5\text{-}HT_{2C}$ (9.01); $5\text{-}HT_6$ (7.21); $5\text{-}HT_7$ (8.22); D_1 (8.45); D_4 (7.33); α_{1A} (7.74); H_1 (7.2); SERT (7.26); NET (7.32)
Quetiapine	6.38	6.41	6.78	6.81	$5\text{-}HT_{2B}$ (7.33); $5\text{-}HT_{2C}$ (5.98); $5\text{-}HT_6$ (6.02); $5\text{-}HT_7$ (6.51); D_1 (6.71); D_4 (5.85); D_5 (7.8); α_{1A} (7.66); α_{1B} (7.84); α_{2A} (5.44); α_{2C} (7.65); H_1 (8.16); H_2 (7.38); M_1 (489); M_3 (5.79)
Brexpiprazole	9.48	8.9	9.21	9.67	α_{1A} (8.42); α_{1B} (9.23); α_{1D} (8.58); α_{2C} (9.77); $5\text{-}HT_{2B}$ (8.72); $5\text{-}HT_7$ (8.43)
Aripiprazole	8.9	8.85	8.57	8.02	$5\text{-}HT_{2B}$ (9.59)
Cariprazine	9.31	10.07	8.59	7.73	$5\text{-}HT_{2B}$ (9.24)
Amisulpiride	8.89	8.62	5.8	5.08	$5\text{-}HT_{2B}$ (7.89); 5-HT7 (7.94)
Blonaserin	9.84	9.3	6.09	9.09	

*The pK_i values shown are taken from several sources, including mean values from the PDSP K_i database (Roth and Driscol, 2016). The values for the receptors: D_2, D_3, $5\text{-}HT_{1A}$, $5\text{-}HT_{2A}$, $5\text{-}HT_{2B}$, $5\text{-}HT_{2C}$ with atypical antipsychotics were from Leggio et al. (2016) or Citrome (2015). The colors indicate: Blue, drugs with higher affinity for D_2 receptors; Orange, drugs with a 5-HT/DA binding profile; Violet, drugs with a D2/3 effects; Green, drugs with partial agonist activities at D_2 receptors. $5\text{-}HT_{2B}$ receptors are a recurrent target of several atypical antipsychotic drugs. Conversely, none of the agents presented above bind at $5\text{-}HT_4$ receptors. M1-M5, muscarinic receptors; σ1, sigma 1 receptors. *in the range of 1 order of magnitude compared to the affinity at D_2 receptors.*

cognitive symptoms, and perhaps D_3 receptor antagonism for the negative symptoms (**Figure 3**).

(iii) The pharmacological analysis of the newer antipsychotic drugs has led to consideration of other targets including $5\text{-}HT_6$, $5\text{-}HT_7$ receptors (Meltzer and Huang, 2008; Mauri et al., 2014) or the intriguing $5\text{-}HT_{2B}$ receptors (Devroye et al., 2016) (**Table 1**). Since the interaction between neurotransmitter systems is extremely complex, actions directed to some targets (e.g., D_2 receptors) might unmask a deleterious involvement of other circuits. For instance, while the $5\text{-}HT_{2C}$ receptor blockade has not been shown to be primarily involved in the antipsychotic drug action, its blockade might be necessary to limit the occurrence of EPS induced by typical neuroleptics (Richtand et al., 2008). The neurobiological process underlying a deleterious involvement of $5\text{-}HT_{2C}$ receptors that follows D_2 receptor blockade is not well understood (De Deurwaerdère et al., 2013). Because of the frequency of co-morbid diseases including mania, anxiety or depression in schizophrenic patients, this analysis further indicated the prescription of other medicines in addition to antipsychotic drugs (Buckley et al., 2009). Most available antipsychotic drugs have

a complex pharmacological profile including adrenergic, muscarinic and histaminergic sites and most of them, especially the newer ones, are also developed for the treatment of bipolar disorder and major depression.

(iv) Very few strategies have tried to avoid the D_2 receptor target because most, if not all trials targeting a single site other than D_2 receptors failed to reach clinical significance (Deutch et al., 1991; Ashby and Wang, 1996; Meltzer and Massey, 2011). Recently, the $5\text{-}HT_{2C}$ receptor agonist vabicanserin has been tested as a monotherapy in the treatment of schizophrenia. This was justified as the $5\text{-}HT_{2C}$ receptor inhibits DA release, at least in the nucleus accumbens, and its preferential agonists are efficacious in several preclinical models of schizophrenia (Rosenzweig-Lipson et al., 2012). Although the strategy of stimulating $5\text{-}HT_{2C}$ receptors should be taken with caution (Di Giovanni and De Deurwaerdère, 2016), it protects at least from the development of obesity due to its anorexigenic property and would be less prone to promoting EPS. Although having an antipsychotic profile, vabicanserin was not more efficacious than risperidone at primary end point, and its development was discontinued (Shen et al., 2014).

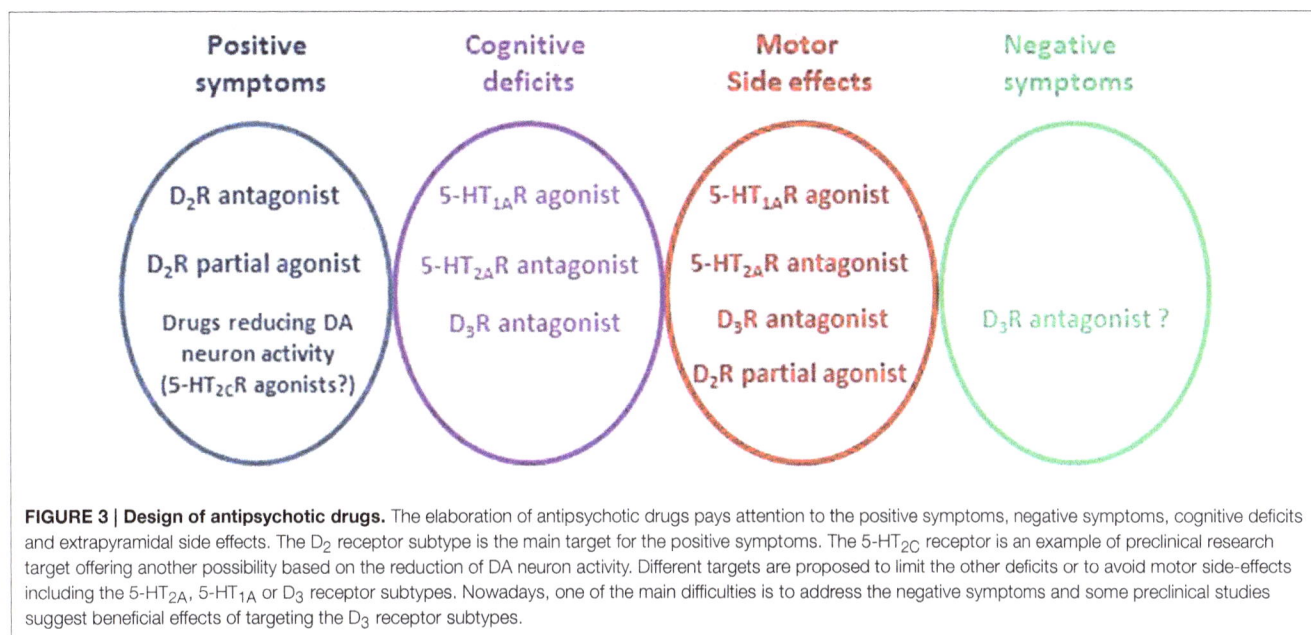

FIGURE 3 | Design of antipsychotic drugs. The elaboration of antipsychotic drugs pays attention to the positive symptoms, negative symptoms, cognitive deficits and extrapyramidal side effects. The D_2 receptor subtype is the main target for the positive symptoms. The 5-HT$_{2C}$ receptor is an example of preclinical research target offering another possibility based on the reduction of DA neuron activity. Different targets are proposed to limit the other deficits or to avoid motor side-effects including the 5-HT$_{2A}$, 5-HT$_{1A}$ or D_3 receptor subtypes. Nowadays, one of the main difficulties is to address the negative symptoms and some preclinical studies suggest beneficial effects of targeting the D_3 receptor subtypes.

Nonetheless, vabicanserin might represent a change of strategy regarding the development of newer antipsychotics, focusing on the activity of the monoaminergic systems rather than on a single site.

Conclusion

After having isolated one target of antipsychotic drugs, namely the D_2 receptor subtype, the search for additional targets is essential for better intervention of the full spectrum of symptoms in schizophrenia. This cannot be achieved by acting on a single target, necessitating the use of a cocktail of drugs or multi-targeted compounds (**Figure 3**). The methodological approach to developing antipsychotic drugs is still conditioned by molecular pharmacology, although new developments in connectomics should prove valuable in the future (Fornito and Bullmore, 2015).

Treatments of Depression
Historical Perspectives of Antidepressant Drugs

Major depression is a severe, highly disabling, psychiatric disorder which is becoming a leading cause of global disease burden, with a growing prevalence of 3–17% in adults and 2.8–5.6% in adolescents (Gururajan et al., 2016; Rantamaki and Yalcin, 2016). Its multifaceted, but poorly understood etiology involves complex interactions between different biological (genetic, epigenetic, neuroendocrine and neuroimmune), psychosocial (personality traits), developmental and environmental (exposure to early life stress) factors.

In the 1950s began a new era in the field of psychopharmacology with the clinical introduction of two antidepressants: iproniazid and imipramine (López-Muñoz and Alamo, 2009). Iproniazid, originally developed for anti-tuberculous purposes, was characterized as MAO inhibitor (MAO-I) by Zeller and Barsky (1952). Its administration improved mood in patients and it was shown to lead to an increase in the brain levels of 5-HT in rodents (Udenfriend et al., 1957). The discovery of the antidepressant effects of iproniazid laid the path for development of more effective MAOIs such as phenelzine, tranylcypromine, isocarboxazid, and other hydrazine and indole derivates (Ban, 2001). The compound, now known as imipramine, was presented by Kuhn in 1957 as the first representative of the tricyclic antidepressants (TCAs) (Brown and Rosdolsky, 2015). In the period between 1960 and 1979, many different TCAs were developed, including amitriptyline, nortriptyline, desipramine, trimipramine, protryptiline, iprindol, dothiepin and clomipramine (Fangmann et al., 2008; López-Muñoz and Alamo, 2009). First tricyclic antidepressants were shown to inhibit the uptake of NA. The modification of the basic dibenzazepine structure of imipramine resulted in the discovery of new cyclic antidepressants during 1970s, including maprotiline and mianserine. The significant therapeutic effects of MAO-Is and TCAs, stimulated an increased interest in the role of monoaminergic system in the etiology of depression.

Fluoxetine, the first selective serotonin reuptake inhibitor (SSRI), came out in 1975 (Wong et al., 1975) and was introduced in 1987. Its unique properties and appropriate clinical efficacy established the SERT as an important target in the treatment of depression (Perez-Caballero et al., 2014). Fluoxetine is, in fact, not highly selective toward the SERT whereas citalopram, escitalopram, fluvoxamine, paroxetine or sertraline block the SERT more selectively (Thomas et al., 1987; Jacquot et al., 2007). Their efficacy is similar to TCAs but SSRIs generally have lower toxicity in comparison with MAO-Is and TCAs.

Mechanisms of Action of Antidepressant Drugs

The neurobiological basis of depression is not fully understood although the monoaminergic theory of depression stipulates 5-HT and NA extracellular deficits in different brain regions. This remains far from to be clear however, except in major depression with suicidal behavior where the levels of tissue 5-HT were found lower compared to levels in age-matched controls (Delgado and Moreno, 2000). In animals, the destruction of either 5-HT or NA systems, or both, does not trigger depressive-like symptoms in some behavioral tests (Page et al., 1999; Cryan et al., 2002, 2005; Delaville et al., 2012). On the other hand, the enhancement of 5-HT and NA neurotransmission with some antidepressant medication results in the improvement of the common symptoms of the disease.

Studies with SSRI and other blockers of monoaminergic reuptake sites indicate that the efficacy of antidepressant drugs entails at least three sequential steps. (1) The blockade of SERT at the level of 5-HT cell bodies enhances somatodendritic 5-HT extracellular levels (Bel and Artigas, 1992; Invernizzi et al., 1992), thereby activating 5-HT$_{1A}$ autoreceptors and reducing the firing rate of 5-HT neurons (Blier and de Montigny, 1990; Adell et al., 1993; Guiard et al., 2005). The blockade of SERT at terminals of 5-HT neurons enhances extracellular levels of 5-HT but this effect is considerably dampened by the decrease in 5-HT neuron firing rate and the stimulation of 5-HT$_{1B}$ autoreceptors located at 5-HT terminals (Invernizzi et al., 1992; Gardier et al., 2003). (2) The desensitization of somatodendritic 5-HT$_{1A}$ receptors in the raphe nuclei upon subchronic administration of SSRI, with the main consequence of magnifying the effects of the SERT blockade on the extracellular levels of 5-HT (Invernizzi et al., 1996; Piñeyro and Blier, 1999). (3) The final step involves modification of 5-HT receptors at 5-HT receptive cells including 5-HT$_{1A}$, 5-HT$_{2A}$ or 5-HT$_{2C}$ receptors (Artigas et al., 2002; Artigas, 2013). These sequential steps take time which may account for the delay between start of treatment with antidepressant drug and clinical effect.

The interaction between 5-HT and NA systems is evident in the mechanism of action of TCAs because most TCAs have a better affinity for the NET compared to the SERT. Numerous studies have provided evidence that α_1 and α_2 receptors exerted complex interactions on 5-HT neurons, α_1 receptor being excitatory. Conversely, 5-HT at least via 5-HT$_{2A}$ receptors inhibits the activity of NA neurons whereas the desensitization of 5-HT$_{2A}$ receptors, also occurring after SSRI, allows for an increase in central NA tone (Piñeyro and Blier, 1999; Hamon and Blier, 2013). Thus, the interaction between the 5-HT and the NA has a pivotal role in the mechanism of action of drugs targeting monoaminergic neurons terminal activity including TCAs, SSRI and MAO-I. Other antidepressant drugs target 5-HT and/or NA receptors (see below), but their mechanisms of action are less well understood. Through the interaction between monoaminergic systems (Hamon and Blier, 2013), DA changes are indirectly involved in the mechanism of action of antidepressants. The DA system is usually not directly targeted in the treatment of depression (nonetheless, see below with the introduction of antipsychotics in major depression).

Amelioration of Antidepressant Drugs Actions

In the last 20 years two main problems with antidepressant treatment have emerged, including a poor or partial response,

i.e., a large proportion of patients not responding well to the therapy (Gumnick and Nemeroff, 2000), and the delay of action of antidepressant drugs usually reached after 2–3 weeks of treatment. The partial response of antidepressant drugs has led to the introduction of new and more effective antidepressants like venlafaxine, which inhibits the reuptake of 5-HT and NA (NSRI), and mirtazapine, which acts primarily as an antagonist of presynaptic α_2-adrenoreceptors (Artigas et al., 2002). A meta-analysis assessed the effects of 12 new-generation antidepressants and showed that mirtazapine, venlafaxine and two SSRIs, escitalopram and sertraline, were more efficacious than other SSRIs (fluoxetine, fluvoxamine and paroxetine), the NSRI duloxetine and the selective NA reuptake inhibitor (SNRI) reboxetine (Cipriani et al., 2009).

The antidepressant effect of MAO-Is is dependent on inhibition of MAO-A but irreversible inhibition of that isoenzyme resulted in adverse hypertensive reactions with foods containing tyramine called "the cheese effect." To avoid this adverse event, a new strategy for the treatment of depression was presented in the form of reversible inhibitors of MAO-A (RIMA), such as moclobemide (Haefely et al., 1992), brofaromine (Davidson, 2003), and befloxatone (Curet et al., 1998). However, the use of MAO-Is today is mostly limited for treating patients with atypical depression, bipolar depression, treatment-resistant depression, or hyperserotonergic responses with SSRIs. In 2009, agomelatine, the first antidepressant that mediates its activity via the melatonergic pathway was approved (San and Arranz, 2008; Millan et al., 2010; Racagni et al., 2011). This antidepressant acts as an antagonist at 5-HT$_{2C}$ receptors and agonist at melatonergic MT$_1$ and MT$_2$ receptors (Millan et al., 2010). In comparison with other standard SSRIs and SNRIs, agomelatine showed similar or even favorable efficacy and tolerability (Kasper et al., 2013). In addition to agomelatine, several other 5-HT$_{2C}$ agents have been reported to display strong anxiolytic/antidepressant properties in animal models and clinical studies (Millan, 2005, 2006; Millan et al., 2005; Di Giovanni and De Deurwaerdère, 2016). A summary of these evolutions has been indicated in the **Table 2**.

The second problem associated with antidepressant treatment is the delay of action of the drugs. Knowledge of the mechanism of action of SSRIs resulted in the proposal to reduce the delay of action by blocking 5-HT$_{1A/1B}$ autoreceptors, thereby lessening the time period needed to produce the massive increase in 5-HT levels at the synaptic cleft (Artigas et al., 1996). However, since the efficacy of SSRI is also associated with postsynaptic 5-HT$_{1A}$ receptors (Blier et al., 1990), which are not desensitized and are required for the benefit of SSRIs, such a blockade might be expected to be counterproductive. Similar augmentation can be achieved by concomitantly blocking 5-HT$_{2C}$ receptors, which indirectly inhibit 5-HT neuronal activity (Cremers et al., 2004, 2007). Clinical trials involving this approach are underway (see Di Giovanni and De Deurwaerdère, 2016). Another monoaminergic possibility to obtain a fast onset of the antidepressant effect is the use of 5-HT$_4$ receptor agonists. These compounds act directly on 5-HT receptive fields in the hippocampus or the cortex and indirectly stimulate 5-HT release. Their pro-cognitive and anxiolytic effects have raised some

TABLE 2 | Pharmacological targets of lead and newer antidepressant drugs from lead compounds.

Lead compounds	Mechanisms of action	New compounds in clinic	Main targets
Imipramine, Fluoxetine	5-HT/NA interaction mostly via blockade of SERT and/or NET + Alteration of monoamine targets and function	SSRI (Escitalopram, Citalopram, Paroxetine...) NSRI (Duoxetine, Venlafaxine) SNRI (Reboxetine) Multi-target drugs (Vortioxetine)	SERT SERT and NET NET SERT/5-HT receptors
Iproniazid	5-HT/NA interaction mostly via inhibition of MAO-A/B (irreversible)	Moclobemide Agomelatine	MAO-A (reversible inhibitor) MT1/MT2 agonist/5-HT$_{2C}$ antagonist

Lead antidepressant drugs and their proposed mechanisms of action as well as newer drugs in clinical use that retain some of their targets. Agomelatine is included, although its 5-HT$_{2C}$ receptor antagonist action was not directly based on a lead drug (Di Giovanni and De Deurwaerdère, 2016).

interest for the treatment of depression (Lucas and Debonnel, 2002; Lucas et al., 2007; Mendez-David et al., 2014).

Future Directions

Newer antidepressants have been developed with more complex pharmacological profile such as vortioxetine (Sanchez et al., 2015). This compound blocks the SERT as well multiple 5-HT receptors (Sanchez et al., 2015; Sagud et al., 2016). This effect is in line with studies reporting that the combination of antidepressants with atypical antipsychotic drugs (olanzapine, risperidone, quetiapine, aripiprazole, paliperidone, ziprazidone, and amisulpride), can boost the effectiveness of depression treatment (Berman et al., 2007; Thase et al., 2007; Bauer et al., 2009; Han et al., 2013). Thus, the monoaminergic system remains an important field for producing newer antidepressant drugs involving refined strategies (Hamon and Blier, 2013; Artigas, 2015). Recently, there has been a growing interest in neuronal plasticity, cholinergic, GABAergic and glutamate neurotransmission, stress and HPA axis, reward system and neuroinflammation as potential underlying mechanisms of depression that go somehow beyond monoaminergic strategies (Artigas, 2015; Dale et al., 2015; Millan et al., 2015a). However, the complexity of the system is such that monoaminergic antidepressant drugs may act on different neurobiological circuits and molecular mechanisms, which might be more important targets.

Obesity and Energy Balance
Historical Perspective

The neurobiological networks involved in food intake and energy balance have been the subjects of many recent studies, in view of the growing evidence for a worldwide problem of obesity. The first anti-obesity drug targeting amine neurotransmitter signaling was amphetamine. Amphetamine, α-methylphenethylamine, member of β-phenylethylamine group of drugs, was synthesized to substitute for ephedrine. Animal and human studies showed that this compound can produce arousal and insomnia. Racemic α-methylphenethylamine, registered by SK&F under the name Benzedrine®, was introduced in 1935 to treat narcolepsy and was also employed for mild depression, post-encephalitic parkinsonism, schizophrenia, alcoholism and other disorders (see (Bett, 1946)). In 1937, SK&F marketed Dexedrine (d-amphetamine), the more potent of the two

isomers which produced euphoria, excitability, hyperactivity and restlessness with hyperthermia. The quick loss of weight in obese subjects treated against narcolepsy with Benzedrine aroused the interest in the use of the sympathomimetics as anti-obese medicines. A clinical study on 162 patients treated with d-amphetamine, which had been performed on a smaller number of subjects, supported its usefulness as appetite depressant (Hawirko and Sprague, 1946). However, d-amphetamine produces addiction (Kiloh and Brandon, 1962). To decrease addictive potential, substituted amphetamines such as phenyl-tertiary-butylamine, phentermine, and fenfluramine (3-trifluoromethyl-N-ethylamphetamine) were synthesized and were approved by FDA between 1959 and 1973 for weight loss.

Mechanism of Action

The hypothalamus is a key structure involved in food intake regulation and energy balance. It receives monoaminergic terminals from several different sources and the roles of the monoamines appear to be different: 5-HT and histamine participate as a satiety factors; DA acts as the main signaling molecule in a reward system, and NA tends to enhance energy expenditure. Animal studies have shown that phenyl-tertiary-butylamine, phentermine, and fenfluramine cause the release of amines from the nerve terminals as well as inhibiting their uptake. While d-amphetamine has higher affinities for DAT and NET than SERT, fenfluramine has a higher affinity for SERT (Garattini, 1995; Kuczenski et al., 1995). In rat, both peripheral and central mechanisms of fenfluramine action have been implicated (Carruba et al., 1986).

Studies with selective ligands of 5-HT receptors *in vivo* have shown that hypophagic effect triggered by d-fenfluramine and its metabolite d-norfenfluramine was mediated by 5-HT acting on 5-HT$_{2C}$ receptors (Vickers et al., 2001) (**Table 3**). Combination of phentermine and fenfluramine, i.e., "Phen-Fen," enables the therapeutically effective dose of appetite suppressants to be decreased. However, the heart valve disease related to a 5-HT$_{2B}$ receptor agonism action and pulmonary hypertension (Vivero et al., 1998; Palmieri et al., 2002) caused the withdrawal of fenfluramine and dexfenfluramine from the U.S. market in 1997. Later meta-analysis of the observational studies indicated that fenfluramine-associated valvular regurgitation was less common that assumed, but still present in 1 out of 8 patients treated for >90 days (Sachdev et al., 2002). The next anti-obesity drug

TABLE 3 | Anti-obesity drugs and mechanisms.

Lead compounds	Mechanisms of action	New compounds in clinic	Main targets
Amphetamine	DAT, NET and release of catecholamines	Sibutramine Reboxetine	NET/SERT (withdrawn) NET
d-fenfluramine	5-HT release and indirect 5-HT$_{2C}$ agonism	Lorcaserin	Preferential 5-HT$_{2C}$ receptor agonist
Antipsychotic drugs	Obesity as side effects via H$_1$ receptor antagonism	Cariprazine, Brexpiprazole, Aripiprazole	Weak to no affinity toward H$_1$ (even 5-HT$_{2C}$) receptors (**Table 1**)

Lead compounds in the field of anti-obesity drugs and their proposed mechanisms of action are shown, together with newer drugs with similar actions. Amphetamine enhances catecholamines release through its action on DAT and NET, which led to the development of drugs that enhanced NA release. D-fenfluramine, chemically derived from amphetamine, loses affinities for DAT and NET in relation to SERT. Conversely, antipsychotic drugs induced weigh gain that has been corrected in newer compounds.

sibutramine (Luque and Rey, 1999), originally developed as an antidepressant, is a potent SERT and NET inhibitor *in vivo* (Luscombe et al., 1990). Animal studies on its mechanisms of action pointed to the activation of β$_1$-adrenoceptors, 5-HT$_{2A/2C}$ receptors and α$_1$-adrenoceptors (Jackson et al., 1997). The compound has been shown in clinical trial to be an efficient therapeutic, although the patients who stopped using the drug quickly regained weight (James et al., 2000), as observed for the substituted amphetamines (Vivero et al., 1998). Sibutramine, having antiatherogenic activities (improvement of insulin resistance, glucose metabolism, dyslipidemia, and inflammation) concomitantly induces a moderate increase in heart rate, a slight increase in blood pressure and may also prolong the QT interval, inducing arrhythmias (Scheen, 2010). Because the hazard ratio for cardiovascular events was significantly increased in sibutramine treated patients, the drug was withdrawn from markets in 2010 (Haslam, 2016).

In 2012, a novel drug, lorcaserin, was approved by FDA for the treatment of obesity. It is a 5-HT$_{2C}$ receptor agonist that is appetite suppressing while free of cardiovascular effects (Gustafson et al., 2013). It has about 15 and 100 times higher affinity for 5-HT$_{2C}$ than for 5-HT$_{2A}$ and 5-HT$_{2B}$ receptor subtypes. This drug stimulates the 5-HT$_{2C}$ receptors located on proopiomelanocortin neurons in the arcuate nucleus resulting in the release of α-melanocyte-stimulating hormone, which suppresses appetite by acting on melanocortin-4-receptors in the paraventricular nucleus (Voigt and Fink, 2015). It probably has other actions in the brain including the decrease in DA release in the nucleus accumbens, dampening goal-directed behavior (Higgins and Fletcher, 2015; Di Giovanni and De Deurwaerdère, 2016).

Histamine and Obesity

The H$_1$ receptor antagonist component of various medications including antipsychotics is suspected to increase body weight (Kroeze et al., 2003; Ratliff et al., 2010). In addition, recent work indicates also that cerebral histaminergic system mediates the anorexic effects of oleoylethanol amide, an endogenous agonist at peroxisome proliferator-activated receptor alpha (PPAR-α) (Provensi et al., 2014). Experimental and preclinical studies employing different animal models have convincingly shown that H$_1$ and H$_3$ receptors play an important role in energy balance and body weight gain, H$_1$ receptor agonists and H$_3$ receptor antagonist/inverse agonists being anorexic drugs (Clineschmidt and Lotti, 1973;

Lecklin et al., 1998; Masaki et al., 2004; Provensi et al., 2014, 2016).

Although much attempt has been done in developing histaminergic agents as anti-obesity treatment, no recent drug with a histaminergic profile reached clinics (Esbenshade et al., 2006; Provensi et al., 2016). Betahistine, registered in Europe in 1970 for the management of vertigo and vestibular pathologies, could be used to achieve anti-obesity action in some conditions (Provensi et al., 2016). This drug, combining weak agonism at H$_1$ receptor and inverse agonism at H$_3$ receptor, stimulates histamine synthesis and release in tuberomammillary nuclei of the posterior hypothalamus (Arrang et al., 1985; Tighilet et al., 2002; Gbahou et al., 2010). On the one hand, only 10% of 281 obese participating to a multicenter randomized placebo controlled trial positively responded to the 12 weeks therapy with betahistine (Barak et al., 2008). On the other hand, betahistine was shown to limit the excess body weight induced by the antipsychotic drug olanzapine (**Table 1**) in a randomized, double blind placebo controlled pilot study involving 36 patients with either schizophrenia or schizoaffective disorders (Barak et al., 2016). In an earlier double blind placebo-controlled study that involved similar number of enrolled patients, betahistine potentiated the anorexic effect of the NET blocker reboxetine in patients receiving olanzapine (Poyurovsky et al., 2013).

Conclusions Regarding Monoamines and Obesity

The study of the mechanism of action of d-fenfluramine led to completely new drugs which is an interesting achievement. Additional data are warranted in the field of the control of energy balance and monoaminergic targets. The reduction of BMI in obese patients with lorcaserin is estimated in the range of 5–10%. This is less compared to the actions of previous drugs amphetamine, d-fenfluramine or sibutramine, but probably safer. Regarding antipsychotic drugs, newer antipsychotics (aripiprazole, cariprazine) display a lower affinity at H$_1$ receptor to prevent weight gain as recommended earlier (Kroeze et al., 2003). A summary has been indicated in **Table 3**.

FROM PATHOPHYSIOLOGY TO TREATMENTS

Parkinson's Disease
Historical Perspectives

PD is a neurological condition characterized by motor impairments including bradykinesia, tremor and rigidity

(Olanow et al., 2009). The symptoms are a consequence of the degeneration of the nigrostriatal DA tract and appear approximately when 30% of DA cells in the SNc are destroyed and/or when striatal tissue DA is reduced by 70% (Burke and O'Malley, 2013). Comorbid diseases are noticed with prevalence ranging from 30 to 45% in the case of anxiety or depression (McDonald et al., 2003). The etiology of the comorbid diseases is still unknown although other neuronal changes have been identified including alterations in 5-HT and NA neurons (Jellinger, 1991; Galati and Di Giovanni, 2010; Delaville et al., 2011). More generally, PD is a synucleopathy characterized histopathologically by the presence of Lewy bodies in multiple brain regions including the SNc and the LC. The lesions of LC NA neurons occur earlier than SNc DA neurons, and can reach a higher extent (Del Tredici et al., 2002; Rommelfanger and Weinshenker, 2007; Delaville et al., 2011). The loss of NA input to the nigrostriatal DA system could be detrimental for the function of DA neurons (Benarroch, 2009), conferring to NA system both a protective role on DA neurons and, consequently a positive influence regarding the outcome of treatments. However, available treatments mostly target DA and not NA-related mechanisms (**Table 4**).

The treatments of PD depend on the stage of the disease. L-DOPA was the first treatment aimed at restoring DA transmission in the brain. This amino acid can cross the blood brain barrier (BBB) and reach the striatum before conversion to DA by AADC. The first trials started in 1961 and L-DOPA still represents the main pharmacological treatment of PD (Lees et al., 2015). Years later it was followed by the administration of DA receptor agonists, and both treatments correspond to the so-called DA replacement therapy. Deep brain stimulation of the subthalamic nucleus is a second therapeutic option in advanced stages of the disease, where patients respond poorly to medication with motor complications and have no psychiatric antecedent (Bronstein et al., 2011). A commonly used option at the onset of the disease, which appears to have few unwanted side-effects, consists in administration of MAO-B inhibitors such as L-deprenyl or rasagiline (Rascol et al., 2011; Hauser et al., 2016).

While the side-effects are still debated in the case of deep brain stimulation of the subthalamic nucleus (Bronstein et al., 2011), long-term pharmacological treatments are associated with severe motor and psychiatric side effects (Bastide et al., 2015).

Mechanisms of Action of Antiparkinsonian Drugs

The therapeutic benefit of L-DOPA and DA receptor agonists has been related to their indirect and direct actions, respectively, at DA receptors. L-DOPA has been shown to enhance extracellular levels of DA in animal models of the disease, using *in vivo* methods or in humans indirectly measured by the displacement of PET ligands binding at DA receptors (de la Fuente-Fernández, 2013; De Deurwaerdère et al., 2016). Since the enzyme AADC is present in most tissues as well as in brain, much of the administered L-DOPA was converted at the periphery to DA, which does not cross the BBB. This problem was ameliorated by the introduction of benserazide or carbidopa, two peripheral AADC inhibitors that do not penetrate the brain

(Cotzias, 1968; Cotzias et al., 1969). The introduction of COMT inhibitors may also increase the efficacy of L-DOPA by limiting its transformation into 3-O-methyl-DOPA, and, perhaps, by limiting the inactivation of central DA (Ries et al., 2010). One of the main side effects of L-DOPA therapy, namely L-DOPA-induced dyskinesia, has been related to the variation of plasma L-DOPA concentrations inherent to its oral administration. The pharmacokinetic challenge is to find a means of smoothing its plasma concentrations. Similarly, a continuous stimulation of DA receptors with agonists is an important criterion, and selective agonists with long-lasting action have been recently synthesized (Butini et al., 2016).

No real progress has been made regarding the pharmacodynamics of L-DOPA: researchers attempted either to boost the ability of L-DOPA to release DA in the striatum during the 1980's and the 90's, or, more recently, to limit the excess of striatal DA release thereby reducing the occurrence of dyskinesia. The danger behind these strategies, which focused on a putative restoration of striatal DA release, magnified by the implantation of grafts aimed at releasing DA into the caudate-putamen of patients, is that nobody knows the extent to which striatal DA release is involved in the benefit and side-effects of peripheral L-DOPA (De Deurwaerdère et al., 2016). We now know that L-DOPA-induced dyskinesia and motor benefit can occur without a measurable enhancement of striatal DA release in animals (Porras et al., 2014), which confirmed earlier data raising doubt about the role of striatal DA in the mechanism of action of L-DOPA (Nakazato and Akiyama, 1989; Fisher et al., 2000).

In humans, the displacement of raclopride binding was observed after the intravenous administration of 3 mg/kg L-DOPA (de la Fuente-Fernández et al., 2004). The authors reported the displacement of ^{11}C-raclopride binding, but indicated also that the presumed levels of extracellular DA produced by the i.v. administration of L-DOPA were lower in patients compared to healthy individuals (de la Fuente-Fernández, 2013). A similar situation occurs in rodent models at comparative, but behaviorally efficacious dosage (Navailles et al., 2010). The conclusion is that the role of striatal DA release may have been overestimated in the benefit and possibly in some side-effects elicited by L-DOPA (De Deurwaerdère et al., 2016).

The overall picture is complicated by the fact that 5-HT neurons are mainly responsible for the release of DA induced by L-DOPA in animal models of the disease. The output of DA is dependent on the integrity of 5-HT neurons (Tanaka et al., 1999; Navailles et al., 2010). Due to the widespread innervation of 5-HT neurons in the brain, the first consequence is that L-DOPA-stimulated DA release occurs widely in the brain (Navailles et al., 2011b; Navailles and De Deurwaerdère, 2012a) (**Figure 4**), and this creates a new balance of central DA chemistry (Navailles and De Deurwaerdère, 2012b). The second consequence is that striatal DA released by L-DOPA is extremely low for at least three reasons: (i) the density of striatal 5-HT fibers is 10 to 20 times lower compared to the natural density of DA fibers; (ii) 5-HT neurons fire around 1 Hz or below and L-DOPA does not enhance the firing rate of 5-HT neurons (Miguelez et al., 2016b); DA neurons normally fire above 4 Hz (Bunney

TABLE 4 | Antiparkinsonian drug treatments and pharmacological target.

Pathophysiology	Drug in the market	Mechanism of action	Efficacy at pharmacological target
Degeneration of SNc DA neurons and striatal DA loss	L-DOPA DA receptor agonists	In part related to DA increase in the brain, possibly outside the striatum Stimulation of $D_{2/3}$ receptors	Unresolved Unresolved
Degeneration of LC NA neurons	None		
Degeneration of neurons—oxidative stress	MAO-B inhibitors (Rasagiline)	Unclear	Unresolved

The table represents brain alterations in Parkinson's disease and the drugs and/or strategies used against these alterations. The full spectrum of the mechanism of action of these drugs may have been misunderstood as no clear efficacy at pharmacological target has been achieved.

et al., 1973; Harden and Grace, 1995); (iii) the intraneuronal and neurochemical organization of striatal DA neurons (low metabolism, high rate of translocation into exocytotic vesicles) is specific to the DA terminals of the striatum and is not encountered in 5-HT terminals (De Deurwaerdère et al., 2016). The apparent higher magnitude of response to L-DOPA in the striatum compared to other brain regions simply corresponds to the stronger loss of clearance in the striatum due to the loss of DAT while the clearance of extracellular DA in extrastriatal regions is in part related to the NET (Navailles et al., 2014) (**Figure 4**).

The mechanism of action of L-DOPA is thus unclear and is likely different from DA agonists. Indeed, the efficacious agonists in the treatment of PD preferentially target the $D_{2/3}$ receptors whereas L-DOPA favors D_1 receptor-mediated mechanisms (Millan, 2010; Butini et al., 2016).

Amelioration of L-DOPA Therapy

There remains scope for improvement in several aspects of L-DOPA therapy in terms of motor side effects, mood disorders, psychiatric side-effects and the evolution of the disease.

It has been proposed that excessive swings of extracellular DA are involved in the dyskinesia induced by L-DOPA (Carta et al., 2007), although this might not occur in the striatum as previously claimed. This possibility is supported by the finding that drugs or conditions that are able to decrease 5-HT neuronal activity reduced L-DOPA-induced dyskinesia (Bastide et al., 2015; De Deurwaerdère et al., 2016). Indeed, the mixed 5-$HT_{1A/1B}$ receptor agonist, $5-HT_{2C}$ ligand, eltoprazine has been shown to reduce L-DOPA-induced dyskinesia in humans and animal models of the disease (Bezard et al., 2013; Svenningsson et al., 2015; Tronci et al., 2015). The efficacy of eltoprazine is not superior to existing treatment such as amantadine (Bezard and Carta, 2015). In terms of new strategies, particular attention has been given to $5-HT_{1A}$ receptor biased agonists, such as NLX-112, which acts preferentially at somatodendritic, rather than post-synaptic, $5-HT_{1A}$ receptors (Iderberg et al., 2015; McCreary et al., 2016). It has also been proposed that SSRIs lower L-DOPA-induced dyskinesia, as a result of their ability to indirectly reduce the firing rate of 5-HT neurons in the DRN (see above for the mechanism of action). The efficacy of SSRIs against L-DOPA-induced dyskinesia in humans is modest (Durif et al., 1995; Mazzucchi et al., 2015), and this is also found in animal models of PD (Fidalgo et al., 2015; Miguelez et al., 2016a).

Indeed, higher doses of SSRIs are required, compared to those effective in normal individuals. This may be due to the action of L-DOPA inside the 5-HT neurons, impairing their normal biochemical processes and altering 5-HT release (Miguelez et al., 2016b), thereby dampening the reactivity of 5-HT neurons to SSRIs administration (Miguelez et al., 2016a). Other strategies that have been tested include D_3 receptor antagonists or partial agonists (Bézard et al., 2003; Visanji et al., 2009). In addition to L-DOPA-induced dyskinesia, the D_3 receptor subtype remains an important target in the treatment of PD with $D_{2/3}$ receptor agonists (pramipexol, piribedil, ropinirole) (Millan, 2010; Leggio et al., 2016; Perez-Lloret and Rascol, 2016) being assessed in the management of impulsive-control disorder consequent to L-DOPA/DA receptor agonist administration (Seeman, 2015). Noradrenergic compounds have also been proposed to limit the occurrence of dyskinesia but the data are unclear (Delaville et al., 2011; Fox, 2013; Bhide et al., 2015; De Deurwaerdère et al., 2016).

The mechanism of action of L-DOPA toward 5-HT neurons also informs the therapeutic strategies for the mood disorders in PD, whose prevalence is higher compared to depressed individuals without PD (McDonald et al., 2003). Nowadays, the use of SSRIs remains a first line treatment in PD but, due to the specific action of L-DOPA on 5-HT neuron activity, the use of SSRIs might not be the best approach (Liu et al., 2013; De Deurwaerdère and Ding, 2016). Other strategies, based on the blockade of post-synaptic 5-HT or NA receptors, MAO-Is, SNRIs or DA receptor agonists, are available. An entire field of research has to be devoted to addressing this question, and also considering that the etiology of mood disorders in Parkinson's disease could be different from classical depression.

The psychotic side effects of DA agonists and L-DOPA have a high prevalence in advanced stage of the disease (Melamed et al., 1996). Historically, these effects have been associated with an excessive DA tone produced by L-DOPA or DA agonists. Interestingly, the $5-HT_{2A}$ receptor inverse agonist primavanserin has been shown to be effective in reducing L-DOPA-induced psychosis (Meltzer et al., 2010; Markham, 2016). It might replace the use of atypical antipsychotics quetiapine or clozapine (Friedman and Factor, 2000; Chang and Fox, 2016). The mechanisms behind the efficacy of primavanserin are, as yet, unclear.

Finally, MAO-B inhibitors L-deprenyl, safinamide, zonisamide or rasagiline have been shown to be efficacious in the treatment of PD either as unique treatment in the early

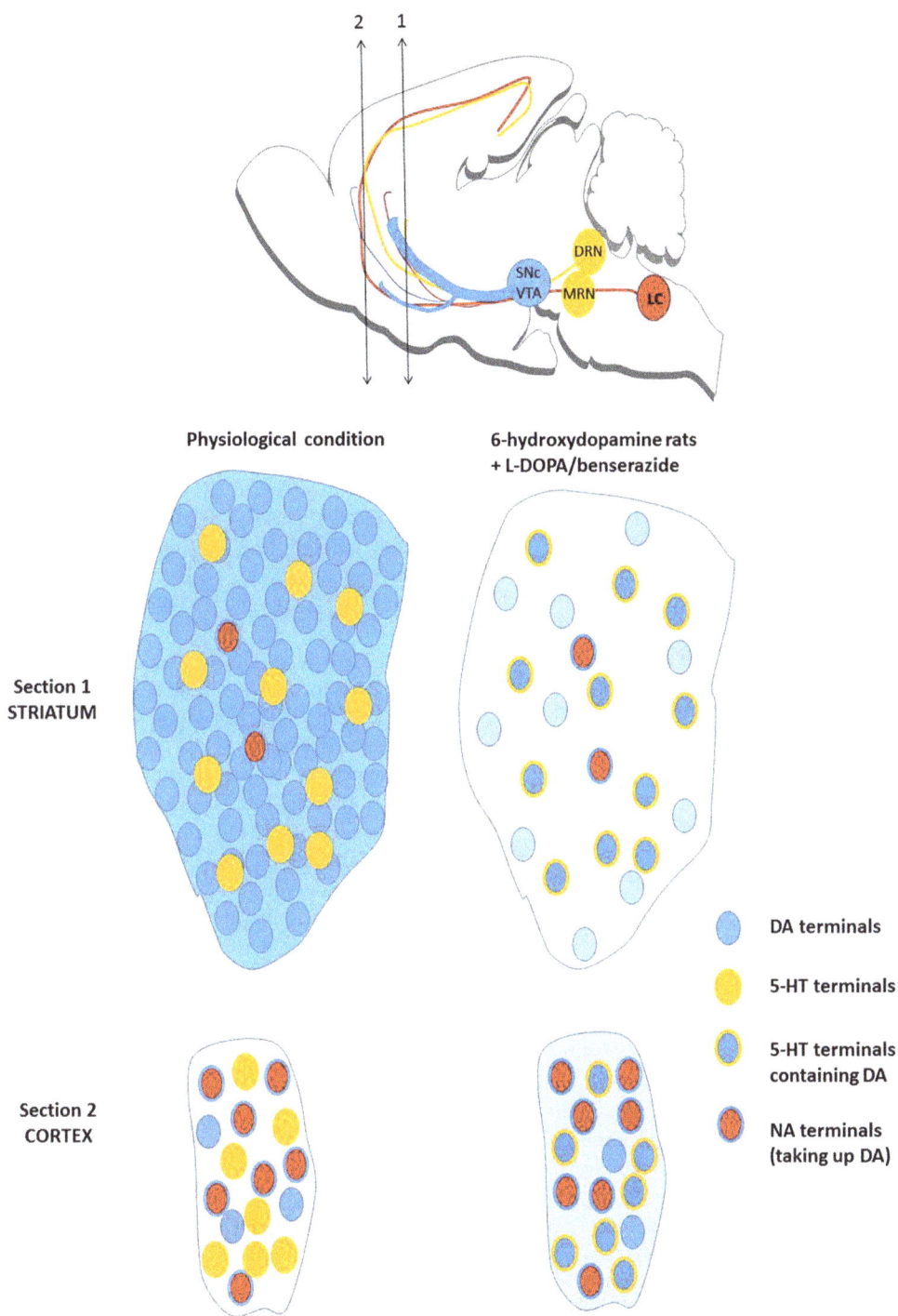

FIGURE 4 | Mechanisms of action of L-DOPA on brain DA release. The upper illustration recalls the origin of ascending fibers for monoamines. The lower displays the normal dopaminergic transmission in the striatum (very dense) and the prefrontal cortex (very low). It includes serotonergic and noradrenergic terminals with their relative density compared to DA terminals. In the 6-hydroxydopamine rat model of PD, the density of dopaminergic fibers drop to less than 10% of the normal situation and the increase in DA release induced by L-DOPA is mostly due to serotonergic terminals. DA reuptake by noradrenergic fibers is low in the striatum due to their poor density. The overall output of striatal DA induced by L-DOPA, identified in the figure by the blue background, is very low compared to the physiological situation without L-DOPA. In the prefrontal cortex, the overall output of DA induced by L-DOPA is higher compared to the physiological situation because the density of serotonergic terminals is higher than the natural density of dopaminergic terminals. The reuptake of DA by NA fibers is magnified in L-DOPA-treated animals. The situation described in the prefrontal cortex is also observed in the hippocampus or the substantia nigra pars reticulata (not shown here) and virtually in most brain regions (De Deurwaerdère and Di Giovanni, 2016; De Deurwaerdère et al., 2016).

stages of the disease or in conjunction with L-DOPA (Youdim et al., 2006; Riederer and Laux, 2011; Fox, 2013; Finberg, 2014). Since MAO-B is not primarily involved in the presynaptic inactivation of DA, it is possible that these compounds act at the glial level during L-DOPA therapy. In this context, L-DOPA has been shown to destroy 5-HT neurons upon chronic exposure in rodents (Navailles et al., 2011a; Stansley and Yamamoto, 2013, 2014), an effect related to an increase in metabolic stress which is blocked by antioxidant drugs including MAO-B inhibitors (Stansley and Yamamoto, 2014). The reduction of oxidative stress by MAO-B inhibitors might also reduce the destruction of DA neurons. MAO-B inhibitors of this type have also been shown to have antiapoptotic actions in a number of model systems (see (Youdim et al., 2006). Thus, the effects of these compounds in PD may be multifactorial.

Conclusion

The mechanisms behind the DA replacement therapy are unclear, because the mechanism of action of L-DOPA is still not understood in terms of its neurochemical effects, which differ from those of DA receptor agonists or MAO-B inhibitors (**Table 4** for a summary). Therefore, the antiparkinsonian agents do not work as it was initially thought and this could explain why no major progress in terms of pharmacodynamics has been made. In the case of L-DOPA, it will be necessary to determine the roles of DA and the brain location of its effects, in order to regionally control DA tone from 5-HT neurons (Navailles and De Deurwaerdère, 2012b; Navailles et al., 2015).

Several models using transgene animals or injection of viral constructs targeting proteins involved in the familial forms of the disease have been raised during recent years (Bezard and Przedborski, 2011). Although these models are still under pathophysiological examination, they might open new ways of treatments, even beyond monoamines.

Drug Addiction
Historical Perspective

The addictive properties of numerous drugs including alcohol and tobacco, the opiates (opium, morphine, heroin) and the psychostimulant drugs amphetamine and cocaine, were recognized before the existence and significance of the DA reward system in the brain was known. Studies of drug addiction received an increased impetus when the primary physiological target in the brain was thought to be determined, namely the DA neurons from the VTA innervating the nucleus accumbens. All drugs of abuse share similar neurobiological property, since they increase DA release in the nucleus accumbens that parallels the reinforcing properties of the drugs (Di Chiara and Imperato, 1988; Di Chiara, 1992; Koob, 1992). While the action of drug of abuse on DA neurons can be viewed as an initiating step, the addiction is a much more complex behavioral disturbance. It involves alterations of neurobiological and humoral mechanisms in sequential steps (Le Moal and Simon, 1991; Koob and Le Moal, 1997, 2008; Koob et al., 2014), and is marked by inter-individual differences, spreading drug addiction as a disease (Deroche-Gamonet et al., 2004; Ahmed, 2010). In spite of the numerous studies focusing on the activity of DA neurons as a possibility to

avoid relapse and to reduce drug intake, it is possible that DA transmission is no longer an appropriate target once addiction is established. At present, no DA drug is given to drug addicts although some substituted drugs targeting the DAT are developed (Hiranita et al., 2014) by analogy with methadone for opiates abuse.

Mechanism of Action

The mechanisms of action of drugs of abuse toward DA neuronal activity differ according to the drug of abuse, and most of them, classically, enhance DA outflow through an increase in impulse flow, whereas psychostimulants promote DA outflow independently from DA neuronal impulse. Gaetano Di Chiara's team has first demonstrated that this distinction was probably fundamental, in view of the control of DA neuronal activity and subsequent behavioral outcomes that can be expected from various targets, particularly 5-HT$_3$ receptors (Carboni et al., 1989). 5-HT$_3$ receptor antagonists counteracted place preference and the enhancement of DA release induced by drugs enhancing DA neuron firing rate. After that discovery (see De Deurwaerdère and Di Giovanni, 2016), 5-HT$_{2A}$ receptor antagonists were shown to counteract the non-exocytotic release of DA induced by amphetamine or 3,4-Methylenedioxymethamphetamine (ecstasy), whereas 5-HT$_{2C}$ receptor agonists inhibited the impulse-dependent release of DA. In parallel, behavioral data have shown that 5-HT$_{2C}$ receptor agonists and 5-HT$_{2A}$ receptor antagonists were capable of dampening the reinforcing properties, the craving and relapse, produced by drugs of abuse, in particular cocaine (Fletcher and Higgins, 2011; Higgins and Fletcher, 2015; Howell and Cunningham, 2015). However, the involvement of DA mechanisms in the benefit of these 5-HT compounds is far from clear, suggesting that the measurement of DA neuronal activity or release is not the most appropriate neurobiological marker of the anti-addictive behavior of therapeutic approaches (De Deurwaerdère and Di Giovanni, 2016).

Other monoaminergic approaches gave promising preclinical results, especially D$_3$ receptor antagonists (Leggio et al., 2016). A better determination of the involvement of other systems in addiction might lead to complete new treatment strategies.

DISEASES WITHOUT CURRENT MONOAMINERGIC TREATMENTS
Epilepsy

Epilepsy is characterized by seizures whose magnitude varies from almost undetectable to intense shaking. Sudden and unprovoked synchrony of bursts of neuronal hyperactivity can be "focal" if it remains confined to the area of origin, or "generalized." The origin of this condition is unknown even though genetic predisposition factors have been identified in some cases. Although it manifests as abnormal neuronal activity, it is possible that glial cells play a substantial role in triggering or maintaining this abnormality (Devinsky et al., 2013). Abnormal astrocytic function has been found in models of epilepsy, including the inability to maintain an appropriate extracellular milieu through different mechanisms (Coulter and Steinhäuser, 2015).

Monoaminergic drugs are not in the armamentarium of anti-epileptic drugs, although they have been the object of numerous articles. The monoamine enhancing antidepressant drugs were contraindicated in patients with epilepsy (Jobe and Browning, 2005). Nevertheless, antidepressants such as SNRIs or SSRIs were commonly prescribed to patients to reduce symptoms of comorbid depression and/or anxiety (Cardamone et al., 2013). Against the initial assumption, preclinical and human studies tend to indicate that SSRIs or SNRIs have an anticonvulsant profile, which can improve seizure outcomes (Cardamone et al., 2013). Moreover, SNRIs and SSRIs could limit the occurrence of seizures in depressed patients rather than increase them (Alper et al., 2007). Additional studies are warranted to evaluate the benefit of monoamine-based antidepressant drugs in clinical praxis (see Strac et al., 2016).

SSRIs and SNRIs, as discussed above, can promote numerous mechanisms other than a simple increase in extracellular monoamine levels (Dale et al., 2015). Indeed, one "pseudo-monoaminergic treatment," namely zonisamide, has received approval for the treatment of epilepsy (Bialer, 2012). Zonisamide interacts with human MAO-B, but not MAO-A (Binda et al., 2011). Similarly, L-deprenyl, the prototypical irreversible MAO-B inhibitor (Ramsay, 2013), has anticonvulsant and antiepileptogenic properties. The mechanisms triggered by these drugs are complex and likely not only related to MAO-B inhibition (Strac et al., 2016).

The roles of individual monoamines and their receptors have been the subject of many studies. To date, no specific target or a combination of specific targets has been approved for epilepsy. In the accompanying paper (Strac et al., 2016), we consider the potential interest of agonistic activity at 5-HT$_{2C}$/D$_2$/α$_2$-adrenergic receptors and antagonistic activity at H$_3$ receptors. It is intriguing that, after years of research, the favorable targets indicated from preclinical studies are those involved in tonic control of neurobiological networks and neuronal activity in the mammalian brain.

Alzheimer's Disease

The oldest of the various hypotheses, proposed in order to explain AD pathogenesis involves the cholinergic system (Sims et al., 1980). Others include the most comprehensive amyloid-β cascade (Karran et al., 2011), glutamate/calcium neurotoxicity (Karran et al., 2011), and hyperphosphorylated tau protein (Li et al., 2007). Recent studies have revealed an association of oxidative imbalance and stress with neuron degeneration (Guidi et al., 2006), and implicated nitric oxide and other reactive nitrogen species (McCann et al., 2005). Accordingly, in addition to the four clinically approved compounds (donepezil, rivastigmine, galantamine, and memantine), that target cholinergic and glutamatergic systems (Parsons et al., 2013), new approaches, focused on the prevention or decline of amyloid cascade events, formation of tangles, oxidative injury, and inflammation, have been proposed for the AD treatment (Ittner and Götz, 2011). It has been suggested that AD patients might benefit from multi-target medication, such as treatment with acetylcholinesterase inhibitors (AChEIs) in combination with memantine (Lopez et al., 2009).

As neuronal degeneration in AD also affects monoaminergic systems (Trillo et al., 2013), dopaminergic and serotonergic dysfunction has been also proposed to be involved (Martorana and Koch, 2014; Claeysen et al., 2015; Šimić et al., 2016), suggesting additional therapeutic targets for AD. Newly synthetized molecules with neuroprotective and multimodal mechanisms of action, currently in different phases of preclinical or clinical investigations (Dias and Viegas, 2014), act not only as AChEI and modulators of Aβ-aggregation (Tonelli et al., 2015), but also at voltage-dependent calcium channels (León and Marco-Contelles, 2011), MAO activity (Bautista-Aguilera et al., 2014), 5-HT$_3$ receptors (Fakhfouri et al., 2012) and N-methyl-D-aspartate (NMDA) receptors (Simoni et al., 2012).

Reduced DA levels in the brain (Storga et al., 1996), cerebrospinal fluid (CSF) (Tohgi et al., 1992) and urine (Liu et al., 2011), as well as lower brain levels of L-DOPA and DOPAC have been found in AD patients (Storga et al., 1996). Individuals with AD also exhibit reduced expression of DA receptors (Kumar and Patel, 2007), DAT, and TH (Joyce et al., 1997) in different brain regions. The COMT Val158Met polymorphism, which affects the COMT activity, has been associated with the risk of AD (Yan et al., 2016). The role of dopaminergic system in AD was confirmed by findings showing that L-DOPA (Martorana et al., 2009), the MAO-B inhibitor l-deprenyl (Filip and Kolibás, 1999), and the D$_2$ agonist rotigotine (Koch et al., 2014), have beneficial effects on cognitive functions in AD patients. The Aβ accumulation seems to be involved in dopaminergic dysfunction, contributing to the extrapyramidal deficits and rapid cognitive decline in AD patients (Preda et al., 2008). Inhibitors of COMT, like tolcapone, reduce Aβ aggregation by stabilizing its monomeric state (Di Giovanni et al., 2010), while the DA receptor agonist apomorphine promotes Aβ degradation and improves memory (Himeno et al., 2011). While most treatments in clinical trials tend to increase DA function, the antipsychotic drugs haloperidol and risperidone have reached the phase IV of clinical trials (Šimić et al., 2016).

Degeneration of NA neurons, observed in the early stages of AD, in mild cognitive impairment, and even in younger individuals with still normal cognitive function, indicates that alterations in noradrenergic system might precede Aβ deposition (Arai et al., 1992; Grudzien et al., 2007; Braak and Del Tredici, 2011). Lower levels of NA in CSF (Liu et al., 1991), TH in the brain, and DBH in the brain and plasma (Iversen et al., 1983; Mustapic et al., 2013) as well as decreased binding of α$_2$ adrenergic receptors (which inhibit the release of NA) in the brain are found in AD patients (Kalaria and Andorn, 1991; Pascual et al., 1992). However, some studies proposed compensatory mechanisms in AD resulting in increased levels of NA (Elrod et al., 1997; Peskind et al., 2005) and TH (Szot et al., 2006).

NA pharmacotherapy has been used primarily to treat different behavioral and psychological symptoms of dementia (BPSD). Propranolol was proposed for the treatment of aggression or agitation (Greendyke et al., 1986; Shankle et al., 1995), and imipramine for treatment of depression in AD

(Reifler et al., 1989). However, NA-enhancing therapy could be also used to treat cognitive impairments in patients with dementia. Combination of the NA prodrug L-DOPS and the NET inhibitor atomoxetine was shown to elevate NA levels, increase expression of brain-derived neurotrophic factor and different enzymes involved in Aβ degradation, resulting in improved spatial memory (Kalinin et al., 2012). Reboxetine is currently tested in clinic (Šimić et al., 2016).

Studies suggest that NA deficiency induces inflammatory response by elevating Aβ deposition and reducing microglial Aβ phagocytosis (Heneka et al., 2002, 2010), thus contributing to AD progression. Moreover, it appears that low DBH activity, associated with -1021C/T DBH regulatory polymorphism, increases the risk for AD in combination with interleukin 1 alpha polymorphisms (Mateo et al., 2006; Combarros et al., 2010). These findings suggest the potential of NA to slow down the neurodegeneration process by stimulating anti-inflammatory responses, microglial migration and phagocytosis, thereby contributing to Aβ clearance. Future studies should evaluate proposed anti-inflammatory and neuroprotective mechanisms of NA pharmacotherapy as therapeutic strategy in AD patients.

Lower number/activity of 5-HT neurons (Aletrino et al., 1992; Meltzer et al., 1998), as well as decreased concentration of 5-HT and its metabolites in the brain (Garcia-Alloza et al., 2005), CSF (Tohgi et al., 1992) and blood platelets (Muck-Seler et al., 2009) suggested a role of the serotonergic system in AD (Terry et al., 2008; Ramirez et al., 2014). A progressive decline in the density of different brain 5-HT receptors was observed in AD patients (Reynolds et al., 1995; Lai et al., 2003; Garcia-Alloza et al., 2004; Kepe et al., 2006; Lorke et al., 2006; Marner et al., 2012), sometimes correlating with the severity of cognitive impairment (Versijpt et al., 2003; Lai et al., 2005). Such changes in the serotonergic system could be also associated with BPSD (Lanari et al., 2006).

The association of 5-HT signaling with accumulation of Aβ plaques (Holm et al., 2010; Cirrito et al., 2011), and improvement in cognitive performance after treatment with 5-HT modulators (Payton et al., 2003; Geldenhuys and Van der Schyf, 2011; Ramirez et al., 2014), point to serotonergic system as a potential target for AD therapy. Both *in vivo* and *in vitro* studies demonstrated the potential of different agonists and/or antagonists of various 5-HT receptors for treating AD, including those affecting 5-HT$_{1A}$, 5-HT$_4$, and 5-HT$_6$ receptors (Meneses, 2013; Ramirez et al., 2014; Šimić et al., 2016; Werner and Covenas, 2016). The development of serotonergic medications which interact with multiple targets (Rezvani et al., 2009; Fakhfouri et al., 2015; Leiser et al., 2015; Stahl, 2015), could be a promising approach for AD treatment. The most advanced clinical trials focus on the 5-HT$_{1A}$ receptor agonists, tandospirone or buspirone, as well as citalopram (Šimić et al., 2016).

Multitarget drug design is also used, targeting enzymes involved in oxidative stress and inflammation, and these strategies are likely to interfere with monoamine tone. This research is presented in the next section.

Ischemic Stroke/Oxidative Stress

Stroke is a vascular disorder that constitutes the second leading cause of death worldwide with higher incidence in elderly people. Inflammation and oxidative stress, accumulated during human aging, negatively influence the vascular damage following a stroke incident (DiNapoli et al., 2008), and the immune system may contribute to the infarct progression (Iadecola and Anrather, 2011). Human brain is highly demanding of oxygen. It accounts for the 20% of the body oxygen consumption. This high demand of energy makes the brain highly dependent on cerebral blood supply and an organ especially susceptible to the deleterious effect of hypoxia. Two different types of stroke occur. Ischemic stroke that occurs in the blood vessels of the brain as a consequence of the formed clots, preventing oxygen arrival to the brain cells and inducing a hypoxic condition. About 80% of all strokes are ischemic. On the other hand, the hemorrhagic stroke occurs when a blood vessel in the brain breaks or ruptures as a consequence of high blood pressure or brain aneurysms, resulting in the blood seeping into the cerebral tissue, causing damage to the brain cells. Actually, the fact that a high percentage of patients having suffered stroke subsequently developed AD, indicates a strong link between these two pathologies. In this context, hypoxia and ischemic injury induce the up-regulation of beta secretase 1 (BACE-1) that increases the β-amyloid formation (Guglielmotto et al., 2009). Increasing evidence suggest that the neurovasculature plays an important role in the onset and progression of neurological disorders like AD (Zlokovic, 2008; Grammas, 2011; Marchesi, 2014). This has led to the concept of "neurovascular unit," integrated by neurons, astrocytes and vascular cells, which constitutes a functional unit able to maintain the homeostasis of the brain's microenvironment (Iadecola, 2010). Different amine oxidases are present in this "neurovascular unit" and they could play an important role under physiological and pathological conditions.

As discussed above, MAOs are involved in the metabolism of biogenic amines. MAO-Is provide additional benefits in neurologic disorders by reducing the formation of neurotoxic products such as hydrogen peroxide and aldehydes, which are derived from MAO activities. In neurodegeneration, MAO-I, especially those containing a propargylamine group, have been reported to possess multiple beneficial activities including neuroprotective, anti-apoptotic and antioxidant properties (Jenner, 2004; Sanz et al., 2004, 2008; Bar-Am et al., 2005).

Another amine oxidase present in cerebrovascular tissue, mainly in endothelial cells constituting the BBB, also plays a role in neurological disorders. Vascular adhesion protein 1 (VAP-1) is a homodimer glycoprotein with enzymatic function that binds leukocytes through its semicarbazide sensitive amine oxidase (SSAO) activity inducing inflammation (Smith et al., 1998; Jalkanen and Salmi, 2008). SSAO/VAP-1 metabolizes only primary amines producing aldehydes, hydrogen peroxide and ammonia, which are able to induce oxidative stress and cellular damage when overproduced (Yu and Deng, 1998). SSAO/VAP-1 is localized at the cell membrane and is released into blood as soluble form that is altered in several human pathologies (Kurkijärvi et al., 1998; Boomsma et al., 2003), including AD (Ferrer et al., 2002; del Mar Hernandez et al., 2005) and cerebral ischemia (Airas et al., 2008). The mediators that induce these alterations in the SSAO/VAP-1 levels are still unknown, but it is believed that increased SSAO/VAP-1 levels may contribute to the physiopathology of these diseases, thus constituting a potential therapeutic target (Conklin et al., 1998; Solé et al., 2008). Actually, human plasma SSAO activity is a strong predictor of parenchymal hemorrhages after tissue plasminogen activator (tPA) treatment in ischemic stroke patients (Hernandez-Guillamon et al., 2010), and plasma SSAO activity, which is also elevated in hemorrhagic stroke patients, predicts their neurological outcome (Hernandez-Guillamon et al., 2012). Considering all these data, SSAO/VAP-1 could mediate the link between stroke and the progression to AD through the alteration of the cerebrovascular function.

In spite of the different cellular localization of both MAO isoforms as well as SSAO/VAP-1, and their different substrate specificities, a cross-talk between these oxidases occurs. It has been described that MAO modulates the behavior of SSAO/VAP-1 (Fitzgerald and Tipton, 2002) and SSAO/VAP-1 may compensate in some extent the deficit in the oxidative deaminating capacity in situations where MAO activity is dysfunctional (Murphy et al., 1991).

Dynamic communication between cells of the neurovascular unit is required for normal brain functioning. The neurovascular unit consists of all major cellular components of the brain including neurons, astrocytes, brain endothelium, pericytes, vascular smooth muscle cells, microglia, and perivascular macrophages. In a situation of hemorrhagic stroke, an alteration of the homeostasis between all components of the neurovascular unit occurs, and the role of amine oxidases, especially the SSAO/VAP-1 activity is increased, contributing through its catalytic activity to the oxidative stress and inflammation (Hernandez-Guillamon et al., 2012). The neurovascular unit disruption may also alter the neuronal monoaminergic transmission. In this context, a pharmacological approach that is able to interact simultaneously with different amine oxidases might be a novel and more effective therapeutic approach (Solé et al., 2015; Sun et al., 2015). The close relationship between AD and stroke and the involvement of SSAO/VAP-1 in both diseases suggests that the synthesis and design of the new multitarget drugs, able to interact with different types of amine oxidases (MAO-A, MAO-B, and SSAO/VAP-1), could provide a useful therapeutic approach that is able to modulate the monoaminergic transmission, to protect the BBB, and hence avoid the progression of both neurological disorders. It should be noted that oxidative stress is recurring feature of several theories of the etiology of neurodegenerative diseases, which might be addressed by reducing hydrogen peroxide formation.

Concluding Remarks

Despite the progress made on the influence of monoamines in the three above-mentioned diseases, no monoamine-based treatments are available at present. In most cases, one emerging strategy would be the use of SSRI or MAO-Is, two approaches that are altering monoaminergic transmission throughout the brain rather than a specific monoaminergic drug targeting the injured tissue. In fact, there are two interconnecting issues: one addressing the regional origin of the disease, and the other addressing the functional consequences away from the dysfunctional site. Assuming that the benefit of antidepressant drugs like SSRI or MAO-I is related to the ultimate reorganization of neurobiological networks, their possible benefit could be related to actions away from the injured sites.

GENERAL CONCLUDING REMARKS

Monoaminergic drugs affect different processes in the brain that control the tone of neurotransmission or/and tissue excitability, and therefore should be studied as future targets for novel therapeutic approaches, not only for depression, but also for schizophrenia, addiction, obesity, PD, epilepsy, AD and stroke. This analysis acknowledges the Neuroscience based Nomenclature proposed by the IUPHAR which is based on the pharmacological profiles of psychotropic drugs rather than the clinical indication (Zohar et al., 2015). Common approaches involve the use of agents acting on monoaminergic transporters, D_2, D_3, $5\text{-HT}_{2B/2C}$, 5-HT_{1A}, 5-HT_{2A}, H_3, or α_2 receptors. All these targets, apart the 5-HT_{2A} receptor, exert widespread influences in the brain and alter multiple brain functions simultaneously. Thus, compounds affecting monoaminergic transmission have numerous consequences for the brain and its neurobiological networks. While researchers are aware that the symptomatic treatment of a disease results from multiple actions on the brain function, the linkages enabling a favorable reorganization of brain function after monoamine-based treatments are still not fully understood.

The search for effective targets in the treatment of brain diseases was facilitated by the serendipitous discoveries of compounds that were efficacious in schizophrenia, depression and obesity. Several new compounds have been developed that retain the original pharmacological targets involved in those therapeutic benefits combined with actions on new targets, identified from subsequent research, whilst aiming to minimize undesirable "off-target" actions. Knowledge of the monoaminergic mechanisms underlying drug efficacy led to the development of drugs with more specific mechanisms of action; lorcaserin, agomelatine, and vortioxetine are interesting achievements in this context. The identification of pathophysiological causes to tailor appropriate therapeutic approaches has been less successful. It has shown some success with PD but not with addiction to drug of abuse. Nonetheless, the failure to improve on current antiparkinsonian therapies confirms that the efficacy of these treatments is not simply related to a compensation of the loss of striatal DA. To some extent, the remarkable clinical success of L-DOPA was serendipitous. It is difficult to implement new monoaminergic treatment strategies in the clinic unless they depend on those currently accepted. This is exemplified by the third group of diseases where the progress regarding the involvement of monoamines in these diseases has not yet resulted in new monoamine-based treatments.

Current attempts to address the full spectrum of action of existing drugs can be improved. It is to be hoped that novel approaches, such as connectomics with polyomic research addressing brain functions, neurobiological networks, monoaminergic systems and their mutual interactions, might offer new perspectives and enhance the current state-of-the-art biological research in these psychiatric and neurological disorders.

AUTHOR CONTRIBUTIONS

All authors contributed to the conception and interpretation of the work and to its critical revision. All authors have approved the final version and may be held accountable for the integrity of this review of current literature.

ACKNOWLEDGMENTS

Support was kindly provided by the EU COST Action CM1103. GD kindly acknowledges MCST R&I 2013-014. PD acknowledges the "Fondation de France" and the Centre National de la Recherche Scientifique."

REFERENCES

Adell, A., Carceller, A., and Artigas, F. (1993). *In vivo* brain dialysis study of the somatodendritic release of serotonin in the Raphe nuclei of the rat: effects of 8-hydroxy-2-(di-n-propylamino)tetralin. *J. Neurochem.* 60, 1673–1681. doi: 10.1111/j.1471-4159.1993.tb13390.x

Ahles, A., and Engelhardt, S. (2014). Polymorphic variants of adrenoceptors: pharmacology, physiology, and role in disease. *Pharmacol. Rev.* 66, 598–637. doi: 10.1124/pr.113.008219

Ahmed, S. H. (2010). Validation crisis in animal models of drug addiction: beyond non-disordered drug use toward drug addiction. *Neurosci. Biobehav. Rev.* 35, 172–184. doi: 10.1016/j.neubiorev.2010.04.005

Airas, L., Lindsberg, P. J., Karjalainen-Lindsberg, M. L., Mononen, I., Kotisaari, K., Smith, D. J., et al. (2008). Vascular adhesion protein-1 in human ischaemic stroke. *Neuropathol. Appl. Neurobiol.* 34, 394–402. doi: 10.1111/j.1365-2990. 2007.00911.x

Aletrino, M. A., Vogels, O. J., Van Domburg, P. H., and Ten Donkelaar, H. J. (1992). Cell loss in the nucleus raphes dorsalis in Alzheimer's disease. *Neurobiol. Aging* 13, 461–468. doi: 10.1016/0197-4580(92)90073-7

Alper, K., Schwartz, K. A., Kolts, R. L., and Khan, A. (2007). Seizure incidence in psychopharmacological clinical trials: an analysis of Food and Drug Administration (FDA) summary basis of approval reports. *Biol. Psychiatry* 62, 345–354. doi: 10.1016/j.biopsych.2006.09.023

Andersson, K. E. (1980). Adrenoceptors–classification, activation and blockade by drugs. *Postgrad. Med. J.* 56(Suppl. 2), 7–16.

Arai, H., Ichimiya, Y., Kosaka, K., Moroji, T., and Iizuka, R. (1992). Neurotransmitter changes in early- and late-onset Alzheimer-type dementia. *Prog. Neuropsychopharmacol. Biol. Psychiatry* 16, 883–890. doi: 10.1016/0278-5846(92)90106-O

Arrang, J. M., Garbarg, M., Quach, T. T., Dam Trung Tuong, M., Yeramian, E., and Schwartz, J. C. (1985). Actions of betahistine at histamine receptors in the brain. *Eur. J. Pharmacol.* 111, 73–84. doi: 10.1016/0014-2999(85)90115-3

Artigas, F. (2013). Serotonin receptors involved in antidepressant effects. *Pharmacol. Ther.* 137, 119–131. doi: 10.1016/j.pharmthera.2012.09.006

Artigas, F. (2015). Developments in the field of antidepressants, where do we go now? *Eur. Neuropsychopharmacol.* 25, 657–670. doi: 10.1016/j.euroneuro.2013.04.013

Artigas, F., Nutt, D. J., and Shelton, R. (2002). Mechanism of action of antidepressants. *Psychopharmacol. Bull.* 36(Suppl. 2), 123–132.

Artigas, F., Romero, L., de Montigny, C., and Blier, P. (1996). Acceleration of the effect of selected antidepressant drugs in major depression by 5-HT1A antagonists. *Trends Neurosci.* 19, 378–383. doi: 10.1016/S0166-2236(96)10037-0

Ashby, C. R. Jr., and Wang, R. Y. (1996). Pharmacological actions of the atypical antipsychotic drug clozapine: a review. *Synapse* 24, 349–394.

Ban, T. A. (2001). Pharmacotherapy of depression: a historical analysis. *J. Neural Transm. (Vienna)* 108, 707–716. doi: 10.1007/s007020170047

Barak, N., Beck, Y., and Albeck, J. H. (2016). A randomized, double-blind, placebo-controlled pilot study of betahistine to counteract olanzapine-associated weight gain. *J. Clin. Psychopharmacol.* 36, 253–256. doi: 10.1097/JCP.0000000000000489

Barak, N., Greenway, F. L., Fujioka, K., Aronne, L. J., and Kushner, R. F. (2008). Effect of histaminergic manipulation on weight in obese adults: a randomized placebo controlled trial. *Int. J. Obes. (Lond).* 32, 1559–1565. doi: 10.1038/ijo.2008.135

Bar-Am, O., Weinreb, O., Amit, T., and Youdim, M. B. (2005). Regulation of Bcl-2 family proteins, neurotrophic factors, and APP processing in the neurorescue activity of propargylamine. *FASEB J.* 19, 1899–1901. doi: 10.1096/fj.05-3794fje

Barnes, N. M., and Sharp, T. (1999). A review of central 5-HT receptors and their function. *Neuropharmacology* 38, 1083–1152. doi: 10.1016/S0028-3908(99)00010-6

Bastide, M. F., Meissner, W. G., Picconi, B., Fasano, S., Fernagut, P. O., Feyder, M., et al. (2015). Pathophysiology of L-dopa-induced motor and non-motor complications in Parkinson's disease. *Prog. Neurobiol.* 132, 96–168. doi: 10.1016/j.pneurobio.2015.07.002

Bauer, M., Pretorius, H. W., Constant, E. L., Earley, W. R., Szamosi, J., and Brecher, M. (2009). Extended-release quetiapine as adjunct to an antidepressant in patients with major depressive disorder: results of a randomized, placebo-controlled, double-blind study. *J. Clin. Psychiatry* 70, 540–549. doi: 10.4088/JCP.08m04629

Bautista-Aguilera, O. M., Esteban, G., Chioua, M., Nikolic, K., Agbaba, D., Moraleda, I., et al. (2014). Multipotent cholinesterase/monoamine oxidase inhibitors for the treatment of Alzheimer's disease: design, synthesis, biochemical evaluation, ADMET, molecular modeling, and QSAR analysis of novel donepezil-pyridyl hybrids. *Drug Des. Devel. Ther.* 8, 1893–1910. doi: 10.2147/DDDT.S69258

Beaulieu, J. M., and Gainetdinov, R. R. (2011). The physiology, signaling, and pharmacology of dopamine receptors. *Pharmacol. Rev.* 63, 182–217. doi: 10.1124/pr.110.002642

Bel, N., and Artigas, F. (1992). Fluvoxamine preferentially increases extracellular 5-hydroxytryptamine in the raphe nuclei: an *in vivo* microdialysis study. *Eur. J. Pharmacol.* 229, 101–103. doi: 10.1016/0014-2999(92)90292-C

Benarroch, E. E. (2009). The locus ceruleus norepinephrine system: functional organization and potential clinical significance. *Neurology* 73, 1699–1704. doi: 10.1212/WNL.0b013e3181c2937c

Berman, R. M., Marcus, R. N., Swanink, R., McQuade, R. D., Carson, W. H., Corey-Lisle, P. K., et al. (2007). The efficacy and safety of aripiprazole as adjunctive therapy in major depressive disorder: a multicenter, randomized, double-blind, placebo-controlled study. *J. Clin. Psychiatry* 68, 843–853. doi: 10.4088/JCP.v68n0604

Bett, W. R. (1946). Benzedrine sulphate in clinical medicine; a survey of the literature. *Postgrad. Med. J.* 22, 205–218. doi: 10.1136/pgmj.22.250.205

Bezard, E., and Carta, M. (2015). Could the serotonin theory give rise to a treatment for levodopa-induced dyskinesia in Parkinson's disease? *Brain* 138(Pt 4), 829–830. doi: 10.1093/brain/awu407

Bézard, E., Ferry, S., Mach, U., Stark, H., Leriche, L., Boraud, T., et al. (2003). Attenuation of levodopa-induced dyskinesia by normalizing dopamine D3 receptor function. *Nat. Med.* 9, 762–767. doi: 10.1038/nm875

Bezard, E., and Przedborski, S. (2011). A tale on animal models of Parkinson's disease. *Mov. Disord.* 26, 993–1002. doi: 10.1002/mds.23696

Bezard, E., Tronci, E., Pioli, E. Y., Li, Q., Porras, G., Björklund, A., et al. (2013). Study of the antidyskinetic effect of eltoprazine in animal models of levodopa-induced dyskinesia. *Mov. Disord.* 28, 1088–1096. doi: 10.1002/mds.25366

Bhide, N., Lindenbach, D., Barnum, C. J., George, J. A., Surrena, M. A., and Bishop, C. (2015). Effects of the beta-adrenergic receptor antagonist Propranolol on dyskinesia and L-DOPA-induced striatal DA efflux in the hemi-parkinsonian rat. *J. Neurochem.* 134, 222–232. doi: 10.1111/jnc.13125

Bialer, M. (2012). Chemical properties of antiepileptic drugs (AEDs). *Adv. Drug Deliv. Rev.* 64, 887–895. doi: 10.1016/j.addr.2011.11.006

Binda, C., Aldeco, M., Mattevi, A., and Edmondson, D. E. (2011). Interactions of monoamine oxidases with the antiepileptic drug zonisamide: specificity of inhibition and structure of the human monoamine oxidase B complex. *J. Med. Chem.* 54, 909–912. doi: 10.1021/jm101359c

Blier, P., and de Montigny, C. (1990). Electrophysiological investigation of the adaptive response of the 5-HT system to the administration of 5-HT1A receptor agonists. *J. Cardiovasc. Pharmacol.* 15(Suppl. 7), S42–S48. doi: 10. 1097/00005344-199001001-00006

Blier, P., de Montigny, C., and Chaput, Y. (1990). A role for the serotonin system in the mechanism of action of antidepressant treatments: preclinical evidence. *J. Clin. Psychiatry* 51(Suppl), 14–20. discussion: 21.

Boomsma, F., Bhaggoe, U. M., van der Houwen, A. M., and van den Meiracker, A. H. (2003). Plasma semicarbazide-sensitive amine oxidase in human (patho)physiology. *Biochim. Biophys. Acta* 1647, 48–54. doi: 10.1016/S1570-9639(03)00047-5

Braak, H., and Del Tredici, K. (2011). The pathological process underlying Alzheimer's disease in individuals under thirty. *Acta Neuropathol.* 121, 171–181. doi: 10.1007/s00401-010-0789-4

Bronstein, J. M., Tagliati, M., Alterman, R. L., Lozano, A. M., Volkmann, J., Stefani, A., et al. (2011). Deep brain stimulation for Parkinson disease: an expert consensus and review of key issues. *Arch. Neurol.* 68, 165. doi: 10.1001/archneurol.2010.260

Brown, W. A., and Rosdolsky, M. (2015). The clinical discovery of imipramine. *Am. J. Psychiatry* 172, 426–429. doi: 10.1176/appi.ajp.2015.14101336

Buckley, P. F., Miller, B. J., Lehrer, D. S., and Castle, D. J. (2009). Psychiatric comorbidities and schizophrenia. *Schizophr. Bull.* 35, 383–402. doi: 10.1093/schbul/sbn135

Bunney, B. S., Aghajanian, G. K., and Roth, R. H. (1973). Comparison of effects of L-dopa, amphetamine and apomorphine on firing rate of rat dopaminergic neurones. *Nat. New Biol.* 245, 123–125. doi: 10.1038/newbio245123a0

Burke, R. E., and O'Malley, K. (2013). Axon degeneration in Parkinson's disease. *Exp. Neurol.* 246, 72–83. doi: 10.1016/j.expneurol.2012.01.011

Butini, S., Nikolic, K., Kassel, S., Brückmann, H., Filipic, S., Agbaba, D., et al. (2016). Polypharmacology of dopamine receptor ligands. *Prog. Neurobiol.* 142, 68–103. doi: 10.1016/j.pneurobio.2016.03.011

Carboni, E., Acquas, E., Frau, R., and Di Chiara, G. (1989). Differential inhibitory effects of a 5-HT3 antagonist on drug-induced stimulation of dopamine release. *Eur. J. Pharmacol.* 164, 515–519. doi: 10.1016/0014-2999(89)90259-8

Cardamone, L., Salzberg, M. R., O'Brien, T. J., and Jones, N. C. (2013). Antidepressant therapy in epilepsy: can treating the comorbidities affect the underlying disorder? *Br. J. Pharmacol.* 168, 1531–1554. doi: 10.1111/bph.12052

Carlsson, A., and Lindqvist, M. (1963). Effect of chlorpromazine or haloperidol on formation of 3-methoxytyramine and normetanephrine in mouse brain. *Acta Pharmacol. Toxicol. (Copenh.)* 20, 140–144. doi: 10.1111/j.1600-0773.1963.tb01730.x

Carruba, M. O., Mantegazza, P., Memo, M., Missale, C., Pizzi, M., and Spano, P. F. (1986). Peripheral and central mechanisms of action of serotoninergic anorectic drugs. *Appetite* 7(Suppl.), 105–113. doi: 10.1016/S0195-6663(86)80056-3

Carta, M., Carlsson, T., Kirik, D., and Björklund, A. (2007). Dopamine released from 5-HT terminals is the cause of L-DOPA-induced dyskinesia in parkinsonian rats. *Brain* 130(Pt 7), 1819–1833. doi: 10.1093/brain/awm082

Chang, A., and Fox, S. H. (2016). Psychosis in Parkinson's disease: epidemiology, pathophysiology, and management. *Drugs* 76, 1093–1118. doi: 10.1007/s40265-016-0600-5

Cipriani, A., Furukawa, T. A., Salanti, G., Geddes, J. R., Higgins, J. P., Churchill, R., et al. (2009). Comparative efficacy and acceptability of 12 new-generation antidepressants: a multiple-treatments meta-analysis. *Lancet* 373, 746–758. doi: 10.1016/S0140-6736(09)60046-5

Cirrito, J. R., Disabato, B. M., Restivo, J. L., Verges, D. K., Goebel, W. D., Sathyan, A., et al. (2011). Serotonin signaling is associated with lower amyloid-beta levels and plaques in transgenic mice and humans. *Proc. Natl. Acad. Sci. U.S.A.* 108, 14968–14973. doi: 10.1073/pnas.1107411108

Citrome, L. (2013). Cariprazine: chemistry, pharmacodynamics, pharmacokinetics, and metabolism, clinical efficacy, safety, and tolerability. *Expert Opin. Drug Metab. Toxicol.* 9, 193–206. doi: 10.1517/17425255.2013.759211

Citrome, L. (2015). The ABC's of dopamine receptor partial agonists - aripiprazole, brexpiprazole and cariprazine: the 15-min challenge to sort these agents out. *Int. J. Clin. Pract.* 69, 1211–1220. doi: 10.1111/ijcp.12752

Claeysen, S., Bockaert, J., and Giannoni, P. (2015). Serotonin: a new hope in Alzheimer's disease? *ACS Chem. Neurosci.* 6, 940–943. doi: 10.1021/acschemneuro.5b00135

Clineschmidt, B. V., and Lotti, V. J. (1973). Histamine: intraventricular injection suppresses ingestive behavior of the cat. *Arch. Int. Pharmacodyn. Ther.* 206, 288–298.

Combarros, O., Warden, D. R., Hammond, N., Cortina-Borja, M., Belbin, O., Lehmann, M. G., et al. (2010). The dopamine beta-hydroxylase -1021C/T polymorphism is associated with the risk of Alzheimer's disease in the Epistasis Project. *BMC Med. Genet.* 11:162. doi: 10.1186/1471-2350-11-162

Conklin, D. J., Langford, S. D., and Boor, P. J. (1998). Contribution of serum and cellular semicarbazide-sensitive amine oxidase to amine metabolism and cardiovascular toxicity. *Toxicol. Sci.* 46, 386–392. doi: 10.1093/toxsci/46.2.386

Cooper, J. R., Bloom, F. E., and Roth, R. H. (2003). *The Biochemical Basis of Neuropharmacology.* New York, NY: Oxford University Press.

Cotzias, G. C. (1968). L-Dopa for Parkinsonism. *N. Engl. J. Med.* 278, 630. doi: 10.1056/NEJM196803142781127

Cotzias, G. C., Papavasiliou, P. S., and Gellene, R. (1969). Modification of Parkinsonism–chronic treatment with L-dopa. *N. Engl. J. Med.* 280, 337–345. doi: 10.1056/NEJM196902132800701

Coulter, D. A., and Steinhäuser, C. (2015). Role of astrocytes in epilepsy. *Cold Spring Harb. Perspect. Med.* 5:a022434. doi: 10.1101/cshperspect.a022434

Cremers, T. I., Giorgetti, M., Bosker, F. J., Hogg, S., Arnt, J., Mørk, A., et al. (2004). Inactivation of 5-HT(2C) receptors potentiates consequences of serotonin reuptake blockade. *Neuropsychopharmacology* 29, 1782–1789. doi: 10.1038/sj.npp.1300474

Cremers, T. I., Rea, K., Bosker, F. J., Wikström, H. V., Hogg, S., Mørk, A., et al. (2007). Augmentation of SSRI effects on serotonin by 5-HT2C antagonists: mechanistic studies. *Neuropsychopharmacology* 32, 1550–1557. doi: 10.1038/sj.npp.1301287

Cryan, J. F., Page, M. E., and Lucki, I. (2002). Noradrenergic lesions differentially alter the antidepressant-like effects of reboxetine in a modified forced swim test. *Eur. J. Pharmacol.* 436, 197–205. doi: 10.1016/S0014-2999(01)01628-4

Cryan, J. F., Valentino, R. J., and Lucki, I. (2005). Assessing substrates underlying the behavioral effects of antidepressants using the modified rat forced swimming test. *Neurosci. Biobehav. Rev.* 29, 547–569. doi: 10.1016/j.neubiorev.2005.03.008

Curet, O., Damoiseau-Ovens, G., Sauvage, C., Sontag, N., Avenet, P., Depoortere, H., et al. (1998). Preclinical profile of befloxatone, a new reversible MAO-A inhibitor. *J. Affect. Disord.* 51, 287–303. doi: 10.1016/S0165-0327(98)00225-0

Dale, E., Bang-Andersen, B., and Sánchez, C. (2015). Emerging mechanisms and treatments for depression beyond SSRIs and SNRIs. *Biochem. Pharmacol.* 95, 81–97. doi: 10.1016/j.bcp.2015.03.011

Davidson, J. R. T. (2003). Pharmacotherapy of social phobia. *Acta Psychiatr. Scand. Suppl.* 108, 65–71. doi: 10.1034/j.1600-0447.108.s417.7.x

Daws, L. C. (2009). Unfaithful neurotransmitter transporters: focus on serotonin uptake and implications for antidepressant efficacy. *Pharmacol. Ther.* 121, 89–99. doi: 10.1016/j.pharmthera.2008.10.004

De Deurwaerdère, P. (2016). Cariprazine: new dopamine biased agonist for neuropsychiatric disorders. *Drugs Today* 52, 97–110. doi: 10.1358/dot.2016.52.2.2461868

De Deurwaerdère, P., and Di Giovanni, G. (2016). Serotonergic modulation of the activity of mesencephalic dopaminergic systems: therapeutic implications. *Prog. Neurobiol.* doi: 10.1016/j.pneurobio.2016.03.004. [Epub ahead of print].

De Deurwaerdère, P., Di Giovanni, G., and Millan, M. J. (2016). Expanding the repertoire of L-DOPA's actions: a comprehensive review of its functional neurochemistry. *Prog. Neurobiol.* doi: 10.1016/j.pneurobio.2016.07.002. [Epub ahead of print].

De Deurwaerdère, P., and Ding, Y. (2016). Antiparkinsonian treatment for depression in Parkinson's disease: are selective serotonin reuptake inhibitors recommended? *Transl. Neurosci. Clin.* 2, 138–149. doi: 10.18679/CN11-6030/R.2016.019

De Deurwaerdère, P., Lagière, M., Bosc, M., and Navailles, S. (2013). Multiple controls exerted by 5-HT2C receptors upon basal ganglia function: from physiology to pathophysiology. *Exp. Brain Res.* 230, 477–511. doi: 10.1007/s00221-013-3508-2

de la Fuente-Fernández, R. (2013). Imaging of dopamine in PD and implications for motor and neuropsychiatric manifestations of PD. *Front. Neurol.* 4:90. doi: 10.3389/fneur.2013.00090

de la Fuente-Fernández, R., Schulzer, M., Mak, E., Calne, D. B., and Stoessl, A. J. (2004). Presynaptic mechanisms of motor fluctuations in Parkinson's disease: a probabilistic model. *Brain* 127(Pt 4), 888–899. doi: 10.1093/brain/awh102

Delaville, C., Chetrit, J., Abdallah, K., Morin, S., Cardoit, L., De Deurwaerdère, P., et al. (2012). Emerging dysfunctions consequent to combined monoaminergic depletions in Parkinsonism. *Neurobiol. Dis.* 45, 763–773. doi: 10.1016/j.nbd.2011.10.023

Delaville, C., Deurwaerdère, P. D., and Benazzouz, A. (2011). Noradrenaline and Parkinson's disease. *Front. Syst. Neurosci.* 5:31. doi: 10.3389/fnsys.2011.00031

Delgado, P. L., and Moreno, F. A. (2000). Role of norepinephrine in depression. *J. Clin. Psychiatry* 61(Suppl. 1), 5–12.

del Mar Hernandez, M., Esteban, M., Szabo, P., Boada, M., and Unzeta, M. (2005). Human plasma semicarbazide sensitive amine oxidase (SSAO), beta-amyloid protein and aging. *Neurosci. Lett.* 384, 183–187. doi: 10.1016/j.neulet.2005.04.074

Del Tredici, K., Rüb, U., De Vos, R. A., Bohl, J. R., and Braak, H. (2002). Where does parkinson disease pathology begin in the brain? *J. Neuropathol. Exp. Neurol.* 61, 413–426. doi: 10.1093/jnen/61.5.413

Deroche-Gamonet, V., Belin, D., and Piazza, P. V. (2004). Evidence for addiction-like behavior in the rat. *Science* 305, 1014–1017. doi: 10.1126/science.1099020

Deutch, A. Y., Moghaddam, B., Innis, R. B., Krystal, J. H., Aghajanian, G. K., Bunney, B. S., et al. (1991). Mechanisms of action of atypical antipsychotic drugs. Implications for novel therapeutic strategies for schizophrenia. *Schizophr. Res* 4, 121–156. doi: 10.1016/0920-9964(91)90030-U

Devinsky, O., Vezzani, A., Najjar, S., De Lanerolle, N. C., and Rogawski, M. A. (2013). Glia and epilepsy: excitability and inflammation. *Trends Neurosci.* 36, 174–184. doi: 10.1016/j.tins.2012.11.008

Devroye, C., Cathala, A., Haddjeri, N., Rovera, R., Vallée, M., Drago, F., et al. (2016). Differential control of dopamine ascending pathways by serotonin2B receptor antagonists: new opportunities for the treatment of schizophrenia. *Neuropharmacology* 109, 59–68. doi: 10.1016/j.neuropharm.2016.05.024

Dias, K. S., and Viegas, C. Jr. (2014). Multi-target directed drugs: a modern approach for design of new drugs for the treatment of alzheimer's disease. *Curr. Neuropharmacol.* 12, 239–255. doi: 10.2174/1570159X1203140511153200

Di Chiara, G. (1992). Reinforcing drug seeking. *Trends Pharmacol. Sci.* 13, 428–429. doi: 10.1016/0165-6147(92)90135-S

Di Chiara, G., and Imperato, A. (1988). Drugs abused by humans preferentially increase synaptic dopamine concentrations in the mesolimbic system of freely moving rats. *Proc. Natl. Acad. Sci. U.S.A.* 85, 5274–5278. doi: 10.1073/pnas.85.14.5274

Di Chiara, G., Tanda, G. L., Frau, R., and Carboni, E. (1992). Heterologous monoamine reuptake: lack of transmitter specificity of neuron-specific carriers. *Neurochem. Int.* 20(Suppl.), 231s–235s.

Di Giovanni, G., and De Deurwaerdère, P. (2016). New therapeutic opportunities for 5-HT2C receptor ligands in neuropsychiatric disorders. *Pharmacol. Ther.* 157, 125–162. doi: 10.1016/j.pharmthera.2015.11.009

Di Giovanni, S., Eleuteri, S., Paleologou, K. E., Yin, G., Zweckstetter, M., Carrupt, P. A., et al. (2010). Entacapone and tolcapone, two catechol O-methyltransferase inhibitors, block fibril formation of alpha-synuclein and beta-amyloid and protect against amyloid-induced toxicity. *J. Biol. Chem.* 285, 14941–14954. doi: 10.1074/jbc.M109.080390

DiNapoli, V. A., Huber, J. D., Houser, K., Li, X., and Rosen, C. L. (2008). Early disruptions of the blood-brain barrier may contribute to exacerbated neuronal damage and prolonged functional recovery following stroke in aged rats. *Neurobiol. Aging* 29, 753–764. doi: 10.1016/j.neurobiolaging.2006.12.007

Durif, F., Vidailhet, M., Bonnet, A. M., Blin, J., and Agid, Y. (1995). Levodopa-induced dyskinesias are improved by fluoxetine. *Neurology* 45, 1855–1858. doi: 10.1212/WNL.45.10.1855

Ebadi, M., and Srinivasan, S. K. (1995). Pathogenesis, prevention, and treatment of neuroleptic-induced movement disorders. *Pharmacol. Rev.* 47, 575–604.

Eisenhofer, G., Kopin, I. J., and Goldstein, D. S. (2004). Catecholamine metabolism: a contemporary view with implications for physiology and medicine. *Pharmacol. Rev.* 56, 331–349. doi: 10.1124/pr.56.3.1

Elrod, R., Peskind, E. R., DiGiacomo, L., Brodkin, K. I., Veith, R. C., and Raskind, M. A. (1997). Effects of Alzheimer's disease severity on cerebrospinal fluid norepinephrine concentration. *Am. J. Psychiatry* 154, 25–30. doi: 10.1176/ajp.154.1.25

Emilien, G., Maloteaux, J. M., Geurts, M., Hoogenberg, K., and Cragg, S. (1999). Dopamine receptors–physiological understanding to therapeutic intervention potential. *Pharmacol. Ther.* 84, 133–156. doi: 10.1016/S0163-7258(99)00029-7

Esbenshade, T. A., Fox, G. B., and Cowart, M. D. (2006). Histamine H3 receptor antagonists: preclinical promise for treating obesity and cognitive disorders. *Mol. Interv.* 6, 77–88, 59. doi: 10.1124/mi.6.2.5

Fakhfouri, G., Mousavizadeh, K., Mehr, S. E., Dehpour, A. R., Zirak, M. R., Ghia, J. E., et al. (2015). From chemotherapy-induced emesis to neuroprotection: therapeutic opportunities for 5-HT3 receptor antagonists. *Mol. Neurobiol.* 52, 1670–1679. doi: 10.1007/s12035-014-8957-5

Fakhfouri, G., Rahimian, R., Ghia, J. E., Khan, W. I., and Dehpour, A. R. (2012). Impact of 5-HT(3) receptor antagonists on peripheral and central diseases. *Drug Discov. Today* 17, 741–747. doi: 10.1016/j.drudis.2012.02.009

Fangmann, P., Assion, H. J., Juckel, G., González, C. A., and López-Muñoz, F. (2008). Half a century of antidepressant drugs: on the clinical introduction of monoamine oxidase inhibitors, tricyclics, and tetracyclics. Part II: tricyclics and tetracyclics. *J. Clin. Psychopharmacol.* 28, 1–4. doi: 10.1097/jcp.0b013e3181627b60

Ferrer, I., Lizcano, J. M., Hernández, M., and Unzeta, M. (2002). Overexpression of semicarbazide sensitive amine oxidase in the cerebral blood vessels in patients with Alzheimer's disease and cerebral autosomal dominant arteriopathy with subcortical infarcts and leukoencephalopathy. *Neurosci. Lett.* 321, 21–24. doi: 10.1016/S0304-3940(01)02465-X

Fidalgo, C., Ko, W. K., Tronci, E., Li, Q., Stancampiano, R., Chuan, Q., et al. (2015). Effect of serotonin transporter blockade on L-DOPA-induced dyskinesia in animal models of Parkinson's disease. *Neuroscience* 298, 389–396. doi: 10.1016/j.neuroscience.2015.04.027

Filip, V., and Kolibás, E. (1999). Selegiline in the treatment of Alzheimer's disease: a long-term randomized placebo-controlled trial. Czech and Slovak Senile Dementia of Alzheimer type study group. *J. Psychiatry Neurosci.* 24, 234–243.

Finberg, J. P. (2014). Update on the pharmacology of selective inhibitors of MAO-A and MAO-B: focus on modulation of CNS monoamine neurotransmitter release. *Pharmacol. Ther.* 143, 133–152. doi: 10.1016/j.pharmthera.2014.02.010

Fisher, A., Biggs, C. S., Eradiri, O., and Starr, M. S. (2000). Dual effects of L-3,4-dihydroxyphenylalanine on aromatic L-amino acid decarboxylase, dopamine release and motor stimulation in the reserpine-treated rat: evidence that behaviour is dopamine independent. *Neuroscience* 95, 97–111. doi: 10.1016/S0306-4522(99)00406-6

Fitoussi, A., Dellu-Hagedorn, F., and De Deurwaerdère, P. (2013). Monoamines tissue content analysis reveals restricted and site-specific correlations in brain regions involved in cognition. *Neuroscience* 255, 233–245. doi: 10.1016/j.neuroscience.2013.09.059

Fitzgerald, D. H., and Tipton, K. F. (2002). Inhibition of monoamine oxidase modulates the behaviour of semicarbazide-sensitive amine oxidase (SSAO). *J. Neural Transm. (Vienna)* 109, 251–265. doi: 10.1007/s007020200021

Fletcher, P. J., and Higgins, G. A. (2011). "Serotonin and reward-related behaviour: focus on 5-HT2C receptors," in *5-HT2C Receptors in the Pathophysiology of CNS Disease*, eds G. Di Giovanni, E. Esposito, and V. Di Matteo (New York, NY: Springer), 293–324. doi: 10.1007/978-1-60761-941-3_15

Fornito, A., and Bullmore, E. T. (2015). Connectomics: a new paradigm for understanding brain disease. *Eur. Neuropsychopharmacol.* 25, 733–748. doi: 10.1016/j.euroneuro.2014.02.011

Fowler, J. S., MacGregor, R. R., Wolf, A. P., Arnett, C. D., Dewey, S. L., Schlyer, D., et al. (1987). Mapping human brain monoamine oxidase A and B with 11C-labeled suicide inactivators and PET. *Science* 235, 481–485. doi: 10.1126/science.3099392

Fox, S. H. (2013). Non-dopaminergic treatments for motor control in Parkinson's disease. *Drugs* 73, 1405–1415. doi: 10.1007/s40265-013-0105-4

Friedman, J. H., and Factor, S. A. (2000). Atypical antipsychotics in the treatment of drug-induced psychosis in Parkinson's disease. *Mov. Disord.* 15, 201–211. doi: 10.1002/1531-8257(200003)15:2<201::AID-MDS1001>3.0.CO;2-D

Gagnon, C., Schatz, R., Otten, U., and Thoenen, H. (1976). Synthesis, subcellular distribution and turnover of dopamine beta-hydroxylase in organ cultures of sympathetic ganglia and adrenal medullae. *J. Neurochem.* 27, 1083–1089. doi: 10.1111/j.1471-4159.1976.tb00312.x

Galati, S., and Di Giovanni, G. (2010). Neuroprotection in Parkinson's disease: a realistic goal? *CNS Neurosci. Ther.* 16, 327–329. doi: 10.1111/j.1755-5949.2010. 00206.x

Garattini, S. (1995). Biological actions of drugs affecting serotonin and eating. *Obes. Res.* 3(Suppl. 4), 463s–470s. doi: 10.1002/j.1550-8528.1995.tb00213.x

Garcia-Alloza, M., Gil-Bea, F. J., Diez-Ariza, M., Chen, C. P., Francis, P. T., Lasheras, B., et al. (2005). Cholinergic-serotonergic imbalance contributes to cognitive and behavioral symptoms in Alzheimer's disease. *Neuropsychologia* 43, 442–449. doi: 10.1016/j.neuropsychologia.2004.06.007

Garcia-Alloza, M., Hirst, W. D., Chen, C. P., Lasheras, B., Francis, P. T., and Ramírez, M. J. (2004). Differential involvement of 5-HT(1B/1D) and 5-HT6 receptors in cognitive and non-cognitive symptoms in Alzheimer's disease. *Neuropsychopharmacology* 29, 410–416. doi: 10.1038/sj.npp.1300330

Gardier, A. M., David, D. J., Jego, G., Przybylski, C., Jacquot, C., Durier, S., et al. (2003). Effects of chronic paroxetine treatment on dialysate serotonin in 5-HT1B receptor knockout mice. *J. Neurochem.* 86, 13–24. doi: 10.1046/j.1471-4159.2003.01827.x

Gbahou, F., Davenas, E., Morisset, S., and Arrang, J. M. (2010). Effects of betahistine at histamine H3 receptors: mixed inverse agonism/agonism *in vitro* and partial inverse agonism *in vivo. J. Pharmacol. Exp. Ther.* 334, 945–954. doi: 10.1124/jpet.110.168633

Geldenhuys, W. J., and Van der Schyf, C. J. (2011). Role of serotonin in Alzheimer's disease: a new therapeutic target? *CNS Drugs* 25, 765–781. doi: 10.2165/ 11590190-000000000-00000

Ghanemi, A., and Hu, X. (2015). Elements toward novel therapeutic targeting of the adrenergic system. *Neuropeptides* 49, 25–35. doi: 10.1016/j.npep.2014.11. 003

Grammas, P. (2011). Neurovascular dysfunction, inflammation and endothelial activation: implications for the pathogenesis of Alzheimer's disease. *J. Neuroinflammation* 8:26. doi: 10.1186/1742-2094-8-26

Greendyke, R. M., Kanter, D. R., Schuster, D. B., Verstreate, S., and Wootton, J. (1986). Propranolol treatment of assaultive patients with organic brain disease. A double-blind crossover, placebo-controlled study. *J. Nerv. Ment. Dis.* 174, 290–294. doi: 10.1097/00005053-198605000-00005

Grudzien, A., Shaw, P., Weintraub, S., Bigio, E., Mash, D. C., and Mesulam, M. M. (2007). Locus coeruleus neurofibrillary degeneration in aging, mild cognitive impairment and early Alzheimer's disease. *Neurobiol. Aging* 28, 327–335. doi: 10.1016/j.neurobiolaging.2006.02.007

Guglielmotto, M., Aragno, M., Autelli, R., Giliberto, L., Novo, E., Colombatto, S., et al. (2009). The up-regulation of BACE1 mediated by hypoxia and ischemic injury: role of oxidative stress and HIF1alpha. *J. Neurochem.* 108, 1045–1056. doi: 10.1111/j.1471-4159.2008.05858.x

Guiard, B. P., Froger, N., Hamon, M., Gardier, A. M., and Lanfumey, L. (2005). Sustained pharmacological blockade of NK1 substance P receptors causes functional desensitization of dorsal raphe 5-HT 1A autoreceptors in mice. *J. Neurochem.* 95, 1713–1723. doi: 10.1111/j.1471-4159.2005.03488.x

Guidi, I., Galimberti, D., Lonati, S., Novembrino, C., Bamonti, F., Tiriticco, M., et al. (2006). Oxidative imbalance in patients with mild cognitive impairment and Alzheimer's disease. *Neurobiol. Aging* 27, 262–269. doi: 10. 1016/j.neurobiolaging.2005.01.001

Gumnick, J. F., and Nemeroff, C. B. (2000). Problems with currently available antidepressants. *J. Clin. Psychiatry* 61(Suppl. 10), 5–15.

Gururajan, A., Clarke, G., Dinan, T. G., and Cryan, J. F. (2016). Molecular biomarkers of depression. *Neurosci. Biobehav. Rev.* 64, 101–133. doi: 10.1016/j. neubiorev.2016.02.011

Gustafson, A., King, C., and Rey, J. A. (2013). Lorcaserin (Belviq): A selective serotonin 5-HT2C agonist in the treatment of obesity. *P T* 38, 525–534.

Haefely, W., Burkard, W. P., Cesura, A. M., Kettler, R., Lorez, H. P., Martin, J. R., et al. (1992). Biochemistry and pharmacology of moclobemide, a prototype RIMA. *Psychopharmacology (Berl)* 106(Suppl.), S6–S14. doi: 10. 1007/BF02246225

Hale, M. W., and Lowry, C. A. (2011). Functional topography of midbrain and pontine serotonergic systems: implications for synaptic regulation of serotonergic circuits. *Psychopharmacology (Berl).* 213, 243–264. doi: 10.1007/ s00213-010-2089-z

Hamon, M., and Blier, P. (2013). Monoamine neurocircuitry in depression and strategies for new treatments. *Prog. Neuropsychopharmacol. Biol. Psychiatry* 45, 54–63. doi: 10.1016/j.pnpbp.2013.04.009

Han, C., Wang, S. M., Kato, M., Lee, S. J., Patkar, A. A., Masand, P. S., et al. (2013). Second-generation antipsychotics in the treatment of major depressive disorder: current evidence. *Expert Rev. Neurother.* 13, 851–870. doi: 10.1586/ 14737175.2013.811901

Harden, D. G., and Grace, A. A. (1995). Activation of dopamine cell firing by repeated L-DOPA administration to dopamine-depleted rats: its potential role in mediating the therapeutic response to L-DOPA treatment. *J. Neurosci.* 15, 6157–6166.

Haslam, D. (2016). Weight management in obesity - past and present. *Int. J. Clin. Pract.* 70, 206–217. doi: 10.1111/ijcp.12771

Hauser, R. A., Abler, V., Eyal, E., and Eliaz, R. E. (2016). Efficacy of rasagiline in early Parkinson's disease: a meta-analysis of data from the TEMPO and ADAGIO studies. *Int. J. Neurosci.* 126, 942–946. doi: 10.3109/00207454.2016. 1154552

Hawirko, L., and Sprague, P. H. (1946). Appetite-depressing drugs in obesity. *Can. Med. Assoc. J.* 54, 26–29.

Heneka, M. T., Galea, E., Gavriluyk, V., Dumitrescu-Ozimek, L., Daeschner, J., O'Banion, M. K., et al. (2002). Noradrenergic depletion potentiates beta - amyloid-induced cortical inflammation: implications for Alzheimer's disease. *J. Neurosci.* 22, 2434–2442.

Heneka, M. T., Nadrigny, F., Regen, T., Martinez-Hernandez, A., Dumitrescu-Ozimek, L., Terwel, D., et al. (2010). Locus ceruleus controls Alzheimer's disease pathology by modulating microglial functions through norepinephrine. *Proc. Natl. Acad. Sci. U.S.A.* 107, 6058–6063. doi: 10.1073/pnas.0909586107

Hensler, J. G., Artigas, F., Bortolozzi, A., Daws, L. C., De Deurwaerdère, P., Milan, L., et al. (2013). Catecholamine/Serotonin interactions: systems thinking for brain function and disease. *Adv. Pharmacol.* 68, 167–197. doi: 10.1016/B978-0-12-411512-5.00009-9

Hernandez-Guillamon, M., Garcia-Bonilla, L., Solé, M., Sosti, V., Parés, M., Campos, M., et al. (2010). Plasma VAP-1/SSAO activity predicts intracranial hemorrhages and adverse neurological outcome after tissue plasminogen activator treatment in stroke. *Stroke* 41, 1528–1535. doi: 10.1161/ STROKEAHA.110.584623

Hernandez-Guillamon, M., Solé, M., Delgado, P., García-Bonilla, L., Giralt, D., Boada, C., et al. (2012). VAP-1/SSAO plasma activity and brain expression in human hemorrhagic stroke. *Cerebrovasc. Dis.* 33, 55–63. doi: 10.1159/ 000333370

Higgins, G. A., and Fletcher, P. J. (2015). Therapeutic potential of 5-ht2c receptor agonists for addictive disorders. *ACS Chem. Neurosci.* 6, 1071–1088. doi: 10. 1021/acschemneuro.5b00025

Himeno, E., Ohyagi, Y., Ma, L., Nakamura, N., Miyoshi, K., Sakae, N., et al. (2011). Apomorphine treatment in Alzheimer mice promoting amyloid-beta degradation. *Ann. Neurol.* 69, 248–256. doi: 10.1002/ana.22319

Hiranita, T., Kohut, S. J., Soto, P. L., Tanda, G., Kopajtic, T. A., and Katz, J. L. (2014). Preclinical efficacy of N-substituted benztropine analogs as antagonists of methamphetamine self-administration in rats. *J. Pharmacol. Exp. Ther.* 348, 174–191. doi: 10.1124/jpet.113.208264

Holm, P., Ettrup, A., Klein, A. B., Santini, M. A., El-Sayed, M., Elvang, A. B., et al. (2010). Plaque deposition dependent decrease in 5-HT2A serotonin receptor in AbetaPPswe/PS1dE9 amyloid overexpressing mice. *J. Alzheimers. Dis.* 20, 1201–1213. doi: 10.3233/JAD-2010-100117

Howell, L. L., and Cunningham, K. A. (2015). Serotonin 5-HT2 receptor interactions with dopamine function: implications for therapeutics in cocaine use disorder. *Pharmacol. Rev.* 67, 176–197. doi: 10.1124/pr.114. 009514

Hoyer, D., Hannon, J. P., and Martin, G. R. (2002). Molecular, pharmacological and functional diversity of 5-HT receptors. *Pharmacol. Biochem. Behav.* 71, 533–554. doi: 10.1016/S0091-3057(01)00746-8

Iadecola, C. (2010). The overlap between neurodegenerative and vascular factors in the pathogenesis of dementia. *Acta Neuropathol.* 120, 287–296. doi: 10.1007/ s00401-010-0718-6

Iadecola, C., and Anrather, J. (2011). The immunology of stroke: from mechanisms to translation. *Nat. Med.* 17, 796–808. doi: 10.1038/nm.2399

Iderberg, H., McCreary, A. C., Varney, M. A., Kleven, M. S., Koek, W., Bardin, L., et al. (2015). NLX-112, a novel 5-HT1A receptor agonist for the treatment of L-DOPA-induced dyskinesia: Behavioral and neurochemical profile in rat. *Exp. Neurol.* 271, 335–350. doi: 10.1016/j.expneurol.2015.05.021

Invernizzi, R., Belli, S., and Samanin, R. (1992). Citalopram's ability to increase the extracellular concentrations of serotonin in the dorsal raphe prevents the drug's effect in the frontal cortex. *Brain Res.* 584, 322–324. doi: 10.1016/0006-8993(92)90914-U

Invernizzi, R., Bramante, M., and Samanin, R. (1996). Role of 5-HT1A receptors in the effects of acute chronic fluoxetine on extracellular serotonin in the frontal cortex. *Pharmacol. Biochem. Behav.* 54, 143–147. doi: 10.1016/0091-3057(95)02159-0

Ittner, L. M., and Götz, J. (2011). Amyloid-beta and tau–a toxic pas de deux in Alzheimer's disease. *Nat. Rev. Neurosci.* 12, 65–72. doi: 10.1038/nrn2967

Iversen, L. L., Rossor, M. N., Reynolds, G. P., Hills, R., Roth, M., Mountjoy, C. Q., et al. (1983). Loss of pigmented dopamine-beta-hydroxylase positive cells from locus coeruleus in senile dementia of Alzheimer's type. *Neurosci. Lett.* 39, 95–100. doi: 10.1016/0304-3940(83)90171-4

Jackson, H. C., Bearham, M. C., Hutchins, L. J., Mazurkiewicz, S. E., Needham, A. M., and Heal, D. J. (1997). Investigation of the mechanisms underlying the hypophagic effects of the 5-HT and noradrenaline reuptake inhibitor, sibutramine, in the rat. *Br. J. Pharmacol.* 121, 1613–1618. doi: 10.1038/sj.bjp.0701311

Jacquot, C., David, D. J., Gardier, A. M., and Sánchez, C. (2007). [Escitalopram and citalopram: the unexpected role of the R-enantiomer]. *Encephale* 33, 179–187. doi: 10.1016/S0013-7006(07)91548-1

Jalkanen, S., and Salmi, M. (2008). VAP-1 and CD73, endothelial cell surface enzymes in leukocyte extravasation. *Arterioscler. Thromb. Vasc. Biol.* 28, 18–26. doi: 10.1161/ATVBAHA.107.153130

James, W. P., Astrup, A., Finer, N., Hilsted, J., Kopelman, P., Rössner, S., et al. (2000). Effect of sibutramine on weight maintenance after weight loss: a randomised trial. STORM Study Group. Sibutramine trial of obesity reduction and maintenance. *Lancet* 356, 2119–2125. doi: 10.1016/S0140-6736(00)03491-7

Jellinger, K. A. (1991). Pathology of Parkinson's disease. Changes other than the nigrostriatal pathway. *Mol. Chem. Neuropathol.* 14, 153–197. doi: 10.1007/BF03159935

Jenner, P. (2004). Preclinical evidence for neuroprotection with monoamine oxidase-B inhibitors in Parkinson's disease. *Neurology* 63(7 Suppl 2), S13–S22. doi: 10.1212/wnl.63.7_suppl_2.s13

Jobe, P. C., and Browning, R. A. (2005). The serotonergic and noradrenergic effects of antidepressant drugs are anticonvulsant, not proconvulsant. *Epilepsy Behav.* 7, 602–619. doi: 10.1016/j.yebeh.2005.07.014

Joyce, J. N., Smutzer, G., Whitty, C. J., Myers, A., and Bannon, M. J. (1997). Differential modification of dopamine transporter and tyrosine hydroxylase mRNAs in midbrain of subjects with Parkinson's, Alzheimer's with parkinsonism, and Alzheimer's disease. *Mov. Disord.* 12, 885–897. doi: 10.1002/mds.870120609

Kalaria, R. N., and Andorn, A. C. (1991). Adrenergic receptors in aging and Alzheimer's disease: decreased alpha 2-receptors demonstrated by [3H]p-aminoclonidine binding in prefrontal cortex. *Neurobiol. Aging* 12, 131–136. doi: 10.1016/0197-4580(91)90051-K

Kalinin, S., Polak, P. E., Lin, S. X., Sakharkar, A. J., Pandey, S. C., and Feinstein, D. L. (2012). The noradrenaline precursor L-DOPS reduces pathology in a mouse model of Alzheimer's disease. *Neurobiol. Aging* 33, 1651–1663. doi: 10.1016/j.neurobiolaging.2011.04.012

Kapur, S., and Remington, G. (1996). Serotonin-dopamine interaction and its relevance to schizophrenia. *Am. J. Psychiatry* 153, 466–476. doi: 10.1176/ajp.153.4.466

Kapur, S., and Seeman, P. (2001). Does fast dissociation from the dopamine d(2) receptor explain the action of atypical antipsychotics?: A new hypothesis. *Am. J. Psychiatry* 158, 360–369. doi: 10.1176/appi.ajp.158.3.360

Karran, E., Mercken, M., and De Strooper, B. (2011). The amyloid cascade hypothesis for Alzheimer's disease: an appraisal for the development of therapeutics. *Nat. Rev. Drug Discov.* 10, 698–712. doi: 10.1038/nrd3505

Kasper, S., Corruble, E., Hale, A., Lemoine, P., Montgomery, S. A., and Quera-Salva, M. A. (2013). Antidepressant efficacy of agomelatine versus SSRI/SNRI: results from a pooled analysis of head-to-head studies without a placebo control. *Int. Clin. Psychopharmacol.* 28, 12–19. doi: 10.1097/YIC.0b013e328359768e

Kepe, V., Barrio, J. R., Huang, S. C., Ercoli, L., Siddarth, P., Shoghi-Jadid, K., et al. (2006). Serotonin 1A receptors in the living brain of Alzheimer's disease patients. *Proc. Natl. Acad. Sci. U.S.A.* 103, 702–707. doi: 10.1073/pnas.0510237103

Kiloh, L. G., and Brandon, S. (1962). Habituation and addiction to amphetamines. *Br. Med. J.* 2, 40–43. doi: 10.1136/bmj.2.5296.40

Kiss, B., Horváth, A., Némethy, Z., Schmidt, E., Laszlovszky, I., Bugovics, G., et al. (2010). Cariprazine (RGH-188), a dopamine D(3) receptor-preferring, D(3)/D(2) dopamine receptor antagonist-partial agonist antipsychotic candidate: *in vitro* and neurochemical profile. *J. Pharmacol. Exp. Ther.* 333, 328–340. doi: 10.1124/jpet.109.160432

Koch, G., Di Lorenzo, F., Bonnì, S., Giacobbe, V., Bozzali, M., Caltagirone, C., et al. (2014). Dopaminergic modulation of cortical plasticity in Alzheimer's disease patients. *Neuropsychopharmacology* 39, 2654–2661. doi: 10.1038/npp.2014.119

Koob, G. F. (1992). Drugs of abuse: anatomy, pharmacology and function of reward pathways. *Trends Pharmacol. Sci.* 13, 177–184. doi: 10.1016/0165-6147(92)90060-J

Koob, G. F., Buck, C. L., Cohen, A., Edwards, S., Park, P. E., Schlosburg, J. E., et al. (2014). Addiction as a stress surfeit disorder. *Neuropharmacology* 76(Pt B), 370–382. doi: 10.1016/j.neuropharm.2013.05.024

Koob, G. F., and Le Moal, M. (1997). Drug abuse: hedonic homeostatic dysregulation. *Science* 278, 52–58. doi: 10.1126/science.278.5335.52

Koob, G. F., and Le Moal, M. (2008). Review. Neurobiological mechanisms for opponent motivational processes in addiction. *Philos. Trans. R. Soc. Lond. B. Biol. Sci.* 363, 3113–3123. doi: 10.1098/rstb.2008.0094

Kroeze, W. K., Hufeisen, S. J., Popadak, B. A., Renock, S. M., Steinberg, S., Ernsberger, P., et al. (2003). H1-histamine receptor affinity predicts short-term weight gain for typical and atypical antipsychotic drugs. *Neuropsychopharmacology* 28, 519–526. doi: 10.1038/sj.npp.1300027

Kuczenski, R., Segal, D. S., Cho, A. K., and Melega, W. (1995). Hippocampus norepinephrine, caudate dopamine and serotonin, and behavioral responses to the stereoisomers of amphetamine and methamphetamine. *J. Neurosci.* 15, 1308–1317.

Kumar, U., and Patel, S. C. (2007). Immunohistochemical localization of dopamine receptor subtypes (D1R-D5R) in Alzheimer's disease brain. *Brain Res.* 1131, 187–196. doi: 10.1016/j.brainres.2006.10.049

Kurkijärvi, R., Adams, D. H., Leino, R., Möttönen, T., Jalkanen, S., and Salmi, M. (1998). Circulating form of human vascular adhesion protein-1 (VAP-1): increased serum levels in inflammatory liver diseases. *J. Immunol.* 161, 1549–1557.

Lai, M. K., Tsang, S. W., Alder, J. T., Keene, J., Hope, T., Esiri, M. M., et al. (2005). Loss of serotonin 5-HT2A receptors in the postmortem temporal cortex correlates with rate of cognitive decline in Alzheimer's disease. *Psychopharmacology (Berl).* 179, 673–677. doi: 10.1007/s00213-004-2077-2

Lai, M. K., Tsang, S. W., Francis, P. T., Esiri, M. M., Hope, T., Lai, O. F., et al. (2003). [3H]GR113808 binding to serotonin 5-HT4 receptors in the postmortem neocortex of Alzheimer disease: a clinicopathological study. *J. Neural Transm. (Vienna)* 110, 779–788. doi: 10.1007/s00702-003-0825-9

Lanari, A., Amenta, F., Silvestrelli, G., Tomassoni, D., and Parnetti, L. (2006). Neurotransmitter deficits in behavioural and psychological symptoms of Alzheimer's disease. *Mech. Ageing Dev.* 127, 158–165. doi: 10.1016/j.mad.2005.09.016

Lecklin, A., Etu-Seppälä, P., Stark, H., and Tuomisto, L. (1998). Effects of intracerebroventricularly infused histamine and selective H1, H2 and H3 agonists on food and water intake and urine flow in Wistar rats. *Brain Res.* 793, 279–288. doi: 10.1016/S0006-8993(98)00186-3

Lees, A. J., Tolosa, E., and Olanow, C. W. (2015). Four pioneers of L-dopa treatment: Arvid Carlsson, Oleh Hornykiewicz, George Cotzias, and Melvin Yahr. *Mov. Disord.* 30, 19–36. doi: 10.1002/mds.26120

Leggio, G. M., Bucolo, C., Platania, C. B. M., Salomone, S., and Drago, F. (2016). Current drug treatments targeting dopamine D3 receptor. *Pharmacol. Ther.* 165, 164–177. doi: 10.1016/j.pharmthera.2016.06.007

Leiser, S. C., Li, Y., Pehrson, A. L., Dale, E., Smagin, G., and Sanchez, C. (2015). Serotonergic regulation of prefrontal cortical circuitries involved in cognitive processing: a review of individual 5-HT receptor mechanisms and concerted effects of 5-HT receptors exemplified by the multimodal antidepressant vortioxetine. ACS Chem. Neurosci. 6, 970–986. doi: 10.1021/cn500340j

Le Moal, M., and Simon, H. (1991). Mesocorticolimbic dopaminergic network: functional and regulatory roles. Physiol. Rev. 71, 155–234.

León, R., and Marco-Contelles, J. (2011). A step further towards multitarget drugs for Alzheimer and neuronal vascular diseases: targeting the cholinergic system, amyloid-beta aggregation and Ca(2+) dyshomeostasis. Curr. Med. Chem. 18, 552–576. doi: 10.2174/092986711794480186

Li, G., Sokal, I., Quinn, J. F., Leverenz, J. B., Brodey, M., Schellenberg, G. D., et al. (2007). CSF tau/Abeta42 ratio for increased risk of mild cognitive impairment: a follow-up study. Neurology 69, 631–639. doi: 10.1212/01.wnl.0000267428.62582.aa

Liu, H., Yang, J. C., Chang, Y. F., Liu, T. Y., and Chi, C. W. (1991). Analysis of monoamines in the cerebrospinal fluid of Chinese patients with Alzheimer's disease. Ann. N. Y. Acad. Sci. 640, 215–218. doi: 10.1111/j.1749-6632.1991.tb00220.x

Liu, J., Dong, J., Wang, L., Su, Y., Yan, P., and Sun, S. (2013). Comparative efficacy and acceptability of antidepressants in Parkinson's disease: a network meta-analysis. PLoS ONE 8:e76651. doi: 10.1371/journal.pone.0076651

Liu, L., Li, Q., Li, N., Ling, J., Liu, R., Wang, Y., et al. (2011). Simultaneous determination of catecholamines and their metabolites related to Alzheimer's disease in human urine. J. Sep. Sci. 34, 1198–1204. doi: 10.1002/jssc.201000799

Lopez, O. L., Becker, J. T., Wahed, A. S., Saxton, J., Sweet, R. A., Wolk, D. A., et al. (2009). Long-term effects of the concomitant use of memantine with cholinesterase inhibition in Alzheimer disease. J. Neurol. Neurosurg. Psychiatr. 80, 600–607. doi: 10.1136/jnnp.2008.158964

López-Muñoz, F., and Alamo, C. (2009). Monoaminergic neurotransmission: the history of the discovery of antidepressants from 1950s until today. Curr. Pharm. Des. 15, 1563–1586. doi: 10.2174/138161209788168001

López-Muñoz, F., Alamo, C., Cuenca, E., Shen, W. W., Clervoy, P., and Rubio, G. (2005). History of the discovery and clinical introduction of chlorpromazine. Ann. Clin. Psychiatry 17, 113–135. doi: 10.1080/10401230591002002

Lorke, D. E., Lu, G., Cho, E., and Yew, D. T. (2006). Serotonin 5-HT2A and 5-HT6 receptors in the prefrontal cortex of Alzheimer and normal aging patients. BMC Neurosci. 7:36. doi: 10.1186/1471-2202-7-36

Lucas, G., and Debonnel, G. (2002). 5-HT4 receptors exert a frequency-related facilitatory control on dorsal raphe nucleus 5-HT neuronal activity. Eur. J. Neurosci. 16, 817–822. doi: 10.1046/j.1460-9568.2002.02150.x

Lucas, G., Rymar, V. V., Du, J., Mnie-Filali, O., Bisgaard, C., Manta, S., et al. (2007). Serotonin(4) (5-HT(4)) receptor agonists are putative antidepressants with a rapid onset of action. Neuron 55, 712–725. doi: 10.1016/j.neuron.2007.07.041

Luque, C. A., and Rey, J. A. (1999). Sibutramine: a serotonin-norepinephrine reuptake-inhibitor for the treatment of obesity. Ann. Pharmacother. 33, 968–978. doi: 10.1345/aph.18319

Luscombe, G. P., Slater, N. A., Lyons, M. B., Wynne, R. D., Scheinbaum, M. L., and Buckett, W. R. (1990). Effect on radiolabelled-monoamine uptake in vitro of plasma taken from healthy volunteers administered the antidepressant sibutramine HCl. Psychopharmacology (Berl). 100, 345–349. doi: 10.1007/BF02244604

Marchesi, V. T. (2014). Alzheimer's disease and CADASIL are heritable, adult-onset dementias that both involve damaged small blood vessels. Cell. Mol. Life Sci. 71, 949–955. doi: 10.1007/s00018-013-1542-7

Markham, A. (2016). Pimavanserin: first global approval. Drugs 76, 1053–1057. doi: 10.1007/s40265-016-0597-9

Marner, L., Frokjaer, V. G., Kalbitzer, J., Lehel, S., Madsen, K., Baare, W. F., et al. (2012). Loss of serotonin 2A receptors exceeds loss of serotonergic projections in early Alzheimer's disease: a combined [11C]DASB and [18F]altanserin-PET study. Neurobiol. Aging 33, 479–487. doi: 10.1016/j.neurobiolaging.2010.03.023

Martorana, A., and Koch, G. (2014). "Is dopamine involved in Alzheimer's disease?". Front. Aging Neurosci. 6:252. doi: 10.3389/fnagi.2014.00252

Martorana, A., Mori, F., Esposito, Z., Kusayanagi, H., Monteleone, F., Codecà, C., et al. (2009). Dopamine modulates cholinergic cortical excitability in Alzheimer's disease patients. Neuropsychopharmacology 34, 2323–2328. doi: 10.1038/npp.2009.60

Masaki, T., Chiba, S., Yasuda, T., Noguchi, H., Kakuma, T., Watanabe, T., et al. (2004). Involvement of hypothalamic histamine H1 receptor in the regulation of feeding rhythm and obesity. Diabetes 53, 2250–2260. doi: 10.2337/diabetes.53.9.2250

Mateo, I., Infante, J., Rodríguez, E., Berciano, J., Combarros, O., and Llorca, J. (2006). Interaction between dopamine beta-hydroxylase and interleukin genes increases Alzheimer's disease risk. J. Neurol. Neurosurg. Psychiatr. 77, 278–279. doi: 10.1136/jnnp.2005.075358

Mauri, M. C., Paletta, S., Maffini, M., Colasanti, A., Dragogna, F., Di Pace, C., et al. (2014). Clinical pharmacology of atypical antipsychotics: an update. EXCLI J. 13, 1163–1191.

Mazzucchi, S., Frosini, D., Ripoli, A., Nicoletti, V., Linsalata, G., Bonuccelli, U., et al. (2015). Serotonergic antidepressant drugs and L-dopa-induced dyskinesias in Parkinson's disease. Acta Neurol. Scand. 131, 191–195. doi: 10.1111/ane.12314

McCann, S. M., Mastronardi, C., de Laurentiis, A., and Rettori, V. (2005). The nitric oxide theory of aging revisited. Ann. N. Y. Acad. Sci. 1057, 64–84. doi: 10.1196/annals.1356.064

McCreary, A. C., Varney, M. A., and Newman-Tancredi, A. (2016). The novel 5-HT1A receptor agonist, NLX-112 reduces L-DOPA-induced abnormal involuntary movements in rat: a chronic administration study with microdialysis measurements. Neuropharmacology 105, 651–660. doi: 10.1016/j.neuropharm.2016.01.013

McDonald, W. M., Richard, I. H., and DeLong, M. R. (2003). Prevalence, etiology, and treatment of depression in Parkinson's disease. Biol. Psychiatry 54, 363–375. doi: 10.1016/S0006-3223(03)00530-4

Melamed, E., Zoldan, J., Friedberg, G., Ziv, I., and Weizmann, A. (1996). Involvement of serotonin in clinical features of Parkinson's disease and complications of L-DOPA therapy. Adv. Neurol. 69, 545–550.

Meltzer, C. C., Smith, G., DeKosky, S. T., Pollock, B. G., Mathis, C. A., Moore, R. Y., et al. (1998). Serotonin in aging, late-life depression, and Alzheimer's disease: the emerging role of functional imaging. Neuropsychopharmacology 18, 407–430. doi: 10.1016/S0893-133X(97)00194-2

Meltzer, H. Y. (1993). New drugs for the treatment of schizophrenia. Psychiatr. Clin. North Am. 16, 365–385.

Meltzer, H. Y. (1999). Treatment of schizophrenia and spectrum disorders: pharmacotherapy, psychosocial treatments, and neurotransmitter interactions. Biol. Psychiatry 46, 1321–1327. doi: 10.1016/S0006-3223(99)00255-3

Meltzer, H. Y., and Huang, M. (2008). In vivo actions of atypical antipsychotic drug on serotonergic and dopaminergic systems. Prog. Brain Res. 172, 177–197. doi: 10.1016/S0079-6123(08)00909-6

Meltzer, H. Y., and Massey, B. W. (2011). The role of serotonin receptors in the action of atypical antipsychotic drugs. Curr. Opin. Pharmacol. 11, 59–67. doi: 10.1016/j.coph.2011.02.007

Meltzer, H. Y., Matsubara, S., and Lee, J. C. (1989a). Classification of typical and atypical antipsychotic drugs on the basis of dopamine D-1, D-2 and serotonin2 pKi values. J. Pharmacol. Exp. Ther. 251, 238–246.

Meltzer, H. Y., Matsubara, S., and Lee, J. C. (1989b). The ratios of serotonin2 and dopamine2 affinities differentiate atypical and typical antipsychotic drugs. Psychopharmacol. Bull. 25, 390–392.

Meltzer, H. Y., Mills, R., Revell, S., Williams, H., Johnson, A., Bahr, D., et al. (2010). Pimavanserin, a serotonin(2A) receptor inverse agonist, for the treatment of parkinson's disease psychosis. Neuropsychopharmacology 35, 881–892. doi: 10.1038/npp.2009.176

Meltzer, H. Y., and Roth, B. L. (2013). Lorcaserin and pimavanserin: emerging selectivity of serotonin receptor subtype-targeted drugs. J. Clin. Invest. 123, 4986–4991. doi: 10.1172/JCI70678

Mendez-David, I., David, D. J., Darcet, F., Wu, M. V., Kerdine-Romer, S., Gardier, A. M., et al. (2014). Rapid anxiolytic effects of a 5-HT(4) receptor agonist are mediated by a neurogenesis-independent mechanism. Neuropsychopharmacology 39, 1366–1378. doi: 10.1038/npp.2013.332

Meneses, A. (2013). 5-HT systems: emergent targets for memory formation and memory alterations. Rev. Neurosci. 24, 629–664. doi: 10.1515/revneuro-2013-0026

Miguelez, C., Navailles, S., De Deurwaerdere, P., and Ugedo, L. (2016a). The acute and long-term L-DOPA effects are independent from changes in the activity of dorsal raphe serotonergic neurons in 6-OHDA lesioned rats. Br. J. Pharmacol. 173, 2135–2146. doi: 10.1111/bph.13447

Miguelez, C., Navailles, S., Delaville, C., Marquis, L., Lagière, M., Benazzouz, A., et al. (2016b). L-DOPA elicits non-vesicular releases of serotonin and dopamine in hemiparkinsonian rats *in vivo*. *Eur. Neuropsychopharmacol.* 26, 1297–1309. doi: 10.1016/j.euroneuro.2016.05.004

Millan, M. J. (2005). Serotonin 5-HT2C receptors as a target for the treatment of depressive and anxious states: focus on novel therapeutic strategies. *Therapie* 60, 441–460. doi: 10.2515/therapie:2005065

Millan, M. J. (2006). Multi-target strategies for the improved treatment of depressive states: Conceptual foundations and neuronal substrates, drug discovery and therapeutic application. *Pharmacol. Ther.* 110, 135–370. doi: 10.1016/j.pharmthera.2005.11.006

Millan, M. J. (2010). From the cell to the clinic: a comparative review of the partial D(2)/D(3)receptor agonist and alpha2-adrenoceptor antagonist, piribedil, in the treatment of Parkinson's disease. *Pharmacol. Ther.* 128, 229–273. doi: 10.1016/j.pharmthera.2010.06.002

Millan, M. J., Brocco, M., Gobert, A., and Dekeyne, A. (2005). Anxiolytic properties of agomelatine, an antidepressant with melatoninergic and serotonergic properties: role of 5-HT2C receptor blockade. *Psychopharmacology (Berl).* 177, 448–458. doi: 10.1007/s00213-004-1962-z

Millan, M. J., Fone, K., Steckler, T., and Horan, W. P. (2014). Negative symptoms of schizophrenia: clinical characteristics, pathophysiological substrates, experimental models and prospects for improved treatment. *Eur. Neuropsychopharmacol.* 24, 645–692. doi: 10.1016/j.euroneuro.2014.03.008

Millan, M. J., Goodwin, G. M., Meyer-Lindenberg, A., and Ögren, S. O. (2015a). 60 years of advances in neuropsychopharmacology for improving brain health, renewed hope for progress. *Eur. Neuropsychopharmacol.* 25, 591–598. doi: 10.1016/j.euroneuro.2015.01.015

Millan, M. J., Goodwin, G. M., Meyer-Lindenberg, A., and Ove Ögren, S. (2015b). Learning from the past and looking to the future: emerging perspectives for improving the treatment of psychiatric disorders. *Eur. Neuropsychopharmacol.* 25, 599–656. doi: 10.1016/j.euroneuro.2015.01.016

Millan, M. J., Marin, P., Kamal, M., Jockers, R., Chanrion, B., Labasque, M., et al. (2010). The melatonergic agonist and clinically active antidepressant, agomelatine, is a neutral antagonist at 5-HT2C receptors. *Int. J. Neuropsychopharmacol.* 14, 768–783. doi: 10.1017/S1461145710001045

Morisset, S., Rouleau, A., Ligneau, X., Gbahou, F., Tardivel-Lacombe, J., Stark, H., et al. (2000). High constitutive activity of native H3 receptors regulates histamine neurons in brain. *Nature* 408, 860–864. doi: 10.1038/35048583

Muck-Seler, D., Presecki, P., Mimica, N., Mustapic, M., Pivac, N., Babic, A., et al. (2009). Platelet serotonin concentration and monoamine oxidase type B activity in female patients in early, middle and late phase of Alzheimer's disease. *Prog. Neuropsychopharmacol. Biol. Psychiatry* 33, 1226–1231. doi: 10.1016/j.pnpbp.2009.07.004

Murphy, D. L., Sims, K. B., Karoum, F., Garrick, N. A., de la Chapelle, A., Sankila, E. M., et al. (1991). Plasma amine oxidase activities in Norrie disease patients with an X-chromosomal deletion affecting monoamine oxidase. *J. Neural Transm. Gen. Sect.* 83, 1–12. doi: 10.1007/BF01244447

Mustapic, M., Presecki, P., Pivac, N., Mimica, N., Hof, P. R., Simic, G., et al. (2013). Genotype-independent decrease in plasma dopamine beta-hydroxylase activity in Alzheimer's disease. *Prog. Neuropsychopharmacol. Biol. Psychiatry* 44, 94–99. doi: 10.1016/j.pnpbp.2013.02.002

Myöhänen, T. T., Schendzielorz, N., and Männistö, P. T. (2010). Distribution of catechol-O-methyltransferase (COMT) proteins and enzymatic activities in wild-type and soluble COMT deficient mice. *J. Neurochem.* 113, 1632–1643. doi: 10.1111/j.1471-4159.2010.06723.x

Nakazato, T., and Akiyama, A. (1989). Effect of exogenous L-dopa on behavior in the rat: an *in vivo* voltammetric study. *Brain Res.* 490, 332–338. doi: 10.1016/0006-8993(89)90250-3

Navailles, S., Bioulac, B., Gross, C., and De Deurwaerdère, P. (2010). Serotonergic neurons mediate ectopic release of dopamine induced by L-DOPA in a rat model of Parkinson's disease. *Neurobiol. Dis.* 38, 136–143. doi: 10.1016/j.nbd.2010.01.012

Navailles, S., Bioulac, B., Gross, C., and De Deurwaerdère, P. (2011a). Chronic L-DOPA therapy alters central serotonergic function and L-DOPA-induced dopamine release in a region-dependent manner in a rat model of Parkinson's disease. *Neurobiol. Dis.* 41, 585–590. doi: 10.1016/j.nbd.2010.11.007

Navailles, S., Carta, M., Guthrie, M., and De Deurwaerdère, P. (2011b). L-DOPA and serotonergic neurons: functional implication and therapeutic perspectives in Parkinson's disease. *Cent. Nerv. Syst. Agents Med. Chem.* 11, 305–320. doi: 10.2174/1871524911106040305

Navailles, S., and De Deurwaerdere, P. (2012a). Contribution of serotonergic transmission to the motor and cognitive effects of high-frequency stimulation of the subthalamic nucleus or levodopa in Parkinson's disease. *Mol. Neurobiol.* 45, 173–185. doi: 10.1007/s12035-011-8230-0

Navailles, S., and De Deurwaerdère, P. (2012b). Imbalanced dopaminergic transmission mediated by serotonergic neurons in L-DOPA-induced dyskinesia. *Parkinsons. Dis.* 2012, 323686. doi: 10.1155/2012/323686

Navailles, S., Di Giovanni, G., and De Deurwaerdère, P. (2015). The 5-HT4 agonist prucalopride stimulates L-DOPA-induced dopamine release in restricted brain regions of the hemiparkinsonian rat *in vivo*. *CNS Neurosci. Ther.* 21, 745–747. doi: 10.1111/cns.12436

Navailles, S., Milan, L., Khalki, H., Di Giovanni, G., Lagière, M., and De Deurwaerdère, P. (2014). Noradrenergic terminals regulate L-DOPA-derived dopamine extracellular levels in a region-dependent manner in Parkinsonian rats. *CNS Neurosci. Ther.* 20, 671–678. doi: 10.1111/cns.12275

Olanow, C. W., Stern, M. B., and Sethi, K. (2009). The scientific and clinical basis for the treatment of Parkinson disease (2009). *Neurology* 72(21 Suppl 4), S1–S136. doi: 10.1212/wnl.0b013e3181a1d44c

Owen, M. J., Sawa, A., and Mortensen, P. B. (2016). Schizophrenia. *Lancet* 388, 86–97. doi: 10.1016/S0140-6736(15)01121-6

Page, M. E., Detke, M. J., Dalvi, A., Kirby, L. G., and Lucki, I. (1999). Serotonergic mediation of the effects of fluoxetine, but not desipramine, in the rat forced swimming test. *Psychopharmacology (Berl).* 147, 162–167. doi: 10.1007/s002130051156

Palmieri, V., Arnett, D. K., Roman, M. J., Liu, J. E., Bella, J. N., Oberman, A., et al. (2002). Appetite suppressants and valvular heart disease in a population-based sample: the HyperGEN study. *Am. J. Med.* 112, 710–715. doi: 10.1016/S0002-9343(02)01123-3

Panula, P., Chazot, P. L., Cowart, M., Gutzmer, R., Leurs, R., Liu, W. L., et al. (2015). International union of basic and clinical pharmacology. XCVIII. Histamine Receptors. *Pharmacol Rev* 67, 601–655. doi: 10.1124/pr.114.010249

Parsons, C. G., Danysz, W., Dekundy, A., and Pulte, I. (2013). Memantine and cholinesterase inhibitors: complementary mechanisms in the treatment of Alzheimer's disease. *Neurotox. Res.* 24, 358–369. doi: 10.1007/s12640-013-9398-z

Pascual, J., Grijalba, B., García-Sevilla, J. A., Zarranz, J. J., and Pazos, A. (1992). Loss of high-affinity alpha 2-adrenoceptors in Alzheimer's disease: an autoradiographic study in frontal cortex and hippocampus. *Neurosci. Lett.* 142, 36–40. doi: 10.1016/0304-3940(92)90614-D

Payton, S., Cahill, C. M., Randall, J. D., Gullans, S. R., and Rogers, J. T. (2003). Drug discovery targeted to the Alzheimer's APP mRNA 5'-untranslated region: the action of paroxetine and dimercaptopropanol. *J. Mol. Neurosci.* 20, 267–275. doi: 10.1385/JMN:20:3:267

Perez-Caballero, L., Torres-Sanchez, S., Bravo, L., Mico, J. A., and Berrocoso, E. (2014). Fluoxetine: a case history of its discovery and preclinical development. *Expert Opin. Drug Discov.* 9, 567–578. doi: 10.1517/17460441.2014.907790

Perez-Lloret, S., and Rascol, O. (2016). Piribedil for the treatment of motor and non-motor symptoms of Parkinson disease. *CNS Drugs.* 30, 703–717. doi: 10.1007/s40263-016-0360-5

Peskind, E. R., Tsuang, D. W., Bonner, L. T., Pascualy, M., Riekse, R. G., Snowden, M. B., et al. (2005). Propranolol for disruptive behaviors in nursing home residents with probable or possible Alzheimer disease: a placebo-controlled study. *Alzheimer Dis. Assoc. Disord.* 19, 23–28. doi: 10.1097/01.wad.0000155067.16313.5e

Piñeyro, G., and Blier, P. (1999). Autoregulation of serotonin neurons: role in antidepressant drug action. *Pharmacol. Rev.* 51, 533–591.

Porras, G., De Deurwaerdere, P., Li, Q., Marti, M., Morgenstern, R., Sohr, R., et al. (2014). L-dopa-induced dyskinesia: beyond an excessive dopamine tone in the striatum. *Sci. Rep.* 4:3730. doi: 10.1038/srep03730

Poyurovsky, M., Fuchs, C., Pashinian, A., Levi, A., Weizman, R., and Weizman, A. (2013). Reducing antipsychotic-induced weight gain in schizophrenia: a double-blind placebo-controlled study of reboxetine-betahistine combination. *Psychopharmacology (Berl).* 226, 615–622. doi: 10.1007/s00213-012-2935-2

Preda, S., Govoni, S., Lanni, C., Racchi, M., Mura, E., Grilli, M., et al. (2008). Acute beta-amyloid administration disrupts the cholinergic control of dopamine release in the nucleus accumbens. *Neuropsychopharmacology* 33, 1062–1070. doi: 10.1038/sj.npp.1301485

Provensi, G., Blandina, P., and Passani, M. B. (2016). The histaminergic system as a target for the prevention of obesity and metabolic syndrome. *Neuropharmacology* 106, 3–12. doi: 10.1016/j.neuropharm.2015.07.002

Provensi, G., Coccurello, R., Umehara, H., Munari, L., Giacovazzo, G., Galeotti, N., et al. (2014). Satiety factor oleoylethanolamide recruits the brain histaminergic system to inhibit food intake. *Proc. Natl. Acad. Sci. U.S.A.* 111, 11527–11532. doi: 10.1073/pnas.1322016111

Racagni, G., Riva, M. A., Molteni, R., Musazzi, L., Calabrese, F., Popoli, M., et al. (2011). Mode of action of agomelatine: synergy between melatonergic and 5-HT2C receptors. *World J. Biol. Psychiatry* 12, 574–587. doi: 10.3109/15622975.2011.595823

Ramirez, M. J., Lai, M. K., Tordera, R. M., and Francis, P. T. (2014). Serotonergic therapies for cognitive symptoms in Alzheimer's disease: rationale and current status. *Drugs* 74, 729–736. doi: 10.1007/s40265-014-0217-5

Ramsay, R. R. (2013). Inhibitor design for monoamine oxidases. *Curr. Pharm. Des.* 19, 2529–2539. doi: 10.2174/1381612811319140004

Rantamaki, T., and Yalcin, I. (2016). Antidepressant drug action– From rapid changes on network function to network rewiring. *Prog. Neuropsychopharmacol. Biol. Psychiatry* 64, 285–292. doi: 10.1016/j.pnpbp.2015.06.001

Rascol, O., Fitzer-Attas, C. J., Hauser, R., Jankovic, J., Lang, A., Langston, J. W., et al. (2011). A double-blind, delayed-start trial of rasagiline in Parkinson's disease (the ADAGIO study): prespecified and *post-hoc* analyses of the need for additional therapies, changes in UPDRS scores, and non-motor outcomes. *Lancet Neurol.* 10, 415–423. doi: 10.1016/S1474-4422(11)70073-4

Ratliff, J. C., Barber, J. A., Palmese, L. B., Reutenauer, E. L., and Tek, C. (2010). Association of prescription H1 antihistamine use with obesity: results from the National Health and Nutrition Examination Survey. *Obesity (Silver. Spring).* 18, 2398–2400. doi: 10.1038/oby.2010.176

Reifler, B. V., Teri, L., Raskind, M., Veith, R., Barnes, R., White, E., et al. (1989). Double-blind trial of imipramine in Alzheimer's disease patients with and without depression. *Am. J. Psychiatry* 146, 45–49. doi: 10.1176/ajp.146.1.45

Remington, G., Foussias, G., Fervaha, G., Agid, O., Takeuchi, H., Lee, J., et al. (2016). Treating negative symptoms in schizophrenia: an update. *Curr Treat Options Psychiatry* 3, 133–150. doi: 10.1007/s40501-016-0075-8

Reynolds, G. P., Mason, S. L., Meldrum, A., De Keczer, S., Parnes, H., Eglen, R. M., et al. (1995). 5-Hydroxytryptamine (5-HT)4 receptors in post mortem human brain tissue: distribution, pharmacology and effects of neurodegenerative diseases. *Br. J. Pharmacol.* 114, 993–998. doi: 10.1111/j.1476-5381.1995.tb13303.x

Rezvani, A. H., Kholdebarin, E., Brucato, F. H., Callahan, P. M., Lowe, D. A., and Levin, E. D. (2009). Effect of R3487/MEM3454, a novel nicotinic alpha7 receptor partial agonist and 5-HT3 antagonist on sustained attention in rats. *Prog. Neuropsychopharmacol. Biol. Psychiatry* 33, 269–275. doi: 10.1016/j.pnpbp.2008.11.018

Richtand, N. M., Welge, J. A., Logue, A. D., Keck, P. E. Jr., Strakowski, S. M., and McNamara, R. K. (2008). Role of serotonin and dopamine receptor binding in antipsychotic efficacy. *Prog. Brain Res.* 172, 155–175. doi: 10.1016/S0079-6123(08)00908-4

Riederer, P., and Laux, G. (2011). MAO-inhibitors in Parkinson's disease. *Exp. Neurobiol.* 20, 1–17. doi: 10.5607/en.2011.20.1.1

Ries, V., Selzer, R., Eichhorn, T., Oertel, W. H., and Eggert, K. (2010). Replacing a dopamine agonist by the COMT-inhibitor tolcapone as an adjunct to L-dopa in the treatment of Parkinson's disease: a randomized, multicenter, open-label, parallel-group study. *Clin. Neuropharmacol.* 33, 142–150. doi: 10.1097/WNF.0b013e3181d99d6f

Rommelfanger, K. S., and Weinshenker, D. (2007). Norepinephrine: the redheaded stepchild of Parkinson's disease. *Biochem. Pharmacol.* 74, 177–190. doi: 10.1016/j.bcp.2007.01.036

Rosenzweig-Lipson, S., Comery, T. A., Marquis, K. L., Gross, J., and Dunlop, J. (2012). 5-HT2C agonists as therapeutics for the treatment of schizophrenia. *Handb. Exp. Pharmacol.* 213, 147–165. doi: 10.1007/978-3-642-25758-2_6

Roth, B. L., and Driscol, J. (2016). *Psychoactive Drug Screening Program Ki Database.* Chapel Hill, NC: University of North Carolina at Chapel Hill and the United States National Institute of Mental Health.

Sachdev, M., Miller, W. C., Ryan, T., and Jollis, J. G. (2002). Effect of fenfluramine-derivative diet pills on cardiac valves: a meta-analysis of observational studies. *Am. Heart J.* 144, 1065–1073. doi: 10.1067/mhj.2002.126733

Sagud, M., Nikolac Perkovic, M., Vuksan-Cusa, B., Maravic, A., Svob Strac, D., Mihaljevic Peles, A., et al. (2016). A prospective, longitudinal study of platelet serotonin and plasma brain-derived neurotrophic factor concentrations in major depression: effects of vortioxetine treatment. *Psychopharmacology (Berl).* 233, 3259–3267. doi: 10.1007/s00213-016-4364-0

San, L., and Arranz, B. (2008). Agomelatine: a novel mechanism of antidepressant action involving the melatonergic and the serotonergic system. *Eur. Psychiatry* 23, 396–402. doi: 10.1016/j.eurpsy.2008.04.002

Sanchez, C., Asin, K. E., and Artigas, F. (2015). Vortioxetine, a novel antidepressant with multimodal activity: review of preclinical and clinical data. *Pharmacol. Ther.* 145, 43–57. doi: 10.1016/j.pharmthera.2014.07.001

Sanz, E., Quintana, A., Battaglia, V., Toninello, A., Hidalgo, J., Ambrosio, S., et al. (2008). Anti-apoptotic effect of Mao-B inhibitor PF9601N [N-(2-propynyl)-2-(5-benzyloxy-indolyl) methylamine] is mediated by p53 pathway inhibition in MPP+-treated SH-SY5Y human dopaminergic cells. *J. Neurochem.* 105, 2404–2417. doi: 10.1111/j.1471-4159.2008.05326.x

Sanz, E., Romera, M., Bellik, L., Marco, J. I., and Unzeta, M. (2004). Indolalkylamines derivatives as antioxidant and neuroprotective agents in an experimental model of Parkinson's disease. *Med. Sci. Monit.* 10, BR477–BR484.

Saura, J., Bleuel, Z., Ulrich, J., Mendelowitsch, A., Chen, K., Shih, J. C., et al. (1996). Molecular neuroanatomy of human monoamine oxidases A and B revealed by quantitative enzyme radioautography and *in situ* hybridization histochemistry. *Neuroscience* 70, 755–774. doi: 10.1016/S0306-4522(96)83013-2

Saura, J., Kettler, R., Da Prada, M., and Richards, J. G. (1992). Quantitative enzyme radioautography with 3H-Ro 41-1049 and 3H-Ro 19-6327 *in vitro*: localization and abundance of MAO-A and MAO-B in rat CNS, peripheral organs, and human brain. *J. Neurosci.* 12, 1977–1999.

Scheen, A. J. (2010). Cardiovascular risk-benefit profile of sibutramine. *Am. J. Cardiovasc. Drugs* 10, 321–334. doi: 10.2165/11584800-000000000-00000

Schendzielorz, N., Oinas, J. P., Myöhänen, T. T., Reenilä, I., Raasmaja, A., and Männistö, P. T. (2013). Catechol-O-methyltransferase (COMT) protein expression and activity after dopaminergic and noradrenergic lesions of the rat brain. *PLoS ONE* 8:e61392. doi: 10.1371/journal.pone.0061392

Schreiber, R., and Newman-Tancredi, A. (2014). Improving cognition in schizophrenia with antipsychotics that elicit neurogenesis through 5-HT(1A) receptor activation. *Neurobiol. Learn. Mem.* 110, 72–80. doi: 10.1016/j.nlm.2013.12.015

Seeman, P. (2015). Parkinson's disease treatment may cause impulse-control disorder via dopamine D3 receptors. *Synapse* 69, 183–189. doi: 10.1002/syn.21805

Seeman, P., Chau-Wong, M., Tedesco, J., and Wong, K. (1975). Brain receptors for antipsychotic drugs and dopamine: direct binding assays. *Proc. Natl. Acad. Sci. U.S.A.* 72, 4376–4380. doi: 10.1073/pnas.72.11.4376

Seeman, P., Lee, T., Chau-Wong, M., and Wong, K. (1976). Antipsychotic drug doses and neuroleptic/dopamine receptors. *Nature* 261, 717–719. doi: 10.1038/261717a0

Shankle, W. R., Nielson, K. A., and Cotman, C. W. (1995). Low-dose propranolol reduces aggression and agitation resembling that associated with orbitofrontal dysfunction in elderly demented patients. *Alzheimer Dis. Assoc. Disord.* 9, 233–237. doi: 10.1097/00002093-199509040-00010

Shen, J. H., Zhao, Y., Rosenzweig-Lipson, S., Popp, D., Williams, J. B., Giller, E., et al. (2014). A 6-week randomized, double-blind, placebo-controlled, comparator referenced trial of vabicaserin in acute schizophrenia. *J. Psychiatr. Res.* 53, 14–22. doi: 10.1016/j.jpsychires.2014.02.012

Šimić, G., Babić Leko, M., Wray, S., Harrington, C. R., Delalle, I., Jovanov-Milošević, N., et al. (2016). Monoaminergic neuropathology in Alzheimer's disease. *Prog. Neurobiol.* doi: 10.1016/j.pneurobio.2016.04.001. [Epub ahead of print].

Simoni, E., Daniele, S., Bottegoni, G., Pizzirani, D., Trincavelli, M. L., Goldoni, L., et al. (2012). Combining galantamine and memantine in multitargeted, new chemical entities potentially useful in Alzheimer's disease. *J. Med. Chem.* 55, 9708–9721. doi: 10.1021/jm3009458

Sims, N. R., Bowen, D. M., Smith, C. C., Flack, R. H., Davison, A. N., Snowden, J. S., et al. (1980). Glucose metabolism and acetylcholine synthesis in relation to neuronal activity in Alzheimer's disease. *Lancet* 1, 333–336. doi: 10.1016/S0140-6736(80)90884-3

Smith, D. J., Salmi, M., Bono, P., Hellman, J., Leu, T., and Jalkanen, S. (1998). Cloning of vascular adhesion protein 1 reveals a novel multifunctional adhesion molecule. *J. Exp. Med.* 188, 17–27. doi: 10.1084/jem.188.1.17

Solé, M., Hernandez-Guillamon, M., Boada, M., and Unzeta, M. (2008). p53 phosphorylation is involved in vascular cell death induced by the catalytic activity of membrane-bound SSAO/VAP-1. *Biochim. Biophys. Acta* 1783, 1085–1094. doi: 10.1016/j.bbamcr.2008.02.014

Solé, M., Minano-Molina, A. J., and Unzeta, M. (2015). Cross-talk between Abeta and endothelial SSAO/VAP-1 accelerates vascular damage and Abeta aggregation related to CAA-AD. *Neurobiol. Aging* 36, 762–775. doi: 10.1016/j.neurobiolaging.2014.09.030

Stahl, S. M. (2015). Modes and nodes explain the mechanism of action of vortioxetine, a multimodal agent (MMA): blocking 5HT3 receptors enhances release of serotonin, norepinephrine, and acetylcholine. *CNS Spectr.* 20, 455–459. doi: 10.1017/S1092852915000346

Stansley, B. J., and Yamamoto, B. K. (2013). L-dopa-induced dopamine synthesis and oxidative stress in serotonergic cells. *Neuropharmacology* 67, 243–251. doi: 10.1016/j.neuropharm.2012.11.010

Stansley, B. J., and Yamamoto, B. K. (2014). Chronic L-dopa decreases serotonin neurons in a subregion of the dorsal raphe nucleus. *J. Pharmacol. Exp. Ther.* 351, 440–447. doi: 10.1124/jpet.114.218966

Storga, D., Vrecko, K., Birkmayer, J. G., and Reibnegger, G. (1996). Monoaminergic neurotransmitters, their precursors and metabolites in brains of Alzheimer patients. *Neurosci. Lett.* 203, 29–32. doi: 10.1016/0304-3940(95)12256-7

Strac, D., Pivac, N., Smolders, I. J., Fogel, W., De Deurwaerdere, P., and Di Giovanni, G. (2016). Monoaminergic mechanisms in epilepsy may offer innovative therapeutic opportunity for monoaminergic multi-target drugs. *Front. Neurosci.* 10:492. doi: 10.3389/fnins.2016.00492

Sun, P., Esteban, G., Inokuchi, T., Marco-Contelles, J., Weksler, B. B., Romero, I. A., et al. (2015). Protective effect of the multitarget compound DPH-4 on human SSAO/VAP-1-expressing hCMEC/D3 cells under oxygen-glucose deprivation conditions: an *in vitro* experimental model of cerebral ischaemia. *Br. J. Pharmacol.* 172, 5390–5402. doi: 10.1111/bph.13328

Svenningsson, P., Rosenblad, C., Af Edholm Arvidsson, K., Wictorin, K., Keywood, C., Shankar, B., et al. (2015). Eltoprazine counteracts l-DOPA-induced dyskinesias in Parkinson's disease: a dose-finding study. *Brain* 138(Pt 4), 963–973. doi: 10.1093/brain/awu409

Szot, P., White, S. S., Greenup, J. L., Leverenz, J. B., Peskind, E. R., and Raskind, M. A. (2006). Compensatory changes in the noradrenergic nervous system in the locus ceruleus and hippocampus of postmortem subjects with Alzheimer's disease and dementia with Lewy bodies. *J. Neurosci.* 26, 467–478. doi: 10.1523/JNEUROSCI.4265-05.2006

Tammimäki, A., Käenmäki, M., Kambur, O., Kulesskaya, N., Keisala, T., Karvonen, E., et al. (2010). Effect of S-COMT deficiency on behavior and extracellular brain dopamine concentrations in mice. *Psychopharmacology (Berl).* 211, 389–401. doi: 10.1007/s00213-010-1944-2

Tanaka, H., Kannari, K., Maeda, T., Tomiyama, M., Suda, T., and Matsunaga, M. (1999). Role of serotonergic neurons in L-DOPA-derived extracellular dopamine in the striatum of 6-OHDA-lesioned rats. *Neuroreport* 10, 631–634. doi: 10.1097/00001756-199902250-00034

Taylor, K. M. (1975). "Brain histamine," in *Biochemistry of Biogenic Amines*, eds L. L. Iversen, S. D. Iversen, and S. H. Snyder (New York, NY: Plenum Press New Yok and London), 327–380. doi: 10.1007/978-1-4684-3171-1_6

Terry, A. V. Jr., Buccafusco, J. J., and Wilson, C. (2008). Cognitive dysfunction in neuropsychiatric disorders: selected serotonin receptor subtypes as therapeutic targets. *Behav. Brain Res.* 195, 30–38. doi: 10.1016/j.bbr.2007.12.006

Thase, M. E., Corya, S. A., Osuntokun, O., Case, M., Henley, D. B., Sanger, T. M., et al. (2007). A randomized, double-blind comparison of olanzapine/fluoxetine combination, olanzapine, and fluoxetine in treatment-resistant major depressive disorder. *J. Clin. Psychiatry* 68, 224–236. doi: 10.4088/JCP.v68n0207

Thomas, D. R., Nelson, D. R., and Johnson, A. M. (1987). Biochemical effects of the antidepressant paroxetine, a specific 5-hydroxytryptamine uptake inhibitor. *Psychopharmacology (Berl).* 93, 193–200. doi: 10.1007/BF00179933

Tighilet, B., Trottier, S., Mourre, C., Chotard, C., and Lacour, M. (2002). Betahistine dihydrochloride interaction with the histaminergic system in the cat: neurochemical and molecular mechanisms. *Eur. J. Pharmacol.* 446, 63–73. doi: 10.1016/S0014-2999(02)01795-8

Tohgi, H., Ueno, M., Abe, T., Takahashi, S., and Nozaki, Y. (1992). Concentrations of monoamines and their metabolites in the cerebrospinal fluid from patients with senile dementia of the Alzheimer type and vascular dementia of the Binswanger type. *J. Neural Transm. Park. Dis. Dement. Sect.* 4, 69–77. doi: 10.1007/BF02257623

Tonelli, M., Catto, M., Tasso, B., Novelli, F., Canu, C., Iusco, G., et al. (2015). Multitarget therapeutic leads for Alzheimer's disease: quinolizidinyl derivatives of Bi- and tricyclic systems as dual inhibitors of cholinesterases and beta-amyloid (Abeta) aggregation. *ChemMedChem* 10, 1040–1053. doi: 10.1002/cmdc.201500104

Torres, G. E., Gainetdinov, R. R., and Caron, M. G. (2003). Plasma membrane monoamine transporters: structure, regulation and function. *Nat. Rev. Neurosci.* 4, 13–25. doi: 10.1038/nrn1008

Trillo, L., Das, D., Hsieh, W., Medina, B., Moghadam, S., Lin, B., et al. (2013). Ascending monoaminergic systems alterations in Alzheimer's disease. Translating basic science into clinical care. *Neurosci. Biobehav. Rev.* 37, 1363–1379. doi: 10.1016/j.neubiorev.2013.05.008

Tronci, E., Fidalgo, C., Stancampiano, R., and Carta, M. (2015). Effect of selective and non-selective serotonin receptor activation on l-DOPA-induced therapeutic efficacy and dyskinesia in parkinsonian rats. *Behav. Brain Res.* 292, 300–304. doi: 10.1016/j.bbr.2015.06.034

Udenfriend, S., Weissbach, H., and Bogdanski, D. F. (1957). Effect of iproniazid on serotonin metabolism *in vivo*. *J. Pharmacol. Exp. Ther.* 120, 255–260.

Versijpt, J., Van Laere, K. J., Dumont, F., Decoo, D., Vandecapelle, M., Santens, P., et al. (2003). Imaging of the 5-HT2A system: age-, gender-, and Alzheimer's disease-related findings. *Neurobiol. Aging* 24, 553–561. doi: 10.1016/S0197-4580(02)00137-9

Vickers, S. P., Dourish, C. T., and Kennett, G. A. (2001). Evidence that hypophagia induced by d-fenfluramine and d-norfenfluramine in the rat is mediated by 5-HT2C receptors. *Neuropharmacology* 41, 200–209. doi: 10.1016/S0028-3908(01)00063-6

Visanji, N. P., Fox, S. H., Johnston, T., Reyes, G., Millan, M. J., and Brotchie, J. M. (2009). Dopamine D3 receptor stimulation underlies the development of L-DOPA-induced dyskinesia in animal models of Parkinson's disease. *Neurobiol. Dis.* 35, 184–192. doi: 10.1016/j.nbd.2008.11.010

Vivero, L. E., Anderson, P. O., and Clark, R. F. (1998). A close look at fenfluramine and dexfenfluramine. *J. Emerg. Med.* 16, 197–205. doi: 10.1016/S0736-4679(97)00289-8

Voigt, J. P., and Fink, H. (2015). Serotonin controlling feeding and satiety. *Behav. Brain Res.* 277, 14–31. doi: 10.1016/j.bbr.2014.08.065

Werner, F. M., and Covenas, R. (2016). Serotonergic drugs: agonists/antagonists at specific serotonergic subreceptors for the treatment of cognitive, depressant and psychotic symptoms in Alzheimer's disease. *Curr. Pharm. Des.* 22, 2064–2071. doi: 10.2174/1381612822666160127113524

Wimalasena, K. (2011). Vesicular monoamine transporters: structure-function, pharmacology, and medicinal chemistry. *Med. Res. Rev.* 31, 483–519. doi: 10.1002/med.20187

Wong, D. T., Bymaster, F. P., Horng, J. S., and Molloy, B. B. (1975). A new selective inhibitor for uptake of serotonin into synaptosomes of rat brain: 3-(p-trifluoromethylphenoxy). N-methyl-3-phenylpropylamine. *J. Pharmacol. Exp. Ther.* 193, 804–811.

Yan, W., Zhao, C., Sun, L., and Tang, B. (2016). Association between polymorphism of COMT gene (Val158Met) with Alzheimer's disease: an updated analysis. *J. Neurol. Sci.* 361, 250–255. doi: 10.1016/j.jns.2016.01.014

Youdim, M. B., Edmondson, D., and Tipton, K. F. (2006). The therapeutic potential of monoamine oxidase inhibitors. *Nat. Rev. Neurosci.* 7, 295–309. doi: 10.1038/nrn1883

Yu, P. H., and Deng, Y. L. (1998). Endogenous formaldehyde as a potential factor of vulnerability of atherosclerosis: involvement of semicarbazide-sensitive amine oxidase-mediated methylamine turnover. *Atherosclerosis* 140, 357–363. doi: 10. 1016/S0021-9150(98)00142-7

Zeller, E. A., and Barsky, J. (1952). *In vivo* inhibition of liver and brain monoamine oxidase by 1-Isonicotinyl-2-isopropyl hydrazine. *Proc. Soc. Exp. Biol. Med.* 81, 459–461. doi: 10.3181/00379727-81-19910

Zlokovic, B. V. (2008). New therapeutic targets in the neurovascular pathway in Alzheimer's disease. *Neurotherapeutics* 5, 409–414. doi: 10.1016/j.nurt.2008. 05.011

Zohar, J., Stahl, S., Moller, H. J., Blier, P., Kupfer, D., Yamawaki, S., et al. (2015). A review of the current nomenclature for psychotropic agents and an introduction to the neuroscience-based nomenclature. *Eur. Neuropsychopharmacol.* 25, 2318–2325. doi: 10.1016/j.euroneuro.2015.08.019

Conflict of Interest Statement: The authors declare that the research was conducted in the absence of any commercial or financial relationships that could be construed as a potential conflict of interest.

5

Key Targets for Multi-Target Ligands Designed to Combat Neurodegeneration

Rona R. Ramsay[1]*, Magdalena Majekova[2], Milagros Medina[3] and Massimo Valoti[4]*

[1] Biomedical Sciences Research Complex, University of St. Andrews, St. Andrews, UK, [2] Department of Biochemical Pharmacology, Institute of Experimental Pharmacology and Toxicology, Slovak Academy of Sciences, Bratislava, Slovakia, [3] Departamento de Bioquímica y Biología Molecular y Celular, Facultad de Ciencias and BIFI, Universidad de Zaragoza, Zaragoza, Spain, [4] Dipartimento di Scienze della Vita, Università degli Studi di Siena, Siena, Italy

Edited by:
Ashok Kumar,
University of Florida, USA

Reviewed by:
Raja S. Settivari,
The Dow Chemical Company, USA
Arianna Bellucci,
University of Brescia, Italy

*Correspondence:
Rona R. Ramsay
rrr@st-andrews.ac.uk
Massimo Valoti
massimo.valoti@unisi.it

HIGHLIGHTS

- Compounds that interact with multiple targets but minimally with the cytochrome P450 system (CYP) address the many factors leading to neurodegeneration.
- Acetyl- and Butyryl-cholineEsterases (AChE, BChE) and Monoamine Oxidases A/B (MAO A, MAO B) are targets for Multi-Target Designed Ligands (MTDL).
- ASS234 is an irreversible inhibitor of MAO A >MAO B and has micromolar potency against the cholinesterases.
- ASS234 is a poor CYP substrate in human liver, yielding the depropargylated metabolite.
- SMe1EC2, a stobadine derivative, showed high radical scavenging property, *in vitro* and *in vivo* giving protection in head trauma and diabetic damage of endothelium.
- Control of mitochondrial function and morphology by manipulating fission and fusion is emerging as a target area for therapeutic strategies to decrease the pathological outcome of neurodegenerative diseases.

Growing evidence supports the view that neurodegenerative diseases have multiple and common mechanisms in their aetiologies. These multifactorial aspects have changed the broadly common assumption that selective drugs are superior to "dirty drugs" for use in therapy. This drives the research in studies of novel compounds that might have multiple action mechanisms. In neurodegeneration, loss of neuronal signaling is a major cause of the symptoms, so preservation of neurotransmitters by inhibiting the breakdown enzymes is a first approach. Acetylcholinesterase (AChE) inhibitors are the drugs preferentially used in AD and that one of these, rivastigmine, is licensed also for PD. Several studies have shown that monoamine oxidase (MAO) B, located mainly in glial cells, increases with age and is elevated in Alzheimer (AD) and Parkinson's Disease's (PD). Deprenyl, a MAO B inhibitor, significantly delays the initiation of levodopa treatment in PD patients. These indications underline that AChE and MAO are considered a necessary part of multi-target designed ligands (MTDL). However, both of these targets are simply symptomatic treatment so if new drugs are to prevent degeneration rather than compensate for loss of neurotransmitters, then oxidative stress and mitochondrial events must also be targeted. MAO inhibitors can protect neurons from apoptosis by mechanisms unrelated to enzyme inhibition. Understanding the involvement of MAO and other proteins in the induction and regulation of the apoptosis in mitochondria will aid progress toward strategies to prevent the loss of neurons. In general, the oxidative stress observed both in PD and AD indicate that antioxidant properties are a desirable part of MTDL molecules. After two or more properties are incorporated into one molecule, the passage from a lead compound to a therapeutic tool is strictly linked to its pharmacokinetic and toxicity. In this context the interaction of any new molecules with cytochrome P450 and other xenobiotic metabolic processes is a crucial point. The present review covers the biochemistry of enzymes targeted in the design of drugs against neurodegeneration and the cytochrome P450-dependent metabolism of MTDLs.

Keywords: multi target designed ligands, mitochondria, oxidative stress, monoamine oxidase, cytochrome P450, neurodegeneration

INTRODUCTION

Neurodegeneration is a complex process that can arise from many different defects or insults. In the last five years at least 80 reviews with "neurodegeneration" in the title have appeared, each covering different aspects of the processes involved. These include protein aggregation, mitochondrial movement, and function, dysregulation of microRNA, iron accumulation, inflammation, defects in proteins such as sirtuins or tau, dysregulation of protein trafficking or breakdown, and oxidative stress (Donmez, 2012; Gascon and Gao, 2012; Schipper, 2012; Sheng and Cai, 2012; Costanzo and Zurzolo, 2013; Butterfield et al., 2014; Moussaud et al., 2014; Rao et al., 2014; Wang X. et al., 2014; Witte et al., 2014; Goedert, 2015; Sankowski et al., 2015). With such complexity, it has proved difficult to identify biomarkers to quantify progression and targets to block to prevent the degeneration. The most obvious physiological symptoms are the loss of neurons in Alzheimer's Disease (AD) and Parkinson's Disease (PD) with the consequently lower neurotransmitter levels, and the formation of protein aggregates in all forms of neurodegeneration. These observations provided the primary targets to date, namely enzymes catalyzing neurotransmitter breakdown (cholinesterases, ChE; monoamine oxidases, MAO; catechol-O-methyltransferase, COMT), prevention of production of amyloid beta (Aβ) by beta-secretase, of protein aggregation, and of oxidative damage known to stress cells to the point of apoptosis (Guzior et al., 2015; Swomley and Butterfield, 2015). Intervention in the potentially damaging outcomes of oxidation stress either by means of upstream (prevention of free radical generation) or downstream (free radical scavenging) antioxidant pathways helps preserve neurons and slow neurodegeneration (Uttara et al., 2009).

Related to oxidative damage and because of their role in the regulation of apoptosis, mitochondria are a current active area of investigation both for generation of reactive oxygen species (ROS) or inefficient energy production that limits defenses against ROS. Recent advances focus on mitochondrial movement, fusion, and fission and interactions with the cytosol (including specific proteins related to neurodegeneration such as the Bax/Bid family and sirtuins) (Eckert et al., 2012; Johri and Beal, 2012). Mitochondria play a central role in the oxidative metabolism of nutrients and ATP synthesis. They also contribute to intracellular second messenger homeostasis (Ca^{2+} and ROS), and are determinant for both cell survival and apoptotic cell coordination (Waagepetersen et al., 2003; Mandemakers et al., 2007; Nunnari and Suomalainen, 2012; Bernardi et al., 2015). Mitochondrial dysfunction is frequently proposed to be involved in neurodegenerative pathogenesis, including PD and AD (Mandemakers et al., 2007; Moreira et al., 2010; Correia et al., 2012a,b; Perier et al., 2012; Perier and Vila, 2012). With their high energy demands neurons are particularly dependent on mitochondrial ATP generation, and are thus intolerant of mitochondrial dysfunction (Lezi and Swerdlow, 2012). This makes the understanding of the mitochondrial mechanisms underlying these pathologies critical for designing more effective strategies to halt or delay disease progression (Correia et al., 2010a,b). An alternative strategy to preserving levels of neurotransmitters by inhibiting breakdown is the pharmacological stimulation of the post-synaptic receptors in the remaining neurons. Most receptors are G-protein coupled receptors (http://www.guidetopharmacology.org/), an area of fast recent progress with the determination of receptor structures, such as the muscarinic acetylcholine receptors (Thal et al., 2016), the availability of cloned receptors for pharmacology and compound screening (Katritch et al., 2013; Melancon et al., 2013), and new methods for assessing the complex function of the receptors (van Unen et al., 2015). Here too, multiple targets are attractive: for example, first-in-class dual M1/M4 agonists now in preclinical development (http://www.heptares.com/pipeline/). Antagonists to histamine receptors are also interesting to prevent the inflammation also thought to contribute to neurodegeneration (Vohora and Bhowmik, 2012; Walter and Stark, 2012). However, a meta-analysis of

---

Abbreviations: AD, Alzheimer's Disease; AChE, acetylcholinesterase; Aβ, amyloid beta; BChE, butyrylcholinesterase; MAO, monoamine oxidase; CYP, cytochrome P450; AIF, apoptosis inducing factor; MTDL, multi-target designed ligand; PD, Parkinson's Disease; ROS, Reactive Oxygen Species; CI Complex I, HLM, human liver mitochondria; RLM, rat liver mitochondria.

placebo-controlled trials for H3 receptor antagonists did not find significant effects on cognition (Kubo et al., 2015). Receptors will not be further mentioned in this article because we focus on intracellular targets.

It is apparent from the above outline that the primary causes of neurodegeneration are not easily defined, and will almost certainly be due to highly individual combinations of factors. This has led to the search for novel compounds that will interact with multiple targets, and have antioxidant properties as part of the desired pharmacologic profile. For the future there will be a need for various combinations of multi-target designed ligands (MTDL) to meet the needs of each individual combination of defects. In this article, we shall describe the background to *in vitro* assessment of compounds to combat neurodegeneration, considering the current targets either for symptomatic treatment (AChE and MAO) or to prevent or reverse deterioration (anti-oxidants or mitochondrial function), and giving examples of compounds from our own work conducted in collaborations facilitated by COST Action CM1103 "Structure-based drug design for diagnosis and treatment of neurological diseases: dissecting and modulating complex function in the monoaminergic systems of the brain."

Screening techniques highlight that many enzymes and receptors interact with a given chemical. This is clear in off-target data-mining (Nikolic et al., 2015; Hughes et al., 2016) and in high throughput screens (Sipes et al., 2013). In the latter project aimed at building a resource of biological pathways of toxicity for various types of chemicals, 976 compounds known as pharmaceuticals, food additives or pesticides were tested for inhibition or activation of enzymes and for binding to monoaminergic transporters and receptors. The most common sub-micromolar interactions were with the cytochrome P450 (CYP) family, transporters, the mitochondrial translocator (benzodiazepine–binding) protein, the dopamine and serotonin reuptake carriers, and the aminergic G-protein coupled receptors, and MAO was also in the top 20 most promiscuous proteins. These results indicate the promise of MTDL for cholinesterase (lower on that list) and MAOs or to include receptor agonism or antagonism into one molecule is not without the drawback of also finding off-target activity. In particular, any effect on the metabolic CYP enzymes must be carefully appraised.

After the identification of the target, be it receptor or enzyme, a variety of empirical and/or *in silico* studies are conducted in order to vary the structure to increase the pharmacological effects of the new compounds. However, good *in vitro* activity may not correspond to a therapeutic effect, unless the molecule also possesses high bioavailability and low toxicity. This means that the new compounds must have good pharmacokinetic properties. The investigation on absorption, distribution, metabolism and excretion properties and toxicological profiling (ADME/Tox) have become an essential step in early drug discovery that has demonstrated a high impact on the successful progression of drug candidates. Growing knowledge of the key roles that pharmacokinetics and drug metabolism play as determinants of *in vivo* drug action, has led many researchers, drug companies and regulatory agencies to include examination of pharmacokinetics and drug metabolism properties as part of their process in the selection of drug candidates. In this context, the role of the CYP isoenzymes is outlined, since it represents a major source of variability toward pharmacokinetics and pharmacological responses in this phase.

In this review we consider the biochemistry of some of the key pharmacological targets of MTDL, giving selected examples from our own expertise. The traditional key targets in Alzheimer's Disease (AD), the ChEs and MAOs, are described first, then the new and diverse potential targets in mitochondrial function for cell survival, followed by an example of targeting the oxidative stress that is seen in a variety of degenerative conditions. Lastly in this overview of metabolic aspects of drug design, the action of the CYP isoenzymes, important for effectiveness of all drugs *in vivo*, on MTDL is described.

ADDRESSING THE PATHOLOGY OF NEURODEGENERATION: THE TARGETS CONSIDERED HERE

Four of the five drugs ever approved to treat symptoms of memory loss and confusion in AD patients are cholinesterase inhibitors. The cholinergic hypothesis of AD posits that the cognitive and behavioral dysfunctions of AD result from deficits in acetylcholine neurotransmission. These early symptoms can be ameliorated by inhibiting the cholinesterases to prolong the presence of acetylcholine in the synapse. However, cholinesterase activities have also been reported correlate with the density of amyloid plaque deposition in the AD brain (Arendt et al., 1992). The mechanism by which AChE and to a lesser extent BChE facilitate plaque deposition is still being investigated (Hou et al., 2014).

The other catabolic enzyme that is inhibited to maintain decreasing neurotransmission is MAO, located on the cytosolic face of the mitochondrial outer membrane where it is attached by a single membrane-spanning helix. To be metabolized by MAO, monoamine neurotransmitters must be taken up into the cells. The two forms, MAO A and MAO B, are co-located in liver mitochondria, but otherwise have very different expression patterns. MAO A is the major form in the intestine and placenta, MAO B in platelets. In the brain, MAO B is expressed in the glia and in serotonergic neurons, whereas MAO A predominates in all other neurons.

Mitochondria produce the majority of energy in all type of cells but particularly in neurons where the energy demand for neurotransmission is high. Deficits in mitochondrial function (i.e., increased oxidative stress, decreased efficiency of the respiratory chain, apoptosis dysfunctions, deregulation of fusion and fission processes) have been found in all neurodegenerative conditions. Understanding the mechanisms underlying these pathologies is critical to designing more effective strategies to halt or delay disease progression (Correia et al., 2010a, 2012a). Each of the mitochondrial functions is closely related to the others and alteration in any of them might develop neurodegeneration, making difficult to discriminate which changes are more critical (Haddad and Nakamura, 2015). Abnormal morphology, altered dynamics, and biochemical dysfunction of mitochondria are usually observed, being often systemic rather than brain-limited (Lezi and Swerdlow, 2012).

Mitochondrial respiratory capacity and efficient ATP production are vital for neuronal survival. In most neurodegenerative conditions mutations accumulate in mitochondrial DNA (encoding 13 proteins essential for respiratory chain function), the enzymatic activity of respiratory chain enzymes is altered and oxidative stress usually increases (Goldberg et al., 2002). Such dysfunctions arise not only as consequence of mutations in mitochondrial DNA but can also be due to mutations in nuclear DNA encoding for proteins either imported to or interacting with the mitochondria. Changes in the mitochondrial membrane potential and the increased reactive oxygen species (ROS) associated with electron transport chain dysfunction have been strongly linked to reduced cell viability (Bird et al., 2014). Although ROS formation is a natural by-product of mitochondrial respiration, overproduction is indicative of cell stress (Murphy, 2009). Antioxidant therapy has therefore long been sought to combat aging as well as neurodegeneration.

Antioxidant compounds can either react with radicals to prevent damage to biological molecules (proteins, lipids or DNA) or can complex metal ions to decrease generation of ROS. Iron ions are the well-established target in AD, playing a key catalytic role in the Fenton reaction (reviewed in Unzeta et al., 2016). Knock out studies have established that loss of Amyloid Precursor Protein (APP) or tau (both AD-linked proteins) results in iron accumulation in the brain. Iron is bound to ferritin, a protein that increases with age and in AD (Bartzokis and Tishler, 2000). Iron is found also in plaques (Meadowcroft et al., 2009). Iron-chelation capability is part of the action spectrum of rasagiline used for treatment of PD (Weinreb et al., 2016) and a highly desirable addition to future MTDL compounds for prevention of neurodegeneration.

Lastly, decreasing the generation of aberrant proteins, preventing their aggregation, and blocking down-stream events are developing targets. The prevention of production of amyloid beta (Aβ) by inhibition of the beta-secretases already has led to candidate small molecule compounds in clinical trials (Yan and Vassar, 2014; Yan et al., 2016). The acceleration of Aβ aggregation by the peripheral site of AChE has long been recognized (Inestrosa et al., 1996; Reyes et al., 1997) and is an important component of effective AChE inhibitors designed to combat AD (Bartolini et al., 2003; Anand and Singh, 2013; Bolea et al., 2013; Bautista-Aguilera et al., 2014a; Hebda et al., 2016). Deleterious intracellular effects of Aβ are also recognized, such as the consequences of Aβ binding to a 17-β-hydroxysteroid dehydrogenase known as Amyloid Binding Alcohol Dehydrogenase (ABAD), a tetrameric mitochondrial enzyme that catalyzes the oxidation of steroids. ABAD is decreased in AD (Lustbader et al., 2004) and missense mutations in its gene (HSD17B10) result in alteration of mitochondria morphology and neurodegeneration in infancy (Yang et al., 2014). The ABAD-Aβ interaction is associated with up-regulation of endophilin, a protein important for membrane-shaping in processes such as synaptic vesicle formation which

might contribute to neuronal sensitivity to ABAD-Aβ complex formation inside neuronal mitochondria (Borger et al., 2013). Drug discovery to prevent the ABAD-Aβ interaction, begun with brain-permeant peptides (Borger et al., 2013), is now moving to small molecules (Valaasani et al., 2014; Benek et al., 2015; Hroch et al., 2015) that will provide information for future incorporation into multi-target compounds.

The aim of MTDL design is to combine features that can interact with two or more of the desired targets (Csermely et al., 2005; Geldenhuys et al., 2011; Hughes et al., 2016). This expands the biological screening required at the early stages for hit discovery and lead optimization. With structures of most targets available, in silico screening is a useful tool for examining large chemical databases (Hughes et al., 2016; Nikolic et al., 2016). Combining known drugs for each target into one molecule has also produced promising compounds by incorporating elements of proven inhibitors for each target into new multi-potent molecules (Bolognesi et al., 2007; Piazzi et al., 2008; Zhu et al., 2009; Kupershmidt et al., 2012; Luo et al., 2013; Sun et al., 2014; Bautista-Aguilera et al., 2014b; Wang L. et al., 2014; Pisani et al., 2016; Weichert et al., 2016; Xie et al., 2016). One example that progressed to clinical trials against AD is ladostigil, designed to inhibit MAOs and ChEs but also incorporating potent anti-apoptotic and neuroprotective activities (Weinreb et al., 2012; Youdim, 2013). The next sections in this review will consider other examples of MTDL in the context of some of these targets of interest for AD drugs.

NEUROTRANSMITTER DEGRADING ENZYMES

Enzyme Inhibitors—Pharmacological Characterization

The development of novel drugs that target enzymes requires an understanding of enzyme mechanism and is deeply informed by detailed knowledge of the protein structure. Understanding how enzymes (or indeed receptors) work is vital for medicinal chemists aiming to design new drugs (Walsh, 2013). In the very first stage of evaluation of new compounds in a biological system, the medicinal chemistry shortcut of IC_{50} measurement is an invaluable tool for comparisons of series of derivatives on a given scaffold and provides useful information for determining a hit or for choice of a lead compound. It is a measurement that can be used for both simple and complex biological systems but it is important to recognize that the meaning of IC_{50} (as opposed to its definition as 50% inhibition of a measured parameter) changes according to the system and the assay conditions. In the context of measurement of a single enzyme activity, IC_{50} is not affinity for a target but simply the concentration of the compound that inhibits the activity by 50% under the specific conditions used. For more informative data on enzyme reversible inhibitors, the K_i (the inhibition constant independent of the substrate concentration used) and the mechanism of inhibition should be determined. For irreversible inhibitors, the rate of inactivation and the concentration dependence are needed (McDonald and Tipton, 2012). It should be recognized that IC_{50} values for reversible and irreversible inhibitors are not directly comparable because of the time element. The initial reversible binding of an inactivating inhibitor can only be compared with reversible inhibitors (or indeed binding constants from docking) if initial rates are measured in an assay where the enzyme is added last to a mixture of substrate and inhibitor.

When comparing alternate targets, care is needed to use conditions for each target that will allow comparison. Selective inhibition of MAO A and MAO B is often desired, but they have different K_M values for their common substrates (the concentration of substrate required to give half the maximum velocity), so are saturated to different degrees at any one concentration. For example, purified human MAO A activity reaches 50% of its maximum at 0.15 mM kynuramine, whereas MAO B reaches 50% of maximum rate with only 0.08 mM kynuramine. With reversible inhibitors,

$E + I \leftrightarrow EI$ but during steady state measurement, when $E + S \leftrightarrow ES \rightarrow E + P$, the concentration of free enzyme (E) available to bind inhibitor is not the total enzyme added but rather a fraction of the total that depends on the substrate concentration used and the relative values of the rate constants. In the steady-state where ES is constant, MAO A assayed with 0.1 mM kynuramine has 60% of free enzyme but MAO B has only 44% available for inhibitor binding. For an inhibitor of both with the same K_i of 0.01 mM, the IC_{50} would be measured as 17 μM for MAO A but 22.5 μM for MAO B despite the fact that the inhibitor bound equally well to both enzymes. Simply using an assay with fixed substrate concentration without taking into account the different K_M values would therefore introduce a 30% bias to the selectivity.

The mechanism of the enzyme can also influence IC_{50} values. This is seen in the kinetic analysis of MAO B where it is clear that there are two forms of the enzyme that can bind the ligand (substrate or inhibitor), namely, the oxidized or the reduced forms, and that these two forms bind ligands with different affinities. Since different substrates give different proportions of these forms during steady-state catalysis, different Ki values for an inhibitor can be obtained from different substrates. Overall, care must be exercised in choice of substrate and of assay conditions to obtain reliable IC_{50} values, but only kinetic constants can be considered meaningful (McDonald et al., 2010; Ramsay et al., 2011). Slow and tight binding inhibitors also require special analysis (Morrison, 1969).

For irreversible inhibition, a time course of the development of the inactive enzyme is essential. The best compounds for specific irreversible inhibition *in vivo* are mechanism-based inhibitors, making use of the catalytic specificity of the target itself. However, sometimes even mechanism-based activation to a reactive product can be catalyzed by more than one enzyme, as seen for the MAO inhibitor tranylcypromine that irreversibly modifies the flavin in MAO after single electron oxidation (Silverman, 1983; Bonivento et al., 2010). Tranylcypromine was recently found to modify also the flavin in the epigenetic histone demethylase enzyme LSD1 (Schmidt and McCafferty, 2007; Binda et al., 2010). For medicinal chemistry screening, irreversible inhibition can be detected as a decrease in the IC_{50} value after 30 min preincubation compared to no preincubation. For example, for MAO B the IC50 for tranylcypromine without preincubation is 4 μM but if preincubated with the enzyme for 30 min before substrate is added, the IC_{50} is 0.074 μM (Malcomson et al., 2015). Proper characterization of mechanism-based inactivation requires measurement of the rate of production of inactive enzyme over time with several inhibitor concentrations to obtain K_I and k_{inact} (Kitz and Wilson, 1962).

Catalysis consists of both binding and kinetics steps. Theoretical screening measuring the sum of the optimal interactions between a compound and a target addresses only binding (and that with limitations depending on the restrictions placed on molecular dynamics). As a result, enzyme IC_{50} values are frequently not in accord with computed binding constants. Although K_i and K_D can be numerically the same if measurements are made in a simple Michaelis-Menten system, they never have the same meaning. Nonetheless, theoretical screening is a useful tool, particularly for large compound libraries and to facilitate repurposing of existing drugs used for other clinical targets (Hughes et al., 2016; Nikolic et al., 2016).

Cholinesterases (AchE, BchE)
AChE/BChE Location, Structure, Activity, Redundancy

AChE is located at neuromuscular junctions and in the central nervous system on the outside of the post-synaptic cell membranes, mainly in a tetrameric form. A Ser-His-Glu catalytic triad in the active site catalyzes the hydrolysis, and anionic and hydrophobic groups in the peripheral anionic site (PAS) contribute to binding a wide range of chemical structures (**Figure 1**). The drug, donepezil, spans both sites with aromatic stacking contributing to the nanomolar binding affinity, as shown in the crystal structure of the human AChE (Cheung et al., 2012). The PAS has a function in allosteric modulation of AChE activity and in increasing amyloid (Inestrosa et al., 2008; Hou et al., 2014).

BChE may also have a role in amyloid plaque formation (Darvesh et al., 2012). It is found mainly in plasma as a soluble monomer secreted by glial cells (Greig et al., 2002). Although the two enzymes share 65% homology and a similar hydrophobic active site structure, they have different specificities in part due to two aromatic residues (Phe295 and Phe297) that constrict the 20 Å long gorge in AChE (Greig et al., 2002; Nicolet et al., 2003). The K_M values and turnover numbers with acetylcholine are 0.1 mM and 6500 s^{-1} for AChE and 0.15 mM and 1433 s^{-1} for BChE (http://www.brenda-enzymes.org). In the normal brain where AChE is localize on the post synaptic membrane it was estimated that 90% of acetylcholine hydrolysis is catalyzed by AChE (Greig et al., 2002). However, BChE is plentiful and secreted by the glial cells so that if AChE is inhibited or is defective as in AChE-knock-out mice, the hydrolysis can be catalyzed by BChE (Mesulam et al., 2002). Thus, in current efforts to design multitarget drugs, reversible inhibition of both AChE and BChE is considered desirable.

Cholinesterase Assay and Inhibitors

Both AChE and BChE can be assayed using acetylthiocholine, but butyrylthiocholine is selective for BChE. The enzymes hydrolyse acetylthiocholine to acetate and thiocholine. Thiocholine reacts with Ellman's reagent (DTNB) to form a mixed dithiol,

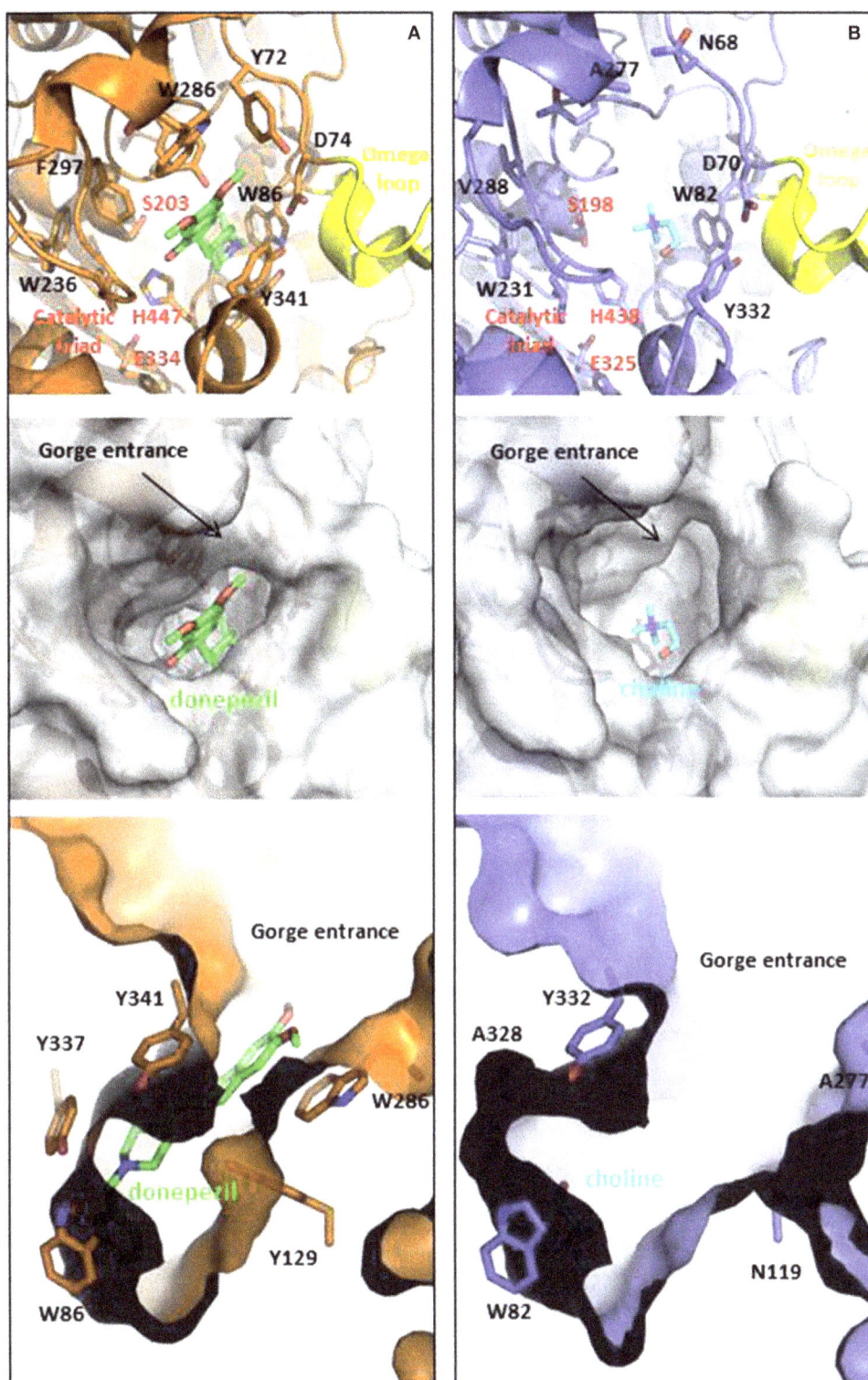

FIGURE 1 | Ligand binding cavities of (A) AChE and (B) BChE. AChE (shown in orange) is in complex with donepezil (shown in CPK colored sticks with carbons in green, PDB ID: 4EY7), while BChE (shown metal blue) is in complex with choline (shown in CPK colored sticks with carbons in light blue, PDB ID: 1P0M). The top panels show the cartoon representations with detail in sticks of relevant residues involved at the gorge entrances, the PAS regions or the catalytic triads (labeled in red), as well as the omega loops colored in yellow. Middle and lower panels show top and lateral views of the ligand binding cavities. The entrance loops are highlighted in pink and yellow respectively. PDB files were obtained from the protein databank and figures were produced using the PyMol software (PyMOL, http://www.pymol.org).

liberating 5-thio-2-nitrobenzoate that absorbs at 412 nm. The molar absorption coefficient is 14,150 M^{-1} cm^{-1}; (Riddles et al., 1979) but it can vary slightly with salt concentration, pH, and temperature (Ellman et al., 1961; Eyer et al., 2003). The K_M for acetylthiocholine (0.025–0.05 mM) is similar for both enzymes although the rate with BChE is slower.

Common drugs inhibiting AChE and BChE are donepezil and tacrine (see **Table 1**) (Camps et al., 2008; Esteban et al., 2014; Wang L. et al., 2014). Carbamates are also reversible inhibitors (e.g., rivastigmine), coumarins, and several natural compounds have also been investigated. Harmine, an endogenous compound from the breakdown of tryptophan is also an inhibitor (He et al., 2015). In the last 5 years most inhibitor development has focused on maintaining a relatively equal inhibitory activity against AChE and BChE with IC_{50} values below μmolar concentrations in a compound that also acts on other targets such as MAO (see below), antioxidant, metal chelation, and preventing protein aggregation (for reviews see: León et al., 2013; Swomley and Butterfield, 2015). Many groups have synthesized and tested a variety of combinations. Here, we consider in detail ASS234, an example from our own work. ASS234 (**Table 1**) with potency similar to tacrine is almost equipotent on human AChE and BChE. ASS234 also has antioxidant properties, inhibits Aβ aggregation, and decreases Aβ-induced apoptosis in cellular studies (Bolea et al., 2013).

The discovery of compounds that combine cholinesterase inhibition with binding to other targets of interest for AD is also underway. For example, the serotonin receptor, 5-HT$_4$, has been linked to memory deficits (Cho and Hu, 2007; Lezoualc'h, 2007; Russo et al., 2009). Stimulation causes release of ACh and increases dopamine, serotonin, and γ-aminobutyric acid (GABA) release, and thus could act synergistically with ChE and MAO inhibition. 5-HT$_4$ stimulation also increases the safer non-amyloidogenic pathway for APP cleavage (Cochet et al., 2013). Agonists or partial agonists have been designed and the first MTDLs with cholinesterase and receptor binding have been designed (Lecoutey et al., 2014; Rochais et al., 2015).

Monoamine Oxidases (MAO A, MAO B)

Neurotransmitter levels influence brain activity and preventing neurotransmitter breakdown has an anti-depressant effect. The monoamines are catabolized by MAO and COMT, inhibitors for which are useful in PD (Talati et al., 2009). Mice treated with MAOI showed significantly higher noradrenaline and serotonin levels in brain and significantly lower metabolites (including DOPAC from dopamine) (Lum and Stahl, 2012). Higher monoamine levels as a result of MAOI are also seen in rats in micro-dialysis experiments (Bazzu et al., 2013; Bolea et al., 2014), and in humans are observed as serotonin toxicity in patients given non-selective MAOI on top of serotonin reuptake inhibitors (SSRIs) (Gillman, 2011). Changes in monoamine levels also have downstream effects on expression and function of receptors and other proteins (Finberg, 2014).

TABLE 1 | AChE and MAO inhibitors and the inhibitory activity of MTDL.

Structure	Compound	AChE (μM)	BChE (μM)	MAO A (nM)	MAO B (nM)	References
	Tacrine	0.205[1]	0.044[1]	–	–	[1]Camps et al., 2008
	Donepezil	0.012[1] 0.011[2]	7.3[1] 6.22[2]	850000[3] Rat	15000[3] Rat	[1]Camps et al., 2008; [2]Esteban et al., 2014; [3]Wang L. et al., 2014
	PF1901N	>100[2]	>100[2]	790[2]	11[2]	[2]Esteban et al., 2014
	ASS234	0.35[4] Eel 0.81[2]	0.46[4] Eel 1.82[2]	5.24[4] 0.17[2]	43350[4] 15830[2]	[2]Esteban et al., 2014; [4]Bolea et al., 2011
	Clorgyline	–	–	0.42[2]	10660[2]	[2]Esteban et al., 2014
	L-Deprenyl	–	–	630[2]	3.0[2]	[2]Esteban et al., 2014

Enzymes activities were measured after 30 min incubation with the inhibitor; inhibition is for the human enzyme unless specified (marked in italics). The – indicates no inhibition.

Altered MAO levels are associated with brain pathology. MAO A/B knockout mice displaying anxiety-like symptoms have greatly elevated monoamine levels (Chen et al., 2004). MAO B, located mainly in glial cells, increases with age and is elevated in AD and PD (Kennedy et al., 2003; Zellner et al., 2012; Woodard et al., 2014; Ooi et al., 2015). Inhibition of MAO B by compounds in cigarette smoke is associated with delayed onset of PD, and the MAO B inhibitor, deprenyl, delays the need to begin levodopa treatment in PD patients. Considering genetic variations, the A allele of the common A644G single nucleotide polymorphism in intron 13 of the MAO B gene is associated with slightly lower platelet MAO B activity and slightly less risk of PD (Liu et al., 2014). For MAO A, a low activity allele is associated with aggression (Gallardo-Pujol et al., 2013), and the high activity that results from the long repeat allele in the promotor region of the gene is associated with depression (Meyer et al., 2006), although a Positron Emission Tomography study found no significant difference in activity MAO A activity in the human brain (Fowler et al., 2015). Inhibition of MAO A has also been shown to decrease the oxidative stress that can result from the hydrogen peroxide and the aldehyde products of MAO catalysis both in heart and brain (Kaludercic et al., 2011; Ooi et al., 2015).

MAO A and MAO B Structure, Activity, Redundancy

MAO A and B share 70% homology and very similar active sites (reviewed in Edmondson et al., 2007). A major influence on substrate and inhibitor specificity is the narrow part ("gate") of the MAO B cavity defined by I199 and Y326 (**Figure 2**). However, the design of selective inhibitors is not simple, although in general MAO A can accommodate bulkier compounds. Simply changing one substituent can alter affinity for one form but not the other. For example, adding a second carbonitrile group to a small furan scaffold, increased the affinity for MAO A by 10-fold but not for MAO B (Juárez-Jiménez et al., 2014) due to a hydrogen bond to asparagine 181 in MAO A. At that position (172 in MAO B) MAO B has a cysteine residue that can contribute to MAO B-selective binding. Structure-function analyses for the design of selective MAO inhibitors has been reviewed recently (Vilar et al., 2012; Patil et al., 2013; Carradori and Petzer, 2015).

Since MAO A and B are located on the X chromosome, human MAO deficiencies were first discovered in males. MAO A deficiency is associated with aggression, but MAO B deficient subjects were mentally normal. The combined deletion found in Norrie disease is associated with severe mental retardation (Brunner et al., 1993; Lenders et al., 1996). Detailed examination of the effects of deletions are now possible through knockout mice, studies that provide insight into the roles of MAO in behavior and development (Shih and Chen, 1999; Bortolato and Shih, 2011). In mice, as in humans, MAO A deficiency is associated with aggression. MAO B deficiency does not perturb monoamine metabolism to any great extent but results in excretion of higher amounts of phenylethylamine. The substrate specificities of the two forms overlap, with MAO A metabolizing serotonin well, MAO B PEA, but both dopamine and noradrenaline. The relative efficiency of catalysis by the two forms is best expressed by the maximum catalytic velocity divided by the K_M, values; these can be found in (Youdim

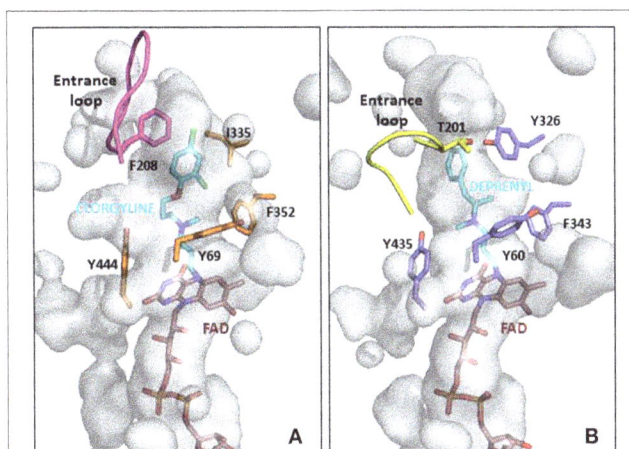

FIGURE 2 | **MAO active site cavities showing the FAD cofactor and the ligand in the crystal structures. (A)** MAO A in complex with clorgyline (PDB ID: 2BXS) and **(B)** MAO B in complex with deprenyl (PDB ID: 2BYB). The FAD cofactors inside the cavities are shown in CPK colored sticks with carbons in pink, the clorgyline and deprenyl ligands are also shown in sticks with carbons in blue, and key residues around the ligand cavity are shown in CPK colored sticks with carbons in orange and metal blue for MAO A and MAO B, respectively. The entrance loops are highlighted in pink and yellow respectively. The PDB files were obtained from the protein databank and figures were produced using PyMOL (http://www.pymol.org).

et al., 2006). In contrast to acetylcholine neurotransmission, the primary termination of the monoamine chemical signal is by reuptake of the monoamines, first into the neuron and then back into the storage vesicles. Inhibition of MAO increases stores of monoamines, for example in PD where inhibition of MAO B slows the breakdown of dopamine (Finberg, 2014).

MAO A/B Assay and Inhibitors

MAO can be assayed using absorbance or fluorescence changes, by radiolabeled product detection, by HPLC separation of the product, or by coupling the second product H_2O_2 to a detection system. The simplest assay is the measurement of the oxidation of kynuramine either continuously by the absorbance change at 314 nm (Weissbach et al., 1960) or in a stopped assay by the fluorescence of the product.

Recombinant human MAO A and MAO B expressed in insect cell membranes is now commercially available but the low activity requires the sensitive coupled assay where H_2O_2 is used by horseradish peroxidase to convert the non-fluorescent dye, N-acetyl-3,7-dihydroxyphenoxazine (Amplex Red), to the fluorescent resorufin (Zhou et al., 1997). As with all coupled assays, considerable care must be taken to check the validity of the assay by ensuring that the enzyme of interest (MAO in this case) is rate limiting. Inhibitors can quench or enhance fluorescence, or may inhibit horseradish peroxidase. These interfering factors must be checked for each type of inhibitor. It should be noted that Amplex Red, N-acetyl-3,7-dihydroxyphenoxazine, a structure similar to the MAO A inhibitor Methylene Blue (Ramsay et al., 2007; Milczek et al., 2011) inhibits MAO A so the dye must be used at 20–50 μM, and not the 200 μM recommend by the assay kit manufacturer. Most substrates (except dopamine) can be used in this continuous coupled assay. The most frequently used is tyramine which has a K_M of 127 μM with MAO A and 107 μM with MAO B (Youdim et al., 2006). However, different laboratories report various values, so the K_M should be checked for each condition used.The discovery of highly selective reversible inhibitors for MAO A or MAO B has been the focus of compound synthesis for antidepressant design in recent years due to reduced side effects and lower drug-drug/food interaction risk. Some effective reversible inhibitors are harmine (K_i = 5 nM) (Kim et al., 1997) used to measure MAO A occupancy in positron emission tomography scans (Sacher et al., 2011) and moclobemide (used in anxiety disorders). Moclobemide, giving 70–78% occupancy of MAO A at clinically effective doses (Sacher et al., 2011), is useful because, as a reversible inhibitor, it does not inactivate the MAO A in the gut wall and so does not potentiate the vascular effects due to tyramine from the intestine. For MAO B, safinamide (K_i = 0.5 μM) (Binda et al., 2007) is in clinical trials for adjunct therapy in PD (Finberg, 2014). Traditional medicinal chemistry approaches, screening of compound libraries, and computational screening continue the search for new scaffolds for reversible inhibitors (Santana et al., 2006; Shelke et al., 2011).

However, irreversible inhibition and the slow turnover rate of MAO allows lower doses compared to reversible inhibitors and thus lower risk of side effects. All the common MAOI used clinically for depression and for PD are irreversible inhibitors (**Table 1**). The mechanism-based inactivation of MAO can be achieved by phenylzines, cyclopropopylamines, and propynamines. The selective irreversible inhibitors clorgyline for MAO A and deprenyl for MAO B both contain the propargyl moiety that after oxidation by MAO A forms a covalent adduct with the N5 of the FAD cofactor (Binda et al., 2002; De Colibus et al., 2005). The propargyl moiety is a useful small entity to add MAOI capability to molecules designed for other targets to give MTDL as describe below. The propargyl group must be oxidized by MAO to generate the reactive species that forms the covalent bond with the enzyme. The rate of inactivation by propargyl compounds for both MAO A and MAO B is around 0.2 min^{-1} with selectivity coming from the binding (Esteban et al., 2014; Malcomson et al., 2015). A further benefit of the propargyl moiety is its association with neuroprotection at levels lower than for inhibition of MAO (Naoi and Maruyama, 2010; Weinreb et al., 2011).

In assessing inhibitors of MAO, a final word of caution must be included regarding the considerable species differences that have been noted for inhibitor binding (Krueger et al., 1995). Happily, the human and rat sensitivities to MAOI are fairly similar but there are clear structural active site differences between the rat and human MAOs (Upadhyay et al., 2008) with implications for drug design (Novaroli et al., 2006; Fierro et al., 2007).

Multi-Target Designed Ligands (MTDL) That Inhibit ChEs and MAOs

One promising MTDL investigated under the auspices of COST Action CM1103 is ASS234 (N-((5-(3-(1-benzylpiperidin-4-yl)propoxy)-1-methyl-1H-indol-2-yl)methyl)-N-methylprop-2-yn-1-amine). The indole group aids MAO A selectivity and

the propynamine (propargyl) group allows for irreversible inhibition. However, by adding a 1-benzylpiperidine fragment (similar to the AChE inhibitor, donepezil), this compound becomes also a reversible inhibitor for AChE and BChE (Bolea et al., 2011). During biological assessment, it became apparent that this compound has neuroprotective properties, by inhibiting Aβ42 and Aβ40 self-aggregation into plaques, and by protecting against depletion of antioxidative enzymes (Bolea et al., 2013). Therefore ASS234 has been patented (PCT/ES070186; WO2011/113988 A1) as a promising compound for the treatment of AD.Many other ChE/MAO targeted MTDL have been designed in the last 5 years, either propargyl-based (Youdim, 2013; Bautista-Aguilera et al., 2014b; Samadi et al., 2015; Weinreb et al., 2015) or coumarins derivatives (Pisani et al., 2011; Patil et al., 2013; Farina et al., 2015; Xie et al., 2015). The challenge will be to add further neuroprotective properties to progress to a disease-modifying drug.

MITOCHONDRIAL HOMEOSTASIS AND APOPTOSIS

Mitochondrial Fusion, Fission, and Trafficking

Mitochondria are dynamic organelles with the ability to divide (fission) and fuse (fusion) as well as to concentrate in particular subcellular locations. Regulation of these processes is crucial for cell health and apoptosis (Hales, 2004, 2010). Fission and fusion play critical roles in maintaining functional mitochondria when cells experience metabolic or environmental stresses, a reason why their improper regulation associates with several human genetic neurodegenerative diseases affecting to neuronal survival and plasticity (Hales, 2010; Youle and van der Bliek, 2012). Fusion is proposed to mitigate stress allowing complementation by mixing contents of partially damaged mitochondria. Fission, besides being required in the creation of new mitochondria, also contributes to quality control by facilitating both removal of damaged mitochondria (mitophagy) and apoptosis under cellular stress situations (Lee et al., 2004). The combined action of several GTPases contributes to the dynamic mitochondrial networks; Drp1/Dnm1 is key in mitochondrial division, mitofusins (Mfn1 and Mfn2) control outer mitochondrial membrane fusion, and OPA1 mediates inner mitochondrial membrane fusion (Griparic et al., 2004, 2007; Ishihara et al., 2006; Cohen et al., 2008). Neurons are more sensitive than other cells to mutations in the genes coding for these proteins, indicating the importance of mitochondrial dynamics for the maintenance of the nervous system integrity (Mandemakers et al., 2007). Deletion of either of the two mitofusins results in unbalanced fission and mitochondrial fragmentation (Koshiba et al., 2004). Mutations in Mfn2 cause the Charcot-Marie-Tooth disease (Züchner et al., 2004), and mutations in OPA1 are associated with genetic forms of blindness (Delettre et al., 2000) (**Figure 3**). A number of other factors contribute to modulate these GTPases activities and changes in their molecular shapes precisely control these processes (Mandemakers et al., 2007). For example, several brain neurodegenerative disorders cause decrease in mitochondrial size

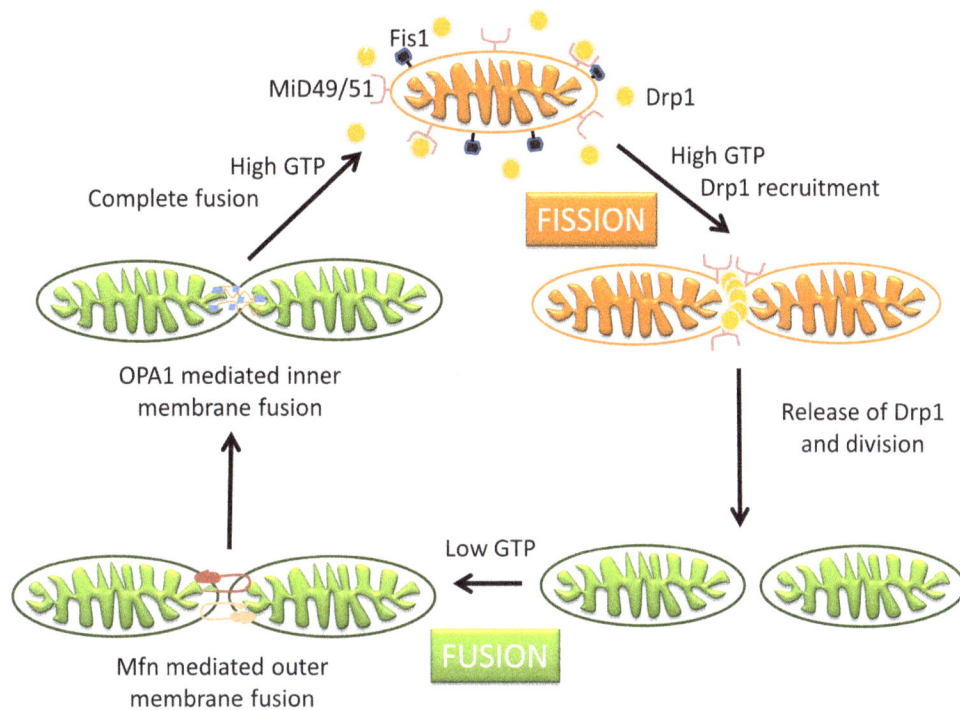

FIGURE 3 | Schematic representation of mitochondrial dynamics. Steady state mitochondrial morphology requires a balance of fission and fusion events. During organelle fission Drp1 is recruited from the cytosol to the outer mitochondrial membrane, where it interacts directly or indirectly with Fis1 forming high molecular weight oligomers on the mitochondrial surface. This leads to constriction of mitochondria and sequential separation of the inner and outer membrane. Once Drp1 is released fission is complete. Fission also allows isolation for mitochondria that cannot be repaired followed by degradation through mitophagy, and is also important for subcellular distribution and transportation of mitochondria based on local energy needs. Mitochondrial fusion is a two-step process that requires outer and inner membrane fusion. Outer membrane fusion is facilitated by mitofusins tethering of adjacent membranes. This is subsequently followed by inner membrane fusion, which is GTP dependent and regulated by OPA1. Fusion allows for functional complementation and repair of damaged mitochondria.

and increased Drp1 translocation to mitochondria, increasing fission events. Treatments inhibiting Drp1 have been shown to restore mitochondrial length, reduce loss of new-born hippocampal neurons, and improve hippocampal-dependent learning and memory after damage (Li et al., 2015; Fischer et al., 2016). Therefore, reducing mitochondrial fission may contribute to rescue from brain injury, and the possibility to regulate the mechanisms of fusion and fission by different mediators in different tissues can represent a potential therapeutic target for related disorders.

Due to their complex structural and molecular features, neurons also require mechanisms for mitochondria trafficking to their distal destinations (presynaptic bouton, axons, synaptic terminals) and anchoring in regions where metabolism is in high demand. Failure to deliver a functional mitochondrion to the appropriate site within a neuron could contribute to neuronal dysfunction. Besides mitochondrial dynamics, the proteins mentioned above are also involved in mitochondrial subcellular positioning in neurons, ensuring a relatively constant mitochondrial population. As an example, membrane bound OPA1 influences mitochondrial elongation and transport in a Mfn1 dependent manner, while its soluble form regulates the tightness of mitochondrial cristae junctions and, therefore, release of apoptotic factors (Frezza et al., 2006) as well as

cristae shape, which in turn, conditions supercomplex assembly (Cogliati et al., 2013). Mitochondria trafficking and anchoring mechanisms also rely on molecular motors (as KIF5 and dynein motors) which recruit mitochondria into stationary pools (Rintoul and Reynolds, 2010; Sheng and Cai, 2012; Sheng, 2014), and ensure neuronal mitochondria are adequately distributed where constant energy supply is crucial. Malfunctioning mitochondria are removed by mitophagy to minimize oxidative damage to the cell, with neurons again facing the challenge of their mitochondria being involved in distal processes located far from the cell body where lysosomes are abundant. The presence of functional lysosomes in axons has been evidenced to contribute to mitophagy of damaged mitochondria, and the local PINK1–Parkin-mediated mitophagy pathway provides rapid neuroprotection against oxidative stress without a requirement for retrograde transport to the soma (Ashrafi et al., 2014).

An imbalance of these processes involved in mitochondria dynamics and homeostasis (fission, fusion, trafficking, and mitophagy) can be detrimental to mitochondrial function, causing decreased respiration, ROS production, and apoptosis. All these are also symptoms caused by a traumatic brain injury, further indicating a prominent role of mitochondria in neuropathophysiology.

Mutations in Mitochondrial Proteins

Mutations in other proteins with primary mitochondrial localization that cause abnormalities of protein conformation (mis-folding or aggregation) also result in neurodegenerative disorders. Examples include the kinase PANK2 involved in coenzyme A biosynthesis and degradation of some neurotransmitters, frataxin implicated in iron metabolism, PINK1 critical to prevent oxidative stress, or pitrilysin metallopeptidase which digests oligopeptides, including the mitochondrial fraction of amyloid-beta (Mandemakers et al., 2007; Brunetti et al., 2015). In addition, mutations in some non-mitochondrial proteins appear to affect mitochondrial function in neurodegeneration (such as superoxide dismutase 1, Parkin, α-synuclein, MAO or the kinase LRRK2), although in general the role of most of these proteins in neurodegeneration must still be elucidated (Nakamura et al., 2011; Schapira and Gegg, 2011; Haddad and Nakamura, 2015).

Apoptosis

Apoptosis is a common type of cell death in neurodegenerative diseases, in which mitochondria make a major contribution to initiation of the death cascade (Petit et al., 1996; Naoi et al., 2006). Fission and fusion rates precisely regulate the number and morphology of mitochondria within a cell, with network fragmentation and cristae remodeling occurring during the early stages of apoptotic cell death (Wang and Youle, 2009; Youle and van der Bliek, 2012). In this context it is not surprising that proteins involved in mitochondrial morphology control also participate in apoptosis, and proteins associated with apoptosis regulation affect mitochondrial ultrastructure. Key apoptotic events in mitochondria include the release of caspase-dependent activators (cytochrome c) and caspase-independent apoptotic factors (the flavoenzyme apoptosis inducing factor, AIF), changes in electron transport, loss of mitochondrial transmembrane potential, altered cellular oxidation-reduction, and participation of pro- and anti- apoptotic Bcl-2 family proteins (Saraste and Pulkki, 2000; Edinger and Thompson, 2004). The different signals that converge on mitochondria to trigger or inhibit these events and their downstream effects delineate several major pathways in cell death (Wang and Youle, 2009).

As an example, AIF is an apoptotic factor that when released from the mitochondria and translocated to nucleus induces chromatin condensation and DNA fragmentation, while also having a vital role in mitochondria healthy cells (Susin et al., 1999; Miramar et al., 2001). Complex I (CI) dysfunction has long been associated with PD. AIF deficiency produces reduced levels of CI subunits, decreased CI activity, and impaired CI-dependent mitochondrial respiration (Vahsen et al., 2004; Urbano et al., 2005; Cheung et al., 2006). Although these AIF linked CI structural alterations have not been shown to cause dopaminergic neurodegeneration, an increase is the susceptibility of these neurons to exogenous PD neurotoxins has been proven (Perier et al., 2010, 2012). The exact role of AIF in intermembrane space of mitochondria of healthy cells has remained a conundrum, but several interesting novelties have been presented in the recent years regarding its redox activity in this organelle (Sevrioukova, 2009, 2011; Ferreira et al., 2014; Villanueva et al., 2015). Recently,

it has also been described that the physical and functional NADH-dependent interaction between AIF and the protein CHCHD4 regulates the correct assembly and maintenance of the respiratory chain complexes (Hangen et al., 2015; Meyer et al., 2015). CHCHD4 participates in mitochondrial protein import and catalyzes oxidative protein folding in cooperation with the sulfhydryl oxidase GFER/ALR/Erv1p (Chacinska et al., 2008; Banci et al., 2009; Fischer et al., 2013; Koch and Schmid, 2014). Upon interaction with NADH, AIF undergoes reduction, with the concomitant dimerization and formation of highly stable charge transfer complexes. Both AIF dimers and charge transfer complexes are proposed to have a physiological function in a model where AIF would act as a sensor of the mitochondrial redox state (Churbanova and Sevrioukova, 2008; Ferreira et al., 2014; Sorrentino et al., 2015). In addition to the interplay with CHCHD4, AIF might also interact at the mitochondria with other proteins yet to be discovered.

Neurons are the cells that suffer larger effects upon deficiency of AIF, probably due to their high energetic dependency on the mitochondrial OXPHOS metabolism. In addition to AIF deficiency being related to different neurodegeneration types (Klein et al., 2002; Joza et al., 2005; van Empel et al., 2005; Cheung et al., 2006; Ishimura et al., 2008), six AIF pathological mutations have also been reported to produce human neurodegenerative diseases, with all patients with AIF mutations showing muscular atrophy, neuropathy and ataxia (Ghezzi et al., 2010; Berger et al., 2011; Rinaldi et al., 2012; Ardissone et al., 2015; Diodato et al., 2015; Kettwig et al., 2015). Thus, AIF appears as an essential protein for post-mitotic neuron survival, cerebellar development, and therefore, neurogenesis (Ishimura et al., 2008). AIF is also one of the proteins described to associate with OPA1 to cooperatively regulate and stabilize the respiratory chain, this interaction being proposed as one of the factors defining mitochondrial morphology (Cheung et al., 2006; Zanna et al., 2008).

The present therapeutics for neurodegenerative diseases are in general symptomatic and lack neuroprotective and neurorestorative properties, being not able to delay disease or modify its neuronal activity. In recent years, the development of multi-target neuroprotective and neurorestorative drugs with simultaneous action on enzymes such as cholinesterase, BChE and MAO A/B activities or being able to enhance the action of proteins intimately associated with mitochondrial biogenesis (Youdim, 2013; Youdim and Oh, 2013). A potential addition for this therapeutic strategy in neurodegenerative diseases is to halt common and progressive pathways for neural injury and cell death. In the current development of neuroprotective drugs, mitochondria are a key target to protect against cell death by preventing mitochondrial permeabilization, Ca^{2+} efflux, membrane potential decline and release of apoptotic factors while also inducing anti-apoptotic pro-survival proteins (Naoi et al., 2007; Weinreb et al., 2012, 2016, 2015). Connections between morphological regulation and the bioenergetics status of mitochondria are reciprocally responsive processes (**Figure 4**), with functional abnormality invoking morphological alterations in many human diseases and genetic defects in mitochondrial fusion/fission genes or insults

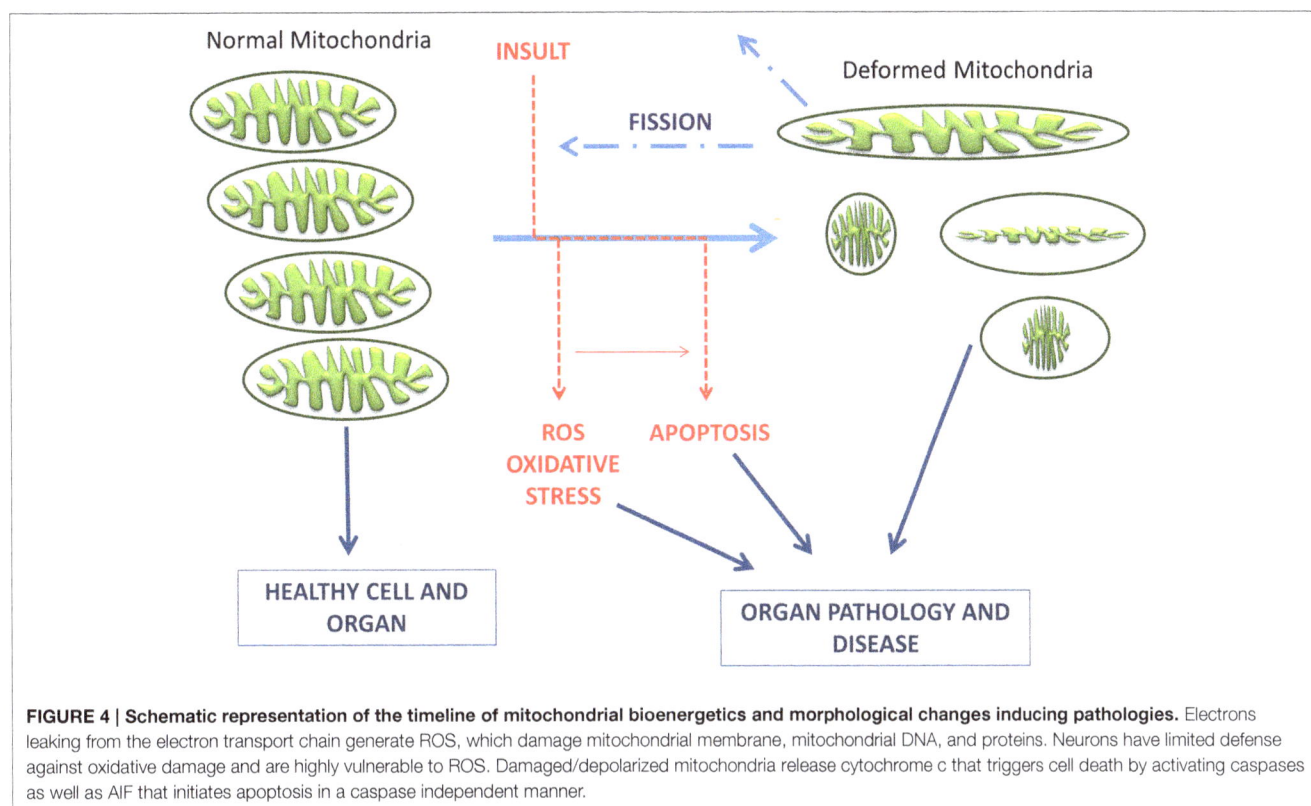

FIGURE 4 | Schematic representation of the timeline of mitochondrial bioenergetics and morphological changes inducing pathologies. Electrons leaking from the electron transport chain generate ROS, which damage mitochondrial membrane, mitochondrial DNA, and proteins. Neurons have limited defense against oxidative damage and are highly vulnerable to ROS. Damaged/depolarized mitochondria release cytochrome c that triggers cell death by activating caspases as well as AIF that initiates apoptosis in a caspase independent manner.

inducing mitochondrial deformation (accompanied by oxidative stress and/or apoptosis) causing human diseases of lethal consequence (Galloway et al., 2012, 2014; Westermann, 2012). In this context, controlling the mitochondrial morphology by manipulating fission and fusion emerges as a future therapeutic strategy to decrease the pathological outcome.

ANTIOXIDANT PROPERTIES IN AN EXAMPLE MTDL

Antioxidant properties, part of a desired pharmacologic profile for MTDLs designed to treat neurodegeneration, are screened by various *in silico*, *in vitro* and *in vivo* methods. Arising from the structure of the parent antioxidant drug stobadine (Horáková et al., 1994; Horáková and Stolc, 1998), several dozen derivatives with a hexahydropyridoindolic scaffold were synthesized and tested for their antioxidant and neuroprotective effect (Rackova et al., 2006; Stolc et al., 2006, 2010; Juranek et al., 2010). The aim of the new design was to use a wide knowledge of the pharmacological actions of stobadine to develop new substances with even higher antioxidant activity and reduced side effects. The screening confirmed the enhancement of the intrinsic radical scavenging activity of the 8-methoxy substituted derivatives, which was predicted for the right position of the electron-donating methoxy group. Several alkoxy-carbonyl substituents at the N2 position were tested to find sufficiently high lipophilicity and lower basicity of

the molecule. From the compounds synthesized and tested (±)-cis-8-methoxy-2,3,4,4a,5,9b-hexahydro-1H-pyrido[4,3-b]indole-2-carboxylic acid ethyl ester (SMe1EC2, **Figure 5**), which showed enhanced antioxidant properties near a lipophilic phase, was chosen for a detailed study.

SMe1EC2 had high intrinsic scavenging activity as measured with 1,1TM-diphenyl-2-picrylhydrazyl (DPPH) (Stefek et al., 2013). The initial velocity of DPPH decolorization by 50 μM SMe1EC2 (0.507 $\pm$ 0.003 optical density(OD)/min) was comparable with that of equimolar trolox (0.494 $\pm$ 0.009 OD/min). The parent compound stobadine at 50 μM concentration was about three times less efficient (0.156 $\pm$ 0.019 OD/min). The high intrinsic activity together with enhanced lipophilicity resulted in significantly higher antioxidant properties in rat brain homogenate or in a cellular model (red cells, macrophage RAW 264.7 cell cultures) when compared with stobadine (Stolc et al., 2006; Stefek et al., 2013; Balcerczyk et al., 2014). In the experiment with red blood cells two types of initiators of the haemolysis were used: hydrophilic AAPH (2,2′-azobis(2-amidinopropane) hydrochloride) and lipophilic t-BuOOH. While the activity of more hydrophilic and basic stobadine surpassed that of SMe1EC2 in AAPH induced haemolysis, SMe1EC2 exceeded stobadine in red blood cells protection when lipophilic t-BuOOH was used (Stefek et al., 2013).

On a tissue level SMe1EC2 was able to recover the field action potential amplitude in CA1 region of rat hippocampal slices after 20 min reoxygenation following 6 min hypoxia to control value

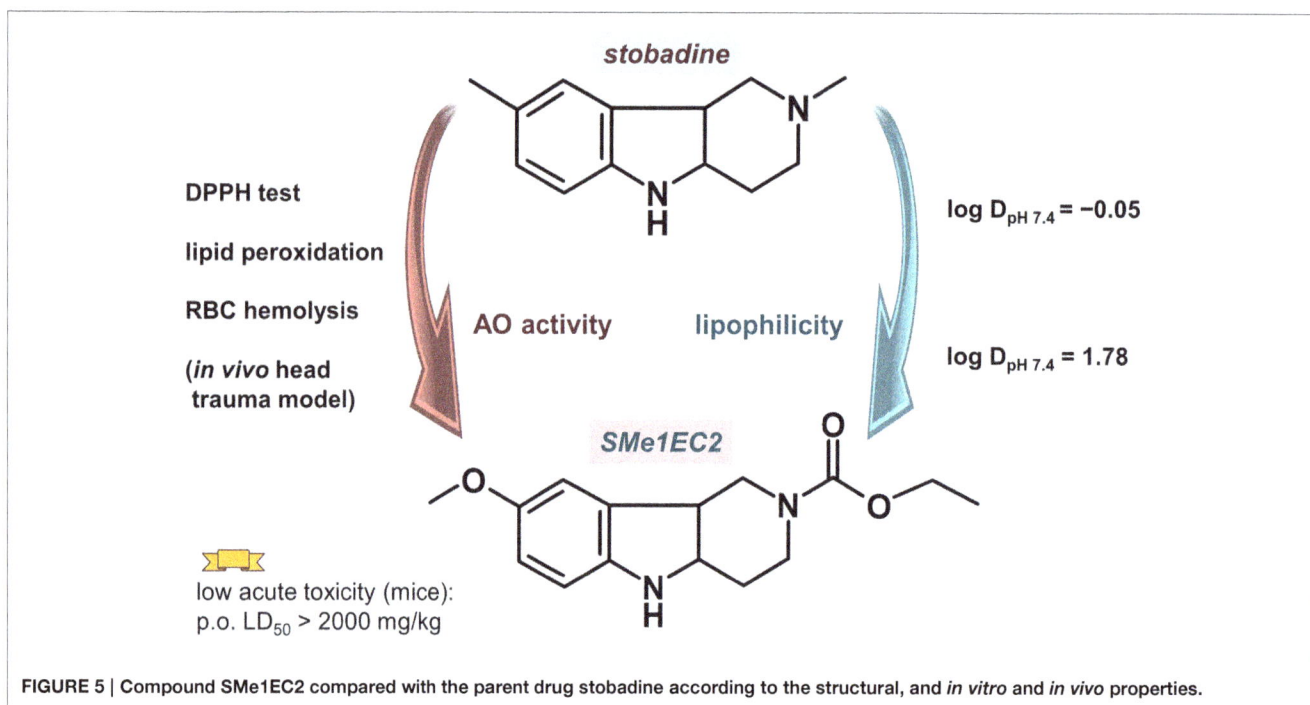

FIGURE 5 | Compound SMe1EC2 compared with the parent drug stobadine according to the structural, and *in vitro* and *in vivo* properties.

(100%) at a concentration of 3 μmol/l (Stolc et al., 2006). The field action potential, created by the pyramidal neurons in the CA1 region after electric stimulation of Schäffer collaterals in the CA3 region and involving excitation of glutamatergic synapses, is an appropriate model for functional status of brain. Neuroprotective effects of the compound were shown also in rat hippocampal slices attacked by Fe^{2+}/ascorbic acid system (Gáspárová et al., 2010). Simultaneously, SMe1EC2 improved functional deficits and edema formation in rat hippocampus exposed to ischemia *ex vivo* after several days of oral treatment of rats (Gáspárová et al., 2009).

In order to estimate the *in vivo* neuroprotective potential of these new hexahydropyridoindoles, an experiment with acute head trauma model in mice has been performed (Stolc et al., 2006, 2010, 2011). There is a close relation between a traumatic head injury and a risk for later development of PD (Witcher et al., 2015; Xu et al., 2015). People aged 55 years and older who were treated in the hospital for traumatic brain injury were 44% more likely to develop PD over the next six years than those who sustained injuries, but not head injuries (Gardner et al., 2015). In the framework of the murine head trauma experiment the drugs were administered i.v. immediately after the trauma in single doses equimolar to 1 mg of stobadine dihydrochloride, and 1 h later the total sensomotoric score was monitored. SMe1EC2 proved to be excellent compound in improvement of a total sensomotoric score (Stolc et al., 2006, 2011), achieving the value 244.33 ± 50.20% ($p = 0.0036$ comparing to placebo) and exceeding such compounds as melatonin, stobadine and SPBN (2-sulfo-α-phenyl-N-tert-butyl-nitrone). During this experiment brain oedema was also evaluated by brain wet weight assessment and brain histology. After triple i.v. administration of 1.14 mg/kg of SMe1EC2 in 1 min, 2 h and 24 h after Acute Head Trauma,

the increase in brain wet weight induced by the trauma and culminating 5 h after the insult was significantly diminished almost to the control level. The reduction of the oedema, occurring especially in glial cells, was also proved histologically. Moreover, the occurrence of subdural bleeding, meningeal bleeding and bleeding in brain chambers throughout the whole follow-up period (168 h) was significantly reduced.

The compound was also tested for cell protection properties in the framework of diabetes-related pathological processes. AD and type 2 diabetes mellitus present many common features (de la Monte and Wands, 2008; Correia et al., 2012c; Ahmad, 2013). Both diseases are connected with malfunctions in glucose metabolism and mitochondria, elevated oxidative stress and activation of pro-inflammatory cytokines. SMe1EC2 enhanced the viability of cultured HT22 neuronal cells exposed to high glucose with simultaneous attenuating of parameters of the oxidations stress (Rackova et al., 2009). The compound also protected rat pancreatic INS-1E β cell cultures against cytotoxic effects of hydrogen peroxide and inhibited profoundly the time-delayed apoptotic changes induced by the attack (Račková et al., 2011).

Besides metabolic disorders related to the high glucose plasma levels, pathologies connected with a high fat diet may also be related to neurodegeneration process (Morris et al., 2010). SMe1EC2 showed also efficiency in treating metabolic high-fat related disorders. In the rat model of hypertriglyceridemia it was shown that higher intake of cholesterol induced an increase in the number of active Na^+/K^+-ATPase molecules in HTG rats, which resulted in the increased retention of sodium. A three-week treatment of animals kept on high cholesterol diet with SMe1EC2 in a dose of 10 mg kg^{-1} day^{-1} normalized the function of renal Na^+/K^+-ATPase to the level comparable in HTG rats fed with the standard diet. For a comparison, fenofibrate in a dose of 100 mg kg^{-1} day^{-1} reversed the function of renal Na$^+$/K$^+$-ATPase only slightly (Mézešová et al., 2012).

Further significant property of SMe1EC2 was its ability to protect endothelium under conditions of experimental diabetes of rats. It significantly decreased endothelaemia of diabetic rats and improved endothelium-dependent relaxation of arteries, slightly decreased ROS-production and increased bioavailability of nitric oxide in the aorta (Sotníková et al., 2011). Overall, the compound attenuated endothelial injury in diabetic animals. Although mechanism of this effect is still not clear, it could represent further positive effect in MTDL potential for treatment of neurodegenerative diseases.

Four ethological tests with rats (open field, elevated plus-maze, light/dark box exploration, forced swim test) were used to obtain information about anxiolytic and antidepressant activity of SMe1EC2 (Sedláčková et al., 2011). The substance was administered intraperitoneally 30 min before the tests at doses of 1, 10, and 25 mg/kg. SMe1EC2 was found to exert anxiolytic activity in elevated plus maze with no affection of locomotor activity in a dose-dependent manner. The middle dose of SMe1EC2 resulted in similar anti-anxiety effect manifested in rats as that of diazepam (dose 2.5 mg/kg). A medium anti-depressant activity was also predicted by combinatorial *in silico* methods (Majekova et al., 2013).

The acute toxicity of SMe1EC2 was assessed in mice after p.o. and i.v. administration. For p.o., it was estimated in GHS scale as 5, a compound with "comparatively low acute toxicity," with the LD$_{50}$ value over 2000 mg/kg. After i.v. administration, the LD$_{50}$ of SMe1EC2 was 181.13 mg/kg (Stolc et al., 2006). The results of prenatal developmental toxicity study were similar: the compound demonstrated neither embryotoxic nor teratogenic effects on rat fetuses and no signs of maternal toxicity were found (Ujhazy et al., 2008).

Compound SMe1EC2 has been revealed to be a potential multi-target drug for neuronal diseases. Apart from its good distribution properties and high intrinsic radical scavenging activity, this is supported by the results of *in vivo* experiments on protection in the process of head trauma and diabetic damage of endothelium.

CYTOCHROME P450

The cytochrome P450 (CYP) family is involved in different steps of therapy from drug efficacy and dose requirement to adverse drug reactions and direct toxicity (Zanger and Schwab, 2013). There are 18 mammalian CYP isoenzymes, which encode 57 genes in the human genome (Nebert et al., 2013). Of these CYP isoenzymes, more than 10 belong to the CYP1, 2, and 3 families and are responsible for the metabolism of more than 80% of xenobiotics and drugs used in therapy. This indicates that the CYP-dependent metabolism is one of the main factors in the regulation of drug concentration at a target level (pharmacokinetic effects) and is indeed involved in the adverse reactions of therapeutic compounds, in drug-drug interaction and their toxic effect. The low substrate specificity

characterizing the CYP metabolism, is associated with the evidence of a large genetic polymorphism of some isoforms, particularly those involved in drug metabolism (i.e., CPY1A2, 2C9, 2C19, 2D6, and 3A4). Multi-allelic genetic polymorphisms, which remarkably depend on ethnicity, (Preissner et al., 2013) lead to distinct pharmacogenetic phenotypes termed as poor, extensive, and ultrarapid metabolizers. The loss of function promotes a reduced clearance with a consequent increase of plasma concentrations, while the gain of function leads to increased clearance and lower drug concentrations, resulting in increase and decrease effect of the drug, respectively, and potentially drug-related toxicity. These effects are not only related to genetic polymorphisms, but CYPs activity is regulated by chemicals and endogenous factors that can be promoted either by the induction or inhibition of some CYP activity. In the liver, most of the xenobiotic-metabolising CYPs are inducible, but one exception is CYP2D6. In general, control of protein expression can be exerted at the transcriptional mRNA, translational and posttranslational level. Posttranslational regulation has been described for CYP1A1, CYP1A2, CYP2E1 and CYP3A4 (Werlinder et al., 2001; Ingelman-Sundberg, 2004; Oesch-Bartlomowicz and Oesch, 2005; Smutny et al., 2013).

Pharmacoepigenomics is a new topic of research in the regulation of xenobiotic metabolizing enzymes. Up to now different studies indicate that DNA methylation and the numerous combinations of post-translational modifications of the histone proteins, are implicated in influencing the expression of genes whose products are engaged in drug metabolism. In addition, the increasing importance of the short regulatory miRNAs, has to be emphasized and initial studies show their involvement in regulating the expression of drug-metabolizing enzymes (Tsuchiya et al., 2006; Pan et al., 2009; Ingelman-Sundberg and Gomez, 2010).

Therefore, pharmacoepigenomics represents the future of research on drug metabolism, while the molecular mechanism of the transcriptional regulation of CYPs has been established and consolidated in several studies. Transcriptional control is of the highest importance and cytosolic receptors sensitive to the concentration of the environmental xenobiotics are crucial, namely the aryl hydrocarbon receptor (AhR), constitutive androgen receptor (CAR), the pregnane X-receptor (PXR), and peroxisome proliferator-activated receptor (PPARα). They regulate CYP forms as follows: CYP1A1, CYP1A2 and CYP2S1 (AhR), CYP2C9, CYP3A4 (PXR), CYP2B6, CYP2C9, CYP3A4 (CAR), and CYP4A family (PPARα) (Waxman, 1999; Ingelman-Sundberg, 2004).

All of these described regulatory mechanisms lead to the first of instances of interindividual variability in drug response, where a clear phenotypic consequence is evident in the population. Another aspect to take in account is the inhibition effects of CYP enzymes promoted by several drugs, chemicals, or diet components. This effect can increase systemic exposure, thereby causing severe toxic effects of the drug or of another concomitantly administered therapeutic compound that is metabolized by the same CYP(s) (Ludwig et al., 1999). The competition between chemicals for CYP activity has resulted in unpredictable pharmacokinetic interactions and can be a cause of drug–drug interactions, a major clinical problem.

Cytochrome P450 in Brain and Its Role in Parkinson's Disease

Most of these studies have been conducted in the liver which is the major organ involved in drug metabolism due to the high concentration of CYP in the endoplasmic reticulum of hepatocytes. However, the CYP families involved in xenobiotic metabolism are also expressed in extrahepatic tissues (i.e., intestine, brain, kidney). Since the expression of the majority of the isoforms appears to be very low compared the predominant expression in liver, and their role in overall total body clearance is lower, the basal expression and up-regulation in peripheral tissues can significantly affect local disposition of drugs or endogenous compounds and thus modify the pharmacological/toxicological effects or affect the distribution of xenobiotics in human body. In the brain, the overall level of CYP is ~0.5–2% of that in liver microsomes (Miksys and Tyndale, 2013) and could play a role in tissue- and/or cell-specific sensitivity to certain drugs or xenobiotics. There have been a number of suggestions that environmental toxins may play a role in the pathogenesis of neurodegenerative disorders by directly damaging neurons or through bioactivation of some toxic compounds via CYPs (Riedl et al., 1999; Shahabi et al., 2008; Miksys and Tyndale, 2009; Ferguson and Tyndale, 2011; Vaglini et al., 2013).

In this context, it is underlined that studies with divergent results are addressed toward the allele mutation of gene that encodes CYP2D6. This isozyme is involved in the metabolism of exogenous drugs and neurotoxins including 1-methyl-4-phenyl-1,2,3,6-tetrahydropyridine (MPTP, a neurotoxin that can cause selective dopaminergic neuronal damage) as well as endogenous compounds including dopamine (Payami et al., 2001). Recently Singh et al. (2014), in a study involving 70 PD patients, showed that a allelic variants of CYP2D6 and glutathione transferase1 were significantly associated with an increase in PD risk, due to a lower capability in the metabolism of neurotoxic compounds such as pesticides. This study is in agreement with the a meta-analysis performed by Lu et al. (2013) that demonstrated that an allele polymorphism of CYP2D6 increases the risk of Parkinson's disease.

On the contrary, other studies did not support an association between PD and mutations of the CYP2D6 and underline that PD is most likely the result of interactions between multiple genetic and environmental factors (Persad et al., 2003; Vilar et al., 2007; Halling et al., 2008). Whatever the cause of PD and other neurodegenerative disease, the knowledge of cytochrome P450 functions and metabolism is pivotal for its key roles in *in vivo* drug action, and why it plays a crucial function in the metabolism of toxic compounds.

Cytochrome P450-Dependent Metabolism of MAO B Inhibitors and ASS234

In the COST Action CM1103, a new family of multi-target molecules able to interact with AChE, as well as with MAO A

and B, was synthesized by Samadi et al. (2011). These compounds bring together the benzylpiperidine and N-propargylamine moieties present in the AChE inhibitor donepezil and the MAO inhibitor PF9601N, respectively. The presence of propargyl moiety in the molecule confers particular susceptibility in terms of CYP-dependent metabolism. It is well-known that the terminal acetylenes can inhibit the CYP isoenzymes by alkylating the P450 prosthetic heme or by binding covalently to the protein with only partial loss of the catalytic activity. Sharma et al. (1996) demonstrated that both deprenyl and clorgyline are irreversible inhibitors of CYP2B1, by a mechanism-based inactivation due to the formation of a reactive intermediate based on their propargyl group. A recent study suggests that deprenyl can also inhibit CYP2B6 (Sridar et al., 2012). This isozyme is involved in the metabolism of Bupropion, an antidepressant often used to Parkinson's disease patients in conjunction with deprenyl, and its inhibition can lead to a potential drug interactions.

However, the inhibition of CYP 2B1 and 2B6 does not promote inhibition of CYP-dependent metabolism of the drug. In fact deprenyl in humans, as well as in experimental animals, is rapidly metabolized by the liver cytochrome CYP system, forming mainly desmethydeprenyl and methamphetamine (Baker et al., 1999; Dragoni et al., 2003b). These two compounds are further metabolized to amphetamine. The CYP-dependent metabolism showed a high hepatic clearance that justifies the low half-life of the drug observed *in vivo* in humans (~0.15 h) (Sridar et al., 2012).

It is important to note that both primary deprenyl metabolites can contribute to the therapeutic effect of the MAO-B inhibitor. Desmethyldeprenyl, a less potent inhibitor of MAO-B than the parent drug both *in vitro* and *in vivo*, is more efficacious in protecting dopamine neurons against oxidative stress damage (Olanow and Tatton, 1999). The other metabolite, methamphetamine, is a more potent inhibitor of presynaptic noradrenaline and dopamine uptake than the parent drug and it has been suggested that this effect contributes to neuroprotection (Szíráki et al., 1994).

These metabolic pathways are also active in the CNS, as observed *in vitro* in microsomal preparations of monkey and mouse brain (Dragoni et al., 2003a). In contrast to deprenyl, PF9601N, the precursor of MTDL compounds studied in the COST CM 1103 project (Bolea et al., 2011), showed significantly lower liver clearance. The *in vivo* treatment of C57BL/6 mice did not modify cytochrome P450 and b5 content, and did not change NADPH-CYP-reductase or CYP2E1, 2A5, 1A1, 2B6, 3A activities. Furthermore, CYP-dependent metabolism of PF9601N by liver microsomes from either control or treated mice gave rise only to the formation of the desmethyl metabolite, FA72 (Dragoni et al., 2007). This desmethyl compound promoted a concentration-dependent inhibition of peroxinitrite oxidation with an IC_{50} value lower than the parent compound and than deprenyl. Furthermore, PF9601N and its metabolite were able to strongly inhibit rat brain neuronal nitric oxide synthase, (NOS) in contrast to observations with deprenyl, which caused a slight decrease of the enzyme activity only at millimolar concentration (Bellik et al., 2010).

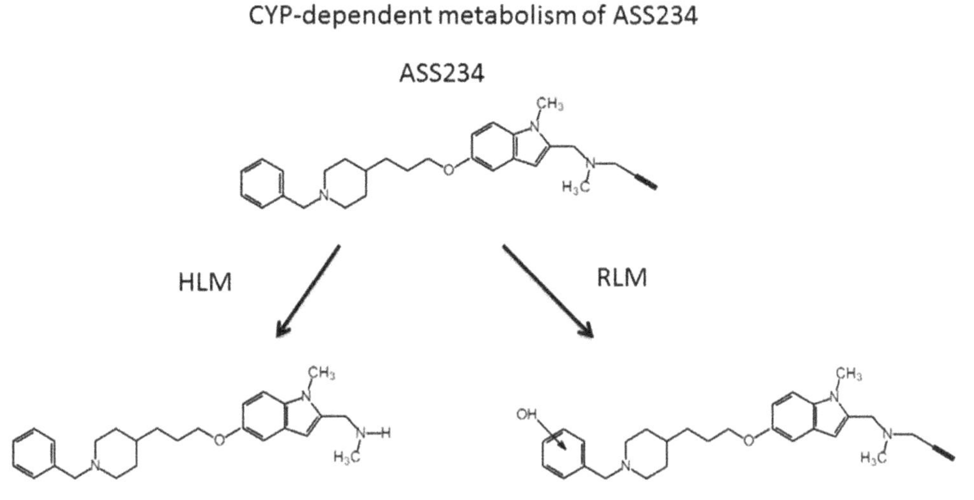

FIGURE 6 | Cytochrome P450-dependent metabolism of ASS234 in human (HLM) and rat (RLM) liver microsomal preparations. ASS234 (25 μM) was incubated at 37°C in phosphate buffer in the presence of microsomes for 30 min.

These observations led us to study the CYP-dependent metabolism of ASS234 (Marco-Contelles et al., 2016). ASS234 was incubated in phosphate buffer with human or rat hepatic microsomal preparations (HLM and RLM, respectively) as previously reported (D'Elia et al., 2009). Samples were analyzed by Agilent UHD Accurate-Mass Q-TOF LC/MS and the experimental data obtained were elaborated using Mass-MetaSite, a computer assisted method for the interpretation of LC–MSMS data that combines prediction of a compound's site of metabolism (SoM) with the processing of MS spectra and rationalization based on fragment analysis (Strano-Rossi et al., 2014). The kinetic analysis indicated that the substrate depletion followed a mono-exponential relationship either in presence of HLM and RLM. RLM metabolized the compound at a higher rate compared to HLM. In fact, after 30 min incubation only 23% of ASS234 was metabolized by human preparations, while RLM preparations were able to metabolized more than the 80% of initial amount (10 μM) of substrate (Simone et al., 2014).

The MS analysis of the products from ASS234 metabolism showed two different pathways as shown in **Figure 6**. The principal metabolite observed with HLM resulted in a compound at $[M-38]^+$ (m/z) indicating the formation of N-depropargylated metabolite, in agreement with that observed for the CYP-dependent metabolism of PF9601N (Dragoni et al., 2007). On the contrary, in RLM preparations, the major metabolite resulted in m/z equal to $[M+16]^+$, which corresponded to the hydroxylated derivative on the benzene ring. Other minor peaks were present in both microsomal preparations and resulted in, as secondary metabolites, the N-demethylated derivatives either on tertiary amine or indole nitrogen. The *in silico* analysis indicated that CYP2D6 and 2C19 are the major CYPs involved in the human metabolism of ASS234 (Simone et al., 2014).

Taken together, this information clearly indicates that ASS234 is a poor CYP(s) substrate in human liver, that the resulting metabolite should be not a MAO inhibitor, but that the inhibition

effect on AChE should remain. Furthermore, in accord with the observations with PF9601N (Dragoni et al., 2007), the ASS234 CYP-dependent metabolite can be a more potent antioxidant and NOS inhibitor than the parent compound.

However, the involvement of CYP2D6 and 2C19, two highly genetic polymorphic cytochrome P450s, require more care due to possible toxic effects of the parent compound having a lower metabolic clearance. Moreover, the evidence that human and rat present two different metabolic behaviors, in terms of velocity and metabolite formation, underlines the differences between species in CYP-dependent metabolism and the danger of attempting to extrapolate results across species.

CONCLUSION

In the last century pharmacological research was driven to discover highly selective drugs. This strategy has failed, in part, because it is seen that the interaction with a single target, either receptor or enzyme, can promote compensatory adaptations in the living organisms leading to a failure of the therapy. These observations and the discovery that different pathologies have common aspects has led to the synthesis of new molecules that can interact with multiple targets with the aim to improved balance of efficacy and safety compared to single targeting drugs.

We have reviewed the major targets for the assessment of MTDL relevant to neurodegenerative diseases, giving examples of compounds generated by our collaborating medicinal chemists in COST Action CM1103. Mitochondria are highlighted as the area of future interest but the many possible targets will have to be refined to those most influential on progression in each specific disease. It is becoming recognized, particularly for mitochondrial function, that the cumulative effect of small inefficiencies can trigger pathology under additional insult such as oxidative stress. Recent advances in cell biology techniques have enabled the study of factors involved in mitochondrial dynamics. The processes vital to mitochondrial health are also vital to neuronal survival and will provide the challenge to discover new tools to prevent neurodegeneration. When single target efficacy is achieved, then new modalities can be added to MTDL for the ultimate prevention of neuropathology.

AUTHOR CONTRIBUTIONS

All authors contributed to the writing of the manuscript. MV and RR integrated and revised it.

REFERENCES

Ahmad, W. (2013). Overlapped metabolic and therapeutic links between Alzheimer and diabetes. *Mol. Neurobiol.* 47, 399–424. doi: 10.1007/s12035-012-8352-z

Anand, P., and Singh, B. (2013). A review on cholinesterase inhibitors for Alzheimer's disease. *Arch. Pharmac. Res.* 36, 375–399. doi: 10.1007/s12272-013-0036-3

Ardissone, A., Piscosquito, G., Legati, A., Langella, T., Lamantea, E., Garavaglia, B., et al. (2015). A slowly progressive mitochondrial encephalomyopathy widens the spectrum of AIFM1 disorders. *Neurology* 84, 2193–2195. doi: 10.1212/WNL.0000000000001613

Arendt, T., Brückner, M. K., Lange, M., and Bigl, V. (1992). Changes in acetylcholinesterase and butyrylcholinesterase in alzheimers-disease resemble embryonic-development - a study of molecular-forms. *Neurochem. Int.* 21, 381–396. doi: 10.1016/0197-0186(92)90189-X

Ashrafi, G., Schlehe, J. S., LaVoie, M. J., and Schwarz, T. L. (2014). Mitophagy of damaged mitochondria occurs locally in distal neuronal axons and requires PINK1 and Parkin. *J. Cell Biol.* 206, 655–670. doi: 10.1083/jcb.201401070

Baker, G. B., Urichuk, L. J., McKenna, K. F., and Kennedy, S. H. (1999). Metabolism of monoamine oxidase inhibitors. *Cell. Mol. Neurobiol.* 19, 411–426. doi: 10.1023/A:1006849732681

Balcerczyk, A., Bartosz, G., Drzewinska, J., Piotrowski, L., Pulaski, L., and Stefek, M. (2014). Antioxidant action of SMe1EC2, the low-basicity derivative of the pyridoindole stobadine, in cell free chemical models and at cellular level. *Interdiscipl. Toxicol.* 7, 27–32. doi: 10.2478/intox-2014-0005

Banci, L., Bertini, I., Cefaro, C., Ciofi-Baffoni, S., Gallo, A., Martinelli, M., et al. (2009). MIA40 is an oxidoreductase that catalyzes oxidative protein folding in mitochondria. *Nat. Struct. Mol. Biol.* 16, 198–206. doi: 10.1038/nsmb.1553

Bartolini, M., Bertucci, C., Cavrini, V., and Andrisano, V. (2003). β-amyloid aggregation induced by human acetylcholinesterase: inhibition studies. *Biochem. Pharmacol.* 65, 407–416. doi: 10.1016/S0006-2952(02)01514-9

Bartzokis, G., and Tishler, T. A. (2000). MRI evaluation of basal ganglia ferritin iron and neurotoxicity in Alzheimer's and Huntingon's disease. *Cell. Mol. Biol (Noisy-le-grand).* 46, 821–833.

Bautista-Aguilera, O. M., Esteban, G., Bolea, I., Nikolic, K., Agbaba, D., Moraleda, I., et al. (2014a). Design, synthesis, pharmacological evaluation, QSAR analysis, molecular modeling and ADMET of novel donepezil-indolyl hybrids as multipotent cholinesterase/monoamine oxidase inhibitors for the potential treatment of Alzheimer's disease. *Eur. J. Med. Chem.* 75, 82–95. doi: 10.1016/j.ejmech.2013.12.028

Bautista-Aguilera, O. M., Samadi, A., Chioua, M., Nikolic, K., Filipic, S., Agbaba, D., et al. (2014b). N-Methyl-N-((1-methyl-5-(3-(1-(2-methylbenzyl)piperidin-4yl).propoxy).-1H- indol-2-yl).methyl)prop-2-yn-1-amine, a New Cholinesterase and Monoamine Oxidase Dual. *J. Med. Chem.* 57, 10455–10463. doi: 10.1021/jm501501a

Bazzu, G., Rocchitta, G., Migheli, R., Alvau, M. D., Zinellu, M., Puggioni, G., et al. (2013). Effects of the neurotoxin MPTP and pargyline protection on extracellular energy metabolites and dopamine levels in the striatum of freely moving rats. *Brain Res.* 1538, 159–171. doi: 10.1016/j.brainres.2013.09.037

Bellik, L., Dragoni, S., Pessina, F., Sanz, E., Unzeta, M., and Valoti, M. (2010). Antioxidant properties of PF9601N, a novel MAO-B inhibitor: assessment of its ability to interact with reactive nitrogen species. *Acta. Biochim. Pol.* 57, 235–239.

Benek, O., Aitken, L., Hroch, L., Kuca, K., Gunn-Moore, F., and Musilek, K. (2015). A direct interaction between mitochondrial proteins and amyloid-beta peptide and its significance for the progression and treatment of Alzheimer's Disease. *Curr. Med. Chem.* 22, 1056–1085. doi: 10.2174/0929867322666150114163051

Berger, I., Ben-Neriah, Z., Dor-Wolman, T., Shaag, A., Saada, A., Zenvirt, S., et al. (2011). Early prenatal ventriculomegaly due to an AIFM1 mutation identified by linkage analysis and whole exome sequencing. *Mol. Genet. Metabolism* 104, 517–520. doi: 10.1016/j.ymgme.2011.09.020

Bernardi, P., Di Lisa, F., Fogolari, F., and Lippe, G. (2015). From ATP to PTP and Back: a dual function for the Mitochondrial ATP Synthase. *Circ. Res.* 116, 1850–1862. doi: 10.1161/CIRCRESAHA.115.306557

Binda, C., Newton-Vinson, P., Hubalek, F., Edmondson, D. E., and Mattevi, A. (2002). Structure of human monoamine oxidase B, a drug target for the treatment of neurological disorders. *Nat. Struct. Biol.* 9, 22–26. doi: 10.1038/nsb732

Binda, C., Valente, S., Romanenghi, M., Pilotto, S., Cirilli, R., Karytinos, A., et al. (2010). Biochemical, Structural, and Biological Evaluation of Tranylcypromine derivatives as inhibitors of Histone Demethylases LSD1 and LSD2. *J. Am. Chem. Soc.* 132, 6827–6833. doi: 10.1021/ja101557k

Binda, C., Wang, J., Pisani, L., Caccia, C., Carotti, A., Salvati, P., et al. (2007). Structures of human monoamine oxidase B complexes with selective noncovalent inhibitors: Safinamide and coumarin analogs. *J. Med. Chem.* 50, 5848–5852. doi: 10.1021/jm070677y

Bird, M. J., Thorburn, D. R., and Frazier, A. E. (2014). Modelling biochemical features of mitochondrial neuropathology. *Biochim. Biophys. Acta.* 1840, 1380–1392. doi: 10.1016/j.bbagen.2013.10.017

Bolea, I., Colivicchi, M. A., Ballini, C., Marco-Contelles, J., Tipton, K. F., Unzeta, M., et al. (2014). Neuroprotective effects of the MAO-B inhibitor, PF9601N, in an *in vivo* model of excitotoxicity. *CNS Neurosci. Ther.* 20, 641–650. doi: 10.1111/cns.12271

Bolea, I., Gella, A., Monjas, L., Perez, C., Rodriguez-Franco, M. I., Marco-Contelles, J., et al. (2013). Multipotent, Permeable Drug ASS234 Inhibits A beta Aggregation, possesses antioxidant properties and protects from a beta-induced Apoptosis *in vitro*. *Curr. Alzheimer Res.* 10, 797–808. doi: 10.2174/15672050113109990151

Bolea, I., Juarez-Jimenez, J., de los Rios, C., Chioua, M., Pouplana, R., Javier Luque, F., et al. (2011). Synthesis, biological evaluation, and molecular modeling of donepezil and N-[(5-(benzyloxy).-1-methyl-1H-indol-2-yl).methyl]-N-methylprop-2-yn-1-amine hybrids as new multipotent cholinesterase/monoamine oxidase inhibitors for the treatment of Alzheimer's Disease. *J. Med. Chem.* 54, 8251–8270. doi: 10.1021/jm200853t

Bolognesi, M. L., Cavalli, A., Valgimigli, L., Bartolini, M., Rosini, M., Andrisano, V., et al. (2007). Multi-target-directed drug design strategy: from a dual binding site acetylcholinesterase inhibitor to a trifunctional compound against Alzheimer's disease. *J. Med. Chem.* 50, 6446–6449. doi: 10.1021/jm701225u

Bonivento, D., Milczek, E. M., McDonald, G. R., Binda, C., Holt, A., Edmondson, D. E., et al. (2010). Potentiation of ligand binding through cooperative effects in monoamine oxidase B. *J. Biol. Chem.* 285, 36849–36856. doi: 10.1074/jbc.M110.169482

ACKNOWLEDGMENTS

This article is based upon work from COST Action CM1103 "Structure-based drug design for diagnosis and treatment of neurological diseases: dissecting and modulating complex function in the monoaminergic systems of the brain," supported by COST (European Cooperation in Science and Technology). The authors thank the participants in COST Action for productive collaborations. MMajekova acknowledges the support of VEGA 2/0033/14, and MMedina the support of MINECO, Spain (BIO2013-42978-P).

Borger, E., Aitken, L., Du, H., Zhang, W., Gunn-Moore, F. J., and Yan, S. S. (2013). Is amyloid binding alcohol dehydrogenase a drug target for treating Alzheimer's disease? *Curr. Alzheimer Res.* 10, 21–29. doi: 10.2174/1567205011310010004

Bortolato, M., and Shih, J. C. (2011). Behavioral outcomes of monoamine oxidase deficiency: preclinical and clinical evidence. *Int. Rev. Neurobiol.* 100, 13–42. doi: 10.1016/b978-0-12-386467-3.00002-9

Brunetti, D., Torsvik, J., Dallabona, C., Teixeira, P., Sztromwasser, P., Fernandez-Vizarra, E., et al. (2015). Defective PITRM1 mitochondrial peptidase is associated with Aβ amyloidotic neurodegeneration. *EMBO Mol. Med.* 8, 176–190 doi: 10.15252/emmm.201505894

Brunner, H. G., Nelen, M., Breakefield, X. O., Ropers, H. H., and Vanoost, B. A. (1993). Abnormal behavior associated with a point mutation in the structural gene for monoamine oxidase-A. *Science* 262, 578–580. doi: 10.1126/science.8211186

Butterfield, D. A., Di Domenico, F., Swomley, A. M., Head, E., and Perluigi, M. (2014). Redox proteomics analysis to decipher the neurobiology of Alzheimer-like neurodegeneration: overlaps in Down's syndrome and Alzheimer's disease brain. *Biochem. J.* 463, 177–189. doi: 10.1042/BJ20140772

Camps, P., Formosa, X., Galdeano, C., Gómez, T., Munoz-Torrero, D., Scarpellini, M., et al. (2008). Novel donepezil-based inhibitors of acetyl- and butyrylcholinesterase and acetylcholinesterase-induced beta-amyloid aggregation. *J. Med. Chem.* 51, 3588–3598. doi: 10.1021/jm8001313

Carradori, S., and Petzer, J. P. (2015). Novel monoamine oxidase inhibitors: a patent review (2012-2014). *Expert Opin. Ther. Pat.* 25, 91–110. doi: 10.1517/13543776.2014.982535

Chacinska, A., Guiard, B., Müller, J. M., Schulze-Specking, A., Gabriel, K., Kutik, S., et al. (2008). Mitochondrial biogenesis, switching the sorting pathway of the intermembrane space receptor Mia40. *J. Biol. Chem.* 283, 29723–22979. doi: 10.1074/jbc.M805356200

Chen, K., Holschneider, D. P., Wu, W. H., Rebrin, I., and Shih, J. C. (2004). A spontaneous point mutation produces monoamine oxidase A/B knock-out mice with greatly elevated monoamines and anxiety-like behavior. *J. Biol. Chem.* 279, 39645–39652. doi: 10.1074/jbc.M405550200

Cheung, E. C., Joza, N., Steenaart, N. A., McClellan, K. A., Neuspiel, M., McNamara, S., et al. (2006). Dissociating the dual roles of apoptosis-inducing factor in maintaining mitochondrial structure and apoptosis. *EMBO J.* 25, 4061–4073. doi: 10.1038/sj.emboj.7601276

Cheung, J., Rudolph, M. J., Burshteyn, F., Cassidy, M. S., Gary, E. N., Love, J., et al. (2012). Structures of Human acetylcholinesterase in complex with pharmacologically important ligands. *J. Med. Chem.* 55, 10282–10286. doi: 10.1021/jm300871x

Cho, S., and Hu, Y. (2007). Activation of 5-HT4 receptors inhibits secretion of beta-amyloid peptides and increases neuronal survival. *Exp. Neurol.* 203, 274–278. doi: 10.1016/j.expneurol.2006.07.021

Churbanova, I. Y., and Sevrioukova, I. F. (2008). Redox-dependent changes in molecular properties of mitochondrial apoptosis-inducing factor. *J. Biol. Chem.* 283, 5622–5631. doi: 10.1074/jbc.M709147200

Cochet, M., Donneger, R., Cassier, E., Gaven, F., Lichtenthaler, S. F., Marin, P., et al. (2013). 5-HT4 receptors constitutively promote the non-amyloidogenic pathway of APP cleavage and interact with ADAM10. *ACS Chem. Neurosci.* 4, 130–140. doi: 10.1021/cn300095t

Cogliati, S., Frezza, C., Soriano, M. E., Varanita, T., Quintana-Cabrera, R., Corrado, M., et al. (2013). Mitochondrial cristae shape determines respiratory chain supercomplexes assembly and respiratory efficiency. *Cell* 155, 160–171. doi: 10.1016/j.cell.2013.08.032

Cohen, M. M., Leboucher, G. P., Livnat-Levanon, N., Glickman, M. H., and Weissman, A. M. (2008). Ubiquitin-proteasome-dependent degradation of a mitofusin, a critical regulator of mitochondrial fusion. *Mol. Biol. Cell.* 19, 2457–2464. doi: 10.1091/mbc.E08-02-0227

Correia, S. C., Carvalho, C., Cardoso, S., Santos, R. X., Santos, M. S., Oliveira, C. R., et al. (2010a). Mitochondrial preconditioning: a potential neuroprotective strategy. *Front. Aging. Neurosci.* 2:138. doi: 10.3389/fnagi.2010.00138

Correia, S. C., Santos, R. X., Cardoso, S., Carvalho, C., Candeias, E., Duarte, A. I., et al. (2012a). Alzheimer disease as a vascular disorder: where do mitochondria fit? *Exp. Gerontol.* 47, 878–886 doi: 10.1016/j.exger.2012.07.006

Correia, S. C., Santos, R. X., Carvalho, C., Cardoso, S., Candeias, E., Santos, M. S., et al. (2012c). Insulin signaling, glucose metabolism and mitochondria:

major players in Alzheimer's disease and diabetes interrelation. *Brain Res.* 1441, 64–78. doi: 10.1016/j.brainres.2011.12.063

Correia, S. C., Santos, R. X., Perry, G., Zhu, X., Moreira, P. I., and Smith, M. A. (2010b). Mitochondria: the missing link between preconditioning and neuroprotection. *J. Alzheimers. Dis.* 20(Suppl. 2), S475–S485. doi: 10.3233/JAD-2010-100669

Correia, S. C., Santos, R. X., Perry, G., Zhu, X., Moreira, P. I., and Smith, M. A. (2012b). Mitochondrial importance in Alzheimer's, Huntington's and Parkinson's diseases. *Adv. Exp. Med. Biol.* 724, 205–221. doi: 10.1007/978-1-4614-0653-2_16

Costanzo, M., and Zurzolo, C. (2013). The cell biology of prion-like spread of protein aggregates: mechanisms and implication in neurodegeneration. *Biochem. J.* 15, 1–17. doi: 10.1042/BJ20121898

Csermely, P., Agoston, V., and Pongor, S. (2005). The efficiency of multi-target drugs: the network approach might help drug design. *Trends Pharmacol. Sci.* 26, 178–182. doi: 10.1016/j.tips.2005.02.007

Darvesh, S., Cash, M. K., Reid, G. A., Martin, E., Mitnitski, A., and Geula, C. (2012). Butyrylcholinesterase is associated with beta-amyloid plaques in the Transgenic APP(SWE)/PSEN1dE9 Mouse Model of Alzheimer Disease. *J. Neuropathol. Exp. Neurol.* 71, 2–14. doi: 10.1097/NEN.0b013e31823cc7a6

De Colibus, L., Li, M., Binda, C., Lustig, A., Edmondson, D. E., and Mattevi, A. (2005). Three-dimensional structure of human monoamine oxidase A (MAO A).: relation to the structures of rat MAO A and human MAO B. *Proc. Natl. Acad. Sci. U.S.A.* 102, 12684–12689. doi: 10.1073/pnas.0505975102

de la Monte, S. M., and Wands, J. R. (2008). Alzheimer's disease is type 3 diabetes - evidence reviewed. *J. Diabetes Sci. Technol.* 2, 1101–1113. doi: 10.1177/193229680800200619

Delettre, C., Lenaers, G., Griffoin, J. M., Gigarel, N., Lorenzo, C., Belenguer, P., et al. (2000). Nuclear gene OPA1, encoding a mitochondrial dynamin-related protein, is mutated in dominant optic atrophy. *Nat. Genet.* 26, 207–210. doi: 10.1038/79936

D'Elia, P., De Matteis, F., Dragoni, S., Shah, A., Sgaragli, G., and Valoti, M. (2009). DP7, a novel dihydropyridine multidrug resistance reverter, shows only weak inhibitory activity on human CYP3A enzyme(s). *Eur. J. Pharmacol.* 614, 7–13. doi: 10.1016/j.ejphar.2009.04.019

Diodato, D., Tasca, G., Verrigni, D., D'Amico, A., Rizza, T., Tozzi, G., et al. (2015). A novel AIFM1 mutation expands the phenotype to an infantile motor neuron disease. *Eur. J. Hum. Genet.* 24, 463–466. doi: 10.1038/ejhg.2015.141

Donmez, G. (2012). The neurobiology of sirtuins and their role in neurodegeneration. *Trends Pharmacol. Sci.* 33, 494–501. doi: 10.1016/j.tips.2012.05.007

Dragoni, S., Bellik, L., Frosini, M., Matteucci, G., Sgaragli, G., and Valoti, M. (2003a). Cytochrome P450-dependent metabolism of l-deprenyl in monkey (Cercopithecus aethiops) and C57BL/6 mouse brain microsomal preparations. *J. Neurochem.* 86, 1174–1180. doi: 10.1046/j.1471-4159.2003.01927.x

Dragoni, S., Bellik, L., Frosini, M., Sgaragli, G., Marini, S., Gervasi, P. G., et al. (2003b). l-Deprenyl metabolism by the cytochrome P450 system in monkey (Cercopithecus aethiops) liver microsomes. *Xenobiotica* 33, 181–195. doi: 10.1080/0049825021000048827

Dragoni, S., Materozzi, G., Pessina, F., Frosini, M., Marco, J. L., Unzeta, M., et al. (2007). CYP-dependent metabolism of PF9601N, a new monoamine oxidase-B inhibitor, by C57BL/6 mouse and human liver microsomes. *J. Pharm. Pharm. Sci.* 10, 473–485. doi: 10.18433/J37P4J

Eckert, G. P., Renner, K., Eckert, S. H., Eckmann, J., Hagl, S., Abdel-Kader, R. M., et al. (2012). Mitochondrial Dysfunction-A Pharmacological Target in Alzheimer's Disease. *Mol. Neurobiol.* 46, 136–150. doi: 10.1007/s12035-012-8271-z

Edinger, A. L., and Thompson, C. B. (2004). Death by design: apoptosis, necrosis and autophagy. *Curr. Opin. Cell. Biol.* 16, 663–669. doi: 10.1016/j.ceb.2004.09.011

Edmondson, D. E., Binda, C., and Mattevi, A. (2007). Structural insights into the mechanism of amine oxidation by monoamine oxidases A and B. *Arch. Biochem. Biophys.* 464, 269–276. doi: 10.1016/j.abb.2007.05.006

Ellman, G. L., Courtney, K. D., Andres, V., and Featherstone, R. M. (1961). A New and Rapid Colorimetric Determination of Acetylcholinesterase Activity. *Biochem. Pharmacol.* 7, 88–95. doi: 10.1016/0006-2952(61)90145-9

Esteban, G., Allan, J., Samadi, A., Mattevi, A., Unzeta, M., Marco-Contelles, J., et al. (2014). Kinetic and structural analysis of the irreversible inhibition of human monoamine oxidases by ASS234, a multi-target compound designed for use in Alzheimer's disease. *Biochim. Biophys. Acta* 1844, 1104–1110. doi: 10.1016/j.bbapap.2014.03.006

Eyer, P., Worek, F., Kiderlen, D., Sinko, G., Stuglin, A., Simeon-Rudolf, V., et al. (2003). Molar absorption coefficients for the reduced Ellman reagent: reassessment. *Anal. Biochem.* 312, 224–227. doi: 10.1016/S0003-2697(02)00506-7

Farina, R., Pisani, L., Catto, M., Nicolotti, O., Gadaleta, D., Denora, N., et al. (2015). Structure-based design and optimization of multitarget-Directed 2H-Chromen-2-one derivatives as potent inhibitors of Monoamine Oxidase B and Cholinesterases. *J. Med. Chem.* 58, 5561–5578. doi: 10.1021/acs.jmedchem.5b00599

Ferguson, C. S., and Tyndale, R. F. (2011). Cytochrome P450 enzymes in the brain: emerging evidence of biological significance. *Trends Pharmacol. Sci.* 32, 708–714. doi: 10.1016/j.tips.2011.08.005

Ferreira, P., Villanueva, R., Martínez-Júlvez, M., Herguedas, B., Marcuello, C., Fernandez-Silva, P., et al. (2014). Structural insights into the coenzyme mediated monomer-dimer transition of the pro-apoptotic apoptosis inducing factor. *Biochemistry* 53, 4204–4215. doi: 10.1021/bi500343r

Fierro, A., Osorio-Olivares, M., Cassels, B. K., Edmondson, D. E., Sepulveda-Boza, S., and Reyes-Parada, M. (2007). Human and rat monoamine oxidase-A are differentially inhibited by (S).-4-alkylthioamphetamine derivatives: insights from molecular modeling studies. *Bioorg. Med. Chem.* 15, 5198–5206. doi: 10.1016/j.bmc.2007.05.021

Finberg, J. P. M. (2014). Update on the pharmacology of selective inhibitors of MAO-A and MAO-B: focus on modulation of CNS monoamine neurotransmitter release. *Pharmacol. Ther.* 143, 133–152. doi: 10.1016/j.pharmthera.2014.02.010

Fischer, M., Horn, S., Belkacemi, A., Kojer, K., Petrungaro, C., Habich, M., et al. (2013). Protein import and oxidative folding in the mitochondrial intermembrane space of intact mammalian cells. *Mol. Biol. Cell.* 24, 2160–2170. doi: 10.1091/mbc.E12-12-0862

Fischer, T. D., Hylin, M. J., Zhao, J., Moore, A. N., Waxham, M. N., and Dash, P. K. (2016). Altered Mitochondrial Dynamics and TBI Pathophysiology. *Front. Syst. Neurosci.* 30, 10:29. doi: 10.3389/fnsys.2016.00029

Fowler, J. S., Logan, J., Shumay, E., Alia-Klein, N., Wang, G. J., and Volkow, N. D. (2015). Monoamine oxidase: radiotracer chemistry and human studies. *J. Label. Compd. Radiopharm.* 58, 51–64. doi: 10.1002/jlcr.3247

Frezza, C., Cipolat, S., Martins de Brito, O., Micaroni, M., Beznoussenko, G. V., Rudka, T., et al. (2006). OPA1 controls apoptotic cristae remodeling independently from mitochondrial fusion. *Cell* 126, 177–189. doi: 10.1016/j.cell.2006.06.025

Gallardo-Pujol, D., Andrés-Pueyo, A., and Maydeu-Olivares, A. (2013). MAOA genotype, social exclusion and aggression: an experimental test of a gene-environment interaction. *Genes Brain Behav.* 12, 140–145. doi: 10.1111/j.1601-183X.2012.00868.x

Galloway, C. A., Lee, H., Brookes, P. S., and Yoon, Y. (2014). Decreasing mitochondrial fission alleviates hepatic steatosis in a murine model of nonalcoholic fatty liver disease. *Am. J. Physiol. Gastrointest. Liver. Physiol.* 307, G632–G641. doi: 10.1152/ajpgi.00182.2014

Galloway, C. A., Lee, H., and Yoon, Y. (2012). Mitochondrial morphology-emerging role in bioenergetics. *Free Radic. Biol. Med.* 53, 2218–2228. doi: 10.1016/j.freeradbiomed.2012.09.035

Gardner, R. C., Burke, J. F., Nettiksimmons, J., Goldman, S., Tanner, C. M., and Yaffe, K. (2015). Traumatic brain injury in later life increases risk for Parkinson Disease. *Ann. Neurol.* 77, 987–995. doi: 10.1002/ana.24396

Gascon, E., and Gao, F. B. (2012). Cause or effect: misregulation of microRNA pathways in neurodegeneration. *Front Neurosci.* 6:48. doi: 10.3389/fnins.2012.00048

Gáspárová, Z., Janega, P., Babal, P., Snirc, V., Stolc, S., Mach, M., et al. (2009). Effect of the new pyridoindole antioxidant SMe1EC2 on functional deficits and oedema formation in rat hippocampus exposed to ischaemia *in vitro*. *Neuro Endocrinol. Lett.* 30, 574–581.

Gáspárová, Z., Ondrejicková, O., Gajdošíková, A., Gajdošík, A., Snirc, V., and Stolc, S. (2010). Oxidative stress induced by the Fe2+/ascorbic acid system or model ischemia *in vitro*: effect of carvedilol and pyridoindole antioxidant SMe1EC2 in young and adult rat brain tissue. *Interdiscipl. Toxicol.* 3, 122–126. doi: 10.2478/v10102-010-0051-x

Geldenhuys, W. J., Youdim, M. B. H., Carroll, R. T., and Van der Schyf, C. J. (2011). The emergence of designed multiple ligands for neurodegenerative disorders. *Progr. Neurobiol.* 94, 347–359. doi: 10.1016/j.pneurobio.2011.04.010

Ghezzi, D., Sevrioukova, I., Invernizzi, F., Lamperti, C., Mora, M., D'Adamo, P., et al. (2010). Severe X-linked mitochondrial encephalomyopathy associated with a mutation in apoptosis-inducing factor. *Am. J. Hum. Genet.* 86, 639–649. doi: 10.1016/j.ajhg.2010.03.002

Gillman, P. K. (2011). Advances pertaining to the pharmacology and interactions of irreversible nonselective monoamine oxidase inhibitors. *J. Clin. Psychopharmacol.* 31, 66–74. doi: 10.1097/JCP.0b013e31820469ea

Goedert, M. (2015). NEURODEGENERATION. Alzheimer's and Parkinson's diseases: the prion concept in relation to assembled A beta, tau, and alpha-synuclein. *Science* 349:1255555. doi: 10.1126/science.1255555

Goldberg, R. N., Kishore, N., and Lennen, R. M. (2002). Thermodinamic quantities for the ionization reactions of buffers. *J. Phys. Chem. Ref. Data* 31, 231–370. doi: 10.1063/1.1416902

Greig, N. H., Lahiri, D. K., and Sambamurti, K. (2002). Butyrylcholinesterase: an important new target in Alzheimer's disease therapy. *Int. Psychogeriatr.* 14, 77–91. doi: 10.1017/S1041610203008676

Griparic, L., Kanazawa, T., and van der Bliek, A. M. (2007). Regulation of the mitochondrial dynamin-like protein Opa1 by proteolytic cleavage. *J. Cell Biol.* 178, 757–764. doi: 10.1083/jcb.200704112

Griparic, L., van der Wel, N. N., Orozco, I. J., Peters, P. J., and van der Bliek, A. M. (2004). Loss of the intermembrane space protein Mgm1/OPA1 induces swelling and localized constrictions along the lengths of mitochondria. *J. Biol. Chem.* 279, 18792–18798. doi: 10.1074/jbc.M400920200

Guzior, N., Wieckowska, A., Panek, D., and Malawska, B. (2015). Recent Development of multifunctional agents as potential drug candidates for the treatment of Alzheimer's Disease. *Curr. Med. Chem.* 22, 373–404. doi: 10.2174/0929867321666141106122628

Haddad, D., and Nakamura, K. (2015). Understanding the susceptibility of dopamine neurons to mitochondrial stressors in Parkinson's disease. *FEBS Lett.* 589(24 Pt A), 3702–3713. doi: 10.1016/j.febslet.2015.10.021

Hales, K. G. (2004). The machinery of mitochondrial fusion, division, and distribution, and emerging connections to apoptosis. *Mitochondrion* 4, 285–308. doi: 10.1016/j.mito.2004.05.007

Hales, K. G. (2010). Mitochondrial fusion and division. *Nat. Educ.* 3:12. Available online at: http://www.nature.com/scitable/topicpage/mitochondrial-fusion-and-division-14264007

Halling, J., Petersen, M. S., Grandjean, P., Weihe, P., and Brosen, K. (2008). Genetic predisposition to Parkinson's disease: CYP2D6 and HFE in the Faroe Islands. *Pharmacogenet. Genomics* 18, 209–212. doi: 10.1097/FPC.0b013e3282f5106e

Hangen, E., Féraud, O., Lachkar, S., Mou, H., Doti, N., Fimia, G. M., et al. (2015). Interaction between AIF and CHCHD4 regulates respiratory chain biogenesis. *Mol. Cell* 58, 1001–1014. doi: 10.1016/j.molcel.2015.04.020

He, D., Wu, H., Wei, Y., Liu, W., Huang, F., Shi, H., et al. (2015). Effects of harmine, an acetylcholinesterase inhibitor, on spatial learning and memory of APP/PS1 transgenic mice and scopolamine-induced memory impairment mice. *Eur. J. Pharmac.* 768, 96–107. doi: 10.1016/j.ejphar.2015.10.037

Hebda, M., Bajda, M., Wieckowska, A., Szalaj, N., Pasieka, A., Panek, D., et al. (2016). Synthesis, molecular modelling and biological evaluation of novel Heterodimeric, multiple ligands targeting Cholinesterases and Amyloid Beta. *Molecules.* 21, 24. doi: 10.3390/molecules21040410

Horáková, L., Sies, H., and Steenken, S. (1994). Antioxidant action of stobadine. *Meth. Enzymol.* 234, 572–580.

Horáková, L., and Stolc, S. (1998). Antioxidant and pharmacodynamic effects of pyridoindole stobadine. *Gen. Pharmacol.* 30, 627–638.

Hou, L. N., Xu, J. R., Zhao, Q. N., Gao, X. L., Cui, Y. Y., Xu, J., et al. (2014). A new motif in the N-terminal of acetylcholinesterase triggers amyloid-β aggregation and deposition. *CNS. Neurosci. Ther.* 20, 59–66. doi: 10.1111/cns.12161

Hroch, L., Aitken, L., Benek, O., Dolezal, M., Kuca, K., Gunn-Moore, F., et al. (2015). Benzothiazoles - Scaffold of Interest for CNS Targeted Drugs. *Curr. Med. Chem.* 22, 730–747. doi: 10.2174/0929867322666141212120631

Hughes, R. E., Nikolic, K., and Ramsay, R. R. (2016). One for all? Hitting multiple Alzheimer's disease targets with one drug. *Front. Neurosci.* 10:177. doi: 10.3389/fnins.2016.00177

Inestrosa, N. C., Alvarez, A., Pérez, C. A., Moreno, R. D., Vicente, M., Linker, C., et al. (1996). Acetylcholinesterase accelerates assembly of amyloid-beta-peptides into Alzheimer's fibrils: possible role of the peripheral site of the enzyme. *Neuron* 16, 881–891. doi: 10.1016/S0896-6273(00)80108-7

Inestrosa, N. C., Dinamarca, M. C., and Alvarez, A. (2008). Amyloid-cholinesterase interactions - Implications for Alzheimer's disease. *FEBS J.* 275, 625–632. doi: 10.1111/j.1742-4658.2007.06238.x

Ingelman-Sundberg, M. (2004). Human drug metabolising cytochrome P450 enzymes: properties and polymorphisms. *Naunyn Schmiedebergs Arch. Pharmacol.* 369, 89–104. doi: 10.1007/s00210-003-0819-z

Ingelman-Sundberg, M., and Gomez, A. (2010). The past, present and future of pharmacoepigenomics. *Pharmacogenomics* 11, 625–627. doi: 10.2217/pgs.10.59

Ishihara, N., Fujita, Y., Oka, T., and Mihara, K. (2006). Regulation of mitochondrial morphology through proteolytic cleavage of OPA1. *EMBO J.* 25, 2966–2977. doi: 10.1038/sj.emboj.7601184

Ishimura, R., Martin, G. R., and Ackerman, S. L. (2008). Loss of apoptosis-inducing factor results in cell-type-specific neurogenesis defects. *J. Neurosci.* 28, 4938–4948. doi: 10.1523/JNEUROSCI.0229-08.2008

Johri, A., and Beal, M. F. (2012). Mitochondrial dysfunction in neurodegenerative diseases. *J. Pharamacol. Exp. Ther.* 342 619–630. doi: 10.1124/jpet.112.192138

Joza, N., Oudit, G. Y., Brown, D., Bénit, P., Kassiri, Z., Vahsen, N., et al. (2005). Muscle-specific loss of apoptosis-inducing factor leads to mitochondrial dysfunction, skeletal muscle atrophy, and dilated cardiomyopathy. *Mol. Cell. Biol.* 25, 10261–10272. doi: 10.1128/MCB.25.23.10261-10272.2005

Juárez-Jiménez, J., Mendes, E., Galdeano, C., Martins, C., Silva, D. B., Marco-Contelles, J., et al. (2014). Exploring the structural basis of the selective inhibition of monoamine oxidase A by dicarbonitrile aminoheterocycles: role of Asn181 and Ile335 validated by spectroscopic and computational studies. *Biochim. Biophys. Acta* 1844, 389–397. doi: 10.1016/j.bbapap.2013.11.003

Juranek, I., Horakova, L., Rackova, L., and Stefek, M. (2010). Antioxidants in treating pathologies involving oxidative damage: an update on medicinal chemistry and biological activity of stobadine and related pyridoindoles. *Curr. Med. Chem.* 17, 552–570. doi: 10.2174/092986710790416317

Kaludercic, N., Carpi, A., Menabò, R., Di Lisa, F., and Paolocci, N. (2011). Monoamine oxidases (MAO). in the pathogenesis of heart failure and ischemia/reperfusion injury. *Biochim. Biophys. Acta* 1813, 1323–1332. doi: 10.1016/j.bbamcr.2010.09.010

Katritch, V., Cherezov, V., and Stevens, R. C. (2013). Structure-function of the G protein-coupled receptor superfamily. *Annu. Rev. Pharmacol. Toxicol.* 53, 531–556. doi: 10.1146/annurev-pharmtox-032112-135923

Kennedy, B. P., Ziegler, M. G., Alford, M., Hansen, L. A., Thal, L. J., and Masliah, E. (2003). Early and persistent alterations in prefrontal cortex MAO A and B in Alzheimer's disease. *J. Neural. Transm.* 110, 789–801.

Kettwig, M., Schubach, M., Zimmermann, F. A., Klinge, L., Mayr, J. A., Biskup, S., et al. (2015). From ventriculomegaly to severe muscular atrophy: expansion of the clinical spectrum related to mutations in AIFM1. *Mitochondrion* 21C, 12–18. doi: 10.1016/j.mito.2015.01.001

Kim, H., Sablin, S. O., and Ramsay, R. R. (1997). Inhibition of monoamine oxidase A by beta-carboline derivatives. *Arch. Biochem. Biophys.* 337, 137–142. doi: 10.1006/abbi.1996.9771

Kitz, R., and Wilson, I. B. (1962). Esters of methanesulfonic acid as irreversible inhibitors of acetylcholinesterase. *J. Biol. Chem.* 237, 3245–3249.

Klein, J. A., Longo-Guess, C. M., Rossmann, M. P., Seburn, K. L., Hurd, R. E., Frankel, W. N., et al. (2002). The harlequin mouse mutation downregulates apoptosis-inducing factor. *Nature* 419, 367–374. doi: 10.1038/nature01034

Koch, J. R., and Schmid, F. X. (2014). Mia40 targets cysteines in a hydrophobic environment to direct oxidative protein folding in the mitochondria. *Nat. Commun.* 5, 3041. doi: 10.1038/ncomms4041

Koshiba, T., Detmer, S. A., Kaiser, J. T., Chen, H., McCaffery, J. M., and Chan, D. C. (2004). Structural basis of mitochondrial tethering by mitofusin complexes. *Science* 305, 858–862. doi: 10.1126/science.1099793

Krueger, M. J., Mazouz, F., Ramsay, R. R., Milcent, R., and Singer, T. P. (1995). Dramatic species differences in the susceptibility of Monoamine-Oxidase-B to a group of powerful inhibitors. *Biochem. Biophys. Res. Commun.* 206, 556–562. doi: 10.1006/bbrc.1995.1079

Kubo, M., Kishi, T., Matsunaga, S., and Iwata, N. (2015). Histamine H3 Receptor Antagonists for Alzheimer's Disease: a systematic review and meta-analysis of Randomized Placebo-controlled trials. *J. Alzheimers Dis.* 48, 667–671. doi: 10.3233/JAD-150393

Kupershmidt, L., Amit, T., Bar-Am, O., Youdim, M. B. H., and Weinreb, O. (2012). The novel multi-target iron chelating-radical scavenging compound M30 possesses beneficial effects on major hallmarks of Alzheimer's disease. *Antiox. Redox Signal.* 17, 860–877. doi: 10.1089/ars.2011.4279

Lecoutey, C., Hedou, D., Freret, T., Giannoni, P., Gaven, F., Since, M., et al. (2014). Design of donecopride, a dual serotonin subtype 4 receptor agonist/acetylcholinesterase inhibitor with potential interest for Alzheimer's disease treatment. *Proc. Natl. Acad. Sci. U.S.A.* 111, E3825–E3830. doi: 10.1073/pnas.1410315111

Lee, Y. J., Jeong, S. Y., Karbowski, M., Smith, C. L., and Youle, R. J. (2004). Roles of the mammalian mitochondrial fission and fusion mediators Fis1, Drp1, and Opa1 in apoptosis. *Mol. Biol. Cell* 15, 5001–5011. doi: 10.1091/mbc.E04-04-0294

Lenders, J. W. M., Eisenhofer, G., Abeling, N., Berger, W., Murphy, D. L., Konings, C. H., et al. (1996). Specific genetic deficiencies of the A and B isoenzymes of monoamine oxidase are characterized by distinct neurochemical and clinical phenotypes. *J. Clin. Invest.* 97, 1010–1019. doi: 10.1172/JCI118492

León, R., Garcia, A. G., and Marco-Contelles, J. (2013). Recent advances in the multitarget-directed ligands approach for the treatment of Alzheimer's disease. *Med. Res. Rev.* 33, 139–189. doi: 10.1002/med.20248

Lezi, E., and Swerdlow, R. H. (2012). Mitochondria in neurodegeneration. *Adv. Exp. Med. Biol.* 942, 269–286. doi: 10.1007/978-94-007-2869-1_12

Lezoualc'h, F. (2007). 5-HT$_4$ receptor and Alzheimer's disease: the amyloid connection. *Exp. Neurol.* 205, 325–329. doi: 10.1016/j.expneurol.2007.02.001

Li, Y., Wang, P., Wei, J., Fan, R., Zuo, Y., Shi, M., et al. (2015). Inhibition of Drp1 by Mdivi-1 attenuates cerebral ischemic injury via inhibition of the mitochondria-dependent apoptotic pathway after cardiac arrest. *Neuroscience* 311, 67–74. doi: 10.1016/j.neuroscience.2015.10.020

Liu, Y., Wang, Z., and Zhang, B. (2014). The relationship between monoamine oxidase B (MAOB). A644G polymorphism and Parkinson disease risk: a meta-analysis. *Ann. Saudi Med.* 34, 12–17. doi: 10.5144/0256-4947.2014.12

Lu, Y., Mo, C., Zeng, Z., Chen, S., Xie, Y., Peng, Q., et al. (2013). CYP2D6*4 allele polymorphism increases the risk of Parkinson's disease: evidence from meta-analysis. *PLoS ONE* 8:e84413. doi: 10.1371/journal.pone.0084413

Ludwig, E., Schmid, J., Beschke, K., and Ebner, T. (1999). Activation of human cytochrome P-450 3A4-catalyzed meloxicam 5'-methylhydroxylation by quinidine and hydroquinidine *in vitro*. *J. Pharmacol. Exp. Ther.* 290, 1–8.

Lum, C. T., and Stahl, S. M. (2012). Opportunities for reversible inhibitors of monoamine oxidase-A (RIMAs). in the treatment of depression. *CNS Spectr.* 17, 107–120. doi: 10.1017/S1092852912000594

Luo, Z., Sheng, J., Sun, Y., Lu, C., Yan, J., Liu, A., et al. (2013). Synthesis and evaluation of multi-target-directed ligands against Alzheimer's Disease based on the fusion of Donepezil and Ebselen. *J. Med. Chem.* 56, 9089–9099. doi: 10.1021/jm401047q

Lustbader, J. W., Cirilli, M., Lin, C., Xu, H. W., Takuma, K., Wang, N., et al. (2004). ABAD directly links A beta to mitochondrial toxicity in Alzheimer's disease. *Science* 304, 448–452. doi: 10.1126/science.1091230

Majekova, M., Stecoza, C. E., Kovacikova, L., and Majek, P. (2013). "The use DRAGON molecular descriptors for the estimation of pharmacologic profile of dibenzothiepine and pyridoindole compounds," in *Pokroky v analytickej chémii*, eds S. Hrouzkova and J. Labuda (Bratislava: STU FCHPT), 504–520.

Malcomson, T., Yelekci, K., Borrello, M. T., Ganesan, A., Semina, E., De Kimpe, N., et al. (2015). cis-cyclopropylamines as mechanism-based inhibitors of monoamine oxidases. *FEBS. J.* 282, 3190–3198. doi: 10.1111/febs.13260

Mandemakers, W., Morais, V. A., and De Strooper, B. (2007). A cell biological perspective on mitochondrial dysfunction in Parkinson disease and other neurodegenerative diseases. *J. Cell. Sci.* 120, 1707–1716. doi: 10.1242/jcs.03443

Marco-Contelles, J., Unzeta, M., Esteban, G., Ramsay, R., Romero, A., Martínez-Murillo, R., et al. (2016). ASS234, as a new multi-target directed Propargylamine for Alzheimer's Disease therapy. *Front. Neurosci.* 10:294. doi: 10.3389/fnins.2016.00294

McDonald, A. G., and Tipton, K. F. (2012). *Enzymes: Irreversible Inhibition*. eLS. doi: 10.1002/9780470015902.a0000601.pub2. Available online at: http://olabout.wiley.com/WileyCDA/Section/id-390001.html

McDonald, G. R., Olivieri, A., Ramsay, R. R., and Holt, A. (2010). On the formation and nature of the imidazoline I(2). binding site on human monoamine oxidase-B. *Pharmacol. Res.* 62, 475–488. doi: 10.1016/j.phrs.2010.09.001

Meadowcroft, M. D., Connor, J. R., Smith, M. B., and Yang, Q. X. (2009). MRI and histological analysis of beta-amyloid plaques in both human Alzheimer's disease and APP/PS1 transgenic mice. *J. Magn. Reson. Imaging* 29, 997–1007. doi: 10.1002/jmri.21731

Melancon, B. J., Tarr, J. C., Panarese, J. D., Wood, M. R., and Lindsley, C. W. (2013). Allosteric modulation of the M1 muscarinic acetylcholine receptor: improving cognition and a potential treatment for schizophrenia and Alzheimer's disease. *Drug Discov. Today* 18, 1185–1199. doi: 10.1016/j.drudis.2013.09.005

Mesulam, M. M., Guillozet, A., Shaw, P., Levey, A., Duysen, E. G., and Lockridge, O. (2002). Acetylcholinesterase knockouts establish central cholinergic pathways and can use butyrylcholinesterase to hydrolyze acetylcholine. *Neuroscience* 110, 627–639. doi: 10.1016/S0306-4522(01)00613-3

Meyer, J. H., Ginovart, N., Boovariwala, A., Sagrati, S., Hussey, D., Garcia, A., et al. (2006). Elevated monoamine oxidase A levels in the brain - An explanation for the monoamine imbalance of major depression. *Arch. Gen. Psychiatry* 63, 1209–1216. doi: 10.1001/archpsyc.63.11.1209

Meyer, K., Buettner, S., Ghezzi, D., Zeviani, M., Bano, D., and Nicotera, P. (2015). Loss of apoptosis-inducing factor critically affects MIA40 function. *Cell. Death. Dis.* 6:e1814. doi: 10.1038/cddis.2015.170

Mézešová, L., Jendruchová-Javorková, V., Vlkovicová, J., Kyselova, Z., Navarová, J., Bezek, S. et al. (2012). Antioxidant SMe1EC2 may attenuate the disbalance of sodium homeostasis in the organism induced by higher intake of cholesterol. *Mol. Cell. Biochem.* 366, 41–48. doi: 10.1007/s11010-012-1281-3

Miksys, S., and Tyndale, R. F. (2009). Brain drug-metabolizing cytochrome P450 enzymes are active *in vivo*, demonstrated by mechanism-based enzyme inhibition. *Neuropsychopharmacology* 34, 634–640. doi: 10.1038/npp.2008.110

Miksys, S., and Tyndale, R. F. (2013). Cytochrome P450-mediated drug metabolism in the brain. *J. Psychiatry Neurosci.* 38, 152–163. doi: 10.1503/jpn.1 20133

Milczek, E. M., Binda, C., Rovida, S., Mattevi, A., and Edmondson, D. E. (2011). *3zyx: Crystal Structure of Human Monoamine Oxidase b in Complex with Methylene Blue and Bearing the Double Mutation i199a-y326a. Protein Data Bank.* Available online at: https://www.ebi.ac.uk/pdbe/entry/pdb/3zyx/biology doi: 10.2210/pdb3zyx/pdb

Miramar, M. D., Costantini, P., Ravagnan, L., Saraiva, L. M., Haouzi, D., Brothers, G., et al. (2001). NADH oxidase activity of mitochondrial apoptosis-inducing factor. *J. Biol. Chem.* 276, 16391–16398. doi: 10.10/4/jbc.M010498200

Moreira, P. I., Carvalho, C., Zhu, X., Smith, M. A., and Perry, G. (2010). Mitochondrial dysfunction is a trigger of Alzheimer's disease pathophysiology. *Biochim. Biophys. Acta* 1802, 2–10. doi: 10.1016/j.bbadis.2009.10.006

Morris, J. K., Bomhoff, G. L., Stanford, J. A., and Geiger, P. C. (2010). Neurodegeneration in an animal model of Parkinson's disease is exacerbated by a high-fat diet. *Am. J. Physiol. Regul. Integr. Comp. Phys.* 299, R1082–R1090. doi: 10.1152/ajpregu.00449.2010

Morrison, J. F. (1969). Kinetics of reversible inhibition of enzyme-catalysed reactions by tight-binding inhibitors. *Biochim. Biophys. Acta* 185, 269–286. doi: 10.1016/0005-2744(69)90420-3

Moussaud, S., Jones, D. R., Moussaud-Lamodière, E. L., Delenclos, M., Ross, O. A., and McLean, P. J. (2014). Alpha-synuclein and tau: teammates in neurodegeneration? *Mol. Neurodegener.* 9:43. doi: 10.1186/1750-1326-9-43

Murphy, M. P. (2009). How mitochondria produce reactive oxygen species. *Biochem. J.* 417, 1–13. doi: 10.1042/BJ20081386

Nakamura, K., Nemani, V. M., Azarbal, F., Skibinski, G., Levy, J. M., Egami, K., et al. (2011). Direct membrane association drives mitochondrial fission by the Parkinson disease-associated protein alpha-synuclein. *J. Biol. Chem.* 286, 20710–20726. doi: 10.1074/jbc.M110.213538

Naoi, M., and Maruyama, W. (2010). Monoamine Oxidase inhibitors as neuroprotective agents in age-dependent neurodegenerative disorders. *Curr. Pharm. Design.* 16, 2799–2817. doi: 10.2174/138161210793176527

Naoi, M., Maruyama, W., Akao, Y., Yi, H., and Yamaoka, Y. (2006). Involvement of type A monoamine oxidase in neurodegeneration: regulation of mitochondrial signaling leading to cell death or neuroprotection. *J. Neural Transm. Suppl.* 71, 67–77. doi: 10.1007/978-3-211-33328-0_8

Naoi, M., Maruyama, W., Yi, H., Akao, Y., Yamaoka, Y., and Shamoto-Nagai, M. (2007). Neuroprotection by propargylamines in Parkinson's disease: intracellular mechanism underlying the anti-apoptotic function and search for clinical markers. *J. Neural Transm. Suppl.* 72, 121–131. doi: 10.1007/978-3-211-73574-9_15

Nebert, D. W., Wikvall, K., and Miller, W. L. (2013). Human cytochromes P450 in health and disease. *Philos. Trans. R. Soc. Lond. Biol. Sci.* 368:20120431. doi: 10.1098/rstb.2012.0431

Nicolet, Y., Lockridge, O., Masson, P., Fontecilla-Camps, J. C., and Nachon, F. (2003). Crystal structure of human butyrylcholinesterase and of its complexes with substrate and products. *J. Biol. Chem.* 278, 41141–41147. doi: 10.1074/jbc.M210241200

Nikolic, K., Mavridis, L., Bautista-Aguilera, O. M., Marco-Contelles, J., Stark, H., do Carmo Carreiras, M., et al. (2015). Predicting targets of compounds against neurological diseases using cheminformatic methodology. *J. Comput. Aided Mol. Des.* 29, 183–198. doi: 10.1007/s10822-014-9816-1

Nikolic, K., Mavridis, L., Djikic, T., Vucicevic, J., Agbaba, D., Yelekci, K., et al. (2016). Drug design for CNS diseases: polypharmacological profiling of compounds using cheminformatic, 3D-QSAR and virtual screening methodologies. *Front. Neurosci.* 10:265. doi: 10.3389/fnins.2016.00265

Novaroli, L., Daina, A., Favre, E., Bravo, J., Carotti, A., Leonetti, F., et al. (2006). Impact of species-dependent differences on screening, design, and development of MAO B inhibitors. *J. Med. Chem.* 49, 6264–6272. doi: 10.1021/jm060441e

Nunnari, J., and Suomalainen, A. (2012). Mitochondria: in sickness and in health. *Cell* 148, 1145–1159. doi: 10.1016/j.cell.2012.02.035

Oesch-Bartlomowicz, B., and Oesch, F. (2005). Phosphorylation of cytochromes P450: first discovery of a posttranslational modification of a drug-metabolizing enzyme. *Biochem. Biophys. Res. Commun.* 338, 446–449. doi: 10.1016/j.bbrc.2005.08.092

Olanow, C. W., and Tatton, W. G. (1999). Ethiology and pathogenesis of Parkinson's disease. *Ann. Rev. Neurosci.* 22, 123–144. doi: 10.1146/annurev. neuro.22.1.123

Ooi, J., Hayden, M. R., and Pouladi, M. A. (2015). Inhibition of excessive monoamine oxidase A/B activity protects against stress-induced neuronal death in Huntington Disease. *Mol. Neurobiol.* 52, 1850–1861. doi: 10.1007/s12035-014-8974-4

Pan, Y. Z., Gao, W., and Yu, A. M. (2009). MicroRNAs regulate CYP3A4 expression via direct and indirect targeting. *Drug Metab. Dispos.* 37, 2112–2117. doi: 10.1124/dmd.109.027680

Patil, P. O., Bari, S. B., Firke, S. D., Deshmukh, P. K., Donda, S. T., and Patil, D. A. (2013). A comprehensive review on synthesis and designing aspects of coumarin derivatives as monoamine oxidase inhibitors for depression and Alzheimer's disease. *Bioorg. Med. Chem.* 21, 2434–2450. doi: 10.1016/j.bmc.2013.02.017

Payami, H., Lee, N., Zareparsi, S., Gonzales McNeal, M., Camicioli, R., Bird, T. D., et al. (2001). Parkinson's disease, CYP2D6 polymorphism, and age. *Neurology* 56, 1363–1370. doi: 10.1212/WNL.56.10.1363

Perier, C., Bové, J., Dehay, B., Jackson-Lewis, V., Rabinovitch, P. S., Przedborski, S., et al. (2010). Apoptosis-inducing factor deficiency sensitizes dopaminergic neurons to parkinsonian neurotoxins. *Ann. Neurol.* 68, 184–192. doi: 10.1002/ana.22034

Perier, C., Bové, J., and Vila, M. (2012). Mitochondria and programmed cell death in Parkinson's disease: apoptosis and beyond. *Antiox. Redox Signal.* 16, 883–895. doi: 10.1089/ars.2011.4074

Perier, C., and Vila, M. (2012). Mitochondrial biology and Parkinson's disease. *Cold Spring Harb. Perspect. Med.* 2:a009332. doi: 10.1101/cshperspect.a009332

Persad, A. S., Stedeford, T., Tanaka, S., Chen, L., and Banasik, M. (2003). Parkinson's disease and CYP2D6 polymorphism in Asian populations: a meta-analysis. *Neuroepidemiology* 22, 357–361. doi: 10.1159/000072926

Petit, P. X., Susin, S. A., Zamzami, N., Mignotte, B., and Kroemer, G. (1996). Mitochondria and programmed cell death: back to the future. *FEBS Lett.* 396, 7–13. doi: 10.1016/0014-5793(96)00988-X

Piazzi, L., Cavalli, A., Colizzi, F., Belluti, F., Bartolini, M., Mancini, F., et al. (2008). Multi-target-directed coumarin derivatives: hAChE and BACE1 inhibitors as potential anti-Alzheimer compounds. *Bioorg. Med. Chem. Lett.* 18, 423–426. doi: 10.1016/j.bmcl.2007.09.100

Pisani, L., Catto, M., Leonetti, F., Nicolotti, O., Stefanachi, A., Campagna, F., et al. (2011). Targeting monoamine oxidases with multipotent ligands: an emerging strategy in the search of new drugs against neurodegenerative diseases. *Curr. Med. Chem.* 18, 4568–4587. doi: 10.2174/092986711797379302

Pisani, L., Farina, R., Soto-Otero, R., Denora, N., Mangiatordi, G. F., Nicolotti, O., et al. (2016). Searching for multi-targeting neurotherapeutics against

Alzheimer's: discovery of potent AChE-MAO B inhibitors through the decoration of the 2H-Chromen-2-one structural motif. *Molecules* 21:362. doi: 10.3390/molecules21030362

Preissner, S. C., Hoffmann, M. F., Preissner, R., Dunkel, M., Gewiess, A., and Preissner, S. (2013). Polymorphic cytochrome P450 enzymes (CYPs) and their role in personalized therapy. *PLoS ONE* 8:e82562. doi: 10.1371/journal.pone.0082562

Račková, L., Cumaoğlu, A., Bağriacik, E. U., Štefek, M., Maechler, P., and Karasu, Ç. (2011). Novel hexahydropyridoindole derivative as prospective agent against oxidative damage in pancreatic β cells. *Med. Chem.* 7, 711–717. doi: 10.2174/157340611797928370

Rackova, L., Snirc, V., Jung, T., Stefek, M., Karasu, C., and Grune, T. (2009). Metabolism-induced oxidative stress is a mediator of glucose toxicity in HT22 neuronal cells. *Free. Radic. Res.* 43, 876–886. doi: 10.1080/10715760903104374

Rackova, L., Snirc, V., Majekova, M., Majek, P., and Stefek, M. (2006). Free radical scavenging and antioxidant activities of substituted hexahydropyridoindoles. Quantitative structure-activity relationships. *J. Med. Chem.* 49, 2543–2548. doi: 10.1021/jm060041r

Ramsay, R. R., Dunford, C., and Gillman, P. K. (2007). Methylene blue and serotonin toxicity: inhibition of monoamine oxidase A (MAO A). confirms a theoretical prediction. *Br. J. Pharmacol.* 152, 946–951. doi: 10.1038/sj.bjp.0707430

Ramsay, R. R., Olivieri, A., and Holt, A. (2011). An improved approach to steady-state analysis of monoamine oxidases. *J. Neural Transm.* 118, 1003–1019. doi: 10.1007/s00702-011-0657-y

Rao, V. K., Carlson, E. A., and Yan, S. S. (2014). Mitochondrial permeability transition pore is a potential drug target for neurodegeneration. *Biochim. Biophys. Acta* 1842, 1267–1272. doi: 10.1016/j.bbadis.2013.09.003

Reyes, A. E., Perez, D. R., Alvarez, A., Garrido, J., Gentry, M. K., Doctor, B. P., et al. (1997). A monoclonal antibody against acetylcholinesterase inhibits the formation of amyloid fibrils induced by the enzyme. *Biochem. Biophys. Res. Commun.* 232, 652–655. doi: 10.1006/bbrc.1997.6357

Riddles, P. W., Blakeley, R. L., and Zerner, B. (1979). Ellman's reagent: 5,5'-dithiobis(2-nitrobenzoic acid).-reexamination. *Anal. Biochem.* 94, 75–81. doi: 10.1016/0003-2697(79)90792-9

Riedl, A. G., Watts, P. M., Brown, C. T., and Jenner, P. (1999). P450 and heme oxygenase enzymes in the basal ganglia and their roles in Parkinson's disease. *Adv. Neurol.* 80, 271–286.

Rinaldi, C., Grunseich, C., Sevrioukova, I. F., Schindler, A., Horkayne-Szakaly, I., Lamperti, C., et al. (2012). Cowchock syndrome is associated with a mutation in apoptosis-inducing factor. *Am. J. Hum. Genet.* 91, 1095–1102. doi: 10.1016/j.ajhg.2012.10.008

Rintoul, G. L., and Reynolds, I. J. (2010). Mitochondrial trafficking and morphology in neuronal injury. *Biochim Biophys Acta* 1802, 143–150. doi: 10.1016/j.bbadis.2009.09.005

Rochais, C., Lecoutey, C., Gaven, F., Giannoni, P., Hamidouche, K., Hedou, D., et al. (2015). Novel multitarget-directed ligands (MTDLs) with acetylcholinesterase (AChE) inhibitory and serotonergic subtype 4 receptor (5-HT4R) agonist activities as potential agents against Alzheimer's disease: the design of donecopride. *J. Med. Chem.* 58, 3172–3187. doi: 10.1021/acs.jmedchem.5b00115

Russo, O., Cachard-Chastel, M., Riviere, C., Giner, M., Soulier, J. L., Berthouze, M., et al. (2009). Design, synthesis, and biological evaluation of New 5-HT(4). receptor agonists: application as amyloid cascade modulators and potential therapeutic utility in Alzheimer's Disease. *J. Med. Chem.* 52, 2214–2225. doi: 10.1021/jm801327q

Sacher, J., Houle, S., Parkes, J., Rusjan, P., Sagrati, S., Wilson, A. A., et al. (2011). Monoamine oxidase A inhibitor occupancy during treatment of major depressive episodes with moclobemide or St. John's wort: an [C-11]-harmine PET study. *J. Psychiatry Neurosci.* 36, 375–382. doi: 10.1503/jpn.100117

Samadi, A., Chioua, M., Bolea, I., de Los Ríos, C., Iriepa, I., Moraleda, I., et al. (2011). Synthesis, biological assessment and molecular modeling of new multipotent MAO and cholinesterase inhibitors as potential drugs for the treatment of Alzheimer's disease. *Eur. J. Med. Chem.* 46, 4665–4678. doi: 10.1016/j.ejmech.2011.05.048

Samadi, A., Marco Contelles, J. L., Bolea Tomas, I., Luque Garriga, F. J., and Unzeta Lopez, M. (2015). *Derivatives of Propargylamine having Neuroprotective Capacity for the Treatment of Alzheimer's and Parkinson's Diseases.* Washington,

DC: Consejo Superior de Investigaciones Cientificas; Universitat Autonoma de Barcelona; Universidad de Barcelona, US20130012522 A1. U.S. Patent and Trademark Office.

Sankowski, R., Mader, S., and Valdés-Ferrer, S. I. (2015). Systemic inflammation and the brain: novel roles of genetic, molecular, and environmental cues as drivers of neurodegeneration. *Front. Cell. Neurosci.* 9:28. doi: 10.3389/fncel.2015.00028

Santana, L., Uriarte, E., González-Díaz, H., Zagotto, G., Soto-Otero, R., and Mendez-Alvarez, E. (2006). A QSAR model for *in silico* screening of MAO-A inhibitors. Prediction, synthesis, and biological assay of novel coumarins. *J. Med. Chem.* 49, 1149–1156. doi: 10.1021/jm0509849

Saraste, A., and Pulkki, K. (2000). Morphologic and biochemical hallmarks of apoptosis. *Cardiovasc. Res.* 45, 528–537. doi: 10.1016/S0008-6363(99)00384-3

Schapira, A. H., and Gegg, M. (2011). Mitochondrial contribution to Parkinson's disease pathogenesis. *Parkinsons Dis.* 2011:159160. doi: 10.4061/2011/159160

Schipper, H. M. (2012). Neurodegeneration with brain iron accumulation Clinical syndromes and neuroimaging. *Biochim Biophys. Acta* 1822, 350–360. doi: 10.1016/j.bbadis.2011.06.016

Schmidt, D. M. Z., and McCafferty, D. G. (2007). trans-2-phenylcyclopropylamine is a mechanism-based inactivator of the histone demethylase LSD1. *Biochemistry* 46, 4408–4416. doi: 10.1021/bi0618621

Sedláčková, N., Ponechalová, V., Ujházy, E., Dubovický, M., and Mach, M. (2011). Anxiolytic activity of pyridoindole derivatives SMe1EC2 and SMe1M2: behavioral analysis using rat model. *Interdiscip. Toxicol.* 4, 211–215. doi: 10.2478/v10102-011-0032-8

Sevrioukova, I. F. (2009). Redox-linked conformational dynamics in apoptosis-inducing factor. *J. Mol. Biol.* 390, 924–938. doi: 10.1016/j.jmb.2009.05.013

Sevrioukova, I. F. (2011). Apoptosis-inducing factor: structure, function, and redox regulation. *Antioxid. Redox Signal.* 14, 2545–2579. doi: 10.1089/ars.2010.3445

Shahabi, H. N., Andersson, D. R., and Nissbrandt, H. (2008). Cytochrome P450 2E1 in the substantia nigra: relevance for dopaminergic neurotransmission and free radical production. *Synapse* 62, 379–388. doi: 10.1002/syn.20505

Sharma, U., Roberts, E. S., and Hollenberg, P. F. (1996). Inactivation of cytochrome P4502B1 by the monoamine oxidase inhibitors R-(-).-deprenyl and clorgyline. *Drug Metab. Dispos.* 24, 669–675.

Shelke, S. M., Bhosale, S. H., Dash, R. C., Suryawanshi, M. R., and Mahadik, K. R. (2011). Exploration of new scaffolds as potential MAO-A inhibitors using pharmacophore and 3D-QSAR based *in silico* screening. *Bioorg. Med. Chem. Lett.* 21, 2419–2424. doi: 10.1016/j.bmcl.2011.02.072

Sheng, Z. H. (2014). Mitochondrial trafficking and anchoring in neurons: New insight and implications. *J. Cell Biol.* 204, 1087–1098. doi: 10.1083/jcb.201312123

Sheng, Z. H., and Cai, Q. (2012). Mitochondrial transport in neurons: impact on synaptic homeostasis and neurodegeneration. *Nat. Rev. Neurosci.* 13, 77–93. doi: 10.1038/nrn3156

Shih, J. C., and Chen, K. (1999). MAO-A and -B gene knock-out mice exhibit distinctly different behavior. *Neurobiology (Bp).* 7, 235–246.

Silverman, R. B. (1983). Mechanism of inactivation of monoamine-oxidase by trans-2-phenylcyclopropylamine and the structure of the enzyme-inactivator adduct. *J. Biol. Chem.* 258, 4766–4769.

Simone, V., Pessina, F., Durante, M., Frosini, M., Marco-Contelles, J., Unzeta, M., et al. (2014). *Interaction of Novel Monoamino Oxidase Inhibitor with Cytochrome P450, Xjenza online, 94.* Available online at: www.xjenza.org

Singh, N. K., Banerjee, B. D., Bala, K., Basu, M., and Chhillar, N. (2014). Polymorphism in cytochrome P450 2D6, Glutathione S-Transferases Pi 1 genes, and organochlorine pesticides in Alzheimer Disease: a case-control study in North Indian Population. *J. Geriatr. Psychiatry Neurol.* 27, 119–127. doi: 10.1177/0891988714522698

Sipes, N. S., Martin, M. T., Kothiya, P., Reif, D. M., Judson, R. S., Richard, A. M., et al. (2013). Profiling 976 ToxCast chemicals across 331 enzymatic and receptor signaling assays. *Chem. Res. Toxicol.* 26, 878–895. doi: 10.1021/tx400021f

Smutny, T., Mani, S., and Pavek, P. (2013). Post-translational and post-transcriptional modifications of pregnane X receptor (PXR) in regulation of the cytochrome P450 superfamily. *Curr. Drug Metab.* 14, 1059–1069. doi: 10.2174/13892002146661312111153307

Sorrentino, L., Calogero, A. M., Pandini, V., Vanoni, M. A., Sevrioukova, I. F., and Aliverti, A. (2015). Key role of the adenylate moiety and integrity of the Adenylate-Binding Site for the NAD(+)/H Binding to mitochondrial apoptosis-inducing factor. *Biochemistry* 54, 6996–7009. doi: 10.1021/acs.biochem.5b00898

Sotníková, R., Nedelčevová, J., Navarová, J., Nosálová, V., Drábiková, K., Szöcs, K., et al. (2011). Protection of the vascular endothelium in experimental situations. *Interdiscip. Toxicol.* 4, 20–26. doi: 10.2478/v10102-011-0005-y

Sridar, C., Kenaan, C., and Hollenberg, P. F. (2012). Inhibition of bupropion metabolism by selegiline: mechanism-based inactivation of human CYP2B6 and characterization of glutathione and peptide adducts. *Drug Metab. Dispos.* 40, 2256–2266. doi: 10.1124/dmd.112.046979

Stefek, M., Milackova, I., Juskova Karasova, M., and Snirc, V. (2013). Antioxidant action of the hexahydropyridoindole SMe1EC2 in the cellular system of isolated red blood cells *in vitro*. *Redox Rep.* 18, 71–75. doi: 10.1179/1351000213Y.0000000043

Stolc, S., Povazanec, F., Bauer, V., Majekova, M., Wilcox, A. L., Snirc, V., et al. (2010). *Pyridoindole Derivatives with Antioxidant Properties: Synthesis, Therapy and Pharmaceutical Remedies.* P 287506. Slovak Republic: Slovak Patent Agency.

Stolc, S., Snirc, V., Gajdosikova, A., Gajdosik, A., Gsparova, Z., Ondrejickova, O., et al. (2011). "Pyridoindoles with antioxidant and neuroprotective actions: a review," in *New frontiers in Molecular Mechanisms in Neurological and Psychiatric Disorders*, Vol. 1, eds E. Babušíková, D. Dobrota, and J. Lehotský (Martin: JLF UK-Ústav lekárskej biochémie), 316–341. ISBN: 978-80-88866-99-2.

Stolc, S., Snirc, V., Majekova, M., Gáspárová, Z., Gajdosíková, A., and Stvrtina, S. (2006). Development of the new group of indole-derived neuroprotective drugs affecting oxidative stress. *Cell. Mol. Neurobiol.* 26, 1495–1504. doi: 10.1007/s10571-006-9037-9

Strano-Rossi, S., Anzillotti, L., Dragoni, S., Pellegrino, R. M., Goracci, L., Pascali, V. L., et al. (2014). Metabolism of JWH-015, JWH-098, JWH-251, and JWH-307 *in silico* and *in vitro*: a pilot study for the detection of unknown synthetic cannabinoids metabolites. *Anal. Bioanal. Chem.* 406, 3621–3636. doi: 10.1007/s00216-014-7793-9

Sun, Q., Peng, D. Y., Yang, S. G., Zhu, X. L., Yang, W. C., and Yang, G. F. (2014). Syntheses of coumarin-tacrine hybrids as dual-site acetylcholinesterase inhibitors and their activity against butylcholinesterase, A-beta aggregation, and beta-secretase. *Bioorg. Med. Chem.* 22, 4784–4791. doi: 10.1016/j.bmc.2014.06.057

Susin, S. A., Lorenzo, H. K., Zamzami, N., Marzo, I., Snow, B. E., Brothers, G. M., et al. (1999). Molecular characterization of mitochondrial apoptosis-inducing factor. *Nature* 397, 441–446. doi: 10.1038/17135

Swomley, A. M., and Butterfield, D. A. (2015). Oxidative stress in Alzheimer disease and mild cognitive impairment: evidence from human data provided by redox proteomics. *Arch. Toxicol.* 89, 1669–1680. doi: 10.1007/s00204-015-1556-z

Sziráki, I., Kardos, V., Patthy, M., Pátfalusi, M., Gaál, J., Solti, M., et al. (1994). Amphetamine-metabolites of deprenyl involved in protection against neurotoxicity induced by MPTP and 2'-methyl-MPTP. *J. Neural. Transm.* 41, 207–219. doi: 10.1007/978-3-7091-9324-2_27

Talati, R., Reinhart, K., Baker, W., White, C. M., and Coleman, C. I. (2009). Pharmacologic treatment of advanced Parkinson's disease: a meta-analysis of COMT inhibitors and MAO-B inhibitors. *Parkinsonism Relat. Disord.* 15, 500–505. doi: 10.1016/j.parkreldis.2008.12.007

Thal, D. M., Sun, B., Feng, D., Nawaratne, V., Leach, K., Felder, C. C., et al. (2016). Crystal structures of the M1 and M4 muscarinic acetylcholine receptors. *Nature* 531, 335–340. doi: 10.1038/nature17188

Tsuchiya, Y., Nakajima, M., Takagi, S., Taniya, T., and Yokoi, T. (2006). MicroRNA regulates the expression of human cytochrome P450 1B1. *Cancer Res.* 66, 9090–9098. doi: 10.1158/0008-5472.CAN-06-1403

Ujhazy, E., Dubovicky, M., Ponechalova, V., Navarova, J., Brucknerova, I., Snirc, V., et al. (2008). Prenatal developmental toxicity study of the pyridoindole antioxidant SMe1EC2 in rats. *Neuro Endocrinol. Lett.* 29, 639–643.

Unzeta, M., Esteban, G., Bolea, I., Fogel, W. A., Ramsay, R. R., Youdim, M. B., et al. (2016). Multi-target directed donepezil-like ligands for Alzheimer's disease. *Front. Neurosci.* 10:205. doi: 10.3389/fnins.2016.00205

Upadhyay, A. K., Wang, J., and Edmondson, D. E. (2008). Comparison of the structural properties of the active site cavities of human and rat monoamine

oxidase A and B in their soluble and membrane-bound forms. *Biochemistry* 47, 526–536. doi: 10.1021/bi7019707

Urbano, A., Lakshmanan, U., Choo, P. H., Kwan, J. C., Ng, P. Y., Guo, K., et al. (2005). AIF suppresses chemical stress-induced apoptosis and maintains the transformed state of tumor cells. *EMBO J.* 24, 2815–2826. doi: 10.1038/sj.emboj.7600746

Uttara, B., Singh, A. V., Zamboni, P., and Mahajan, R. T. (2009). Oxidative stress and neurodegenerative diseases: a review of upstream and downstream antioxidant therapeutic options. *Curr. Neuropharmacol.* 7, 65–74. doi: 10.2174/157015909787602823

Vaglini, F., Viaggi, C., Piro, V., Pardini, C., Gerace, C., Scarselli, M., et al. (2013). Acetaldehyde and parkinsonism: role of CYP450 2E1. *Front. Behav. Neurosci.* 7:71. doi: 10.3389/fnbeh.2013.00071

Vahsen, N., Candé, C., Briere, J. J., Benit, P., Joza, N., Larochette, N., et al. (2004). AIF deficiency compromises oxidative phosphorylation. *EMBO J.* 23, 4679–4689. doi: 10.1038/sj.emboj.7600461

Valaasani, K. R., Sun, Q., Hu, G., Li, J., Du, F., Guo, Y., et al. (2014). Identification of human ABAD inhibitors for rescuing A-beta-mediated mitochondrial dysfunction. *Curr. Alzheimer Res.* 11, 128–136. doi: 10.2174/1567205011666140130150108

van Empel, V. P., Bertrand, A. T., van der Nagel, R., Kostin, S., Doevendans, P. A., Crijns, H. J., et al. (2005). Downregulation of apoptosis-inducing factor in harlequin mutant mice sensitizes the myocardium to oxidative stress-related cell death and pressure overload-induced decompensation. *Circ. Res.* 96, e92–e101. doi: 10.1161/01.res.0000172081.30327.28

van Unen, J., Woolard, J., Rinken, A., Hoffmann, C., Hill, S. J., Goedhart, J., et al. (2015). A perspective on studying G-Protein-Coupled receptor signaling with resonance energy transfer biosensors in living organisms. *Mol. Pharmacol.* 88, 589–595. doi: 10.1124/mol.115.098897

Vilar, R., Coelho, H., Rodrigues, E., Gama, M. J., Rivera, I., Taioli, E., et al. (2007). Association of A313 G polymorphism (GSTP1*B) in the glutathione-S-transferase P1 gene with sporadic Parkinson's disease. *Eur. J. Neurol.* 14, 156–161. doi: 10.1111/j.1468-1331.2006.01590.x

Vilar, S., Ferino, G., Quezada, E., Santana, L., and Friedman, C. (2012). Predicting monoamine oxidase inhibitory activity through ligand-based models. *Curr. Top. Med. Chem.* 12, 2258–2274. doi: 10.2174/156802612805219987

Villanueva, R., Ferreira, P., Marcuello, C., Usón, A., Miramar, M. D., Peleato, M. L., et al. (2015). Key residues regulating the reductase activity of the human mitochondrial apoptosis inducing factor. *Biochemistry* 54, 5175–5184. doi: 10.1021/acs.biochem.5b00696

Vohora, D, and Bhowmik, M. (2012). Histamine H3 receptor antagonists/inverse agonists on cognitive and motor processes: relevance to Alzheimer's disease, ADHD, schizophrenia, and drug abuse. *Front. Syst. Neurosci.* 6:72. doi: 10.3389/fnsys.2012.00072

Waagepetersen, H. S., Sonnewald, U., and Schousboe, A. (2003). Compartmentation of glutamine, glutamate, and GABA metabolism in neurons and astrocytes: functional implications. *Neuroscientist* 9, 398–403. doi: 10.1177/1073858403254006

Walsh, C. T. (2013). "Why enzymes as drug targets?," in *Evaluation of Enzyme Inhibitors in Drug Discovery: A Guide for Medicinal Chemists and Pharmacologists*," 2nd Edn., ed R. A. Copeland (Chichester: John Wiley & Sons, Inc.), 1–23. doi: 10.1002/9781118540398

Walter, M., and Stark, H. (2012). Histamine receptor subtypes: a century of rational drug design. *Front. Biosci.* 1:279. doi: 10.2741/s279

Wang, C., and Youle, R. J. (2009). The role of mitochondria in apoptosis*. *Annu. Rev. Genet.* 43, 95–118. doi: 10.1146/annurev-genet-102108-134850

Wang, L., Esteban, G., Ojima, M., Bautista-Aguilera, O. M., Inokuchi, T., Moraleda, I., et al. (2014). Donepezil + propargylamine + 8-hydroxyquinoline hybrids as new multifunctional metal-chelators, ChE and MAO inhibitors for the potential treatment of Alzheimer's disease. *Eur. J. Med. Chem.* 80, 543–561. doi: 10.1016/j.ejmech.2014.04.078

Wang, X., Huang, T., Bu, G., and Xu, H. (2014). Dysregulation of protein trafficking in neurodegeneration. *Mol. Neurodegener.* 9:31. doi: 10.1186/1750-1326-9-31

Waxman, D. J. (1999). P450 gene induction by structurally diverse xenochemicals: central role of nuclear receptors CAR, PXR, and PPAR. *Arch. Biochem. Biophys.* 369, 11–23. doi: 10.1006/abbi.1999.1351

Weichert, D., Stanek, M., Hübner, H., and Gmeiner, P. (2016). Structure-guided development of dual β2 adrenergic/dopamine D2 receptor agonists. *Bioorg. Med. Chem.* 24, 2641–2653. doi: 10.1016/j.bmc.2016.04.028

Weinreb, O., Amit, T., Bar-Am, O., and Youdim, M. B. (2012). Ladostigil: a novel multimodal neuroprotective drug with cholinesterase and brain-selective monoamine oxidase inhibitory activities for Alzheimer's disease treatment. *Curr. Drug Targets* 13, 483–494. doi: 10.2174/138945012799 499794

Weinreb, O., Amit, T., Bar-Am, O., and Youdim, M. B. (2016). Neuroprotective effects of multifaceted hybrid agents targeting MAO, cholinesterase, iron and β-amyloid in aging and Alzheimer's disease. *Br. J. Pharmacol.* 173, 2080–2094. doi: 10.1111/bph.13318

Weinreb, O., Amit, T., Riederer, P., Youdim, M. B. H., and Mandel, S. A. (2011). Neuroprotective profile of the multitarget drug rasagiline in Parkinson's disease. *Int. Rev. Neurobiol.* 100, 127–149. doi: 10.1016/B978-0-12-386467-3. 00007-8

Weinreb, O., Badinter, F., Amit, T., Bar-Am, O., and Youdim, M. B. (2015). Effect of long-term treatment with rasagiline on cognitive deficits and related molecular cascades in aged mice. *Neurobiol. Aging* 36, 2628–2636. doi: 10.1016/j.neurobiolaging.2015.05.009

Weissbach, H., Smith, T. E., Daly, J. W., Witkop, B., and Udenfriend, S. (1960). A rapid spectrophotometric assay of Monoamine Oxidase based on the rate of disappearance of kynuramine. *J. Biol. Chem* 235, 1160–1163.

Werlinder, V., Backlund, M., Zhukov, A., and Ingelman-Sundberg, M. (2001). Transcriptional and post-translational regulation of CYP1A1 by primaquine. *J. Pharmacol. Exp. Ther.* 297, 206–214.

Westermann, B. (2012). Bioenergetic role of mitochondrial fusion and fission. *Biochim. Biophys. Acta* 1817, 1833–1838. doi: 10.1016/j.bbabio.2012. 02.033

Witcher, K. G., Eiferman, D. S., and Godbout, J. P. (2015). Priming the Inflammatory Pump of the CNS after Traumatic Brain Injury. *Trends Neurosci.* 38, 609–620. doi: 10.1016/j.tins.2015.08.002

Witte, M. E., Mahad, D. J., Lassmann, H., and van Horssen, J. (2014). Mitochondrial dysfunction contributes to neurodegeneration in multiple sclerosis. *Trends Mol. Med.* 20, 179–187. doi: 10.1016/j.molmed.2013. 11.007

Woodard, C. M., Campos, B. A., Kuo, S. H., Nirenberg, M. J., Nestor, M. W., Zimmer, M., et al. (2014). iPSC-derived dopamine neurons reveal differences between monozygotic twins discordant for Parkinson's disease. *Cell Reports.* 9, 1173–1182. doi: 10.1016/j.celrep.2014.10.023

Xie, S. S., Lan, J. S., Wang, X., Wang, Z. M., Jiang, N., Li, F., et al. (2016). Design, synthesis and biological evaluation of novel donepezil-coumarin hybrids as multi-target agents for the treatment of Alzheimer's disease. *Bioorg. Med. Chem.* 24, 1528–1539. doi: 10.1016/j.bmc.2016.02.023

Xie, S. S., Wang, X., Jiang, N., Yu, W., Wang, K. D. G., Lan, J. S., et al. (2015). Multi-target tacrine-coumarin hybrids: cholinesterase and monoamine oxidase B inhibition properties against Alzheimer's disease. *Eur. J. Med. Chem.* 95, 153–165. doi: 10.1016/j.ejmech.2015.03.040

Xu, L., Ryu, J., Nguyen, J. V., Arena, J., Rha, E., Vranis, P., et al. (2015). Evidence for accelerated tauopathy in the retina of transgenic P301S tau mice exposed to repetitive mild traumatic brain injury. *Exp. Neurol.* 273, 168–176. doi: 10.1016/j.expneurol.2015.08.014

Yan, R., Fan, Q., Zhou, J., and Vassar, R. (2016). Inhibiting BACE1 to reverse synaptic dysfunctions in Alzheimer's disease. *Neurosci. Biobehav. Rev.* 65, 326–340. doi: 10.1016/j.neubiorev.2016.03.025

Yan, R., and Vassar, R. (2014). Targeting the beta secretase BACE1 for Alzheimer's disease therapy. *Lancet Neurol.* 13, 319–329. doi: 10.1016/S1474-4422(13)70276-X

Yang, S. Y., He, X. Y., Isaacs, C., Dobkin, C., Miller, D., and Philipp, M. (2014). Roles of 17 beta-hydroxysteroid dehydrogenase type 10 in neurodegenerative disorders. *J. Steroid Biochem. Mol. Biol.* 143, 460–472. doi: 10.1016/j.jsbmb.2014.07.001

Youdim, M. B. (2013). Multi target neuroprotective and neurorestorative anti-Parkinson and anti-Alzheimer drugs ladostigil and m30 derived from rasagiline. *Exp. Neurobiol.* 22, 1–10. doi: 10.5607/en.2013.22.1.1

Youdim, M. B. H., Edmondson, D., and Tipton, K. F. (2006). The therapeutic potential of monoamine oxidase inhibitors. *Nat. Rev. Neurosci.* 7, 295–309. doi: 10.1038/nrn1883

Youdim, M. B., and Oh, Y. J. (2013). Promise of neurorestoration and mitochondrial biogenesis in Parkinson's disease with multi target drugs: an alternative to stem cell therapy. *Exp. Neurobiol.* 22, 167–172. doi: 10.5607/en.2013.22.3.167

Youle, R. J., and van der Bliek, A. M. (2012). Mitochondrial fission, fusion, and stress. *Science* 337, 1062–1065. doi: 10.1126/science.1219855

Zanger, U. M., and Schwab, M. (2013). Cytochrome P450 enzymes in drug metabolism: regulation of gene expression, enzyme activities, and impact of genetic variation. *Pharmacol. Ther.* 138, 103–141. doi: 10.1016/j.pharmthera.20 12.12.007

Zanna, C., Ghelli, A., Porcelli, A. M., Karbowski, M., Youle, R. J., Schimpf, S., et al. (2008). OPA1 mutations associated with dominant optic atrophy impair oxidative phosphorylation and mitochondrial fusion. *Brain* 131, 352–367. doi: 10.1093/brain/awm335

Zellner, M., Baureder, M., Rappold, E., Bugert, P., Kotzailias, N., Babeluk, R., et al. (2012). Comparative platelet proteome analysis reveals an increase of monoamine oxidase-B protein expression in Alzheimer's disease but not in non-demented Parkinson's disease patients. *J. Proteomics* 75, 2080–2092. doi: 10.1016/j.jprot.2012.01.014

Zhou, M. J., Diwu, Z. J., PanchukVoloshina, N., and Haugland, R. P. (1997). A stable nonfluorescent derivative of resorufin for the fluorometric determination of trace hydrogen peroxide: applications in detecting the activity of phagocyte NADPH oxidase and other oxidases. *Anal. Biochem.* 253, 162–168. doi: 10.1006/abio.1997.2391

Zhu, Y., Xiao, K., Ma, L., Xiong, B., Fu, Y., Yu, H., et al. (2009). Design, synthesis and biological evaluation of novel dual inhibitors of acetylcholinesterase and beta-secretase. *Bioorg. Med. Chem.* 17, 1600–1613. doi: 10.1016/j.bmc.2008. 12.067

Züchner, S., Mersiyanova, I. V., Muglia, M., Bissar-Tadmouri, N., Rochelle, J., Dadali, E. L., et al. (2004). Mutations in the mitochondrial GTPase mitofusin 2 cause Charcot-Marie-Tooth neuropathy type 2A. *Nat. Genet.* 36, 449–451. doi: 10.1038/ng1341

Conflict of Interest Statement: The authors declare that the research was conducted in the absence of any commercial or financial relationships that could be construed as a potential conflict of interest.

Multiple Targeting Approaches on Histamine H₃ Receptor Antagonists

6

Mohammad A. Khanfar[1,2†], Anna Affini[1†], Kiril Lutsenko[1†], Katarina Nikolic[3],
Stefania Butini[4] and Holger Stark[1*]

[1] Stark Lab, Institut fuer Pharmazeutische and Medizinische Chemie, Heinrich-Heine-Universitaet Duesseldorf, Duesseldorf, Germany, [2] Faculty of Pharmacy, The University of Jordan, Amman, Jordan, [3] Department of Pharmaceutical Chemistry, Faculty of Pharmacy, University of Belgrade, Belgrade, Serbia, [4] Department of Biotechnology, Chemistry, and Pharmacy, European Research Centre for Drug Discovery and Development, University of Siena, Siena, Italy

With the very recent market approval of pitolisant (Wakix®), the interest in clinical applications of novel multifunctional histamine H₃ receptor antagonists has clearly increased. Since histamine H₃ receptor antagonists in clinical development have been tested for a variety of different indications, the combination of pharmacological properties in one molecule for improved pharmacological effects and reduced unwanted side-effects is rationally based on the increasing knowledge on the complex neurotransmitter regulations. The polypharmacological approaches on histamine H₃ receptor antagonists on different G-protein coupled receptors, transporters, enzymes as well as on NO-signaling mechanism are described, supported with some lead structures.

Keywords: multiple targeting, GPCR, enzymes, NO, histamine, transporter

Edited by:
Giuseppe Di Giovanni,
University of Malta, Malta

Reviewed by:
Peter McCormick,
University of Barcelona, Spain
Wladyslaw Lason,
Polish Academy of Sciences, Poland

*Correspondence:
Holger Stark
stark@hhu.de

[†] These authors have contributed equally to this work.

INTRODUCTION

The idea of synthesizing multiple targeting compounds arises from the fact that the paradigm "one drug—one target" or "single-target drug" is not sufficiently meeting the need for the treatment of a large number of complex diseases caused by multifunctional pathophysiological processes. Since central nervous system (CNS) disorders are characterized by diverse physiological dysfunctions and deregulations of a complex network of signaling pathways, optimal multipotent drugs should simultaneously and specifically modulate selected groups of biological targets. Polypharmacology is a new scientific area focused on discovery, development, and pharmacological study of Multiple Targeting Designed Ligands (MTDL) able to simultaneously modify the activities of several interacting pharmacological targets (Hopkins, 2008).

This emerging approach suggests that multifactorial CNS diseases such as depression (Millan, 2014), schizophrenia (Ye et al., 2014), Parkinson's disease (PD) and Alzheimer's disease (AD; Youdim and Buccafusco, 2005; Leon et al., 2013) can be treated with higher efficacy, lower toxicity, less drug-drug interactions, and also with unified pharmacokinetic profile if a single drug molecule is able to simultaneously interact with multiple targets (Anighoro et al., 2014; Huang et al., 2015).

Despite the positive effects of MTDL, there are several potential disadvantages, which need to be taken into consideration. In order to identify multiple targeting hits, a more detailed and extensive pharmacological characterization of current drug-target interactions is needed (Peters, 2013). In most previous cases, the need for a polypharmacology to reach a therapeutic effect is discovered retrospectively. After finding a lead compound for a specific group of targets, the optimization of complex structure-activity relationships (SAR) profile is one of the first challenging tasks from a medicinal chemistry point of view. Most importantly, simultaneous targeting of several receptors may lead to a wider and sometimes unpredictable spectrum of biological activities such as side effects. Therefore, a balance between polypharmacological benefits and potential drawbacks brought by promiscuous scaffolds needs to be evaluated at least as carefully as with all other candidates, but based on a more complex behavior (Anighoro et al., 2014). Herein we describe the current implementation of target-oriented polypharmacological approaches with histamine H_3 receptor (H_3R) ligands based on research findings (**Figure 1**).

H_3R is a member of transmembrane class A of G protein–coupled receptors (GPCR) family (Arrang et al., 1983; Schwartz et al., 1991). It influences several intracellular pathways through its coupling to $G\alpha_{i/o}$ (Bongers et al., 2007). Analysis of H_3R mRNA in rat (Héron et al., 2001) and human (Jin and Panula, 2005) brains showed that H_3R is largely expressed on the histaminergic neurons of the CNS (located presynaptically and postsynaptically; Jadhav and Singh, 2013). As auto-receptor, H_3R plays an important role in histamine biosynthesis and release and as hetero-receptor in the modulation of different neurotransmitters release (e.g., acetylcholine, noradrenaline, dopamine, GABA, glutamate, and serotonin; Schlicker et al., 1989, 1990). A lower level of H_3R is distributed in the peripheral nervous system and is responsible for the regulation of sympathetic effector systems and pain sensation (Héron et al., 2001). Therefore, modulation of the H_3R can potentially prevent the activation of the negative feedback mechanism leading to increased neurotransmitter release. Consequently, targeting of H_3R with antagonist/inverse agonist may have therapeutic applications in CNS-related disorders, such as depression, schizophrenia, PD, and AD (Esbenshade et al., 2008; Gemkow et al., 2009; Chazot, 2010; Raddatz et al., 2010; Lin et al., 2011; Ghasemi and Tavakoli, 2012) as well as in inflammatory and gastrointestinal diseases (Vuyyuru et al., 1995; Ceras et al., 2012). Recently, several substances have entered late clinical phases

for the treatment of several CNS disorders (Sander et al., 2008; Panula et al., 2015).

H_3R/H_1R

The drug Betahistine (*N*-methyl-2-(2-pyridyl)ethanamine), indicated for the treatment of vestibular Morbus Menière, can be considered as the first MTDL in this category by working as an agonist at histamine H_1 receptor (H_1R) and antagonist at H_3R (Lian et al., 2014, 2016; Møller et al., 2015). The H_3R antagonism leads to inhibition of vestibular neurotransmission, central vasodilatation with potential antipsychotic effects, whereas the H_1R agonism have an immune-regulatory effect (Dagli et al., 2008; Zhou et al., 2013).

Currently, the main focus on polypharmacological targeting of H_3R/H_1R is to develop dual agonist or dual antagonist ligands. Dual acting H_3/H_1 receptor (H_3R/H_1R) antagonists were synthesized for the treatment of allergic diseases. These diseases are associated with the degranulation of the mast cell and histamine release which can activate H_1R and consequently stimulates phospholipase C that ultimately liberate inositol-1,4,5-trisphosphate and Ca^{2+}; thereby improves mucus secretion and vasodilatation (McLeod et al., 1999; Bakker et al., 2002).

H_1R antagonists play a key role in the treatment of allergic rhinitis; however, there are several limitations to their clinical use. The first generation of H_1R antagonists (e.g., Diphenhydramine, Chlorpheniramine) show sedative effects whereas second generation H_1R blockers (e.g., Loratadine, Mizolastine) have poor penetration to the CNS, thus generating non-sedating antihistaminic activity (Cowart et al., 2004; Stark et al., 2004). However, the second generation H_1R blockers

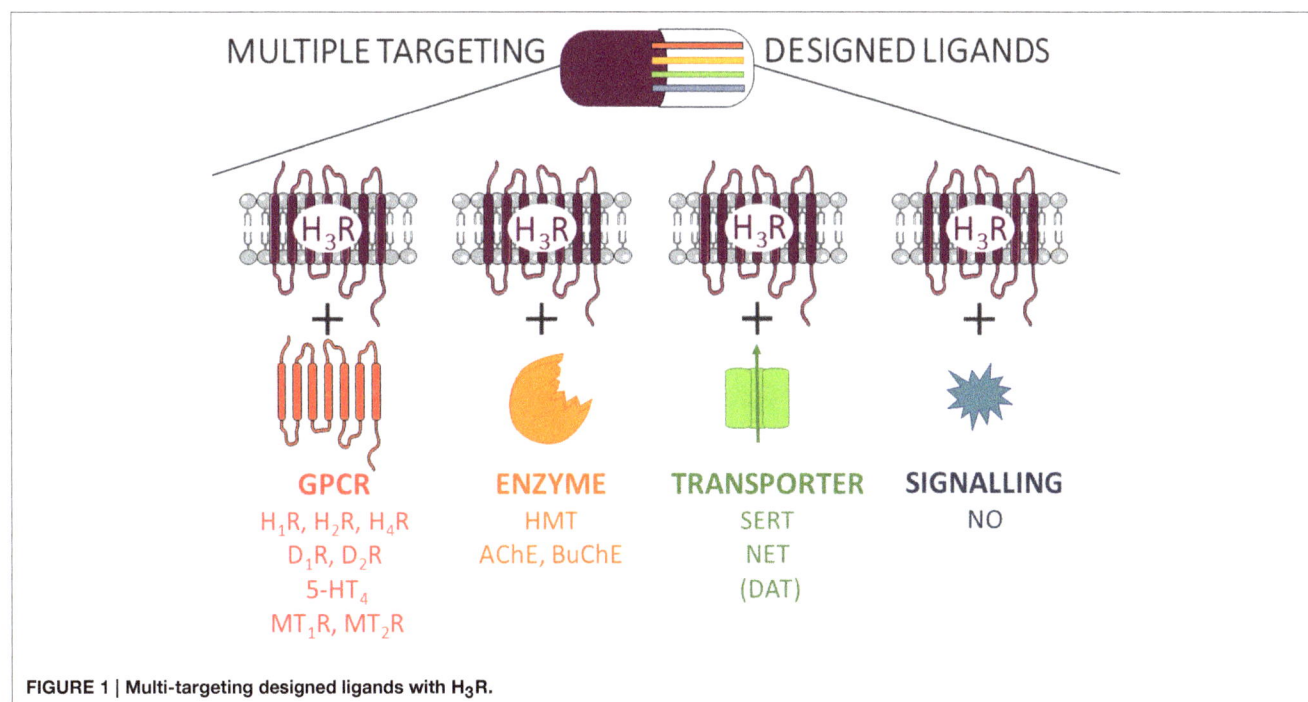

FIGURE 1 | Multi-targeting designed ligands with H_3R.

are often combined with α-adrenergic agonists to stimulate normal vascular tone and to reduce nasal congestion. Such combination is associated with serious cardiac side effects (QT time prolongation, ventricular arrhythmia).

These findings have encouraged several research groups to consider if other histamine receptor subtypes may contribute to the histamine-induced nasal congestion. Several studies confirmed that H_3R may play an important role in histamine-induced nasal congestion because the vasodilatation is caused by activation of H_3R in peripheral post-sympathetic ganglionic neurons (Hey et al., 1992). The activation of the H_3R hetero-receptors located on neighboring noradrenergic neurons (Berlin et al., 2011) modulates the release of the neurotransmitter noradrenaline in the nasal blood vessel. Therefore, a compound that antagonizes H_1R on one hand and inhibits H_3R on the other hand may treat allergic diseases without having nasal congestion.

Based on first and second generations of H_3R antagonists, imidazole and non-imidazole H_3R/H_1R ligands were designed. Several imidazole-derivatives taking Chlorphenamine 1 (hH_1R K_i = 2 nM) as an additional pharmacophore for the introduction of H_1R antagonist activity show dual H_3R/H_1R inhibitory affinity (Wieland et al., 1999). Limited variations of the linker in both sides of the aliphatic amino moiety provided compounds with good H_3R binding affinity. Like all aminergic GPCR, H_1R, and H_3R contain an aspartate residue in the transmembrane domain III, that is involved in electrostatic interaction with protonated amino functionality (Wieland et al., 1999). Therefore, replacement of the basic amino linker by a neutral linker such as amide or urea, resulted in activity loss on the H_1R. However, incorporating a tertiary amine led to the synthesis of the most potent dual inhibitor in that series (compound 2, Figure 2) that

displays affinities at low nanomolar concentration range for both H_1R and H_3R.

Further structural optimization was conducted by replacing the imidazole ring with different heterocycles in order to avoid potential interactions with CYP450 enzymes. In one of the trials, the non-imidazole heterocycles were combined with a benzothiazole structure (Walczyński et al., 1999). In vitro results of this series from guinea pig ileum system showed increasing H_3R antagonist potency in the presence of an alkyl-substituted azepane (compound 3, Figure 2). However, this compound showed weak H_1R antagonist activity, with pA_2 value of 5.77. A similar approach was applied in designing H_3R/H_1R dual inhibitors by combining nitrogen-containing heterocycles, with a benzylphthalazinone (GSK-1004723), compound 4 (Figure 2), or a quinoline structure (GSK-835726) (Slack et al., 2011; Daley-Yates et al., 2012), and WO-094643 (Norman, 2011). Compounds 4 and GSK-835726 were potent H_3R/H_1R antagonists in vitro and in vivo systems. Compound 3 has a major advantage associated with its long duration of action ($t_{1/2}$ of 1.2–1.5 h, Table 1) which allows once a day intranasal dosing for the treatment of allergic rhinitis. GSK–1004723 completed phase II of clinical trials for the treatment of allergic rhinitis.

H_3R/H_2R

Limited efforts have been conducted so far for the designing of dual H_3R/H_2R ligands. However, guanidine-based histamine H_2R ligands demonstrate additional H_3R antagonist potencies. Recently, Buschauer et al. investigated dimeric carbamoylguanidine derivatives for the synthesis of potent H_2R agonists (Kagermeier et al., 2015). Compounds containing two imidazole moieties, display selectivity for H_3R and H_2R in

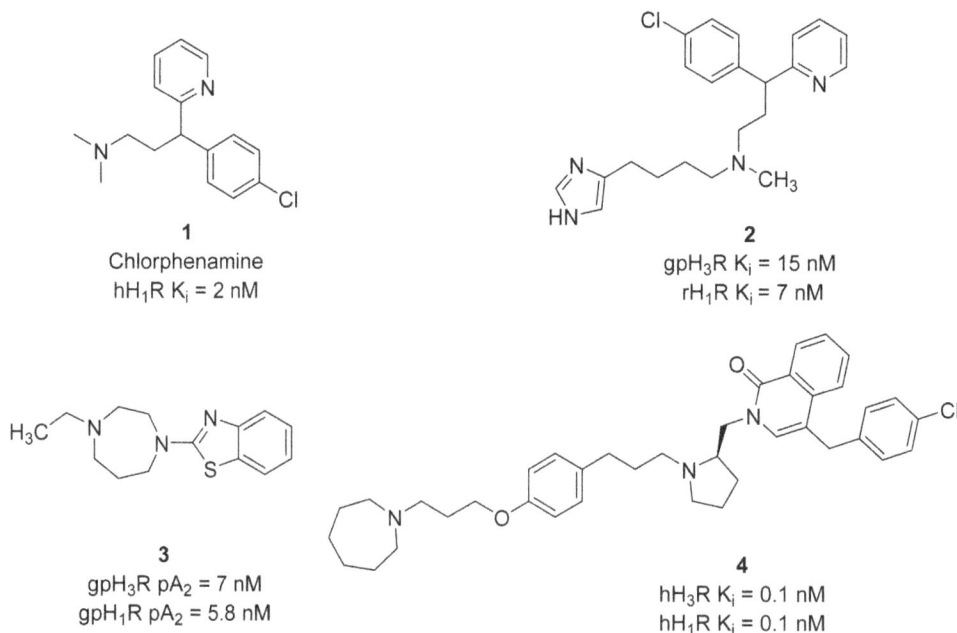

1
Chlorphenamine
hH_1R K_i = 2 nM

2
gpH_3R K_i = 15 nM
rH_1R K_i = 7 nM

3
gpH_3R pA_2 = 7 nM
gpH_1R pA_2 = 5.8 nM

4
hH_3R K_i = 0.1 nM
hH_1R K_i = 0.1 nM

FIGURE 2 | Structures and biological activities of selected H_3R/H_1R ligands.

TABLE 1 | Selected pharmacokinetic data of preclinical candidates (Ly et al., 2008; Slack et al., 2011; Daley-Yates et al., 2012).

Code	$C_{max\ blood}$	$C_{max\ brain}$	$t_{0.5}$	F	Cl	Vss	K_{off}	K_{on}
4	–	–	1.2–1.5 h	–	–	–	$0.007 \pm 0.001\ min^{-1}$	$4.76 \pm 0.69 \times 10^8$
GSK-835726	0.747 µM	–	15.5 h	–	–	–	$0.802 \pm 0.010\ min^{-1}$	$3.04 \pm 0.14 \times 10^9$
26	1 µM	1 µM	16.1 ± 0.9 h	93%	10.2 ± 1.0 mL/min/k	13.0 ± 1.2 L/kg	–	–

radioligand competition binding studies, whereas compound 5 (**Figure 3**) shows high H_2R affinity with simultaneous high H_3R inhibitory affinity. Since the brain penetration of these compounds is quite low, they can mostly be used on cells and isolated tissues.

H_3R/H_4R

Similarly, dual targeting is also often applied on histamine H_3R and H_4 receptors (H_4R). Because of the relative high H_4R homology with H_3R (37% in entire sequence, 68% within transmembrane domains) many potent histamine H_3R ligands containing imidazole moieties (**6–8**; **Figure 4**) show off-target affinity at H_4R (Neumann et al., 2013). The human H_4R is the last receptor subtype that has been identified in the histamine receptor family (Corrêa and Fernandes, 2015). The H_4R is mainly located on cells of hematopoietic origin and, therefore, may be a promising target for the treatment of inflammatory diseases like allergic rhinitis, asthma, and pruritus (Thurmond et al., 2008). The expression of H_4R in the CNS is a controversial topic because immunostaining methods are critically discussed and inconsistent mRNA screening results were obtained (Panula et al., 2015). Dual H_3R/H_4R ligands could be promising targets for pain and cancer since it is likely that these two targets contribute to the development of pain sensation and itching as well as cell-proliferation-associated effects (Medina and Rivera, 2010). However, further investigation is required to fully understand and evaluate their functions for therapeutic applications.

Clobenpropit (**7**), a potent reference H_3R antagonist, was identified as a template for dual H_3R/H_4R ligands. Variations in substituents of the phenyl moiety as well as in the length of the alkyl chain between the central core isothiourea and the lipophilic aromatic residue were performed (Lim et al., 2009). Elongation of the spacer and introduction of bulky groups in the east part of these molecules such as diphenyl residue led to moderate affinity for both H_3R and H_4R. Nevertheless, most of these compounds showed moderate to high affinity at both H_3R and H_4R in a similar concentration range [human H_3 receptor (hH_3R) $K_i = 2.5–79.4$, hH_4R $K_i = 1.6–158.4$]. Compounds with a halogen substituent at the 4-position of the benzyl moiety showed the best binding affinities at both receptors. Further structural modifications were performed to expand the SAR on imidazole-containing histamine receptor ligands. Changing the polarity of the central core isothiourea by introducing different moieties such as amide, carbamate, urea, ester, ketone, and ethers was exploited (Kottke et al., 2011). Amide derivatives were unsuccessful because they had poor

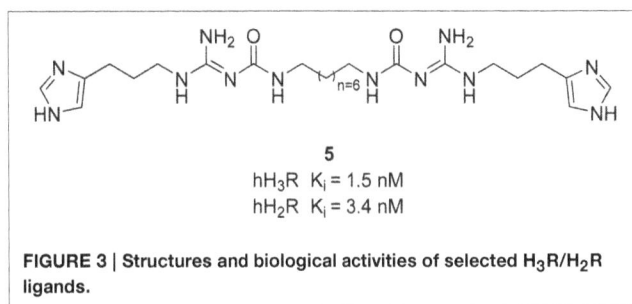

5
hH_3R K_i = 1.5 nM
hH_2R K_i = 3.4 nM

FIGURE 3 | Structures and biological activities of selected H_3R/H_2R ligands.

affinity at the hH_3R. In contrast, all the other moieties bound to both receptors in a comparable concentration range, showing that these central cores of the alkyl imidazole can be used as a lead structure for dual acting H_3R/H_4R ligands. Among the carbamate series, the presence of a cycloalkyl moiety in the east part is important to have K_i values for both receptors below 200 nM. Cyclohexylmethyl derivative **9** (**Figure 4**) is the most potent H_3R/H_4R antagonist in that series (Wicek et al., 2011). It must be stressed that the affinity is not the only criteria for the MTDL selection. Some compounds may have similar affinities, but different efficacies. In this respect, replacing the carbamate function with a thioether group led to the synthesis of a potent dual H_3R antagonist and H_4R partial agonist **10** (**Figure 4**). These compounds are potent dual H_3R/H_4R ligands that can be optimized for further pre-clinical trials; however, no further work has been reported. Therefore, efficacy and not only affinity data has to be considered for the pharmacological profile evaluation of new drugs.

H_3R AND NON-HISTAMINERGIC GPCRs

In addition to combined properties with other histamine receptor subtypes, other aminergic GPCRs have also been addressed with polypharmacology targeting of H_3R. Dopamine is an important neurotransmitter in the human brain. It affects almost all mental functions, such as movement control, motivation, emotion, learning, and memory. Dysregulations of dopamine neurotransmitter system of the CNS may cause schizophrenia and related mood disorders (Schlicker et al., 1993; Witkin and Nelson, 2004). Neuroleptics used for the treatment of schizophrenia usually inhibit dopamine D_2-like receptors and other aminergic receptors, such as serotonin $5-HT_{2A}$ receptor, dopamine D_1 receptor (D_1R) receptors, and other serotonin receptor subtypes (Remington, 2003). The most important side effects of these neuroleptics are extrapyramidal side effects and weight gain problems

(Vuyyuru et al., 1995; Deng et al., 2010; Lian et al., 2016). These side effects are related to their antagonistic properties at the dopamine D_2-like and H_1R, respectively (Kroeze et al., 2003; Von Coburg et al., 2009). Additionally, schizophrenic patients usually showed a significantly high level of N-methylhistamine in cerebral cerebrospinal fluid (Ligneau et al., 2007). There are several studies showing an interaction between histamine H_3R and dopamine D_2 receptors (D_2R) as well as H_3R and D_1R as oligomeric hetero-receptors (Humbert-Claude et al., 2007; Ferrada et al., 2008). Furthermore, H_3R inverse agonists/antagonists showed a reduction of undesirable side effects like weight gain, somnolence, and cognitive impairment in several rodent models of schizophrenia while displaying a significant inhibitory activity (Ligneau et al., 2007). Combining the known H_3R antagonists pharmacophore 4-(3-piperidinopropoxy)phenyl with known neuroleptics may provide novel multi-acting antipsychotic drugs with an improved

pharmacological profile and reduced side effects by decreasing H_1R affinity and introducing H_3R activity while maintaining D_2R/D_3R affinity (Humbert-Claude et al., 2007; Von Coburg et al., 2009). For this approach 4-(3-piperidinopropoxy)phenyl was linked to several known neuroleptics. Resulting compounds showed high H_3R affinity with K_i values between 4.90 nM and 42 pM while simultaneously reduced the H_1R affinity by a factor of 10–600 as off-target and maintained the D_2-like receptor subtypes affinity (**Figure 5**; Deng et al., 2010). Compound **11** (**Figure 5**) with a good overall profile and high H_3R affinity was synthesized by merging 4-(3-piperidinopropoxy)phenyl fragment with amitriptyline **12** (**Figure 5**). This compound was selected for an early *in vivo* screening for central H_3R antagonist potency on male Swiss mice. To determine the *in vivo* potency, an increase in N-methylhistamine level in the brain 90 min after the oral application of the compound was measured (Von Coburg et al., 2009). Unfortunately, this compound seems to be

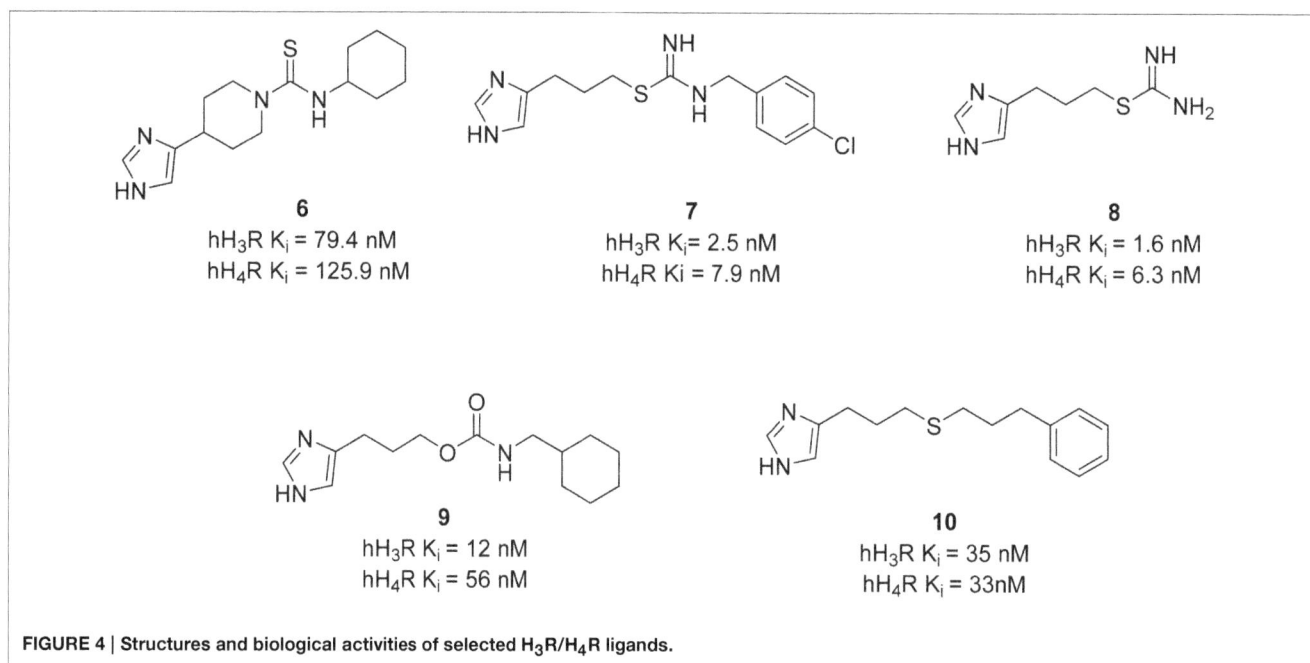
FIGURE 4 | Structures and biological activities of selected H_3R/H_4R ligands.

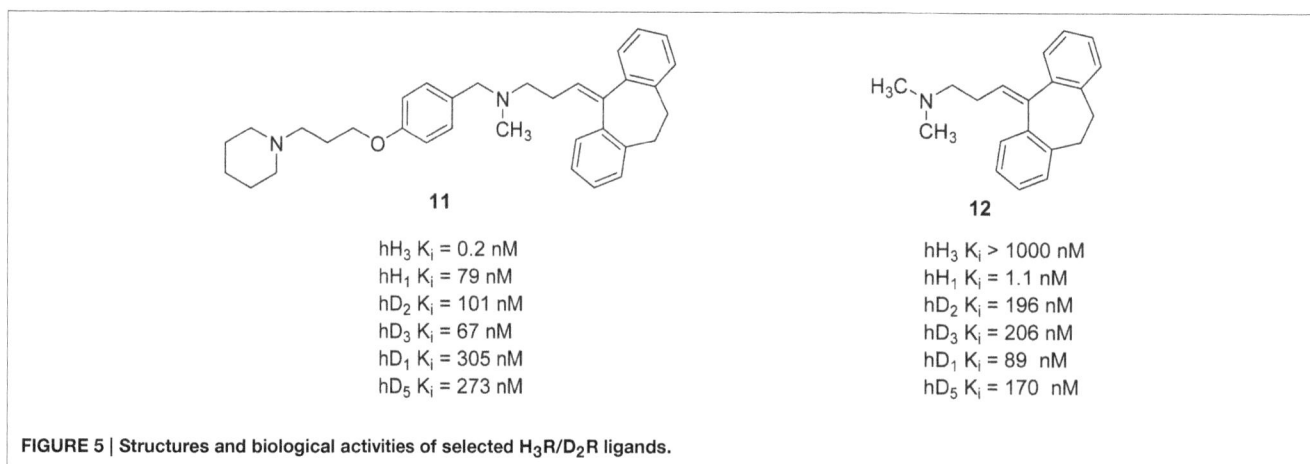
FIGURE 5 | Structures and biological activities of selected H_3R/D_2R ligands.

inactive (ED_{50} > 10 mg/kg p.o.) with unclear reasons mostly for absorption, distribution, or metabolism.

Using pharmacophore-based virtual screening, Lepailleur et al. identified an interesting additional target activity while analyzing the screening hits (Lepailleur et al., 2014). A series of tricyclic derivatives have high serotonin 5-HT$_4$ receptor (5-HT$_4$R) affinity. There is a connection between different serotonin receptor subtypes, especially on 5-HT$_{1A}$R, 5-HT$_4$R, and 5-HT$_6$R and emerging AD therapies (Sabbagh, 2009; Mangialasche et al., 2010; Herrmann et al., 2011) and other degenerative disorders connected to an impaired cholinergic function (Esbenshade et al., 2008; Sander et al., 2008; Gemkow et al., 2009). 5-HT$_4$R provide symptomatic alleviation of cognitive impairments and neuroprotection by reducing amyloid-β (βA) generation and toxicity (Lezoualc'h, 2007). 5-HT$_4$R activation improves cognitive processes such as learning and memory (Lelong et al., 2001, 2003; Levallet et al., 2009; Hotte et al., 2012). Combined with the beneficial effects of H$_3$R on neurodegenerative diseases, dual targeting of H$_3$R and 5-HT$_4$R would therapeutically be useful. One of the identified hits, compound **13** (**Figure 6**) showed high affinities with K_i values of 41.6 nM at H$_3$R and 208 nM at 5-HT$_4$R and significant selectivity over 5-HT$_{1A}$R and 5-HT$_6$R. Compound **13** was able to reverse the scopolamine-induced cognitive impairment partially at 1 mg/kg and completely at 3 mg/kg in a spatial working memory experiment (Klinkenberg and Blokland, 2011). Scopolamine is a nonselective muscarinic antagonist, which partially blocks the cholinergic neurotransmission and is used to examine the cognitive enhancing effects of potential compounds (Snyder et al., 2005; Fredrickson et al., 2008). These results reveal the potential of combined H$_3$R antagonist/5-HT$_4$R agonist profiles in one multi-targeting compound to modify symptomatic effects in Alzheimer's disease.

Recently, different combinations between melatonin and another neuroprotection agent, e.g., curcurmin derivatives, have shown that melatonin may have a therapeutic potential in the treatment of cognitive disorders and neurodegenerative pathologies like AD (Chojnacki et al., 2014). Different H$_3$R antagonists also showed neuroprotective actions (Brioni et al., 2011). Therefore, the synthesis of ligands able to bind at both H$_3$R and melatonin receptors could be useful for the treatment of the diseases mentioned above. Pala et al. have

synthesized compounds that can interact simultaneously with the H$_3$R and melatonin T$_1$ receptor (MT$_1$R) and melatonin T$_2$ receptor (MT$_2$R; Pala et al., 2014). Melatonin is a methoxyindole-derived hormone secreted mainly by the pineal gland. The activation of MT$_1$R and MT$_2$R is not only important for the regulation of cardiac rhythms, but also for having antioxidant and neuroprotective effects (Srinivasan et al., 2006). For the synthesis of this melatonergic/histaminergic ligands the classical pharmacophore showed for potent H$_3$R antagonists such as Ciproxifan and its analogs, was combined with an anilinoethylamide to have comparable binding affinity with the indol-3-ylrthylamide moiety of the melatonin (**Figure 7**). The length of the alkyl chain influences more the binding affinities at hMT$_1$R and hMT$_2$R than that at hH$_3$R. Compounds with a short spacer such as a propyl or ethyl chain did not show affinity toward both MT$_1$R and MT$_2$R. One good dual acting ligand was obtained by elongating the alkyl chain between the imidazole ring and the melatonin moiety with a pentyl linker. The introduction of a six methylene unit improved the K_i values for both hMT$_1$R and hMT$_2$R. The elongation of the spacer can store the imidazole in a more peripheral region of the melatonin receptors. In that region, negative interactions with positively charged amino groups are weakened. Therefore, compounds (**14**, **15**; **Figure 7**) able to bind to both melatonin and histamine H$_3$R with affinity in the micromolar concentration range were designed. The optimization of these ligands can be the next step for discovering new multiple targeting compounds that belong to the new melatonin-histamine combination.

H$_3$R AND TRANSPORTERS

Selective serotonin reuptake inhibitors (SSRI) have been the drugs of choice to treat depression. However, the efficacy of these drugs is noticeable only after weeks of treatment and do not improve cognitive functions of depressive patients, which prompt many physicians to co-prescribe stimulants with SSRI to provide subjective relief. H$_3$R antagonists produce wakefulness in animals without releasing dopamine or producing behavioral activation. Such activation has been avoided due to the risk of allowing patients to act on their suicidal ideation (Menza et al., 2000; Stahl, 2001). Combined H$_3$R/SERT inhibition would provide symptomatic relief for the fatigue during the first weeks of treatment and afford immediate relief from some of the symptoms of depression with possible concurrent cognitive enhancement (Schlicker et al., 1998; Barbier et al., 2007; Nikolic et al., 2014).

Until now, most of the medicinal chemistry effort to develop new dual H$_3$R/SERT inhibitors was conducted by Johnson & Johnson Pharmaceutical Research and Development group. Their effort was started with the identification of lead compounds with desirable SERT affinity, which could then be used as a template to introduce H$_3$R antagonist activity. Two SSRI templates were designated, the first based on fluoxetine, which is the third most prescribed antidepressant drug (**16**, **Figure 8**; Wong et al., 1995), and the second based on the hexahydropyrroloisoquinoline scaffold represented

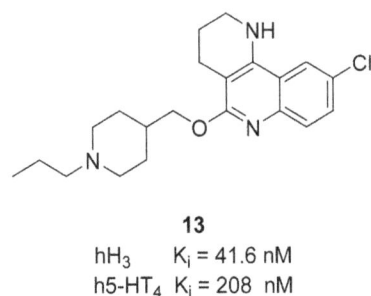

FIGURE 6 | Structure and biological activity of the selected H$_3$R/5-HT$_4$ ligand.

13
hH$_3$ K_i = 41.6 nM
h5-HT$_4$ K_i = 208 nM

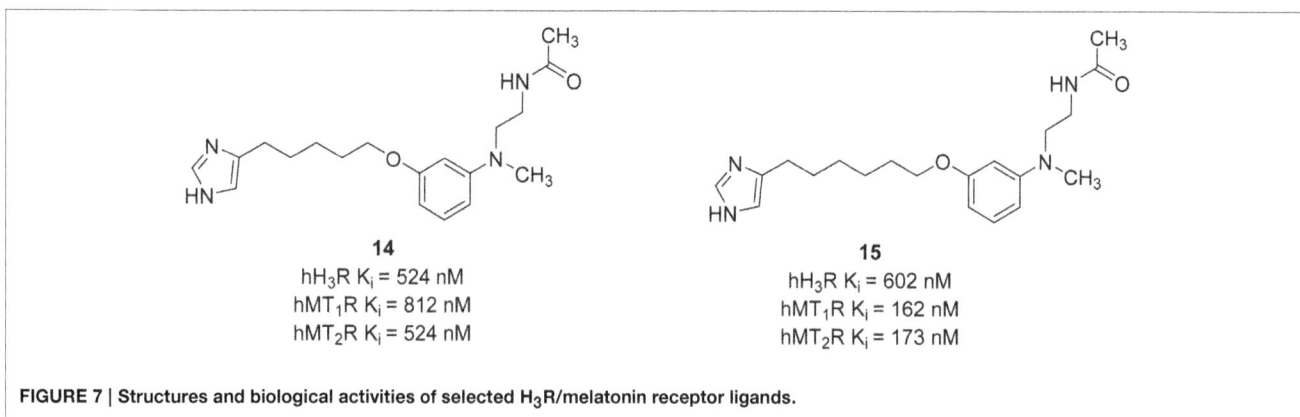

FIGURE 7 | Structures and biological activities of selected H₃R/melatonin receptor ligands.

by JNJ-7925476 (**17, Figure 8**), identified by high-throughput screening (Aluisio et al., 2008). Four templates of potent and selective H₃R antagonists were considered to develop dual H₃R/SERT inhibitors evaluated pre-clinically (**18–21, Figure 8**; Letavic et al., 2006). Starting from fluoxetine template, the tertiary benzyl amines of **18–21** were replaced with the fluoxetine template, so that the known SSRI would serve as both, the lipophilic core and one of the basic amines. Several H₃ amine side moieties were initially 3- or 4-substituted on both phenylene rings of fluoxetine (rings A and B). All the regioisomers had high affinity for the hH₃R, but the 3-piperidinyl-propyloxy derivative provided the highest affinity for both the rat serotonin transporter (rSERT) and human serotonin transporter (hSERT) (e.g., compound **22, Figure 8**; Stocking et al., 2007). The 4-(trifluoromethyl) substituted phenoxy (B) ring derivatives have no discrepancy between rSERT and hSERT, however, a decrease in affinity for hSERT over rSERT was observed for the unsubstituted derivatives. Electron donating substituents on B ring is associated with 5 to 30-fold decrease in hSERT affinity, however, electron withdrawing substituents displayed a good correlation between rSERT and hSERT (Stocking et al., 2007).

The same approach was applied for designing of hexahydropyrroloisoquinolines-derived dual H₃R antagonists and SERT inhibitors. The overlap of the H₃R antagonist **17** and SERT inhibitor **16** was pictured as exemplified in compound **23** (**Figure 8**). This approach generated a series of high affinity H₃R antagonists with the SERT affinity dependent on aryl ring (A) substitution. Nevertheless, unlike the fluoxetine scaffold, most simple substitutions on the aryl ring (A) of the hexahydropyrroloisoquinoline scaffold provided similar rSERT and hSERT affinity (Keith et al., 2007c). On the other hand, the hydroxyl and the heterocyclic derivatives displayed a slightly higher affinity for rSERT than hSERT. Two high affinity compounds, the 4-methoxy derivative and the 3-pyridyl derivatives demonstrated good *in vivo* activities in serotonin potentiated head twitch model for SERT inhibition and blockade of imetit-induced drinking model for the H₃R inhibition. However, this series showed unsatisfactory pharmacokinetics with low oral bioavailability, long t₁/₂ and a slow onset of action. In addition, these structures still retained affinity for the

dopamine transporter (DAT; Keith et al., 2007c). Consequently, simpler templates from hexahydropyrroloisoquinoline were attempted, initially, by removal of the fused pyrrolidine ring and one chiral center to obtain the tetrahydroisoquinolines (Letavic et al., 2007a). Structural optimization of tetrahydroisoquinolines derivatives was conducted using a large number of amines in order to improve the binding affinity at H₃R, varying the physical properties of the resulting compounds and maintaining SERT affinity (Keith et al., 2007b). Several modifications were attempted on the pendant piperidine ring; morpholine and substituted piperidines usually resulted in high affinity compounds. Replacing the piperidine with piperazine afforded compounds that have variable affinity for the hH₃R, depending greatly on the basicity of the terminal nitrogen. For example, small alkyl substituents on the piperazine provided compounds with high affinity for the H₃R, but decreasing the basicity of the terminal nitrogen by addition of bulky groups lowered the affinity for the H₃R. Among the large number of derivatives that were synthesized, compound **24** (**Figure 8**), which was afforded by removal of the pyrrolidine ring of **23** together with the replacement of the piperidine ring with a morpholine, has improved rat pharmacokinetics and improved pharmacodynamics with a head twitch response (Keith et al., 2007a).

Further simplification was conducted by removing one carbon on the tetrahydroisoquinoline, which deleted the last remaining stereocenter to provide the benzyl amine derivatives (e.g., **25, Figure 8**). The benzylic carbon of tetrahydroisoquinolines was replaced with an oxygen in order to improve overall physical properties (Letavic et al., 2007b). The 3-piperidinyl-propyloxy derivatives were not used in this series; instead, they used the alkyne and amide side chains corresponding to the known H₃R antagonists **19** and **21**. The later modification was important to avoid any potential metabolic problems associated with 1,4-hydroxyquinone. The SAR of alkynes was generally similar to that of the tetrahydroisoqinolines and most of the compounds have high affinity toward H₃R and SERT. Selected compounds had good brain penetration in rat with brain levels of above 1 μM when dosed at 10 mg/kg p.o. (Letavic et al., 2007b). The benzamides benzyl amine derivatives were very potent with good selectivity over the norepinephrine transporter (NET) and

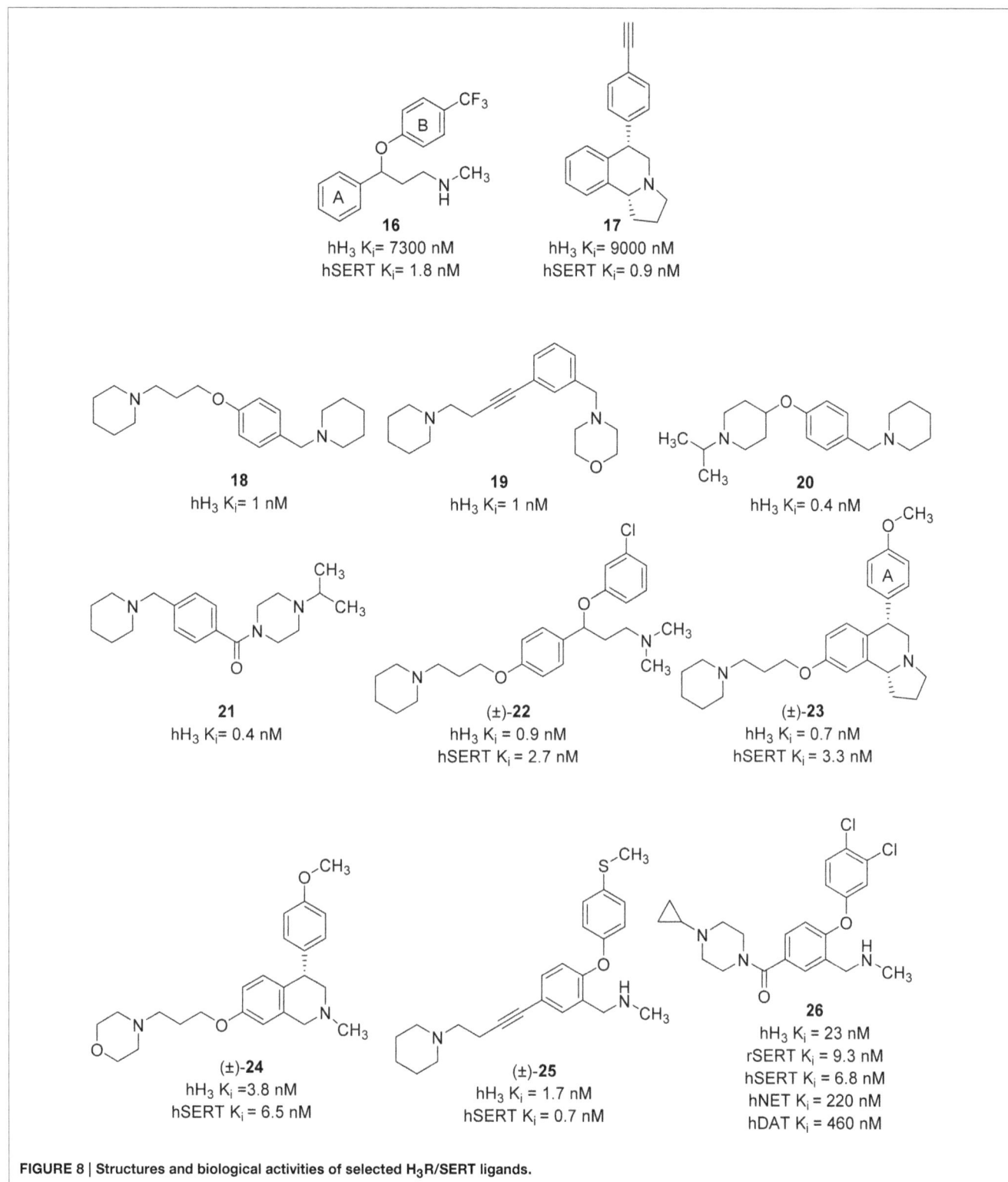

FIGURE 8 | Structures and biological activities of selected H₃R/SERT ligands.

DAT. One of the compounds, **26** (**Figure 8**), was extensively profiled *in vivo* and was found to have good rat pharmacokinetic and pharmacodynamics properties (**Table 1**; Ly et al., 2008). Although not yet tested on humans, inhibition of the H₃R makes

it an attractive combination with SERT blockade in order to create a novel antidepressant treatment.

The serotonin/norepinephrine reuptake inhibitor (SNRI) duloxetine **27** (**Figure 9**) is used in therapeutic off-label treatment

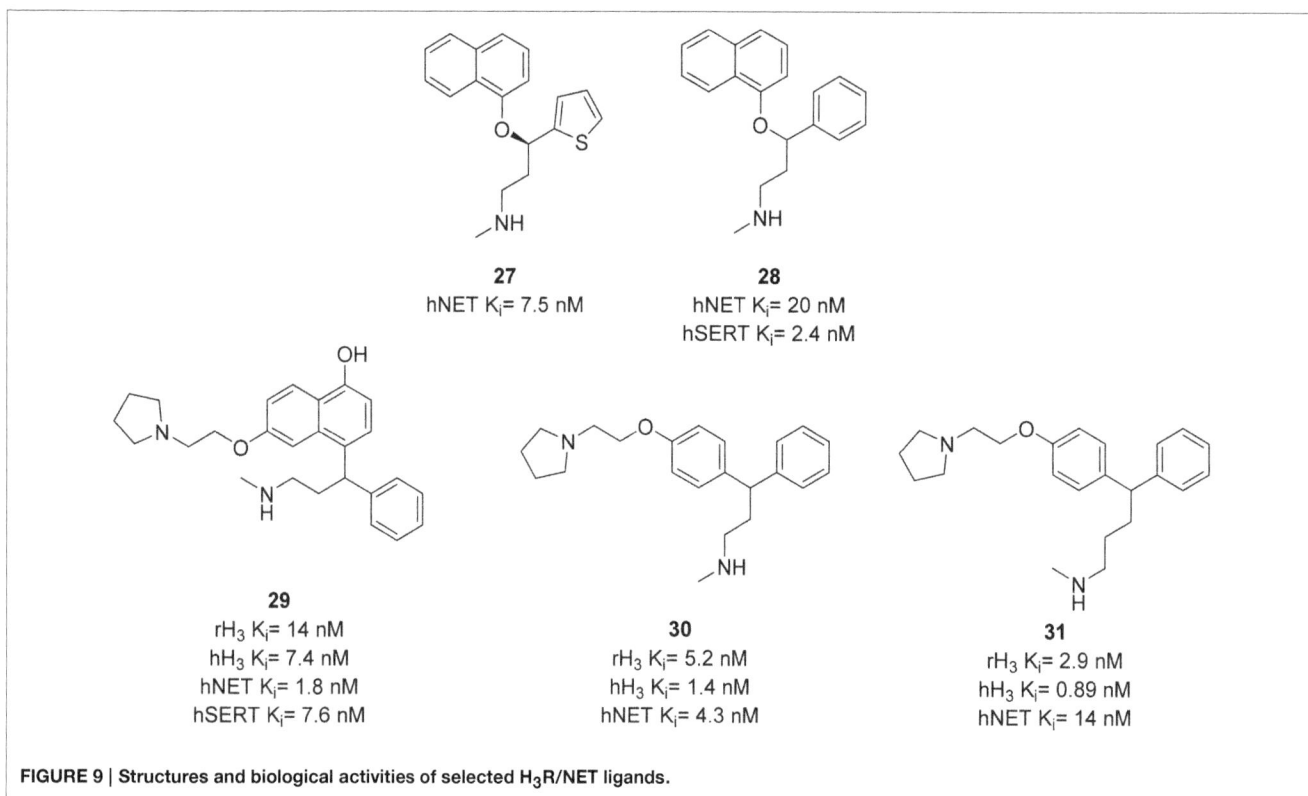

FIGURE 9 | Structures and biological activities of selected H₃R/NET ligands.

of neuropathic pain (Fishbain et al., 2006). The inhibition of NE uptake is essential for the pain efficacy (Leventhal et al., 2007). H₃R antagonists Thioperamide 6 and GSK-189254 28 (**Figure 9**) have been reported to be active in models of pain (Farzin et al., 1994; Medhurst et al., 2008). Using these results Altenbach et al. designed a series of molecules combining pharmacophores of H₃R antagonism and NET inhibition in one molecule. An H₃R pharmacophore was linked to duloxetine analogs, cf. **28** (**Figure 9**). Resulting compounds **29–31** (**Figure 9**) showed low nanomolar affinity at H₃R and NET, where **29** additionally had SERT affinity (K_i = 7.6 nM) comparable to that of **28** (K_i = 2.4 nM; Bymaster et al., 2003). This affinity was reduced to $K_i >$ 70 nM in compounds **30**, and **31** providing a better selectivity. Compound **29** was also found to be potent in osteoarthritis pain model in rats with efficacies of 70 and 93% at doses of 3 and 10 mg/kg, respectively (Anighoro et al., 2014).

H₃R AND ENZYMES

Histamine level in the CNS is controlled not only by the receptors but also by the inactivating enzyme histamine N-methyltransferase (HMT; Parsons and Ganellin, 2006). Ligands with dual inhibitory activities on both H₃R and HMT could increase intersynaptic histamine levels in the CNS and may lead to beneficial procognitive effects in psychiatric and neurodegenerative diseases (Apelt et al., 2002; Sander et al., 2008). Even if they have low or missing *in vivo* activity, such ligands could greatly enhance histaminergic neurotransmission *via* inhibition of

histamine H₃ auto-receptors and reduce the catabolic rate for histamine degradation *via* HMT inhibition (Grassmann et al., 2003).

Most of the HMT inhibitors have a 4-aminoquinoline moiety in common (e.g., tacrine, **32, Figure 10**). Therefore, the synthetic effort to develop novel and dual H₃R\HMT inhibitors started from coupling of different 4-aminoquinolines with different spacers to the piperidine, the basic component that is essential for binding at the H₃R. Variation of the spacer structure provides two different series of compounds. The first series have an alkylene spacer separating the basic center from the 4-aminoquinoline. These compounds showed potent HMT inhibitory activities with moderate to high H₃R affinity. The second series, which possessed a p-phenoxypropyl spacer, showed a strong inhibitory activity on HMT and the H₃R affinity, exceeding that of the first series. One of the compounds, FUB 836 (**33, Figure 10**), combines a high H₃R affinity with a high HMT inhibitory activity and exhibited high H₃R selectivity when compared to H₁R and H₂R (Apelt et al., 2002). Similar approach was applied in designing H₃R/HMT dual inhibitors by combining imidazole heterocycle, which is an integral part of potent H₃R antagonists, with several aromatic carbo- or heterocyclic structures (e.g., aminoquinoline or tetrahydroacridine moieties) of standard HMT inhibitors by different alkyl and alkenyl spacers. One interesting compound, **34** (**Figure 10**), showed a high H₃R affinity with a high HMT inhibitory activity (Grassmann et al., 2003). Replacing imidazole head with a piperidine ring accompanied by a methylation of the amino functionality improved the inhibitory activity against HMT

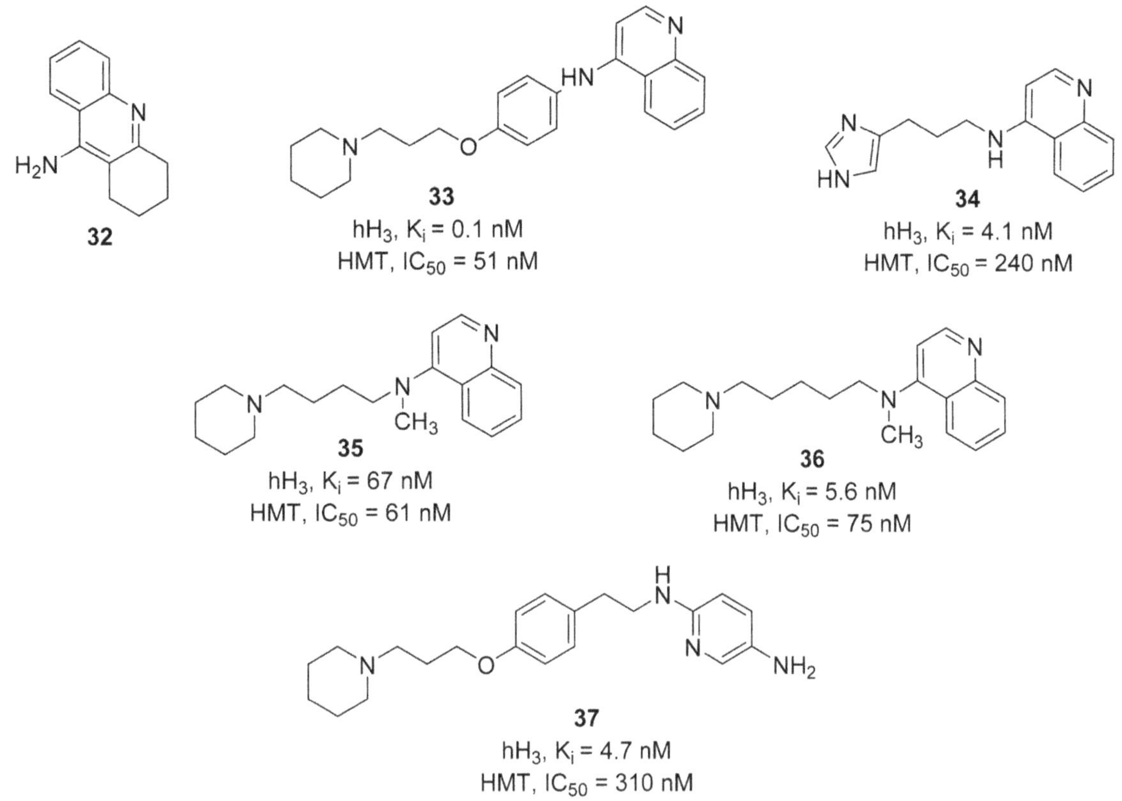

FIGURE 10 | Structures and biological activities of selected H₃R/HMT ligands.

(e.g., compounds **35** and **36**; **Figure 10**; Grassmann et al., 2004).

Another approach was attempted on FUB 836 (**33**) by replacing the aminoquinoline with different heterocycles (e.g., nitro- or amino-substituted pyridines, quinolines, benzothiazole, or pyrroline) in order to improve its dual H₃R/HMT affinities. In contrast to the aminoquinoline, the reported compounds showed moderate to good dual affinities. Whereas, some compounds showed potent HMT inhibitors, they only showed a moderate H₃R affinity and *vice versa* (Apelt et al., 2005). The most potent compound in this series was 4-(3-piperidinopropyl)phenylether with substituted alkylaminopyridine (**37, Figure 10**).

Tacrine (**32**) mentioned above is an acetylcholinesterase (AChE) inhibitor. Together with the symptomatically acting *N*-methyl-D-aspartate (NMDA) blocker memantine, tacrine represents the only therapeutic treatment of AD currently available. AD is a complex neurodegenerative disorder and the most common form of dementia. Patients show a degeneration of cholinergic neutrons in the basal forebrain according to cholinergic hypothesis and aggregation of βA through an interaction with the peripheral anionic site (PAS) of the AChE (Davies and Maloney, 1976; Giacobini, 2000). H₃R antagonists showed an ability to increase acetylcholine (ACh) but unlike the AChE, H₃R antagonist will raise acetylcholine levels mostly in the brain, since H₃R is mainly located in the CNS (Clapham and Kilpatrick, 1992; Darras et al., 2014). Therefore, the combination

of both activities in a single molecule may offer the desired therapeutic effect with fewer unpleasant side effects considering acetylcholine release in the periphery (Fang et al., 2015; Guzior et al., 2015).

Using available crystal structure information and applying pharmacophore modeling and docking simulations Bembenek et al. proposed compound **38** (**Figure 11**) and similar structures to have activity on both AChE and H₃R. Moreover, the used models suggest a possible interaction for this series of compounds with the PAS of the AChE (Bembenek et al., 2008). Some additional *in vitro* an *in vivo* studies with these compounds could be of interest to verify the calculated results. In 2008 Morini et al. introduced a class of symmetric and asymmetric 4,4′−biphenyl H₃R antagonists with a moderate ability to inhibit rat brain cholinesterase (Morini et al., 2008). This class is characterized by a rigid biphenyl scaffold and displays nanomolar binding affinities at human and rodent H₃R. The compound **39** (**Figure 11**) showed low nanomolar affinity to the H₃R and low micromolar activity to inhibit AChE. Docking the compound **39** into the catalytic cavity of mouse AChE showed similarity to the binding mode, earlier reported for **38**, confirming that more rigid and bulky biphenyl scaffolds are tolerated by the AChE active site. Interaction with PAS of the AChE is suggested for **39** as well as for **38**. In 2012 Bajda et al. presented a new class of diether derivatives of homo substituted piperidine with **40** (**Figure 11**) being the most active compound,

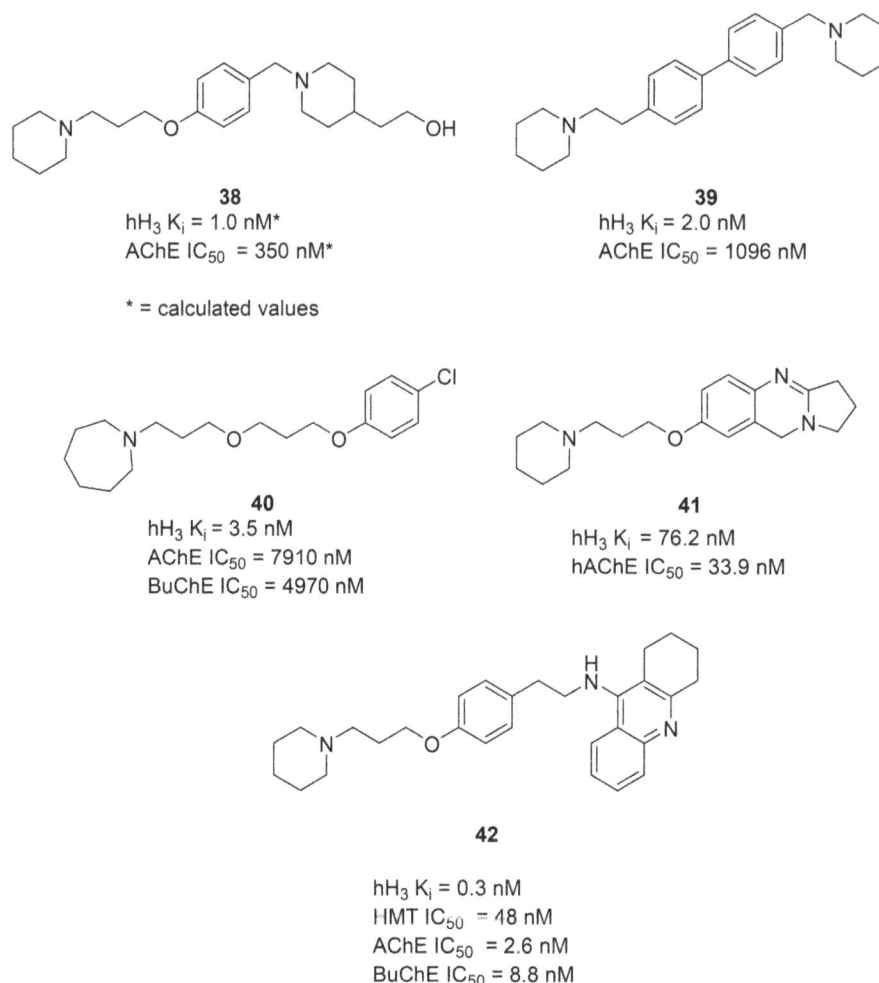

38
hH$_3$ K$_i$ = 1.0 nM*
AChE IC$_{50}$ = 350 nM*

* = calculated values

39
hH$_3$ K$_i$ = 2.0 nM
AChE IC$_{50}$ = 1096 nM

40
hH$_3$ K$_i$ = 3.5 nM
AChE IC$_{50}$ = 7910 nM
BuChE IC$_{50}$ = 4970 nM

41
hH$_3$ K$_i$ = 76.2 nM
hAChE IC$_{50}$ = 33.9 nM

42
hH$_3$ K$_i$ = 0.3 nM
HMT IC$_{50}$ = 48 nM
AChE IC$_{50}$ = 2.6 nM
BuChE IC$_{50}$ = 8.8 nM

FIGURE 11 | Structures and biological activities of selected H$_3$R/AChE ligands.

showing low nanomolar affinity for the hH$_3$R and micromolar inhibitory potency toward both cholinergic receptors (Bajda et al., 2012). In 2014 Darras et al. presented new tetracyclic nitrogen-bridge headed compounds showing balanced affinities as hAChE inhibitor and hH$_3$R antagonist with UW-MD-71 (**41, Figure 11**). It showed the best activity in two digit nanomolar area for both targets and greater than 200-fold selectivity over the other histamine receptor subtypes. This compound was tested on acquisition, consolidation and retrieval in a model of dizocilpine-induced amnesia. Test results indicated that using multiple targeting ligands lead to pharmacological and behavioral profiles different from interaction with the respective single target ligands. Furthermore, a potential applicability in the modulation of the memory impairment could be shown (Khan et al., 2016).

In 2006, Petroianu et al. tested several compounds, containing structural features of tacrine (**32**) for their inhibitory activities on AChE and Butyrylcholinesterase (BuChE; Petroianu et al., 2006). These compounds have previously shown combined H$_3$R antagonist and HMT inhibitory potencies (Apelt et al., 2002; Grassmann et al., 2003). From this series of compounds

FUB833 (**42, Figure 11**) was the most promising four-target compound, showing subnanomolar affinity for hH$_3$R, low nanomolar IC$_{50}$ values for both cholinesterases and good affinity for HMT. These compounds have shown only moderate effects under *in vivo* conditions (Apelt et al., 2002). Furthermore, these new compounds might serve as novel important tools for further pharmacological investigations on histaminergic neurotransmission and its regulatory processes.

H$_3$R AND NO-RELEASING MOLECULES

Nitric oxide (NO) is an endogenous messenger, displaying a variety of actions in our body (Kerwin et al., 1995). NO is a key messenger in cardiovascular, immune, central, and peripheral nervous systems (Szabo, 2010). Released in the CNS after stimulation of excitatory NMDA, it diffuses in the adjacent presynaptic nerve terminal and astrocytes. There it activates the soluble guanylate cyclase (sGC) implying a number of physiological roles like gastro-protective effect, control of food intake and learning and formation of memory. H$_3$R antagonists have also shown positive effects concerning learning and memory (Miyazaki et al., 1997; Komater et al., 2005). Combining H$_3$R antagonists with NO-releasing moiety could synergistically contribute to a curative effect in pathologies like memory and learning disorders. Bertinaria et al. synthesized and tested some H$_3$R antagonists with NO-donor properties by coupling H$_3$R antagonist SKF 91486 (**43, Figure 12**) with the furoxan system (1,2,5-oxadiazole 2-oxide), which is able to release NO under the action of thiol cofactors like cysteine (Schönafinger, 1999). Resulting compounds had similar or greater potency as SKF 91486 (**43**). Derivative **44** (**Figure 12**) showed additional NO-dependent muscle relaxation (Bertinaria, 2003; Bertinaria et al., 2003). Another potent compound **45** is derived from Imoproxifan **46** (**Figure 12**) by replacing the oxime moiety with a five-membered NO-donor furoxan ring (Tosco et al., 2005). As a further development, a new class of NO-donor H$_3$R antagonists with non-basic (thio)ether linker and furoxan (**47**) or nitrooxy (**48**) NO-donor moieties is introduced (**Figure 12**). These compounds are more appropriate to enter the CNS due to a better lipophilic-hydrophilic balance (Tosco et al., 2004).

H$_3$R AND DIFFERENT ANTISEIZURE PHARMACOPHORES

Epilepsy is a common human brain disorder, affecting more than 60 million people worldwide. There is a need to discover an effective and safer antiepileptic drugs (AED) since Phenytoin

(**49**) and recent AEDs like Loreclezole (**50**), Remacemide (**51**), and Safinamide (**52**) (**Figure 13**) only show efficacy within a maximum of 60–80% of patients and are responsible for many unwanted side-effects, such as headache, nausea, anorexia, ataxia, hepatotoxicity, drowsiness, gastrointestinal disturbance, gingival hyperplasia, attention deficit, und cognitive problems leading to additional discomfort (Sadek et al., 2014). There are indices for histamine receptors to improve the development of convulsions (Kasteleijn-Nolst Trenité et al., 2013). Seizure threshold can be increased and seizure susceptibility to electrically and chemically induced seizures can be decreased via activation of the central histaminergic system (Zhu et al., 2007; Bhowmik et al., 2012). Pitolisant has been tested in clinical trial phase II for patients suffering from photosensitive epilepsy. Supported by these results Sadek et al. designed some multiple-target ligands by combining the known 3-piperidinopropoxy or (3-piperidinopropoxy)aryl H$_3$R pharmacophore with different AEDs on the market (**49–52**) leading to a small series of compounds (**53–56, Figure 13**; Sadek et al., 2014). These compounds showed moderate to good affinity to H$_3$R with K$_i$ values in the range of 562–0.24 nM and were tested in vivo for their anticonvulsive effect against maximum electroshock (MES)-induced and pentylenetetrazole (PTZ)-kindled convulsions in rats having phenytoin (**55**) as the reference AED. Surprisingly the compound with the lowest in vitro potency (**55**) was the only one to show the ability to reduce convulsions in both in vivo models being administered at 10 mg/kg intraperitoneally. Still the results are controversial and need new epilepsy models to elucidate the pharmacological profile of the current multiple targeting class in

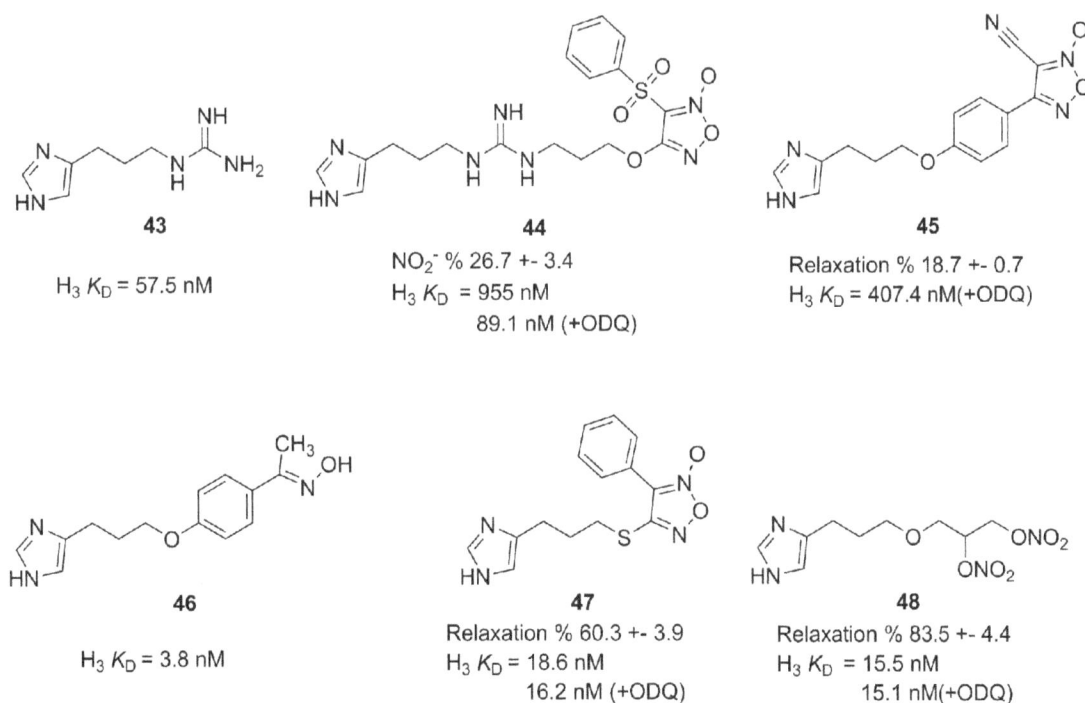

FIGURE 12 | Structures and biological activities of selected H$_3$R/NO-donor ligands.

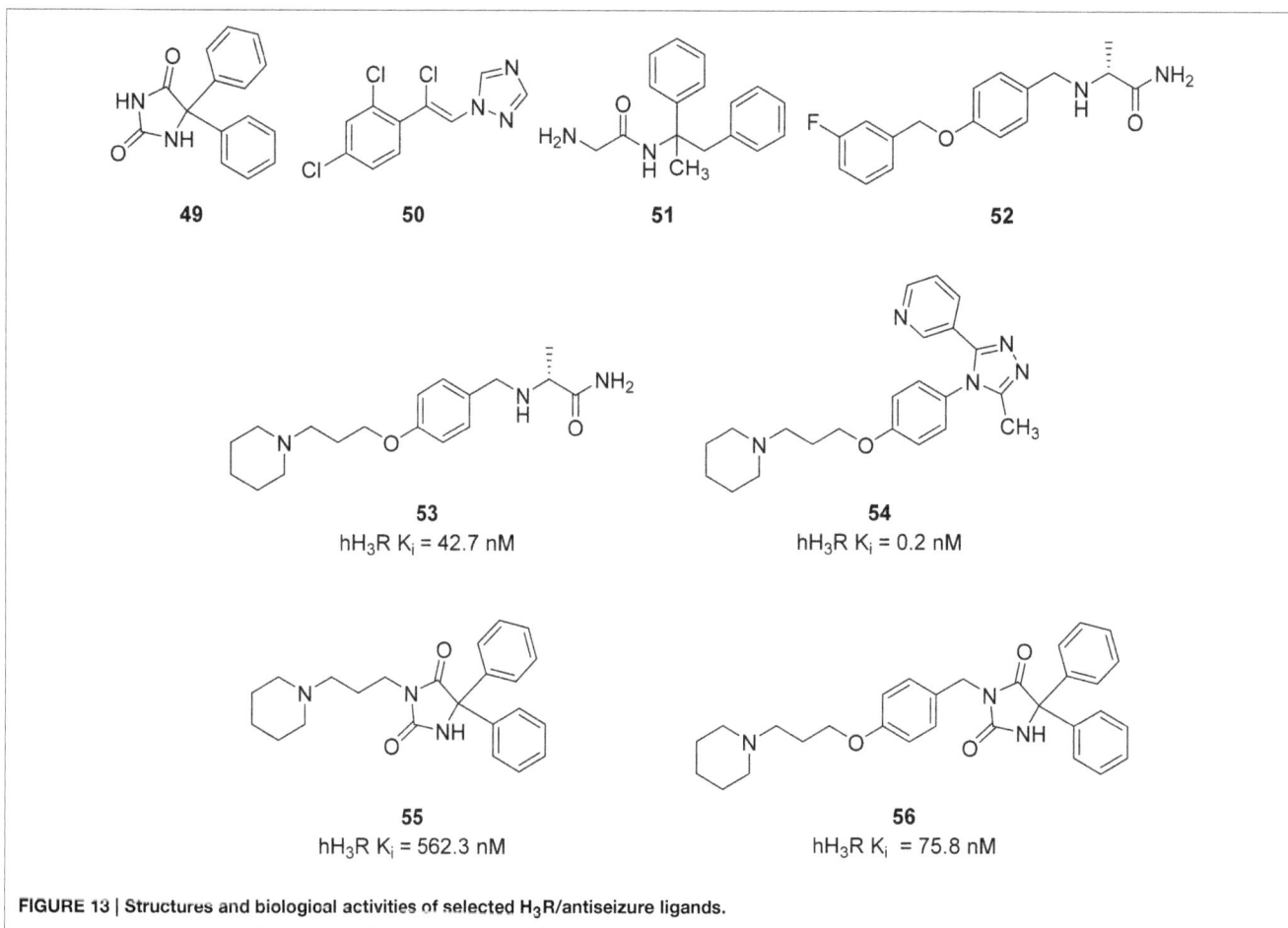

FIGURE 13 | Structures and biological activities of selected H₃R/antiseizure ligands.

order to develop suitable and clinically useful AEDs (Bertinaria, 2003).

CONCLUSION

Several combinations of different H₃R pharmacophores with pharmacophoric elements of other histamine subtypes, other aminergic GPCRs, other transporters, other enzymes, and other disease-modifying elements have been described. The increasing knowledge on the complex interaction of the different signaling pathways as well as on the complex mechanism of central disorders, give promises for the development of optimized drugs with synergistic pharmacological properties at multiple targets and also reduced side effects. The different leads for MTDLs described here, are very early or at best preclinical candidates.

Therefore, a lot of work on improvements has to be performed before these designed multiple targeting approaches will get into clinical trials.

AUTHOR CONTRIBUTIONS

All authors listed, have made substantial, direct and intellectual contribution to the work, and approved it for publication.

ACKNOWLEDGMENTS

Support was kindly provided by the EU COST Actions CM1103, CM1207, and CA15135 as well by DFG INST 208/664-1 FUGG and Ol16112039.

REFERENCES

Aluisio, L., Lord, B., Barbier, A. J., Fraser, I. C., Wilson, S. J., Boggs, J., et al. (2008). *In-vitro* and *in-vivo* characterization of JNJ-7925476, a novel triple monoamine uptake inhibitor. *Eur. J. Pharmacol.* 587, 141–146. doi: 10.1016/j.ejphar.2008.04.008

Anighoro, A., Bajorath, J., and Rastelli, G. (2014). Polypharmacology:challenges and opportunities in epigenetic

drug discovery. *J. Med. Chem.* 57, 7874–7887. doi: 10.1021/jm50 06463

Apelt, J., Grassmann, S., Ligneau, X., Pertz, H. H., Ganellin, C. R., Arrang, J. M., et al. (2005). Search for histamine H3 receptor antagonists with combined inhibitory potency at N-tau-methyltransferase: Ether derivatives. *Pharmazie* 60, 97–106.

Apelt, J., Ligneau, X., Pertz, H. H., Arrang, J. M., Ganellin, C. R., Schwartz, J. C., et al. (2002). Development of a new class of nonimidazole histamine H(3) receptor ligands with combined inhibitory histamine N-methyltransferase activity. *J. Med. Chem.* 45, 1128–1141. doi: 10.1021/jm0110845

Arrang, J. M., Garbarg, M., and Schwartz, J. C. (1983). Auto-inhibition of brain histamine release mediated by a novel class (H3) of histamine receptor. *Nature* 302, 832–837. doi: 10.1038/302832a0

Bajda, M., Kuder, K. J., Lażewska, D., Kieć-Kononowicz, K., Więckowska, A., Ignasik, M., et al. (2012). Dual-acting diether derivatives of piperidine and homopiperidine with histamine H3 receptor antagonistic and anticholinesterase activity. *Arch. Pharm. (Weinheim)* 345, 591–597. doi: 10.1002/ardp.201200018

Bakker, R. A., Timmerman, H., and Leurs, R. (2002). Histamine receptors: Specific ligands, receptor biochemistry, and signal transdution. *Clin. Allergy Immunol.* 17, 27–64.

Barbier, A. J., Aluisio, L., Lord, B., Qu, Y., Wilson, S. J., Boggs, J. D., et al. (2007). Pharmacological characterization of JNJ-28583867, a histamine H(3) receptor antagonist and serotonin reuptake inhibitor. *Eur. J. Pharmacol.* 576, 43–54. doi: 10.1016/j.ejphar.2007.08.009

Bembenek, S. D., Keith, J. M., Letavic, M. A., Apodaca, R., Barbier, A. J., Dvorak, L., et al. (2008). Lead identification of acetylcholinesterase inhibitors-histamine H3 receptor antagonists from molecular modeling. *Bioorg. Med. Chem.* 16, 2968–2973. doi: 10.1016/j.bmc.2007.12.048

Berlin, M., Boyce, C. W., and de Lera Ruiz, M. (2011). Histamine H3 receptor as a drug discovery target. *J. Med. Chem.* 54, 26–53. doi: 10.1021/jm100064d

Bertinaria, M. (2003). H3 receptor ligands: new imidazole H3-antagonists endowed with NO-donor properties. *Farmaco* 58, 279–283. doi: 10.1016/S0014-827X(03)00023-5

Bertinaria, M., Stilo, A. D., Tosco, P., Sorba, G., Poli, E., Pozzoli, C., et al. (2003). [3-(1H-Imidazol-4-yl)propyl]guanidines containing furoxan moieties. *Bioorg. Med. Chem.* 11, 1197–1205. doi: 10.1016/S0968-0896(02)00651-X

Bhowmik, M., Khanam, R., and Vohora, D. (2012). Histamine H3 receptor antagonists in relation to epilepsy and neurodegeneration: a systemic consideration of recent progress and perspectives. *Br. J. Pharmacol.* 167, 1398–1414. doi: 10.1111/j.1476-5381.2012.02093.x

Bongers, G., Bakker, R. A., and Leurs, R. (2007). Molecular aspects of the histamine H3 receptor. *Biochem. Pharmacol.* 73, 1195–1204. doi: 10.1016/j.bcp.2007.01.008

Brioni, J. D., Esbenshade, T. A., Garrison, T. R., Bitner, S. R., and Cowart, M. D. (2011). Discovery of histamine H3 antagonists for the treatment of cognitive disorders and Alzheimer's disease. *J. Pharmacol. Exp. Ther.* 336, 38–46. doi: 10.1124/jpet.110.166876

Bymaster, F. P., Beedle, E. E., Findlay, J., Gallagher, P. T., Krushinski, J. H., Mitchell, S., et al. (2003). Duloxetine (Cymbalta), a dual inhibitor of serotonin and norepinephrine reuptake. *Bioorg. Med. Chem. Lett.* 13, 4477–4480. doi: 10.1016/j.bmcl.2003.08.079

Ceras, J., Cirauqui, N., Pérez-Silanes, S., Aldana, I., Monge, A., and Galiano, S. (2012). Novel sulfonylurea derivatives as H3 receptor antagonists. Preliminary SAR studies. *Eur. J. Med. Chem.* 52, 1–13. doi: 10.1016/j.ejmech.2012.02.049

Chazot, P. L. (2010). Therapeutic potential of histamine H3 receptor antagonists in dementias. *Drug News Perspect.* 2, 99–103. doi: 10.1358/dnp.2010.23.2.1475899

Chojnacki, J. E., Liu, K., Yan, X., Toldo, S., Selden, T., Estrada, M., et al. (2014). Discovery of 5-(4-Hydroxyphenyl)-3-oxo-pentanoic acid [2-(5-methoxy-1H-indol-3-yl)-ethyl]-amide as a neuroprotectant for Alzheimer's disease by hybridizayion of curcumin and melatonin. *Chem. Neurosci.* 5, 690–699. doi: 10.1021/cn500081s

Clapham, J., and Kilpatrick, G. J. (1992). Histamine H3 receptors modulate the release of [3H]-acetylcholine from slices of rat entorhinal cortex: evidence for the possible existence of H3 receptor subtypes. *Br. J. Pharmacol.* 107, 919–923. doi: 10.1111/j.1476-5381.1992.tb13386.x

Corrêa, M. F., and Fernandes, J. P. D. S. (2015). Histamine H4 receptor ligands: future applications and state of art. *Chem. Biol. Drug Des.* 85, 461–480. doi: 10.1111/cbdd.12431

Cowart, M., Altenbach, R., Black, L., Faghih, R., Zhao, C., and Hancock, A. A. (2004). Medicinal chemistry and biological properties of non-imidazole histamine H3 antagonists. *Mini Rev. Med. Chem.* 4, 979–992. doi: 10.2174/1389557043403215

Dagli, M., Goksu, N., Eryilmaz, A., Mocan Kuzey, G., Bayazit, Y., Gun, B. D., et al. (2008). Expression of histamine receptors (H1, H2, and H3) in the rabbit endolymphatic sac: an immunohistochemical study. *Am. J. Otolaryngol.* 29, 20–23. doi: 10.1016/j.amjoto.2006.12.003

Daley-Yates, P., Ambery, C., Sweeney, L., Watson, J., Oliver, A., and McQuade, B. (2012). The efficacy and tolerability of two novel H(1)/H(3) receptor antagonists in seasonal allergic rhinitis. *Int. Arch. Allergy Immunol.* 158, 84–98. doi: 10.1159/000329738

Darras, F. H., Pockes, S., Huang, G., Wehle, S., Strasser, A., Wittmann, H. J., et al. (2014). Synthesis, biological evaluation, and computational studies of Tri- and tetracyclic nitrogen-bridgehead compounds as potent dual-acting AChE inhibitors and hH3 receptor antagonists. *ACS Chem. Neurosci.* 5, 225–242. doi: 10.1021/cn4002126

Davies, P., and Maloney, A. J. (1976). Selective loss of central cholinergic neurons in Alzheimer's disease. *Lancet* 308, 1403.

Deng, C., Weston-Green, K., and Huang, X. F. (2010). The role of histaminergic H1 and H3 receptors in food intake: a mechanism for atypical antipsychotic-induced weight gain? *Prog. Neuropsychopharmacol. Biol. Psychiatry* 34, 1–4. doi: 10.1016/j.pnpbp.2009.11.009

Esbenshade, T. A., Browman, K. E., Bitner, R. S., Strakhova, M., Cowart, M. D., and Brioni, J. D. (2008). The histamine H3 receptor: an attractive target for the treatment of cognitive disorders. *Br. J. Pharmacol.* 154, 1166–1181. doi: 10.1038/bjp.2008.147

Fang, J., Li, Y., Liu, R., Pang, X., Li, C., Yang, R., et al. (2015). Discovery of multitarget-directed ligands against Alzheimer's disease through systematic prediction of chemical -protein interactions. *J. Chem. Inf. Model.* 55, 149–164. doi: 10.1021/ci500574n

Farzin, D., Asghari, L., and Nowrouzi, M. (1994). Rodent antinociception following acute treatment with different histamine receptor agonists and antagonists. *Pharmacol. Biochem. Behav.* 111, 751–760.

Ferrada, C., Ferré, S., Casadó, V., Cortés, A., Justinova, Z., Barnes, C., et al. (2008). Interactions between histamine H3 and dopamine D2 receptors and the implications for striatal function. *Neuropharmacology* 55, 190–197. doi: 10.1016/j.neuropharm.2008.05.008

Fishbain, D., Berman, K., and Kajdasz, D. K. (2006). Duloxetine for neuropathic pain based on recent clinical trials. *Curr. Pain Headache Rep.* 10, 199–204. doi: 10.1007/s11916-006-0046-7

Fredrickson, A., Snyder, P. J., Cromer, J., Thomas, E., Lewis, M., and Maruff, P. (2008). The use of effect sizes to characterize the nature of cognitive change in psychopharmacological studies: an example with scopolamine. *Hum. Psychopharmacol.* 23, 425–436. doi: 10.1002/hup.942

Gemkow, M. J., Davenport, A. J., Harich, S., Ellenbroek, B. A., Cesura, A., and Hallett, D. (2009). The histamine H3 receptor as a therapeutic drug target for CNS disorders. *Drug Discov. Today* 14, 509–515. doi: 10.1016/j.drudis.2009.02.011

Ghasemi, J. B., and Tavakoli, H. (2012). Improvement of the prediction power of the CoMFA and CoMSIA models on histamine H3 antagonists by different variable selection methods. *Sci. Pharm.* 80, 547–566. doi: 10.3797/scipharm.1204-19

Giacobini, E. (2000). Cholinesterase inhibitors stabilize Alzheimer's disease. *Ann. N.Y. Acad. Sci.* 920, 321–327. doi: 10.1111/j.1749-6632.2000.tb06942.x

Grassmann, S., Apelt, J., Ligneau, X., Pertz, H. H., Arrang, J. M., Ganellin, C. R., et al. (2004). Search for histamine H(3) receptor ligands with combined inhibitory potency at histamine N-methyltransferase: omega-piperidinoalkanamine derivatives. *Arch. Pharm.* 337, 533–545. doi: 10.1002/ardp.200400897

Grassmann, S., Apelt, J., Sippl, W., Ligneau, X., Pertz, H. H., Zhao, Y. H., et al. (2003). Imidazole derivatives as a novel class of hybrid compounds with inhibitory histamine N-methyltransferase potencies and histamine hH3 receptor affinities. *Bioorg. Med. Chem.* 11, 2163–2174. doi: 10.1016/S0968-0896(03)00120-2

Guzior, N., Wieckowska, A., Panek, D., and Malawska, B. (2015). Recent development of multifunctional agents as potential drug candidates for the treatment of Alzheimer's disease. *Curr. Med. Chem.* 22, 373–404. doi: 10.2174/0929867321666141106122628

Héron, A., Rouleau, A., Cochois, V., Pillot, C., Schwartz, J. C., and Arrang, J. M. (2001). Expression analysis of the histamine H3 receptor in developing rat tissues. *Mech. Dev.* 105, 167–173. doi: 10.1016/S0925-4773(01)00389-6

Herrmann, N., Chau, S. A., and Kircanski, L. K. (2011). Current and emerging drug treatment options for Alzheimer's disease: a systematic review. *Drugs* 71, 2031–2065. doi: 10.2165/11595870-000000000-00000

Hey, J. A., Del Prado, M., Egan, R. W., Kreutner, W., and Chapman, R. W. (1992). Inhibition of sympathetic hypertensive responses in the guinea-pig by prejunctional histamine H3-receptors. *Br. J. Pharmacol.* 107, 347–351. doi: 10.1111/j.1476-5381.1992.tb12749.x

Hopkins, A. L. (2008). Network pharmacology: the next paradigm in drug discovery. *Nat. Chem. Biol.* 4, 682–690. doi: 10.1038/nchembio.118

Hotte, M., Dauphin, F., Freret, T., Boulouard, M., and Levellat, G. (2012). A biphasic and brain-region selective down-regulation of cyclic adenosine monophosphate concentrations supports object recognition in the rat. *PLoS ONE* 7:e32244. doi: 10.1371/journal.pone.0032244

Huang, G., Nimczick, M., and Decker, M. (2015). Rational modification of the biological profile of GPCR ligands through combination with other biologically active moieties: GPCR ligand combinations. *Arch. Pharm. (Weinheim)* 348, 531–540. doi: 10.1002/ardp.201500079

Humbert-Claude, M., Morisset, S., Gbahou, F., and Arrang, J. M. (2007). Histamine H3 and dopamine D2 receptor-mediated [35S]GTPγ[S] binding in rat striatum: evidence for additive effects but lack of interactions. *Biochem. Pharmacol.* 73, 1172–1181. doi: 10.1016/j.bcp.2007.01.006

Jadhav, H. R., and Singh, M. (2013). Histamine H3 receptor function and ligands: recent developments. *Mini Rev. Med. Chem.* 13, 47–57. doi: 10.2174/138955713804484695

Jin, C. Y., and Panula, P. (2005). The laminar histamine receptor system in human prefrontal cortex suggests multiple levels of histaminergic regulation. *Neuroscience* 132, 137–149. doi: 10.1016/j.neuroscience.2004.12.017

Kagermeier, N., Werner, K., Keller, M., Baumeister, P., Seifert, R., Buschauer, A., et al. (2015). Dimeric carbamoylguanidine-type histamine H2 receptor ligands: a new class of potent and selective agonists. *Bioorg. Med. Chem.* 23, 3957–3969. doi: 10.1016/j.bmc.2015.01.012

Kasteleijn-Nolst Trenité, D., Parain, D., Genton, P., Masnou, P., Schwartz, J.-C., and Hirsch, E. (2013). Efficacy of the histamine 3 receptor (H3R) antagonist pitolisant (formerly known as tiprolisant; BF2.649) in epilepsy: dose-dependent effects in the human photosensitivity model. *Epilepsy Behav.* 28, 66–70. doi: 10.1016/j.yebeh.2013.03.018

Keith, J. M., Gomez, L. A., Barbier, A. J., Wilson, S. J., Boggs, J. D., Lord, B., et al. (2007a). Pyrrolidino-tetrahydroisoquinolines bearing pendant heterocycles as potent dual H3 antagonist and serotonin transporter inhibitors. *Bioorg. Med. Chem. Lett.* 17, 4374–4377. doi: 10.1016/j.bmcl.2007.03.043

Keith, J. M., Gomez, L. A., Letavic, M. A., Ly, K. S., Jablonowski, J. A., Seierstad, M., et al. (2007b). Dual serotonin transporter/histamine H3 ligands: optimization of the H3 pharmacophore. *Bioorg. Med. Chem. Lett.* 17, 702–706. doi: 10.1016/j.bmcl.2006.10.089

Keith, J. M., Gomez, L. A., Wolin, R. L., Barbier, A. J., Wilson, S. J., Boggs, J. D., et al. (2007c). Pyrrolidino-tetrahydroisoquinolines as potent dual H3 antagonist and serotonin transporter inhibitors. *Bioorg. Med. Chem. Lett.* 17, 2603–2607. doi: 10.1016/j.bmcl.2007.01.106

Kerwin, J. F., Lancaster, J. R., and Feldman, P. L. (1995). Nitric oxide: a new paradigm for second messengers. *J. Med. Chem.* 38, 4343–4362. doi: 10.1021/jm00022a001

Khan, N., Saad, A., Nurulain, S. M., Darras, F. H., Decker, M., and Sadek, B. (2016). The dual-acting H3 receptor antagonist and AChE inhibitor UW-MD-71 dose-dependently enhances memory retrieval and reverses dizocilpine-induced memory impairment in rats. *Behav. Brain. Res.* 297, 155–164. doi: 10.1016/j.bbr.2015.10.022

Klinkenberg, I., and Blokland, A. (2011). The validity of scopolamine as a pharmacological model for cognitive impairment: a review of animal behavioral studies. *Neurosci. Biobehav. Rev.* 34, 1307–1350. doi: 10.1016/j.neubiorev.2010.04.001

Komater, V. A., Buckley, M. J., Browman, K. E., Pan, J. B., Hancock, A. A., Decker, M. W., et al. (2005). Effects of histamine H3 receptor antagonists in two models of spatial learning. *Behav. Brain Res.* 159, 295–300. doi: 10.1016/j.bbr.2004.11.008

Kottke, T., Sander, K., Weizel, L., Schneider, E. H., Seifert, R., and Stark, H. (2011). Receptor-specific functional efficacies of alkyl imidazoles as dual

histamine H3/H4 receptor ligands. *Eur. J. Pharmacol.* 654, 200–208. doi: 10.1016/j.ejphar.2010.12.033

Kroeze, W. K., Hufeisen, S. J., Popadak, B. A., Renock, S. M., Steinberg, S., Ernsberger, P., et al. (2003). H1-histamine receptor affinity predicts short-term weight gain for typical and atypical antipsychotic drugs. *Neuropsychopharmacology* 28, 519–526. doi: 10.1038/sj.npp.1300027

Lelong, V., Dauphin, F., and Boulouard, M. (2001). RS 67333 and D-cycloserine accelerate learning acquisition in the rat. *Neuropharmacology* 41, 517–522. doi: 10.1016/S0028-3908(01)00085-5

Lelong, V., Lhonneur, L., Dauphin, F., and Boulouard, M. (2003). BIMU 1 and RS 67333, two 5-HT4 receptor agonists, modulate spontaneous alternation deficits induced by scopolamine in the mouse. *Naunyn Schmiedebergs Arch. Pharmacol.* 367, 621–628. doi: 10.1007/s00210-003-0743-2

Leon, R., Garcia, A. G., and Marco-Contelles, J. (2013). Recent advances in the multitarget-directed ligands approach for the treatment of Alzheimer's disease. *Med. Res. Rev.* 33, 139–189. doi: 10.1002/med.20248

Lepailleur, A., Freret, T., Lemaître, S., Boulouard, M., Dauphin, F., Hinschberger, A., et al. (2014). Dual histamine H3R/serotonin 5-HT4R ligands with antiamnesic properties: pharmacophore-based virtual screening and polypharmacology. *J. Chem. Inf. Model.* 54, 1773–1784. doi: 10.1021/ci500157n

Letavic, M. A., Barbier, A. J., Dvorak, C. A., and Carruthers, N. I. (2006). Recent medicinal chemistry of the histamine H3 receptor. *Prog. Med. Chem.* 44, 181–206. doi: 10.1016/S0079-6468(05)44405-7

Letavic, M. A., Keith, J. M., Jablonowski, J. A., Stocking, E. M., Gomez, L. A., Ly, K. S., et al. (2007a). Novel tetrahydroisoquinolines are histamine H3 antagonists and serotonin reuptake inhibitors. *Bioorg. Med. Chem. Lett.* 17, 1047–1051. doi: 10.1016/j.bmcl.2006.11.036

Letavic, M. A., Stocking, E. M., Barbier, A. J., Bonaventure, P., Boggs, J. D., Lord, B., et al. (2007b). Benzylamine histamine H(3) antagonists and serotonin reuptake inhibitors. *Bioorg. Med. Chem. Lett.* 17, 4799–4803. doi: 10.1016/j.bmcl.2007.06.061

Levallet, G., Hotte, M., Boulouard, M., and Dauphin, F. (2009). Increased particulate phosphodiesterase 4 in the prefrontal cortex supports 5-HT4 receptor-induced improvement of object recognition memory in the rat. *Psychopharmacology* 202, 125–139. doi: 10.1007/s00213-008-1283-8

Leventhal, L., Smith, V., Hornby, G., Andree, T. H., Brandt, M. R., and Rogers, K. F. (2007). Differential and synergistic effects of selective norepinephrine and serotonin reuptake inhibitors in rodent models of pain. *J. Pharmacol. Exp. Ther.* 320, 1178–1185. doi: 10.1124/jpet.106.109728

Lezoualc'h, F. (2007). 5-HT4 receptor and Alzheimer's disease: the amyloid connection. *Exp. Neurol.* 205, 325–329. doi: 10.1016/j.expneurol.2007.02.001

Lian, J., Huang, X. F., Pai, N., and Deng, C. (2014). Betahistine ameliorates olanzapine-induced weight gain through modulation of histaminergic, NPY and AMPK pathways. *Psychoneuroendocrinology* 48, 77–86. doi: 10.1016/j.psyneuen.2014.06.010

Lian, J., Huang, X. F., Pai, N., and Deng, C. (2016). Ameliorating antipsychotic-induced weight gain by betahistine: mechanisms and clinical implications. *Pharmacol. Res.* 106, 51–63. doi: 10.1016/j.phrs.2016.02.011

Ligneau, X., Landais, L., Perrin, D., Piriou, J., Uguen, M., Denis, E., et al. (2007). Brain histamine and schizophrenia: potential therapeutic applications of H3-receptor inverse agonists studied with BF2.649. *Biochem. Pharmacol.* 73, 1215–1224. doi: 10.1016/j.bcp.2007.01.023

Lim, H. D., Istyastono, E. P., van de Stolpe, A., Romeo, G., Gobbi, S., Schepers, M., et al. (2009). Clobenpropit analogs as dual activity ligands for the histamine H3 and H4 receptors: synthesis, pharmacological evaluation, and cross-target QSAR studies. *Bioorg. Med. Chem.* 17, 3987–3994. doi: 10.1016/j.bmc.2009.04.007

Lin, J., Sergeeva, O. A., and Haas, H. L. (2011). Histamine H3 receptors and sleep-wake regulation. *J. Pharmacol. Exp. Ther.* 336, 17–23. doi: 10.1124/jpet.110.170134

Ly, K. S., Letavic, M. A., Keith, J. M., Miller, J. M., Stocking, E. M., Barbier, A. J., et al. (2008). Synthesis and biological activity of piperazine and diazepane amides that are histamine H3 antagonists and serotonin reuptake inhibitors. *Bioorg. Med. Chem. Lett.* 18, 39–43. doi: 10.1016/j.bmcl.2007.11.016

Mangialasche, F., Solomon, A., Winblad, B., Mecocci, P., and Kivipelto, M. (2010). Alzheimer's disease: clinical trials and drug development. *Lancet Neurol.* 9, 702–716. doi: 10.1016/S1474-4422(10)70119-8

McLeod, R. L., Mingo, G. G., Herczku, C., DeGennaro-Culver, F., Kreutner, W., Egan, R. W., et al. (1999). Combined Histamine H1 and H3 receptor blockade produces nasal degongestion in an experimental model of nasal congestion. *Am. J. Rhinol.* 13, 391–399. doi: 10.2500/1050658997813 67483

Medhurst, S. J., Collins, S. D., Billinton, A., Bingham, S., Dalziel, R. G., Brass, A., et al. (2008). Novel histamine H3 receptor antagonists GSK189254 and GSK334429 are efficacious in surgically-induced and virally-induced rat models of neuropathic pain. *Pain* 138, 61–69. doi: 10.1016/j.pain.2007.11.006

Medina, V. A., and Rivera, E. S. (2010). Histamine receptors and cancer pharmacology. *Br. J. Pharmacol.* 161, 755–767. doi: 10.1111/j.1476-5381.2010.00961.x

Menza, M. A., Kaufman, K. R., and Castellanos, A. (2000). Modafinil augmentation of antidepressant treatment in depression. *J. Clin. Psychiatry* 61, 378–381. doi: 10.4088/JCP.v61n0510

Millan, M. J. (2014). On "polypharmacy" and multi-target agents, complementary strategies for improving the treatment of depression: a comparative appraisal. *Int. J. Neuropsychopharmacol.* 17, 1009–1037. doi: 10.1017/S1461145712001496

Miyazaki, S., Onodera, K., Imaizumi, M., and Timmerman, H. (1997). Effects of clobenpropit (VUF-9153), a histamine H3-receptor antagonist, on learning and memory, and on cholinergic and monoaminergic systems in mice. *Life Sci.* 61, 355–361. doi: 10.1016/S0024-3205(97)00406-2

Møller, M. N., Kirkeby, S., Vikeså, J., Nielsen, F. C., and Caye-Thomasen, P. (2015). Expression of histamine receptors in the human endolymphatic sac: the molecular rationale for betahistine use in Menieres disease. *Eur. Arch. Otorhinolaryngol.* doi: 10.1007/s00405-015-3731-5. [Epub ahead of print].

Morini, G., Comini, M., Rivara, M., Rivara, S., Bordi, F., Plazzi, P. V., et al. (2008). Synthesis and structure-activity relationships for biphenyl H3 receptor antagonists with moderate anti-cholinesterase activity. *Bioorg. Med. Chem.* 16, 9911–9924. doi: 10.1016/j.bmc.2008.10.029

Neumann, D., Beermann, S., Burhenne, H., Glage, S., Hartwig, C., and Seifert, R. (2013). The dual H3/4R antagonist thioperamide does not fully mimic the effects of the "standard" H4R antagonist JNJ 7777120 in experimental murine asthma. *Naunyn Schmiedebergs Arch. Pharmacol.* 386, 983–990. doi: 10.1007/s00210-013-0898-4

Nikolic, K., Filipic, S., Agbaba, D., and Stark, H. (2014). Procognitive properties of drugs with single and multitargeting H 3 receptor antagonist activities. *CNS Neurosci. Ther.* 20, 613–623. doi: 10.1111/cns.12279

Norman, P. (2011). New H1/H3 antagonists for treating allergic rhinitis: WO2010094643. *Expert. Opin. Ther. Pat.* 21, 425–429. doi: 10.1517/13543776.2011.536533

Pala, D., Scalvini, L., Lodola, A., Mor, M., Flammini, L., Barocelli, E., et al. (2014). Synthesis and characterization of new bivalent agents as melatonin- and histamine H3-ligands. *Int. J. Mol. Sci.* 15, 16114–16133. doi: 10.3390/ijms150916114

Panula, P., Chazot, P. L., Cowart, M., Gutzmer, R., Leurs, R., Liu, W. L., et al. (2015). International union of basic and clinical pharmacology. XCVIII. Histamine Receptors. *Pharmacol. Rev.* 67, 601–655. doi: 10.1124/pr.114.0 10249

Parsons, M. E., and Ganellin, C. R. (2006). Histamine and its receptors. *Br. J. Pharmacol.* 147, S127–S135. doi: 10.1038/sj.bjp.0706440

Peters, J. U. (2013). Polypharmacology - Foe or friend? *J. Med. Chem.* 56, 8955–8971. doi: 10.1021/jm400856t

Petroianu, G., Arafat, K., Sasse, B. C., and Stark, H. (2006). Multiple enzyme inhibitions by histamine H3 receptor antagonists as potential procognitive agents. *Pharmazie* 61, 179–182.

Raddatz, R., Tao, M., and Hudkins, R. L. (2010). Histamine H3 antagonists for treatment of cognitive deficits in CNS diseases. *Curr. Top. Med. Chem.* 10, 153–169. doi: 10.2174/156802610790411027

Remington, G. (2003). Understanding antipsychotic "atypicality": a clinical and pharmacological moving target. *J. Psychiatry Neurosci.* 28, 275–284.

Sabbagh, M. N. (2009). Drug development for Alzheimer's disease: where are we now and where are we headed? *Am. J. Geriatr. Pharmacother.* 7, 167–185. doi: 10.1016/j.amjopharm.2009.06.003

Sadek, B., Schwed, J. S., Subramanian, D., Weizel, L., Walter, M., Adem, A., et al. (2014). Non-imidazole histamine H3 receptor ligands incorporating antiepileptic moieties. *Eur. J. Med. Chem.* 77, 269–279. doi: 10.1016/j.ejmech.2014.03.014

Sander, K., Kottke, T., and Stark, H. (2008). Histamine H3 receptor antagonists go to clinics. *Biol. Pharm. Bull.* 31, 2163–2181. doi: 10.1248/bpb.31.2163

Schlicker, E., Betz, R., and Göthert, M. (1998). Histamine H3 receptor-mediated inhibition of serotonin release in the rat brain cortex. *Naunyn Schmiedebergs Arch. Pharmacol.* 337, 588–590.

Schlicker, E., Fink, K., Detzner, M., and Göthert, M. (1993). Histamine inhibits dopamine release in the mouse striatum via presynaptic H3 receptors. *J. Neural Transm. Gen. Sect.* 93, 1–10. doi: 10.1007/BF01244933

Schlicker, E., Fink, K., Göthert, M., Hoyer, D., Molderings, G., Roschke, I., et al. (1989). The pharmacological properties of the presynaptic serotonin autoreceptor in the pig brain cortex conform to the 5-HT1D receptor subtype. *Naunyn Schmiedebergs Arch. Pharmacol.* 340, 45–51. doi: 10.1007/BF00169206

Schlicker, E., Schunack, W., and Göthert, M. (1990). Histamine H3 receptor-mediated inhibition of noradrenaline release in pig retina discs. *Naunyn Schmiedeberg Arch. Pharmacol.* 342, 497–501. doi: 10.1007/BF00169035

Schönafinger, K. (1999). Heterocyclic NO prodrugs. *Farmaco* 54, 316–320. doi: 10.1016/S0014-827X(99)00031-2

Schwartz, J. C., Arrang, J. M., Garbarg, M., Pollard, H., and Ruat, M. (1991). Histaminergic transmission in the mammalian brain. *Physiol. Rev.* 71, 1–21.

Slack, R. J., Russell, L. J., Hall, D. A., Luttmann, M. A., Ford, A. J., Saunders, K. A., et al. (2011). Pharmacological characterization of GSK1004723, a novel, long-acting antagonist at histamine H1 and H3 receptors. *Br. J. Pharmacol.* 164, 1627–1641. doi: 10.1111/j.1476-5381.2011.01285.x

Snyder, P. J., Bednar, M. M., Cromer, J. R., and Maruff, P. (2005). Reversal of scopolamine-induced deficits with a single dose of donepezil, an acetylcholinesterase inhibitor. *Alzheimers Dement.* 1, 126–135. doi: 10.1016/j.jalz.2005.09.004

Srinivasan, V., Pandi-Perumal, S. R., Cardinali, D. P., Poeggeler, B., and Hardeland, R. (2006). Melatonin in Alzheimer's disease and other neurodegenerative disorders. *Behav. Brain. Funct.* 2, 1–23. doi: 10.1186/1744-9081-2-15

Stahl, M. (2001). "Commentary on the limitation of antidepressants in current use," in *Antidepressants: Milestones in Drug Therapy MDT*, ed B. E. Leonard (Basel; Boston, MA; Berlin: Birkhäuser Basel), 31–43.

Stark, H., Kathmann, M., Schlicker, E., Schunack, W., Schlegel, B., and Sippl, W. (2004). Medicinal chemical and pharmacological aspects of imidazole-containing histamine H3 receptor antagonists. *Mini Rev. Med. Chem.* 4, 965–977. doi: 10.2174/1389557043403107

Stocking, E. M., Miller, J. M., Barbier, A. J., Wilson, S. J., Boggs, J. D., McAllister, H. M., et al. (2007). Synthesis and biological evaluation of diamine-based histamine H3 antagonists with serotonin reuptake inhibitor activity. *Bioorg. Med. Chem. Lett.* 17, 3130–3135. doi: 10.1016/j.bmcl.2007.03.034

Szabo, C. (2010). Gaseotransmitters: new frontiers for translational science. *Sci. Transl. Med.* 2, 1–7. doi: 10.1126/scitranslmed.3000721

Thurmond, R. L., Gelfand, E. W., and Dunford, P. J. (2008). The role of histamine H1 and H4 receptors in allergic inflammation: the search for new antihistamines. *Nat. Rev. Drug. Discov.* 7, 41–53. doi: 10.1038/nrd2465

Tosco, P., Bertinaria, M., Di Stilo, A., Cena, C., Sorba, G., Fruttero, R., et al. (2005). Furoxan analogues of the histamine H3-receptor antagonist imoproxifan and related furazan derivatives. *Bioorg. Med. Chem.* 13, 4750–4759. doi: 10.1016/j.bmc.2005.05.004

Tosco, P., Bertinaria, M., Di Stilo, A., Marini, E., Rolando, B., Sorba, G., et al. (2004). A new class of NO-donor H3-antagonists. *Farmaco* 59, 359–371. doi: 10.1016/j.farmac.2003.12.008

Von Coburg, Y., Kottke, T., Weizel, L., Ligneau, X., and Stark, H. (2009). Potential utility of histamine H3 receptor antagonist pharmacophore in antipsychotics. *Bioorg. Med. Chem. Lett.* 19, 538–542. doi: 10.1016/j.bmcl.2008. 09.012

Vuyyuru, L., Schubert, M. L., Harrington, L., Arimura, A., and Makhlouf, G. M. (1995). Dual inhibitory pathways link antral somatostatin and histamine secretion in human, dog, and rat stomach. *Gastroenterology* 109, 1566–1574. doi: 10.1016/0016-5085(95)90645-2

Walczyński, K., Guryn, R., Zuiderveld, O. P., and Timmerman, H. (1999). Non-imidazole histamine H3 ligands. Part, I. Synthesis of 2-(1-piperazinyl)- and 2-(hexahydro-1H-1,4-diazepin-1-yl)benzothiazole derivatives as H3-antagonists with H1 blocking activities. *Farmaco* 54, 684–694. doi: 10.1016/S0014-827X(99)00081-6

Wicek, M., Kottke, T., Ligneau, X., Schunack, W., Seifert, R., Stark, H., et al. (2011). N-Alkenyl and cycloalkyl carbamates as dual acting histamine

H3 and H4 receptor ligands. *Bioorganic. Med. Chem.* 19, 2850–2858. doi: 10.1016/j.bmc.2011.03.046

Wieland, K., Laak, A. M., Smit, M. J., Kuhne, R., Timmerman, H., and Leurs, R. (1999). Mutational analysis of the antagonist-binding site of the histamine H1 receptor. *J. Biol. Chem.* 274, 29994–30000. doi: 10.1074/jbc.274.42.29994

Witkin, J. M., and Nelson, D. L. (2004). Selective histamine H3 receptor antagonists for treatment of cognitive deficiencies and other disorders of the central nervous system. *Pharmacol. Ther.* 103, 1–20. doi: 10.1016/j.pharmthera.2004.05.001

Wong, D. T., Bymaster, F. P., and Engleman, E. A. (1995). Prozac (fluoxetine, Lilly 110140), the first selective serotonin uptake inhibitor and an antidepressant drug: twenty years since its first publication. *Life Sci.* 57, 411–441. doi: 10.1016/0024-3205(95)00209-O

Ye, N., Song, Z., and Zhang, A. (2014). Dual ligands targeting dopamine D2 and serotonin 5-HT1A receptors as new antipsychotical or anti-Parkinsonian agents. *Curr. Med. Chem.* 21, 437–457. doi: 10.2174/0929867311320660 60300

Youdim, M. B., and Buccafusco, J. J. (2005). Multi-functional drugs for various CNS targets in the treatment of neurodegenerative disorders. *Trends Pharmacol. Sci.* 26, 27–35. doi: 10.1016/j.tips.2004. 11.007

Zhou, L., Zhou, W., Zhang, S., Liu, B., Leng, Y., Zhou, R., et al. (2013). Changes in histamine receptors (H1, H2, and H3) expression in rat medial vestibular nucleus and flocculus after unilateral labyrinthectomy: histamine receptors in vestibular compensation. *PLoS ONE* 8:e66684. doi: 10.1371/journal.pone.0066684

Zhu, Y. Y., Zhu-Ge, Z. B., Wu, D. C., Wang, S., Liu, L. Y., Ohtsu, H., et al. (2007). Carnosine inhibits pentylenetetrazol-induced seizures by histaminergic mechanisms in histidine decarboxylase knock-out mice. *Neurosci. Lett.* 416, 211–216. doi: 10.1016/j.neulet.2007.01.075

Conflict of Interest Statement: The authors declare that the research was conducted in the absence of any commercial or financial relationships that could be construed as a potential conflict of interest.

7

Drug Design for CNS Diseases: Polypharmacological Profiling of Compounds using Cheminformatic, 3D-QSAR and Virtual Screening Methodologies

Katarina Nikolic[1]*, Lazaros Mavridis[2], Teodora Djikic[3], Jelica Vucicevic[1], Danica Agbaba[1], Kemal Yelekci[3] and John B. O. Mitchell[4]

[1] Department of Pharmaceutical Chemistry, Faculty of Pharmacy, University of Belgrade, Belgrade, Serbia, [2] School of Biological and Chemical Sciences, Queen Mary University of London, London, UK, [3] Department of Bioinformatics and Genetics, Faculty of Engineering and Natural Sciences, Kadir Has University, Istanbul, Turkey, [4] EaStCHEM School of Chemistry and Biomedical Sciences Research Complex, University of St Andrews, St Andrews, UK

HIGHLIGHTS

- Many CNS targets are being explored for multi-target drug design
- New databases and cheminformatic methods enable prediction of primary pharmaceutical target and off-targets of compounds
- QSAR, virtual screening and docking methods increase the potential of rational drug design

Edited by:
Rona R. Ramsay,
University of St Andrews, UK

Reviewed by:
Elizabeth Yuriev,
Monash University, Australia
Janez Mavri,
National Institute of Chemistry,
Slovenia

*Correspondence:
Katarina Nikolic
knikolic@pharmacy.bg.ac.rs

The diverse cerebral mechanisms implicated in Central Nervous System (CNS) diseases together with the heterogeneous and overlapping nature of phenotypes indicated that multitarget strategies may be appropriate for the improved treatment of complex brain diseases. Understanding how the neurotransmitter systems interact is also important in optimizing therapeutic strategies. Pharmacological intervention on one target will often influence another one, such as the well-established serotonin-dopamine interaction or the dopamine-glutamate interaction. It is now accepted that drug action can involve plural targets and that polypharmacological interaction with multiple targets, to address disease in more subtle and effective ways, is a key concept for development of novel drug candidates against complex CNS diseases. A multi-target therapeutic strategy for Alzheimer's disease resulted in the development of very effective Multi-Target Designed Ligands (MTDL) that act on both the cholinergic and monoaminergic systems, and also retard the progression of neurodegeneration by inhibiting amyloid aggregation. Many compounds already in databases have been investigated as ligands for multiple targets in drug-discovery programs. A probabilistic method, the Parzen-Rosenblatt Window approach, was used to build a "predictor" model using data collected from the ChEMBL database. The model can be used to predict both the primary pharmaceutical target and off-targets of a compound based on its structure. Several multi-target ligands were selected for further study, as compounds with possible additional beneficial pharmacological activities. Based on all these findings, it is concluded that multipotent ligands targeting AChE/MAO-A/MAO-B and also D_1-R/D_2-R/5-HT$_{2A}$-R/H$_3$-R are promising novel drug candidates with improved efficacy and beneficial neuroleptic and procognitive activities in treatment of Alzheimer's and related neurodegenerative diseases. Structural information for drug targets permits docking and virtual screening and exploration of the molecular determinants of binding, hence facilitating the design of multi-targeted drugs. The crystal structures and models of enzymes of the monoaminergic and cholinergic systems have been used to investigate the structural origins of target selectivity and to identify molecular determinants, in order to design MTDLs.

Keywords: multi-target drugs, CNS disease, QSAR, rational drug design, cheminformatic, virtual screening, virtual docking

POLYPHARMACOLOGY OF COMPOUNDS AGAINST CNS DISEASES

Traditional drug discovery methods have mainly been based on development of selective agents for a specific target able to modulate its activity and the pathophysiology of the disease. This approach in now generally recognized as too simplistic for designing effective drugs to address complex multifactorial diseases, characterized by diverse physiological dysfunctions caused by dysregulation of complex networks of proteins (Anighoro et al., 2014). Modern drug design of multitarget ligands able to specifically modulate a network of interacting targets and show unique polypharmacological profiles is becoming increasingly important in drug discovery for multifactorial pathologies such as complex central nervous system (CNS) diseases (Hopkins, 2008; Mestres and Gregori-Puigjaneİą, 2009; Boran and Iyengar, 2010; Peters, 2013; Anighoro et al., 2014).

The most significant advantages of the use of multitarget drugs over other therapeutic strategies, such as polypharmaceutical or single-targeted therapy, are: improved efficacy as result of synergistic or additive effects caused by simultaneous and specific interactions with chosen palette of biological targets; better distribution in target tissue for simultaneous action on multiple targets; accelerated therapeutic efficacy in terms of initial onset and achievement of full effect; treatment of broader therapeutic range of symptoms; predictable pharmacokinetic profile and mitigated drug-drug interactions; lower incidence of molecule-based side effects; increased therapeutic interval of doses as result of lower risk of acute and delayed toxicity; better quality of treatment; improved patient compliance and tolerance; and lower incidence of target-based resistance as result of modulation of multiple targets (Millan, 2006, 2014; Anighoro et al., 2014). The main challenge in drug discovery of MTDLs is to develop an efficient methodology for the design of novel multipotent

drugs able to interact only with one additional target and without significant affinities for other related targets.

The polypharmacological design of CNS drugs is challenging because of the complex pathophysiological mechanisms of brain diseases, interactions of neurotransmitter systems and observed ligand cross-reactivities (Roth et al., 2004). Since multipotent ligands could also interact with off-targets and cause target-based adverse effects, a major objective in polypharmacology is to rationally design multi-target drugs able to specifically modulate only a group of desired targets while minimizing interactions with off-targets and avoiding interactions with anti-targets (Anighoro et al., 2014; Millan, 2014). Multi-Target Designed Ligands (MTDL) contain the primary pharmacophore elements for each target which could be separated by a linker (conjugate MTDLs), could touch at one point (fused), or could be combined by using commonalities in the structures of underlying pharmacophores (merged) (Besnard et al., 2012; Millan, 2014).

Smaller and relatively rigid structures of highly merged MTDLs result in better physicochemical, pharmacokinetic and pharmacological profiles (Besnard et al., 2012; Millan, 2014). For the rationally designed MTDLs, activities against the targets and pharmacokinetic profiles are predicted. Based on the results obtained, the most promising MTDLs are selected for further modifications and studies (Hajjo et al., 2010; Besnard et al., 2012; Hajjo et al., 2012; Zhang et al., 2013; Nikolic et al., 2015a).

Several previous studies confirmed that multifactorial pathologies, such as cerebral mechanisms implicated in neurological and psychiatric diseases (Threlfell et al., 2004; Dai et al., 2007; Garduno-Torres et al., 2007; Humbert-Claude et al., 2007; Gemkow et al., 2009) and neurodegenerative disorders (Goedert and Spillantini, 2006), are often polygenic and involve the dysregulation of very complex networks of proteins. The diverse cerebral mechanisms implicated in CNS diseases together with the heterogeneous and overlapping nature of phenotypes indicated that multitarget strategies may be appropriate for improved treatment of complex brain diseases. Both the activity and the side effects of CNS drugs are characterized by a complex pattern of biological activities on multiple targets and a complex mechanism of action (Roth et al., 2004; Lipina et al., 2012, 2013). Understanding how the neurotransmitter systems interact is also important in optimizing therapeutic strategies. Pharmacological intervention on the dopamine system will often influence the

Abbreviations: MTDL, multi-target designed ligands; QSAR, quantitative structure-activity relationship; AD, Alzheimer's disease; PD, Parkinson's disease; AChE, acetylcholinesterase; BuChE, butyrylcholinesterase; MAO, monoamine oxidase; Aβ, amyloid beta; 5-HT, serotonin receptor; D-R, dopamine receptor; H-R, histamine receptor; GPCRs, G protein–coupled receptors; HMT, histamine N-methyltransferase; SERT, serotonin transporter; AMPK, 5''-adenosine monophosphate-activated protein kinase.

serotonin or glutamate neurotransmitter systems. Interactions of the neurotransmitter systems, such as the dopamine-glutamate interaction (Carlsson and Carlsson, 1990; Millan, 2005) and the serotonin-dopamine interaction (Di Giovanni et al., 2008; Di Matteo et al., 2008), are also very important factors in design of multitargeted ligands with specific cross-reactivity and optimized neuropharmacological effects (Youdim and Buccafusco, 2005). Therefore, a more efficient polypharmacological strategy for treatment of complex CNS diseases is based on drug interactions with multiple targets, to address disease in more subtle and effective ways while avoiding side effects arising from interaction with defined antitargets and off-targets (Lu et al., 2012; Anighoro et al., 2014). Thus, polypharmacology is now recognized as a key pharmacological concept for development of novel drug candidates against complex CNS diseases.

As a result of the multitarget approach (Morphy and Rankovic, 2005; León et al., 2013; Anighoro et al., 2014; Millan, 2014) many CNS drugs with improved efficacy compared to their lead compounds have been developed and examined. Monoamine reuptake inhibitors with serotonin 5-HT_{2C} antagonistic properties were developed as novel class of antidepressants (Millan, 2006; Meltzer et al., 2012; Quesseveur et al., 2012). Dopamine receptors are G protein–coupled receptors (GPCRs), distinct in pharmacology, amino acid sequence, distribution, and physiological function. Based on their effector-coupling profiles dopamine receptors are organized into two families, the D_1-like (D_1, D_5) and D_2-like (D_2, D_3, D_4) receptors (Brunton et al., 2011).

The physiological processes under dopaminergic control include reward, emotion, cognition, memory, and motor activity. Therefore, dysregulation of the dopaminergic system is critical in a number of disease states, including Parkinson's disease, Tourette's syndrome, bipolar depression, schizophrenia, attention deficit hyperactivity disorder, and addiction/substance abuse (Brunton et al., 2011). Dopamine receptor antagonists are a mainstay in the pharmacotherapy of schizophrenia.

Since the pathophysiology of schizophrenia and related diseases involves deregulation of the dopamine, serotonin and glutamate neurotransmitter systems (Witkin and Nelson, 2004; Esbenshade et al., 2008; Brunton et al., 2011), therapeutic effects of typical and atypical neuroleptics are mostly mediated by inhibition of dopamine D_1/D_2-like receptors and other related aminergic receptors (**Table 1**). Blockade of dopamine D_2 and serotonin 5-HT_{2A} receptors is the main mechanism of action of atypical antipsychotics (Remington, 2003). Furthermore, interaction with various dopamine (D_1, D_3, D_4), serotonin (5-HT_{1A}, 5-HT_{1D}, 5-HT_{2A}, 5-HT_{2C}, 5-HT_6, and 5-HT_7), and histamine H_3 receptors may produce additional antipsychotic or procognitive effects (Reynolds, 2004; Esbenshade et al., 2008; Coburg et al., 2009) by indirectly modulating the mesolimbic dopaminergic neurons (Amato, 2015).

A significant improvement in schizophrenia therapy came in the early 2000s with the use of aripiprazole acting as a dopamine D_2-like partial agonist with partial agonistic properties on serotonergic 5-HT_{1A} and 5-HT_{2A} receptors (Buckley, 2003; Kiss et al., 2010; Johnson et al., 2011). Dopamine D_2/D_3 antagonists, with 5-HT_{2A} antagonistic and 5-HT_{1A} partial agonistic activities, were proposed as drug candidates for

schizophrenia therapy (Roth et al., 2004; Lipina et al., 2012, 2013). The efficient polypharmacological profile of aripiprazole and related antipsychotics resulted in the development of cariprazine and pardoprunox as drug candidates, which are currently in clinical trials (Ye et al., 2014).

Despite selective D_1 antagonism not being accepted on its own as an effective antipsychotic principle (**Table 1**; Tauscher et al., 2004; Sedvall and Karlsson, 2006), moderate antagonistic activity at D_1-receptors has been confirmed to be responsible for atypical neuroleptic clozapine effectiveness against treatment-resistant schizophrenia (Tauscher et al., 2004). Based on the polypharmacological profiles of recently approved antipsychotic drugs, it could be concluded that optimal and balanced modulation of D_1/D_2-like receptors - as well as interaction with serotonin and histamine H_3 receptors - should provide the most favorable neuroleptic effect. The successfully developed effective MTDLs with optimal polypharmacological profile for CNS diseases (**Table 1**) are experimental proof of the polypharmacological concept. Polypharmacological approaches are therefore likely to be extensively applied for rational design of ligands with optimal multitarget profile and for discovery of multipotent drug candidates with improved efficacy and safety in therapy of complex brain diseases.

Novel procognitive agents were developed as histamine H_3R antagonists/inverse agonists with inhibition of acetylcholine esterase (AChE), monoamine oxidase (MAO), histamine N-methyltransferase (HMT), or serotonin transporter (SERT) (Ligneau et al., 1998; Apelt et al., 2002, 2005; Grassmann et al., 2003, 2004; Petroianu et al., 2006; Decker, 2007; Esbenshade et al., 2008; Sander et al., 2008; Coburg et al., 2009; Bajda et al., 2011; Nikolic et al., 2015a). Rasagiline and ladostigil, drugs currently used as selective MAO-B inhibitors in therapy of PD, contain the propargylamine scaffold and therefore exert significant neuroprotective activity. Thus, phase II clinical trials of rasagiline (www.clinicaltrials.gov/ct2/show/NCT00104273) and ladostidil (www. clinicaltrials.gov/ct2/show/NCT01354691) in therapy of AD were proposed, and subsequently successfully completed. A multi-target therapeutic strategy for Alzheimer's disease resulted in the development of very effective MTDLs that act on both the cholinergic and monoaminergic systems, and also retard the neurodegenerative progress by inhibiting amyloid aggregation. Multi-target inhibitors of acetylcholine esterase and MAO (AChE/BuChE/MAO-A/MAO-B) were effective drug candidates for therapy of neurodegenerative Alzheimer's (AD) and Parkinson's diseases (PD) (Pérez et al., 1999; Marco-Contelles et al., 2006, 2009; Bolea et al., 2011; León et al., 2013; Bautista-Aguilera et al., 2014a,c; Nikolic et al., 2015b).

Besides the difficulties of effective modulation of the CNS targets, the need to design drugs that are able to reach the targets in the brain increases the complexity of CNS drug discovery. This is mainly due to the blood-brain barrier (BBB) protection system between the blood capillaries of the brain and brain tissue (Pardridge, 2005). The BBB enables selective access of required nutrients and hormones, while removing waste and preventing or reducing penetration of xenobiotics (Pardridge, 2005). Therefore, a major challenge in CNS drug discovery is to build and apply relationships between chemical structure and brain exposure (Rankovic and Bingham, 2013; Rankovic,

TABLE 1 | Polypharmacological profiles of drugs and drug candidates affecting the dopaminergic system.

Compound	Targets
 Aripiprazole (Johnson et al., 2011)	D_2, D_3, 5-HT$_{2B}$, D_4, 5-HT$_{2A}$, 5-HT$_{1A}$, 5-HT$_7$, α_{1A}, H_1 receptors (Buckley, 2003; Shapiro et al., 2003)
 Amitriptyline (Coburg et al., 2009)	D_1, D_5, D_2, D_3, H_1 receptors (Ligneau et al., 2000)
 Chlorpromazine (Bourne, 2001)	D_1, D_5, D_2, D_3, D_4, 5-HT$_{2a}$ receptors (Rajagopalan et al., 2014)
 Clozapine (Coburg et al., 2009)	D_1, D_5, D_2, D_3, D_4, 5-HT$_{2A}$, H_1 receptors (Ligneau et al., 2000; Bourne, 2001; Rajagopalan et al., 2014)
 Chlorprothixene (Coburg et al., 2009)	D_1, D_5, D_2, D_3, D_4, H_1 receptors (Ligneau et al., 2000)
 Fluphenazine (Coburg et al., 2009)	D_1, D_5, D_2, D_3, D_4, H_1 receptors (Ligneau et al., 2000)

(Continued)

TABLE 1 | Continued

Compound	Targets
 Haloperidol (Bourne, 2001)	D_1, D_5, D_2, D_3, D_4, 5-HT$_{2A}$ receptors (Hamacher et al., 2006)
 SCH 23390 (Bourne, 2001)	D_1, D_5, D_2, D_3, D_4, 5-HT$_{2A}$, 5-HT, α_{2A} receptors (Wu et al., 2005)
 SCH 39166 (Wu et al., 2005)	D_1, D_5, D_2, 5-HT, α_{2A} receptors
 13 (Coburg et al., 2009)	D_1, D_5, D_2, D_3, D_4, H_1, H_3 receptors (Ligneau et al., 2000; Bourne, 2001; Hamacher et al., 2006; Rajagopalan et al., 2014)

2015a). Total brain concentration (Cb) is now recognized as being only a portion of the non-specific binding to brain tissue, while the unbound brain concentration (Cu,b) is defined as the drug concentration at the target sites and is a measure of *in vivo* drug efficacy. Finally, receptor occupancy (RO) is direct measure of target engagement (Rankovic, 2015b). Lipophilicity of CNS drugs is generally considered the most critical physicochemical parameter for improved penetration and potency. Higher lipophilicity causes low solubility, high plasma protein binding, and increased metabolic and toxicity risks in CNS drugs (Leeson and Springthorpe, 2007). Furthermore, hydrogen bond molecular parameters are the dominant descriptors for unbound drug brain concentrations (Leeson and Davis, 2004). Reducing the HBD (Hydrogen Bond Donor) count of a molecule is one of the most successful strategies used in the optimization of brain exposure (Weiss et al., 2012). In CNS drug discovery, aqueous solubility is also considered in combination with the previously described parameters. Most of the CNS drugs with low safety risk are very soluble compounds, displaying aqueous solubility of more than 100 μM (Alelyunas et al., 2010). Generally, fine-tuning physicochemical properties for optimal brain exposure is now an essential method in CNS drug discovery (**Table 2**). Further studies of CNS property space and development of predictive models for brain exposure should result in the formation of a general methodology with a wide applicability domain in CNS drug design.

3D-QSAR STUDY OF MULTITARGET COMPOUNDS FOR CNS DISEASES

QSAR (*Quantitative Structure-Activity Relationship*) modeling has progressed from analysis of small series of congeners using

TABLE 2 | Developing CNS property space for optimal brain exposure (Rankovic and Bingham, 2013; Rankovic, 2015b).

CNS property space
TPSA < 60 Å^2, pKa < 8 and HBD count < 2 are minimizing P-gp recognition (Hitchcock, 2012; Desai et al., 2013)
TPSA (25–60 Å^2); at least one N atom; linear chains outside of rings (2–4); HBD (0–3); volume (740–970 Å^3); SAS (460–580 Å^2) → ↑BBB penetration (Ghose et al., 2012)
Optimal cLogP <3 (Gleeson, 2008)
cLogP < 4 and TPSA 40–80 Å^2 → ↑Cu,b (Raub et al., 2006) PSA < 90 Å^2; HBD < 3; cLogP 2–5; cLogD (pH 7.4) 2–5; and MW < 500 → ↑BBB penetration (Hitchcock and Pennington, 2006)
MW < 450; cLogP < 5; HBD < 3; HBA < 7; RB < 8; H-bonds < 8; pKa 7.5–10.5; PSA < 60–70 Å^2. → ↑BBB penetration (Pajouhesh and Lenz, 2005)

TPSA, topological polar surface area; Å^2, square angstrom; Å^3, qubic angstrom; HBD, hydrogen-bond donors; P-gp, P-glycoprotein; BBB, blood-brain bariere; HBA, hydrogen-bond acceptors; MW, molecular weight; PSA, polar surface area; cLogP, partition coefficient; cLogD, distribution coefficient; RB, rotatable bonds; Cu,b, unbound drug concentrations in brain; ↓, decreased; ↑, increased.

basic regressions to applications on very large and diverse data sets using a variety of statistical and machine learning methods. Today's QSAR practice widely uses ligand based theoretical approaches for modeling the physical, biological and pharmacological properties of compounds, and forms a crucial initial step in drug discovery. Together with structure-based methods, statistically based QSAR techniques are essential tools in lead optimization within several leading drug discovery groups (Cramer, 2012; Cherkasov et al., 2014).

Modern QSAR methodologies started with a 1962 publication by the Hansch group (Hansch et al., 1962), and further developed with the exploration of series of congeners (Craig, 1971; Topliss, 1972; Hansch et al., 1973). Steric effects of substituents were successfully described by five shape descriptors for substituents (Verloop et al., 1976). Electrostatic interaction energies in a series of superimposed 3D-conformations of analogs were effectively included in CoMFA (*Comparative Molecular Field Analysis*) and other 3D-QSAR methods (Cramer et al., 1988). In CoMFA, steric and electrostatic molecular fields of ligands are calculated and correlated with bioactivities by use of PLS (*Partial Least Squares*) (Wold et al., 1984). Based on the CoMFA approach, the CoMSIA method (*Molecular Similarity Indices in a Comparative Analysis*) was developed (Klebe et al., 1994), encompassing the steric, electrostatic, hydrogen bonding and hydrophobic effects of ligands. The main limitation of CoMFA/CoMSIA and other 3D-QSAR methods relates to their being applicable only to static structures of chemical analogs, while neglecting the dynamical nature of the ligands (Acharya et al., 2011).

Molecular field generating software, such as GRID (Goodford, 1985) and PHASE (Dixon et al., 2006), historically applied pharmacophoric constraints to facilitate 3D-QSAR modeling, considering multiple conformations. The new generation of 3D-descriptors, such as GRIND/GRIND-2/GRID-PP (*Grid-Independent Descriptor*), are alignment free descriptors derived from the *Molecular Interaction Fields* (MIF) of the series and designed to retain the chemical characteristics of the ligands examined. The GRIND descriptors so obtained are provided by programs from Molecular Discovery (Pastor et al., 2000; Durán et al., 2009) and used for advanced multivariate analyses and 3D-QSAR modeling.

Some novel 3D-QSAR approaches based on ligand-based 3D-QSAR models and complementary drug target fields are included in the AFMoC (Gohlke and Klebe, 2002) and QMOD (Varela et al., 2012) programs. The QSAR study of multitarget compounds involves QSAR modeling for each target activity individually, study of all developed QSAR models as part in a network of interrelated models, and design of novel multipotent compounds (Cherkasov et al., 2014). Combinations of the QSAR approach and related theoretical methods, such as virtual screening and docking, are very useful in the study and design of multitarget ligands with unique polypharmacological profiles (**Figure 1**; Ning et al., 2009; Zheng et al., 2010; Besnard et al., 2012; Kupershmidt et al., 2012; Bolea et al., 2013; Bautista-Aguilera et al., 2014c). Based on the developed QSAR models, analogs of a multitarget lead are designed with enhanced activity on the targets and optimal polypharmacological and safety profiles as drug candidates for further study. Recently developed QSAR approaches were the only *in silico* methodologyies able to distinguish between antagonists and agonists of olfactory receptors (ORs), a superfamily of G-protein coupled receptors (Don and Riniker, 2014).

Several successful cases of reported 3D-QSAR studies used in CNS drugs discovery have been listed in **Table 3**. In this chapter we provide an overview of some of them. For example, polypharmacological profiles of *in silico* generated analogs of donepezil, an approved acetylcholinesterase inhibitor drug, were evaluated by a QSAR study. More than 75% of the ligand-target predictions were confirmed by *in vitro* testing (Besnard et al., 2012). Pathophysiology of Alzheimer's disease (AD) includes extracellular deposition of amyloid β peptide (Aβ)-containing plaques, progressive loss of cholinergic neurons, metal dyshomeostasis, mitochondrial dysfunction, neuroinflammation, oxidative stress and increased MAO enzyme activity. Furthermore, levels of neurotransmitters such as dopamine, noradrenaline, and serotonin are significantly decreased in AD patients (Reinikainen et al., 1990). MAO-A/B inhibitors could increase the levels of dopamine, noradrenaline, and serotonin in the CNS. Therefore, MAO-A/B inhibitors have also been proposed as potential drugs for AD (Youdim et al., 2006).

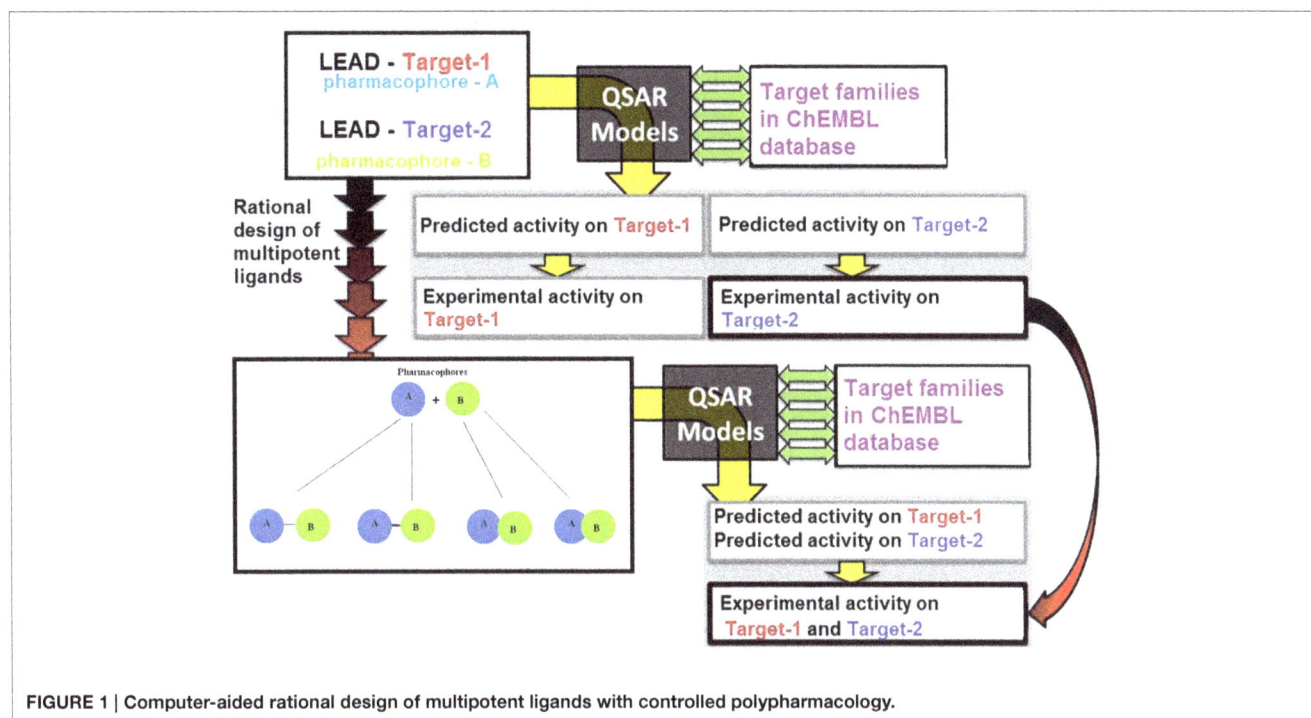

FIGURE 1 | Computer-aided rational design of multipotent ligands with controlled polypharmacology.

TABLE 3 | Reported 3D-QSAR studies used in CNS drug discovery.

Drug target	CNS disease	3D-QSAR method	Software package	References
MAO-A, MAO-B, AChE, BuChE	AD	GRID based 3D-QSAR modeling (Goodford, 1985; Pastor et al., 2000; Durán et al., 2009)	Pentacle www.moldiscovery.com	Bautista-Aguilera et al., 2014a,b
AChE	AD	Molecular field based 3D-QSAR modeling (Dixon et al., 2006)	PHASE www.schrodinger.com	Lakshmi et al., 2013
AChE, BuChE	AD	CoMFA based 3D-QSAR modeling Wold et al. (1984)	Tripos Sybyl www.tripos.com	Li et al., 2013
AChE	AD	3D multi-target QSAR (Prado-Prado et al., 2012)	DRAGON http://www.talete.mi.it/ MARCH-INSIDE (MARkovian CHemicals IN SIlico DEsign)	González-Díaz et al., 2012
H₃-R, HMT, AChE, BuChE	AD, PD, depression, schizophrenia	Molecular field and GRID based 3D-QSAR modeling (Goodford, 1985; Pastor et al., 2000; Dixon et al., 2006; Durán et al., 2009)	PHASE www.schrodinger.com Pentacle www.moldiscovery.com	Nikolic et al., 2015a

Multimodal brain permeable drugs affecting a few brain targets involved in the disease pathology, such as MAO and ChE enzymes, iron accumulation and amyloid-β generation/aggregation, were extensively examined as an essential therapeutic approach in AD treatment (Zheng et al., 2010; Bautista-Aguilera et al., 2014b). For instance, hybrid compound **M30D** contains the important pharmacophores from three drugs: tacrine, rivastigmine (ChEIs) and rasagiline/ladostigil (MAO-B inhibitor) (Zheng et al., 2010), while **ASS234** and **MBA236** contain the pharmacophores of the drugs donepezil (ChEIs) and clorgiline (MAO-A inhibitor) (Bolea et al., 2011). Pharmacophore and 3D-QSAR studies of donepezil and clorgiline derivatives inhibiting both AChE/BuChE and MAO-A/B were successfully applied for lead optimization work and for design of **ASS234**, **MBA236**

and related ligands with optimal polypharmacological and pharmacokinetic profiles (Bautista-Aguilera et al., 2014a,b,c). The propargylamine moiety in the MAO-inhibiting pharmacophore of rasagiline, ladostigil or clorgiline is responsible for their neuroprotective-neurorestorative effects. Therefore, the propargylamine moiety was used as the main chemical scaffold responsible for MAO inhibition in the designed **M30D**, **ASS234**, and **MBA236** hybrids (**Figure 2**). Hybrid compound **ASS234** acted as an 11-fold less potent MAO-A inhibitor and 54-fold more potent MAO-B inhibitor than the reference compound clorgiline, while **MBA236** was nine times more potent as an MAO-A inhibitor and 6-fold more potent for MAO-B than reference compound **ASS234**. Inhibition of the ChEs by the hybrid **MBA236** is in the micromolar range, slightly better than compound **ASS234** for AChEs while slightly poorer for BuChE (**Table 4**; Bautista-Aguilera et al., 2014b). The Multi-Target Designed Ligand **M30D** was found to be a highly potent inhibitor of MAO-A with moderate MAO-B inhibiting activity. Also, **M30D** was a more potent AChE inhibitor than rivastigmine, while rivastigmine was a much stronger BuChE inhibitor than **M30D** (**Table 4**; Zheng et al., 2010). Further to their MAO/ChE inhibitory properties, **ASS234** and **M30D** exert beneficial pharmacological effects in therapy of AD by inhibiting Aβ plaque formation and aggregation and, by blocking AChE-mediated Aβ1-40/Aβ1-42 aggregation (Kupershmidt et al., 2012; Bolea et al., 2013).

CHEMINFORMATICS METHODS FOR ON-TARGET AND OFF-TARGET BIOACTIVITY PREDICTION

The prediction of interactions between druglike organic molecules and proteins is a ubiquitous goal at the interface of biology and chemistry. The problem is approached from various different directions and with diverse purposes in mind. Much of this section will discuss the use of cheminformatics

methods to identify likely interactions between ligands, as the organic molecules are collectively called, and proteins. Such predictions may have many uses in terms of understanding the likely bioactivities of molecules and both cellular and molecular functions of proteins.

The prediction of pharmaceutically relevant molecular properties has been the default problem addressed by cheminformatics throughout its history. The most obvious application, and a useful source of financial support, for cheminformatics research has been drug discovery. The label "drug discovery," however, obscures the complexity of a variety of distinct questions. One objective, early in the drug discovery pipeline, is the identification of lead compounds, molecules possessing modest pharmacological activity that are starting points for chemical modifications enhancing their potency, selectivity and bioavailability. Subsequently, lead optimization will require Quantitative Structure-Activity Relationship (QSAR) studies to understand which modifications will best enhance affinity while, for instance, maximizing solubility and avoiding regions of chemical space likely to lead to toxicity.

Protein target predictions (Bender et al., 2007; Lounkine et al., 2012) allow us to link molecular interactions to biological effects, and hence to identify and rationalize the bioactivities of compounds. Since many molecules interact promiscuously with several targets as well as different ligands interacting with the same target (**Figure 3**), we must predict off-target as well as on-target interactions. Protein-ligand interactions, other than those with the expected pharmacological protein target, can help to identify opportunities for drug repurposing (Kinnings et al., 2011; Napolitano et al., 2013), where a drug developed for one disease is able to treat a different condition. Such compounds have the advantage of already having been optimized for bioavailability and non-toxicity. More adventurously, polypharmacology (Chen et al., 2009) is possible, where deliberate use is made of the drug's ability to hit two targets,

TABLE 4 | IC50 values for the inhibitory effects of test compounds on the enzymatic activity of MAO-A, MAO-B, AChE, and BuChE.

Compound	MAO-A	MAO-B	AChE	BuChE
MBA236[a]	6.3 ± 0.4 nM	183.6 ± 7.4 nM	2.8 ± 0.1 μM	4.9 ± 0.2 μM
ASS234[a]	58.2 ± 1.2 nM	1.2 ± 0.1 μM	3.4 ± 0.2 μM	3.3 ± 0.2 μM
Clorgiline[a]	4.7 ± 0.2 nM	65.8 ± 1.6 μM	**	**
M30D[b]	7.7 ± 0.7 nM	7.9 ± 1.3 μM	0.5 ± 0.1 μM	44.9 ± 6.1 μM

[a]Bautista-Aguilera et al. (2014b).
[b]Zheng et al. (2010).
**Inactive at 100 μM (highest concentration tested).

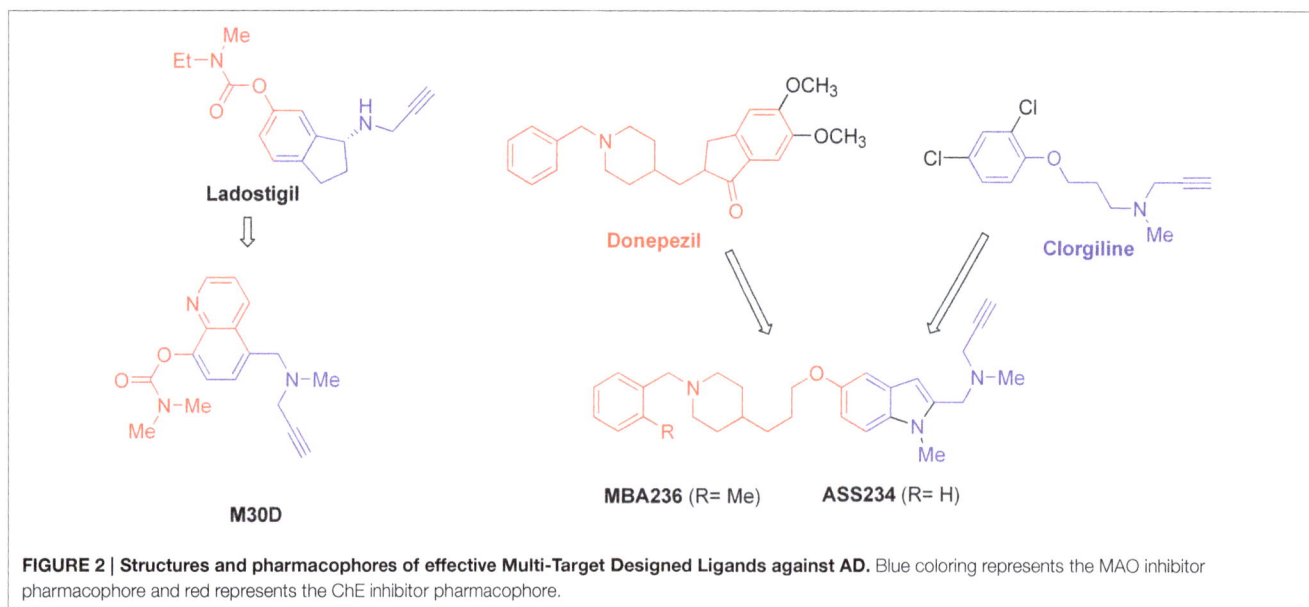

FIGURE 2 | Structures and pharmacophores of effective Multi-Target Designed Ligands against AD. Blue coloring represents the MAO inhibitor pharmacophore and red represents the ChE inhibitor pharmacophore.

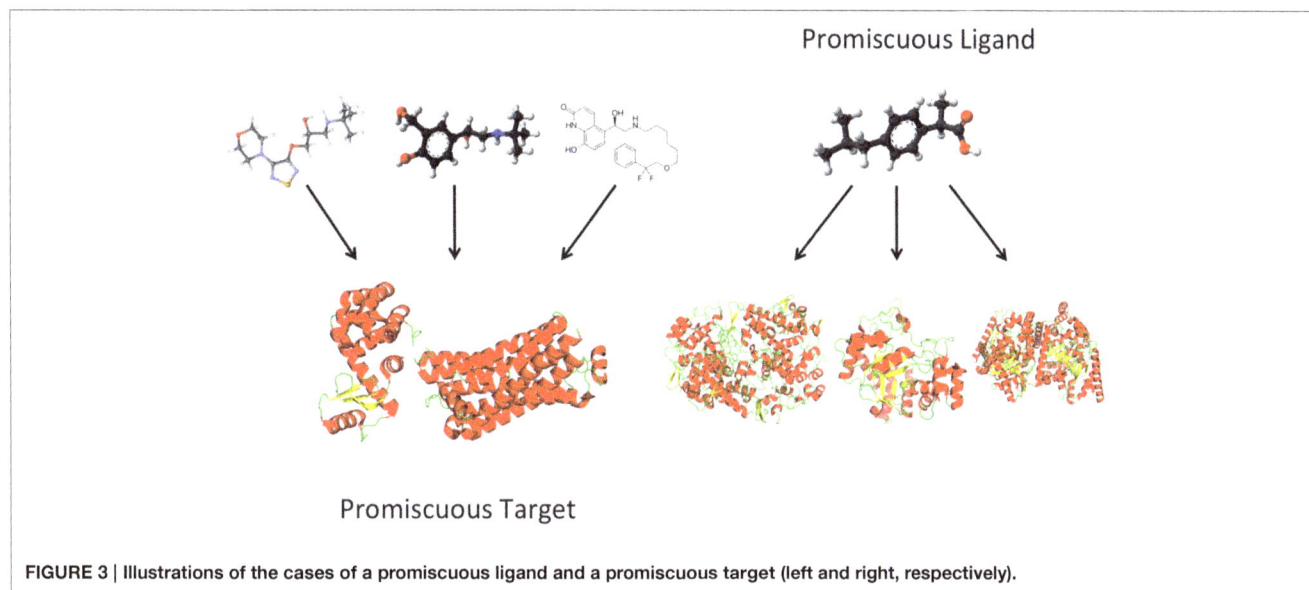

FIGURE 3 | Illustrations of the cases of a promiscuous ligand and a promiscuous target (left and right, respectively).

permitting more subtle modulation of its effect on a disease. Just as importantly, off-target prediction can identify likely side-effects (Lounkine et al., 2012) and adverse drug reactions (Bender et al., 2007).

Similarity-Based Methods

One of the core methodologies of cheminformatics is the use of molecular similarity to predict bioactivity. In the simplest single-target cases, an *in silico* library of chemical structures is compared with those chemical structures known to possess bioactivity against that protein. Molecules are usually represented by one of the many sets of fingerprints or descriptors (Steinbeck et al., 2003; Bender et al., 2004) that distil various chemical, topological and physicochemical properties of a molecular structure into a string of tens to hundreds of bits. This exercise is predicated on the Similar Property Principle, that structures close together in the vector space defined by the descriptors should possess similar chemical or biochemical properties. Thus, proximity in an arbitrary chemical space is used as a proxy for likely similarity of properties. This is an extremely common approach for lead identification.

Adaptation of Similarity Approaches to Off-Target Prediction

We have created our own similarity-based procedure that has two significant modifications and is particularly suitable for use on multi-target problems with some missing data. This workflow has been applied in our work to two specific problems: the identification of performance-enhancing molecules that should be prohibited in sports (Mavridis and Mitchell, 2013), and predicting multi-target bioactivities of potential polypharmacological compounds for treatment of neurological diseases (Nikolic et al., 2015b).

The first methodological modification is that we do not base our search on single known actives, but rather on families of compounds. We define our families on the twin criteria of bioactivity against a particular protein family and cluster membership (Mavridis et al., 2013) of structurally similar ligands. For each target, we obtain one or often more *refined families*, as we call them, of compounds sharing both a structural scaffold and a target-specific bioactivity in common.

Our second modification was to devise a quantitative method of estimating the probability that a given query molecule is associated with a particular bioactivity-scaffold combination defining one specific *refined family*. This allows us to make comparable predictions across both on-target and off-target activities based on the current 1,715,667 compounds and 10,774 targets in the ChEMBL database (Gaulton et al., 2012). Doing this requires us to create a common scale for the different affinity measures reported in the literature, (IC50, Ki, Kd, EC50, ED50, potency, activity, inhibition) relevant to bioactivity. We applied a number of rules in order to generate sets of molecules experimentally reported to be bioactive, given affinities defined using the eight different measures, separating these from sets of inactive molecules. Those empirical rules were derived by considering the distributions of the different affinity measures amongst reported active and inactive compounds. Subsequently, we use the Parzen-Rosenblatt (PR) (Rosenblatt, 1956; Parzen, 1962) kernel density estimation method to transform Tanimoto similarities into probabilities of family membership.

Our study of molecules related to doping in sport (Steinbeck et al., 2003) used protein target prediction to predict athletic performance-enhancing properties. In it, we demonstrated that the freely available ChEMBL database can be clustered into bioactivity-based refined families of ligands, using our clustering algorithm PFClust (Mavridis and Mitchell, 2013). These refined families consist of distinct sets of compounds, each set with its own molecular scaffold. For example, we separated the ligands for the beta-2 adrenergic receptor, a target hit by many beta blockers, into two distinct families with each ligand generating a high probability of belonging to just one or other of the two groups and a lower score for the alternative refined family, as shown in **Figure 4**. The use of such structurally distinct refined families significantly improved our method's performance in cross-validation, to the extent of giving encouraging concordance with experiment. Overall, two thirds of our test cases in cross-validation had the correct refined family as the number one prediction, and seven eighths had this "correct" family among the top four hits. We sometimes found many different scaffolds for one target; for the androgen receptor ligands PFClust generated 126 different refined families. Even where we have no experimental data, we can still undertake predictions of the likely bioactivity. We identified the protein targets corresponding to seven of the World Anti-Doping Agency's defined prohibited classes of compounds; we found a mixture of expected and surprising protein targets. Many of the apparently unexpected targets, however, turned out to have published biochemically or clinically validated links to the relevant bioactivities.

We recently studied (Nikolic et al., 2015b) multi-target ligands intended to interact with MAO A and B; acetylcholinesterase (AChE) and butyrylcholinesterase (BuChE); or with histamine N-methyltransferase (HMT) and histamine H3-receptor (H$_3$R). These enzymes are all potential drug targets for neurological conditions, including depression, Alzheimer's disease, obsessive disorders, and Parkinson's disease. Three groups of dual or multi-target compounds facilitated the generation of 3D-QSAR models for activity against the aforementioned protein targets. The first set of ligands consisted of novel carbonitrile–aminoheterocyclic compounds, designed to inhibit both MAO A and B. Amongst these, dicarbonitrile aminofuran derivatives were generally more selective MAO A inhibitors. The second group included acetylene-, indol-, piperidine- and pyridine-derivatives, which exhibited polypharmacology against MAO A/B, AChE, and BuChE. These agents are putative multitarget compounds against Alzheimer's disease. The third set of ligands contained multipotent histamine H3R antagonists that can concurrently inhibit HMT, and are therefore two-target procognitive compounds with potential therapeutic application against several psychiatric and neurodegenerative diseases. We used the Parzen–Rosenblatt kernel approach to build probabilistic models for both primary targets and off-targets, using data collected from the ChEMBL (Nikolic et al., 2015b) and DrugBank (Knox et al., 2011) databases. The cheminformatics-based target identifications agreed with four 3D-QSAR models for the various receptors, and with *in vitro* assays for serotonin 5-HT$_{1A}$ and 5HT$_{2A}$ receptor binding of the most promising ligand. As a result of this work, this and several other multi-target ligands were chosen for further investigation of their possible additional beneficial pharmacological activities.

Ain et al. (2014) used both protein and ligand descriptors to model the multi-target inhibitory profiles of serine proteinase inhibitors. They built separate sets of Random Forest (Breiman, 2001) models, some using only ligand descriptors, which they called "QSAR models," and others built using also protein descriptors, namely "proteochemometric (PCM) models". Across 12,625 inhibitors and 67 targets, they found that the models including protein descriptors performed substantially better than ligand-only ones, in terms of both R^2 (0.64 v 0.35) and root mean squared error (0.66 v 1.05 log units). They found that both the binding site amino acids and the protein sequence corresponded to important protein descriptors in their models.

Relationship to Protein Structure Prediction

Ain et al.'s finding that the best models require protein information (Ain et al., 2014) is particularly interesting. We recently asked *why* sequence-based protein function prediction methods work so effectively. For example, De Ferrari et al. obtained 98% prediction accuracy for enzyme function, based on transferring annotations from a query sequence's nearest neighbor of known function (De Ferrari et al., 2012). We have recently demonstrated that the majority of the predictive power of such sequence signature-based methods comes from the wealth of evolutionary information contained in the whole sequence, and only a small part of the predictive ability emanates from the many fewer functionally essential conserved residues (Beattie et al., 2015). In the context of polypharmacology and off-target interactions, structure-based methods of protein function prediction (Laskowski et al., 2005; Pal and Eisenberg, 2005; Cuff et al., 2011) are also highly relevant. Unexpected ligand-target interactions can be discovered by cross-docking the library of compounds into the active sites of the known structures of the various proteins (Favia et al., 2008; Patel et al., 2015). This methodology, however, requires an experimental protein structure, or at least a high-quality structural model, for the target, and is computationally much more expensive than cheminformatics.

As well as predicting interactions with a protein's major functional site, which we term orthosteric, it is also possible to predict allosteric ligand function. For example, van Westen et al. predicted allosteric behavior of compounds based on structural and chemical descriptors and data from ChEMBL (van Westen et al., 2014). As well as such predictions of allosteric molecules, it is also important to be able to predict which proteins will be amendable to allosteric proteins and which residues or clefts may be involved. We have recently used a Random Forest model to predict the presence of allosteric binding sites on proteins, based on structure, solvent accessibility and predicted binding affinity (Chen et al., 2016). Other predictions of allostery are derived from reduced models of protein dynamics, for instance using normal mode analysis (Panjkovich and Daura, 2012) or modeling energy flow within the protein structure (Erman, 2011).

VIRTUAL SCREENING OF MULTITARGET COMPOUNDS FOR CNS DISEASES

Virtual Screening (VS) is widely used in drug discovery to reduce the enormous compound collections to a more manageable number for further synthesis and biological *in vitro* testing (Alvarez, 2004). The application of computational technologies has allowed medicinal chemists to develop new drugs in a time and cost-effective manner. Two generally accepted VS methods used in Computer Aided Drug Design (CADD) are classified as Ligand-Based Virtual Screening (LB-VS) and Structure-Based Virtual Screening (SB-VS) (**Figure 5**; Wilson

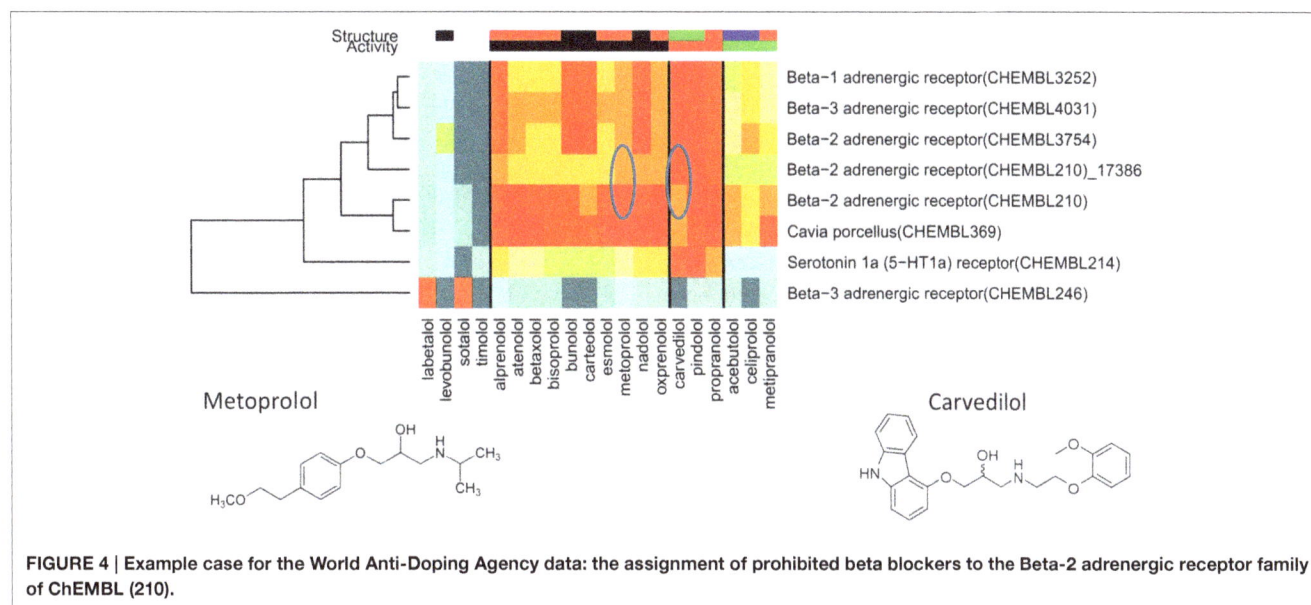

FIGURE 4 | Example case for the World Anti-Doping Agency data: the assignment of prohibited beta blockers to the Beta-2 adrenergic receptor family of ChEMBL (210).

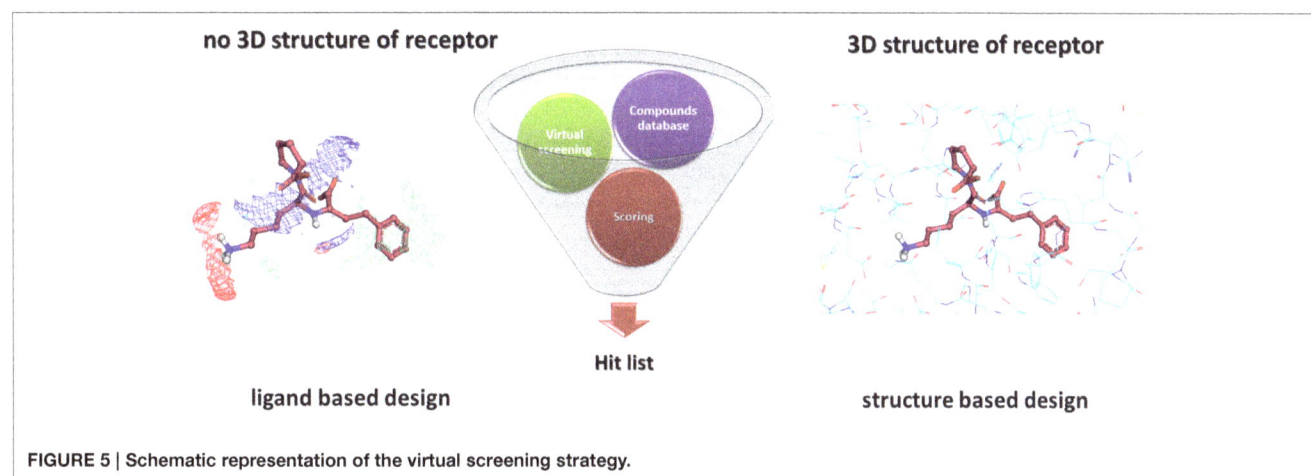

FIGURE 5 | Schematic representation of the virtual screening strategy.

and Lill, 2011). Ligand-based VS approaches are often applied when no structural information about the target protein is available and analyze the physicochemical similarity between large compound databases and known active molecules. On the other hand, the structure-based VS approach applies different modeling techniques, often including docking, to mimic the binding interaction of ligands to a biomolecular target. In both VS approaches, structures from virtual libraries or commercial databases are compared to the template and scored. In recent years, besides the individual application of ligand- and structure-based VS methods, combined techniques have also been proposed (Sperandio et al., 2008; Wilson and Lill, 2011). Even though docking is the most widely used approach in early phase drug discovery, a recent study has shown that ligand-based virtual screening methods in general yield a higher fraction of potent hits (Ripphausen et al., 2010). It is also important to note that hits with low nanomolar potency are rarely identified by VS (Eckert and Bajorath, 2007). However, compounds for further chemical exploration are predominantly provided.

Ligand-based VS applies two-dimensional (e.g., 2D-fingerprint) or three-dimensional (e.g., 3D-pharmacophore) searches between large compound databases and already known active molecules. This technique essentially neglects the target structure and allows a prioritization of molecules based on the Similar Property Principle, the assumption that compounds with similar descriptors tend to exhibit similar biological activity (Koeppen et al., 2011). Typically, topology-based descriptors of the known active compounds and the potential bioactive hits are compared to quantify molecular similarity. A major problem related to similarity methods is their bias toward input molecules and difficulty in making decision which structure to use as input (Venkatraman et al., 2010).

Beside similarity searching, the ligand-based pharmacophore method is also applied in VS. Pharmacophore models are usually built by using a set of structurally and functionally diverse ligands. This method is not only used to identify novel hit compounds, but also for profiling and anti-target modeling to avoid side-effects resulting from off-target activity (Schuster,

2010). However, ligand-based virtual screening is often applied in combination with structure-based approaches to identify potential hit molecules.

In contrast to ligand-based approaches, which allow the identification of chemically similar ligands, SBVS offers the possibility of discovering ligands with new scaffolds or chemical functional groups. SBVS categories, such as shape similarity, structure-based pharmacophores and docking, require knowledge of the three-dimensional structure of target protein. Structures for target proteins are usually obtained by X-ray crystallography or nuclear magnetic resonance (NMR) spectroscopy. In cases when this information does not exist, which is common in membrane receptors such as GPCRs, homology models can be used instead (Cavasotto, 2011). Structure-based pharmacophore models are developed on the basis of the active site and can be used to screen a compound database. Such pharmacophores are obtained by investigating all possible interaction sites in a binding pocket (Leach et al., 2010). Energy-based and geometry-based methods are applied to identify potentially important interaction sites and translate them into pharmacophore features. Typically, a binding pocket has a higher number of potential interaction sites than are normally observed actually being used in protein-ligand complexes.

The combination of the structure- and ligand-based VS strategies also occurs in many CADD studies (Drwal and Griffith, 2013). Sequential, parallel or hybrid combinations of VS techniques take into account all available chemical and biological information and thereby mitigate the drawbacks of each individual method (**Figure 6**; Hein et al., 2010; Wilson and Lill, 2011). Most of the recently published CADD studies apply a *sequential* VS approach (Khan et al., 2010; Weidlich et al., 2010; Drwal et al., 2011; Banoglu et al., 2012). In this approach ligand- and structure-based strategies are used in the VS protocol to gradually filter the large databases until the number of remaining potential hit compounds is small enough for biological testing. In *parallel combination* of VS methods, ligand- and structure-based strategies are run independently. Top ranked hit compounds are selected by a consensus aproach and processed for further biological testing. Benchmarking studies with retrospective analysis of performance have shown that successful application of parallel methods in VS is possible (Tan et al., 2008; Swann et al., 2011; Svensson et al., 2012). The *Hybrid VS approach* integrates ligand- and structure-based methods into one technique (protein-ligand pharmacophores) in order to enhance the accuracy of performance (Chen et al., 2010; Postigo et al., 2010; Spitzer et al., 2010; Drwal et al., 2011; Planesas et al., 2011).

During the last decade, many virtual screening methods have been developed and applied to discover novel potent ligands for the treatment of various neurological diseases. Several successful cases of reported virtual screening studies used to identify promising hits for CNS drugs discovery have been listed in **Table 5**. In this chapter we provide an overview of some of them that are significant from the polypharmacological point of view.

Lepailleur and co-workers applied pharmacophore-based virtual screening in combination with similarity based clustering method and molecular docking to identify dual

H_3R antagonist/$5HT_4R$ agonists (Lepailleur et al., 2014). Novel ligands would have potential for treatment of neurodegenerative diseases such as Alzheimer's disease. A three-dimensional pharmacophore model was constructed based on a set of six H3R antagonists developed by different pharmaceutical companies, using Catalyst software implemented in Discovery Studio 3.5 (Accelrys Inc., San Diego, CA, USA). This model was used as a search query for virtual screening of the CERMN chemical library (*www.cermn.unicaen.fr*) with a focus on serotonin (5-HT) "privileged structures". Binding experiments confirmed that benzo[h]-[1,6]naphthyridine ligands selected by this VS approach exert high affinity for both H3 and 5-HT_4 receptors. Recently, Bottegoni et al. carried out a virtual ligand screening protocol to identify fragments that display considerable activity at both β-secretase 1 (BACE-1) and glycogen synthase kinase 3β (GSK-3β) (Bottegoni et al., 2015). Discovery of multitarget drugs which are able to modulate BACE-1 and GSK-3 β activity simultaneously represents a promising strategy in the treatment of Alzheimer's disease. In this study, a VS approach based on docking simulations and Tanimoto similarity analysis was applied on the ZINC database (*www.zinc.docking.org*). Top ranked compounds selected by VS were tested *in vitro* and one with activitiy in the low-micromolar range at both enzymes was identified as a hit. Potential acetylcholinesterase inhibitors were also discovered using a virtual screening approach, in combination with molecular docking (Lu et al., 2011). Three-dimensional pharmacophore models were constructed based on a set of known AChE inhibitors. Virtual screening performed on the National Cancer Institute (NCI) compound database obtained nine new inhibitors that can block both catalytic and peripheral anionic sites of AChE. Designing or identifying dual-acting inhibitors that block both AChE binding sites is essential in preventing the degradation of acetylcholine in the brain and in protection of neurons from Abeta (Aβ) toxicity.

Finally it can be concluded that most of the recent successfully performed drug discovery studies used a sequential combination of ligand and structure-based virtual screening techniques, with particular focus on pharmacophore models and the docking approach.

Docking of Multi-Target Compounds for Neurodegenerative Diseases

Docking is a computational technique that predicts the preferred orientation of one molecule toward the other (Lengauer and Rarey, 1996). It is widely utilized as a hit identification and lead optimization tool, before compound synthesis, if the structure of the target is reliably known (Kitchen et al., 2004). In this chapter, the focus will be on some of the most commonly used docking software (**Table 6**).

Ligand-protein docking samples the conformations of small molecules—igands—in binding sites of proteins, and scoring functions are used to evaluate which of these conformations best fits the protein binding site (Warren et al., 2006). Thus, it calculates and ranks the complexes resulting from the association between a certain ligand and a target protein of known three-dimensional structure (Sousa et al., 2006). Initially

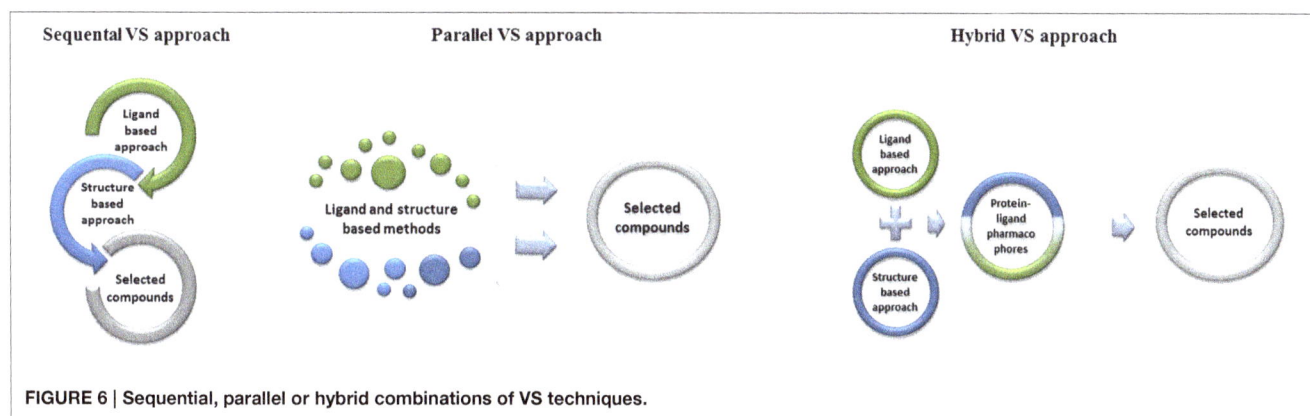

FIGURE 6 | Sequential, parallel or hybrid combinations of VS techniques.

TABLE 5 | Reported virtual screening studies used in CNS drug discovery.

Compounds	CNS diseases	Virtual screening method	Software package	References
BACE1 (beta-secretase 1) inhibitors	AD	SB approach based on pharmacophore model and molecular docking	LigandScout 1.03 www.inteligand.com GOLD 3.2 www.ccdc.cam.ac.uk	Vijayan et al., 2009
NK3 receptor antagonists	Schizophrenia; depression; anxiety	Sequential similarity analysis followed by CoMFA	ROCS 2.4.1. and 3.0 www.eyesopen.com	Geldenhuys et al., 2010
AChE inhibitors	AD	LB approach based on pharmacophore model and molecular docking	Discovery Studio 2.5.5 www.accelrys.com LibDock (Diller and Merz, 2001)	Lu et al., 2011
Human DOPA Decarboxylase Inhibitors	PD	SB approach based on pharmacophore model and molecular docking	MOE; Dovis 2.0; (Jiang et al., 2008) AutoDock Vina http://vina.scripps.edu/	Daidone et al., 2012
Histamine H_3 receptor ligands	PD; AD; epilepsy; sleeping disorders	LB and structure-based virtual fragment screening	FLAP www.moldiscovery.com	Sirci et al., 2012
MAO-B inhibitors	PD	LB virtual screening based on scaffold hopping approach	vROCS 3.0 www.eyesopen.com	Geldenhuys et al., 2012
SERT (serotonin transporter) Inhibitors	Depression	LB virtual screening based on two- and three-dimensional similarities; flexibile docking	JChem www.chemaxon.com Discovery studio	Gabrielsen et al., 2014
BuChE inhibitors	AD	LB virtual screening based on two- and three-dimensional similarities	LiSiCA	Lešnik et al., 2015
Serotonine 5-HT_6 antagonists	AD; schizophrenia; obesity	LB virtual approach based on two-dimensional similarities and pharmacophore model	InstJChem; JChemForExcel; www.chemaxon.com Phase-program www.schrodinger.com	Dobi et al., 2015
H_3R antagonist/5HT_4R agonist	AD	LB approach based on pharmacophore model similarity based clustering method and molecular docking	Discovery Studio 3.5 www.accelrys.com LibMCS http://www.chemaxon.com/jchem/doc/user/LibMCS.html Glide Induced-Fit Docking http://www.schrodinger.com/Induced-Fit/	Lepailleur et al., 2014
BACE-1/GSK-3 β activity	AD	SB approach based on molecular docking followed by Tanimoto ligand similarity	Monte Carlo stochastic optimizer implemented in ICM (Abagyan and Totrov, 1994)	Bottegoni et al., 2015

rigid docking was used, where both target and compound were rigid. However, advances in both software and computer power mean that full flexibility on the ligand can now be allowed, and this approach is the most popular now. There are three general kinds of algorithms formulated to apply ligand flexibility: systematic methods, random or stochastic methods, and simulation methods. Systematic search algorithms explore all the degrees of freedom in a molecule, random search

TABLE 6 | Recent docking studies employed to identify potential inhibitors for neurological targets.

Compounds	CNS diseases	Software package	References
MAO-A inhibitors	Depression	AutoDock http://autodock.scripps.edu/	Evranos-Aksoz et al., 2015
Metallothionein-III inhibitors	AD	Discovery Studio 2.5.5 www.accelrys.com	Roy et al., 2015
Sirtuin inhibitors	AD	GLIDE http://www.schrodinger.com/Glide	Karaman and Sippl, 2015
MAO-A, MAO-B, AChE, BuChE inhibitors	AD	GLIDE http://www.schrodinger.com/Glide	Bautista-Aguilera et al., 2014b,c
AMPK2 inhibitors	Stroke	AutoDock, FlexX http://autodock.scripps.edu/ https://www.biosolveit.de/FlexX/	Park et al., 2014
MAO- B inhibitors	PD, AD	AutoDock, GOLD, LibDock	Yelekci et al., 2013
Dopamine transporter inhibitors	ADHD, PD, depression and addiction	MOE https://www.chemcomp.com/	Schmitt et al., 2010

algorithms explore the conformational space by applying random changes to a single ligand or a group of ligands, and simulation methods utilize a different approach to the docking process such as molecular dynamics (MD) or energy minimization methods (Sousa et al., 2006). Also, many scoring functions have been reported over the years, and classified as force-field-based, empirical, and knowledge-based. The first category uses available force fields to calculate the direct interactions between protein and ligand atoms (frequently comprising the non-covalent energy terms covering the electrostatic energy, the van der Waals (vdW), and hydrogen bonding). Secondly, an empirical scoring function calculates the fitness of protein—ligand binding by summing up the contributions of various individual terms, each representing a significant energetic factor in protein—ligand binding. The third type of method utilizes pairwise statistical potentials between protein and ligand, based on the occurrence frequencies of particular atom-atom interaction frequencies in databases of protein-ligand complex structures (Mitchell et al., 1999). Recently, methods that bring pharmacophore and structure—activity relationship (SAR) analysis into protein—ligand interaction assessment have been introduced, representing new trends in this field (Hu and Lill, 2014).

Today, there are numerous docking software packages available, based on different search algorithms and scoring functions. None of the existing docking programs and scoring functions is uniquely excellent and the improvements are still continuing. The best way is to apply several docking programs in order to reduce the artifacts. The three widely used software tools are CDOCKER (Wu et al., 2003), GOLD (Jones et al., 1995) and AutoDock (Morris et al., 1998, 2009).

The usage of docking tools in discovery of novel compounds for neurodegenerative diseases could be explained through the example of our study on MAO -A and B inhibitors. The crystal structure of human MAO-A (hMAO-A) complexed with the reversible inhibitor harmine (PDB 2Z5X) (Son et al., 2008) and the crystal structure of human MAO-B (hMAO-B) co-crystallized with the reversible inhibitor safinamide (PDB 2V5Z) (Binda et al., 2007) were extracted from the Protein Data Bank (PDB) (Berman et al., 2000; http://www.rcsb.org) for protein setup. Studies were carried out on only one

subunit of the enzymes. Each structure was cleaned of all water molecules and inhibitors and all non-interacting ions were removed before being used in the docking studies. For each protein, all hydrogens were added and the protein is minimized using the Discovery Studio protocol (accelrys.com), assigning a CHARMM force field. Missing hydrogen atoms were added on the basis of the protonation state of the titratable residues at a pH of 7.4. Ionic strength was set to 0.145 and the dielectric constant was set to 10. Molecular models of the inhibitors were built and optimized using SPARTAN 10.0. Docking was performed using AutoDock 4.2. For coordinates of the binding pocket, the N5 atom of the FAD molecule was taken, and the chosen region covers the entire binding site and its neighboring residues. Compounds were docked in both MAO-A and MAO-B and the selectivity was compared. To study the binding pose of these compounds, several representative ligands were chosen, the important interactions were visualized in the Accelrys Visualization 4.5. program. Analysis of binding modes revealed that aromatic groups of these compounds in hydrophobic cage of MAO-A and MAO-B enzymes were important for affinity (**Figures 7**, **8**; Evranos-Aksoz et al., 2015).

CONCLUDING REMARKS

Extensive use of computational methods such as data mining, cheminformatics, QSAR modeling, virtual screening and docking, provide a time and cost efficient drug discovery processes.

These methods have become an integral part of drug discovery. A wide range of computational tools is being developed and used to obtain hits that are more likely to give potential clinical candidates. However, despite their success, both ligand- and structure-based techniques face challenges and limitations that should be considered during application. In recent years, integration of various cheminformatic, QSAR, virtual screening and docking protocols has become very popular, since it enhances their strength and applicability. This chapter focuses on various computation methodologies successfully applied in CNS drug discovery processes, such as

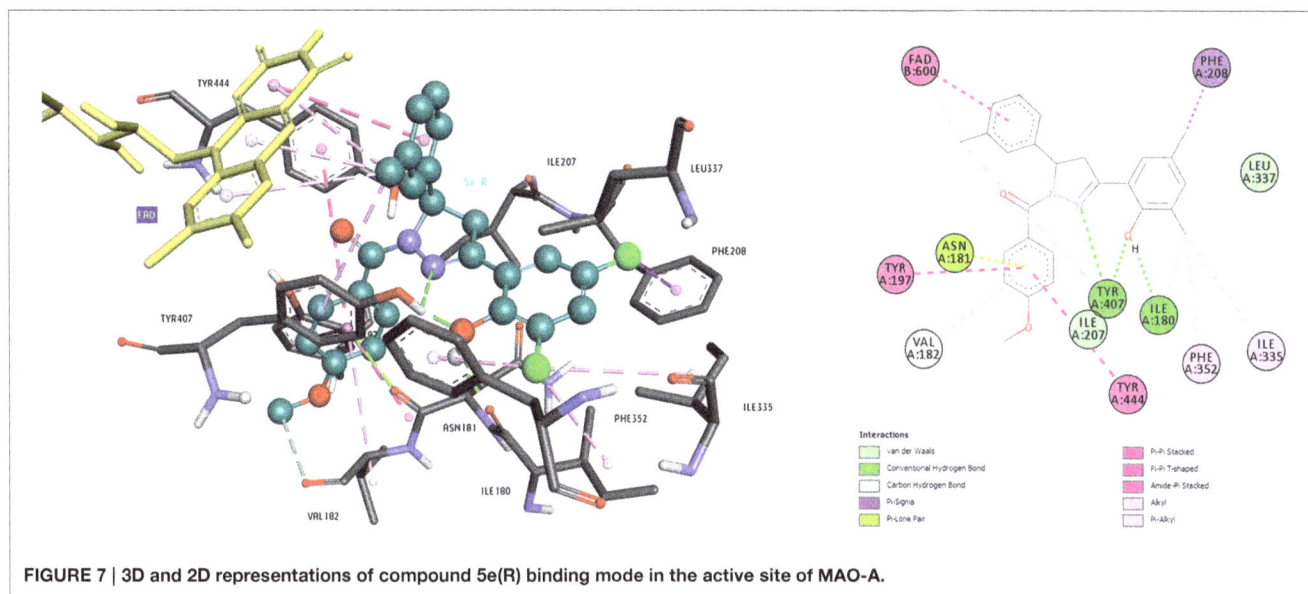

FIGURE 7 | 3D and 2D representations of compound 5e(R) binding mode in the active site of MAO-A.

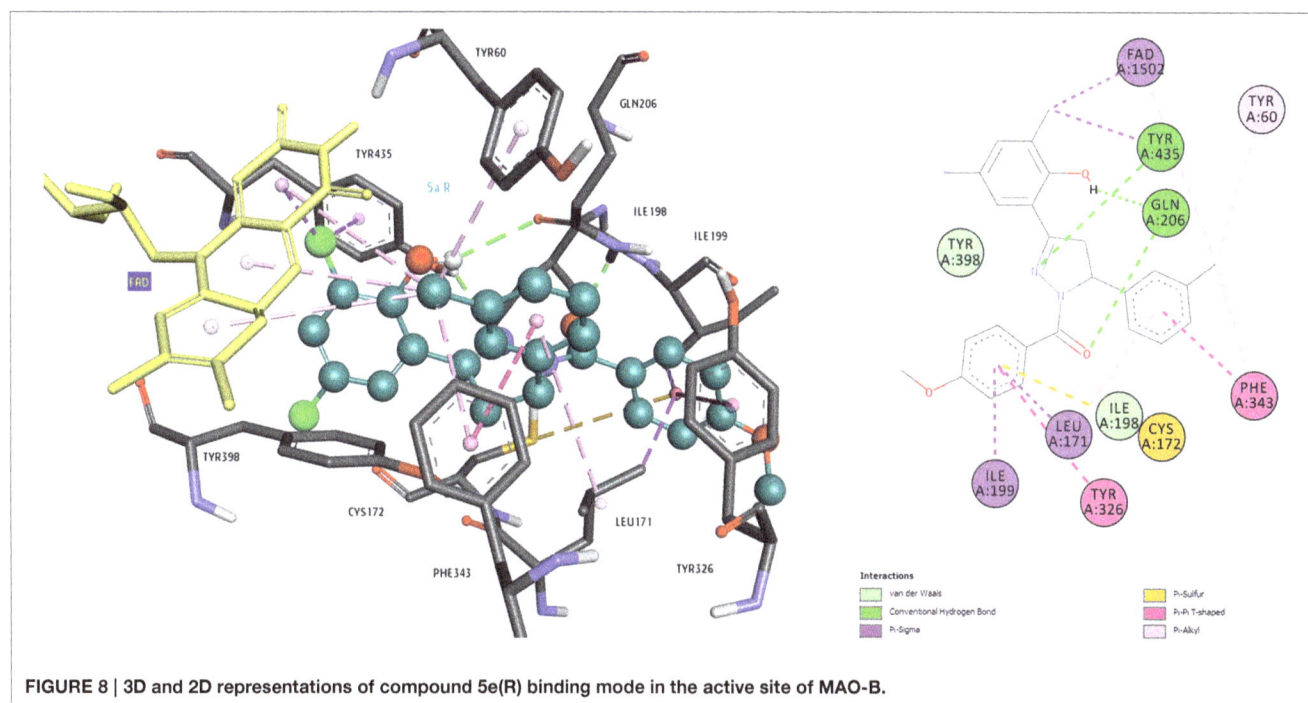

FIGURE 8 | 3D and 2D representations of compound 5e(R) binding mode in the active site of MAO-B.

design of novel donepezil–indolyl hybrids, N-Methyl-N-((1-methyl-5-(3-(1-(2-methylbenzyl)piperidin-4-yl)propoxy)-1H-indol-2-yl)methyl)prop-2-yn-1-amine, and donepezil-pyridyl hybrids, as multitarget inhibitors of acetylcholine esterase and MAO (AChE/BuChE/MAO-A/MAO-B) that were effective drug candidates for therapy of neurodegenerative Alzheimer's (AD) and Parkinson's diseases (PD).

Detailed analysis of the recently reported case studies revealed that the majority of them use a sequential combination of ligand and structure-based virtual screening techniques, with particular focus on pharmacophore models and the docking approach.

AUTHOR CONTRIBUTIONS

All authors contributed to the conception and interpretation of the work and to its critical revision. All authors have approved the final version and may be held accountable for the integrity of this review of current literature.

ACKNOWLEDGMENTS

Support was kindly provided by the EU COST Action CM1103. DA, KN, and JV kindly acknowledge national project number 172033 and OI1612039 supported by the Ministry of the Republic of Serbia. TD and KY kindly acknowledge "Training in Neurodegeneration, Therapeutics, Intervention and Neurorepair" project number 608381 funded by Marie Skłodowska-Curie action, funding scheme: FP7-MC-ITN.

REFERENCES

Abagyan, R., and Totrov, M. (1994). Biased probability Monte Carlo conformational searches and electrostatic calculations for peptides and proteins. *J. Mol. Biol.* 235, 983–1002. doi: 10.1006/jmbi.1994.1052

Acharya, C., Coop, A., Polli, J. E., and Mackerell, A. D. Jr. (2011). Recent advances in ligand based drug design: relevance and utility of the conformationally sampled pharmacophore approach. *Curr. Comput. Aided Drug Des.* 7, 10–22. doi: 10.2174/157340911793743547

Ain, Q. U., Mendez-Lucio, O., Ciriano, I. C., Malliavin, T., van Westen, G. J. P., and Bender, A. (2014). Modelling ligand selectivity of serine proteases using integrative proteochemometric approaches improves model performance and allows the multi-target dependent interpretation of features. *Integr. Biol.* 6, 1023–1033. doi: 10.1039/c4ib00175c

Alelyunas, Y. W., Empfield, J. R., McCarthy, D., Spreen, R. C., Bui, K., Pelosi-Kilby, L., et al. (2010). Experimental solubility profiling of marketed CNS drugs, exploring solubility limit of CNS discovery candidate. *Bioorg. Med. Chem. Lett.* 20, 7312–7316. doi: 10.1016/j.bmcl.2010.10.068

Alvarez, J. C. (2004). High-throughput docking as a source of novel drug leads. *Curr. Opin. Chem. Biol.* 8, 365–370. doi:10.1016/j.cbpa.2004.05.001

Amato, D. (2015). Serotonin in antipsychotic drugs action. *Behav. Brain Res.* 277C, 125–135. doi: 10.1016/j.bbr.2014.07.025

Anighoro, A., Bajorath, J., and Rastelli, G. (2014). Polypharmacology: challenges and opportunities in drug discovery. *J. Med. Chem.* 57, 7874–7887. doi: 10.1021/jm5006463

Apelt, J., Grassmann, S., Ligneau, X., Pertz, H. H., Ganellin, C. R., Arrang, J. M., et al. (2005). Search for histamine H3 receptor antagonists with combined inhibitory potency at Ntau-methyltransferase: ether derivatives. *Pharmazie* 60, 97–106.

Apelt, J., Ligneau, X., Pertz, H. H., Arrang, J. M., Ganellin, C. R., Schwartz, J. C., et al. (2002). Development of a new class of nonimidazole histamine H(3) receptor ligands with combined inhibitory histamine N-methyltransferase activity. *J. Med. Chem.* 45, 1128–1141. doi: 10.1021/jm0110845

Bajda, M., Guzior, N., Ignasik, M., and Malawska, B. (2011). Multi-target-directed ligands in Alzheimer's disease treatment. *Curr. Med. Chem.* 18, 4949–4975. doi: 10.2174/092986711797535245

Banoglu, E., ÇaliÅ§kan, B., Luderer, S., Eren, G., Özkan, Y., Altenhofen, W., et al. (2012). Identification of novel benzimidazole derivatives as inhibitors of leukotriene biosynthesis by virtual screening targeting 5-lipoxygenase-activating protein (FLAP). *Bioorg. Med. Chem.* 20, 3728–3374. doi:10.1016/j.bmc.2012.04.048

Bautista-Aguilera, O. M., Esteban, G., Bolea, I., Nikolic, K., Agbaba, D., Moraleda, I., et al. (2014a). Design, synthesis, pharmacological evaluation, QSAR analysis, molecular modeling and ADMET of novel donepezil–indolyl hybrids as multipotent cholinesterase/monoamine oxidase inhibitors for the potential treatment of Alzheimer's disease. *Eur. J. Med. Chem.* 75, 82–95. doi: 10.1016/j.ejmech.2013.12.028

Bautista-Aguilera, O. M., Esteban, G., Chioua, M., Nikolic, K., Agbaba, D., Moraleda, I., et al. (2014c). Multipotent cholinesterase/monoamine oxidase inhibitors for the treatment of Alzheimer's disease: design, synthesis, biochemical evaluation, ADMET, molecular modeling, and QSAR analysis of novel donepezil-pyridyl hybrids. *Drug Des. Dev. Ther.* 8, 1893–1910. doi: 10.2147/DDDT.S69258

Bautista-Aguilera, O. M., Samadi, A., Chioua, M., Nikolic, K., Filipic, S., Agbaba, D., et al. (2014b). N-Methyl-N-((1-methyl-5-(3-(1-(2-methylbenzyl)piperidin-4-yl)propoxy)-1H-indol-2-yl)methyl)prop-2-yn-1-amine, a new cholinesterase and monoamine oxidase dual inhibitor *J. Med. Chem.* 57, 10455–10463. doi: 10.1021/jm501501a

Beattie, K. E., De Ferrari, L., and Mitchell, J. B. O. (2015). Why do sequence signatures predict enzyme mechanism? Homology versus chemistry. *Evol. Bioinform.* 11, 267–274. doi: 10.4137/ebo.s31482

Bender, A., Mussa, H. Y., Glen, R. C., and Reiling, S. (2004). Molecular similarity searching using atom environments, information-based feature selection and a naive bayesian classifier. *J. Chem. Inf. Comput. Sci.* 44, 170–178. doi: 10.1021/ci034207y

Bender, A., Scheiber, J., Glick, M., Davies, J. W., Azzaoui, K., Hamon, J., et al. (2007). Analysis of pharmacology data and the prediction of adverse drug reactions and off-target effects from chemical structure. *ChemMedChem.* 2, 861–873. doi: 10.1002/cmdc.200700026

Berman, H. M., Westbrook, J., Feng, Z., Gilliland, G., Bhat, T. N., Weissig, H., et al. (2000). The protein data bank. *Nucleic Acids Res.* 28, 235–242. doi: 10.1093/nar/28.1.235

Besnard, J., Ruda, G. F., Setola, V., Abecassis, K., Rodriguiz, R. M., Huang, X. P., et al. (2012). Automated design of ligands to polypharmacological profiles. *Nature* 492, 215–220. doi: 10.1038/nature11691

Binda, C., Wang, J., Pisani, L., Caccia, C., Carotti, A., Salvati, P., et al. (2007). Structures of human monoamine oxidase B complexes with selective noncovalent inhibitors: safinamide and coumarin analogs. *J. Med. Chem.* 50, 5848–5852. doi: 10.1021/jm070677y

Bolea, I., Gella, A., Monjas, L., Pérez, C., Rodríguez-Franco, M. I., Marco-Contelles, J., et al. (2013). Multipotent, permeable drug ASS234 inhibits Aβ aggregation, possesses antioxidant properties and protects from Abeta-induced apoptosis *in vitro*. *Curr. Alzh. Res.* 10, 797–808. doi: 10.2174/15672050113109990151

Bolea, I., Juarez-Jimenez, J., de los Rios, C., Chioua, M., Pouplana, R., Luque, F. J., et al. (2011). Synthesis, biological evaluation, and molecular modeling of donepezil and N-[(5-(Benzyloxy)-1-methyl-1H-indol-2-yl)methyl]-nmethylprop-2-yn-1-amine hybrids as new multipotent cholinesterase/monoamine oxidase inhibitors for the treatment of Alzheimer's disease. *J. Med. Chem.* 54, 8251–8270. doi: 10.1021/jm200853t

Boran, A. D. W., and Iyengar, R. (2010). Systems approaches to polypharmacology and drug discovery. *Curr. Opin. Drug Disc.* 13, 297–309.

Bottegoni, G., Veronesi, M., Bisignano, P., Kacker, P., Favia, A. D., and Cavalli, A. (2015). Development and application of a virtual screening protocol for the identification of multitarget fragments. *ChemMedChem.* doi: 10.1002/cmdc.201500521. [Epub ahead of print].

Bourne, J. A. (2001). SCH 23390: the first selective dopamine D1-like receptor antagonist. *CNS Drug. Rev.* 7, 399–414. doi: 10.1111/j.1527-3458.2001.tb00207.x

Breiman, L. (2001). Random forests. *Mach. Learn.* 45, 5–32. doi: 10.1023/a:1010933404324

Brunton, L., Chabner, B., and Knollman, B. (2011). *Goodman and Gilman's the Pharmacological Basis of Therapeutics.* The McGraw-Hill Companies, Inc.

Buckley, P. F. (2003). Aripirazole: efficacy and tolerability profile of a novel-acting atypical antipsychotic. *Drug. Today* 39, 145–151. doi: 10.1358/dot.2003.39.2.799421

Carlsson, M., and Carlsson, A. (1990). Interactions between glutamatergic and monoaminergic systems within the basal ganglia - implications for schizophrenia and Parkinson 's disease. *Trends Neurosci.* 13, 272–276.

Cavasotto, C. N. (2011). Homology models in docking and high-throughput docking. *Curr. Top Med. Chem.* 11, 1528–1534. doi: 10.2174/156802611795860951

Chen, A. S. Y., Westwood, N. J., Brear, P., Rogers, G. W., Mavridis, L., and Mitchell, J. B. O. (2016). A random forest model for predicting allosteric and functional sites on proteins. *Mol. Inf.* 35, 125–136. doi: 10.1002/minf.201500108

Chen, B., Wild, D., and Guha, R. (2009). PubChem as a source of polypharmacology. *J. Chem. Inf. Model.* 49, 2044–2055. doi: 10.1021/ci9001876

Chen, Z., Tian, G., Wang, Z., Jiang, H., Shen, J., and Zhu, W. (2010). Multiple pharmacophore models combined with molecular docking: a reliable way for efficiently identifying novel PDE4 inhibitors with high structural diversity. *J. Chem. Inf. Model.* 50, 615–625. doi: 10.1021/ci9004173

Cherkasov, A., Muratov, E. N., Fourches, D., Varnek, A., Baskin, I. I., Cronin, M., et al. (2014). QSAR modeling: where have you been? Where are you going to? *J. Med. Chem.* 57, 4977–5010. doi: 10.1021/jm4004285

Coburg, Y., Kottke, T., Weizel, L., Ligneau, X., and Stark, H. (2009). Potential utility of histamine H3 receptor antagonist pharmacophore in antipsychotics. *Bioorg. Med. Chem. Lett.* 19, 538–542. doi: 10.1016/j.bmcl.2008.09.012

Craig, P. N. (1971). Interdependence between physical parameters and selection of substituent groups for correlation studies. *J. Med. Chem.* 14, 680–684.

Cramer, R. D. (2012). The inevitable QSAR renaissance. *J. Comp. Aided Mol. Des.* 26, 35–38. doi: 10.1007/s10822-011-9495-0

Cramer, R. D., Patterson, D. E., and Bunce, J. D. (1988). Comparative molecular field analysis (CoMFA). 1. Effect of shape on binding of steroids to carrier proteins. *J. Am. Chem. Soc.* 110, 5959–5967. doi: 10.1021/ja00226a005

Cuff, A., Redfern, O., Dessailly, B., and Orengo, C. A. (2011). "Exploiting protein structures to predict protein functions," in *Protein Function Prediction for Omics Era*, ed D. Kihara (Dordrecht: Springer Netherlands), 107–123.

Dai, H., Fu, Q., Shen, Y., Hu, W., Zhang, Z., Timmerman, H., et al. (2007). The histamine H3 receptor antagonist clobenpropit enhances GABA release to protect against NMDA induced excitotoxicity through the cAMP/protein kinase A pathway in cultured cortical neurons. *Eur. J. Pharmacol.* 563, 117–123. doi:10.1016/j.ejphar.2007.01.069

Daidone, F., Montioli, R., Paiardini, A., Cellini, B., Macchiarulo, A., Giardina, G., et al. (2012). Identification by virtual screening and *in vitro* testing of human DOPA decarboxylase inhibitors. *PLoS ONE* 7:e31610. doi: 10.1371/journal.pone.0031610

Decker, M. (2007). Recent advances in the development of hybrid molecules/designed multiple compounds with antiamnesic properties. *Mini-Rev. Med. Chem.* 7, 221–229. doi: 10.2174/138955707780059817

De Ferrari, L., Aitken, S., van Hemert, J., and Goryanin, I. (2012). EnzML: multi-label prediction of enzyme classes using InterPro signatures. *BMC Bioinformatics* 13:61. doi: 10.1186/1471-2105-13-61

Desai, P. V., Sawada, G. A., Watson, I. A., and Raub, T. J. (2013). Integration of *in silico* and *in vitro* tools for scaffold optimization during drug discovery: predicting P-glycoprotein efflux. *Mol. Pharmaceut.* 10, 1249–1261. doi: 10.1021/mp300555n

Di Giovanni, G., Di Matteo, V., Pierucci, M., and Esposito, E. (2008). Serotonin-dopamine interaction: electrophysiological evidence. *Prog. Brain Res.* 172, 45–71. doi: 10.1016/S0079-6123(08)00903-5

Diller, D. J., and Merz, K. M. (2001). High throughput docking for library design and library prioritization. *Proteins* 43, 113–124. doi: 10.1002/1097-0134(20010501)43:2<113::AID-PROT1023>3.0.CO;2-T

Di Matteo, V., Di Giovanni, G., Pierucci, M., and Esposito, E. (2008). Serotonin control of central dopaminergic function: focus on *in vivo* microdialysis studies. *Prog. Brain Res.* 172, 7–44. doi: 10.1016/S0079-6123(08)00902-3

Dixon, S. L., Smondyrev, A. M., and Rao, S. N. (2006). PHASE: a novel approach to pharmacophore modeling and 3D database searching. *Chem. Biol. Drug Des.* 67, 370–372. doi: 10.1111/j.1747-0285.2006.00384.x

Dobi, K., Flachner, B., Pukáncsik, M., Máthé, E., Bognár, M., Szaszkó, M., et al. (2015). Combination of pharmacophore matching, 2D similarity search, and *in vitro* biological assays in the selection of potential 5-HT6 antagonists from large commercial repositories. *Chem. Biol. Drug Des.* 86, 864–880. doi: 10.1111/cbdd.12563

Don, C. G., and Riniker, S. (2014). Scents and sense: *in silico* perspectives on olfactory receptors. *J. Comp. Chem.* 35, 2279–2287. doi: 10.1002/jcc.23757

Drwal, M. N., Agama, K., Wakelin, L. P., Pommier, Y., and Griffith, R. (2011). Exploring DNA topoisomerase I ligand space in search of novel anticancer agents. *PLoS ONE* 6:25150. doi: 10.1371/journal.pone.0025150

Drwal, M. N., and Griffith, R. (2013). Combination of ligand- and structure-based methods in virtual screening. *Drug Discov. Today Technol.* 10, e395–e401. doi: 10.1016/j.ddtec.2013.02.002

Durán, A., Zamora, I., and , Pastor, M. (2009). Suitability of GRIND-based principal properties for the description of molecular similarity and ligand-based virtual screening. *J. Chem. Inf. Model.* 49, 2129–2138. doi: 10.1021/ci900228x

Eckert, H., and Bajorath, J. (2007). Molecular similarity analysis in virtual screening: foundations, limitations and novel approaches. *Drug Discov. Today* 12, 225–233. doi:10.1016/j.drudis.2007.01.011

Erman, B. (2011). Relationships between ligand binding sites, protein architecture and correlated paths of energy and conformational fluctuations. *Phys. Biol.* 8:056003. doi: 10.1088/1478-3975/8/5/056003

Esbenshade, T. A., Browman, K. E., Bitner, R. S., Strakhova, M., Cowart, M. D., and Brioni, J. D. (2008). The histamine H3 receptor: an attractive target for the treatment of cognitive disorders. *Brit. J. Pharmacol.* 154, 1166–1181. doi: 10.1038/bjp.2008.147

Evranos-Aksoz, B., Baysal, Äř., Yabanoğlu-Çiftçi, S., Djikic, T., Yelekçi, K., Uçar, G., et al. (2015). Synthesis and screening of human Monoamine Oxidase-A inhibitor effect of new 2-pyrazoline and hydrazine derivatives. *Arch. Pharm. Chem. Life Sci.* 348, 1–14. doi: 10.1002/ardp.201500212

Favia, A. D., Nobeli, I., Glaser, F., and Thornton, J. M. (2008). Molecular docking for substrate identification: the short-chain dehydrogenases/reductases. *J. Mol. Biol.* 375, 855–874. doi: 10.1016/j.jmb.2007.10.065

Gabrielsen, M., Kurczab, R., Siwek, A., Wolak, M., Ravna, A. W., Kristiansen, K., et al. (2014). Identification of novel serotonin transporter compounds by virtual screening. *J. Chem. Inf. Model.* 54, 933–943. doi: 10.1021/ci400742s

Garduno-Torres, B., Treviño, M., Gutiérrez, R., and Arias-Montaño, J. A. (2007). Presynaptic histamine H3 receptors regulate glutamate, but not GABA release in rat thalamus. *Neuropharmacology* 52, 527–535. doi:10.1016/j.neuropharm.2006.08.001

Gaulton, A., Bellis, L. J., Bento, P. A., Chambers, J., Davies, M., Hersey, A., et al. (2012). ChEMBL: a large-scale bioactivity database for drug discovery. *Nucleic Acids Res.* 40, D1100–D1107. doi: 10.1093/nar/gkr777

Geldenhuys, W. J., Funk, M. O., Van der Schyf, C. J., and Carroll, R. T. (2012). A scaffold hopping approach to identify novel monoamine oxidase B inhibitors. *Bioorg. Med. Chem. Lett.* 22, 1380–1383. doi: 10.1016/j.bmcl.2011.12.056

Geldenhuys, W. J., Kuzenko, S. R., and Simmons, M. A. (2010). Virtual screening to identify novel antagonists for the G protein-coupled NK3 receptor. *J. Med. Chem.* 53, 8080–8088. doi:10.1021/jm1010012

Gemkow, M. J., Davenport, A. J., Harich, S., Ellenbroek, B. A., Cesura, A., and Hallett, D. (2009). The histamine H3 receptor as a therapeutic drug target for CNS disorders. *Drug Discov. Today* 14, 509–515. doi: 10.1016/j.drudis.2009.02.011

Ghose, A. K., Herbertz, T., Hudkins, R. L., Dorsey, B. D., and Mallamo, J. P. (2012). Knowledge-based, central nervous system (CNS) lead selection and lead optimization for CNS drug discovery. *ACS Chem. Neurosci.* 3, 50–68. doi: 10.1021/cn200100h

Gleeson, M. P. (2008). Generation of a set of simple, interpretable ADMET rules of thumb. *J. Med. Chem.* 51, 817–834. doi: 10.1021/jm701122q

Goedert, M., and Spillantini, M. G. A. (2006). A century of Alzheimer's disease. *Science* 314, 777–781. doi: 10.1126/science.1132814

Gohlke, H., and Klebe, G. (2002). DrugScore meets CoMFA: adaptation of fields for molecular comparison (AFMoC) or how to tailor knowledge-based pair-potentials to a particular protein. *J. Med. Chem.* 45, 4153–4170. doi: 10.1021/jm020808p

González-Díaz, H., Prado-Prado, F., and Ubeira, F. M. (2012). Predicting antimicrobial drugs and targets with the MARCH-INSIDE approach. *Curr. Top. Med Chem.* 8, 1676–1690. doi: 10.2174/156802608786786543

Goodford, P. J. (1985). A computational procedure for determining energetically favorable binding sites on biologically important macromolecules. *J. Med. Chem.* 28, 849–857.

Grassmann, S., Apelt, J., Ligneau, X., Pertz, H. H., Arrang, J. M., Ganellin, C. R., et al. (2004). Search for histamine H(3) receptor ligands with combined inhibitory potency at histamine N-methyltransferase: omega-piperidinoalkanamine derivatives. *Arch. Pharm. (Weinheim)* 337, 533–545. doi: 10.1002/ardp.200400897

Grassmann, S., Apelt, J., Sippl, W., Ligneau, X., Pertz, H. H., Zhao, Y. H., et al. (2003). Imidazole derivatives as a novel class of hybrid compounds with inhibitory histamine N-methyltransferase potencies and histamine H3 receptor affinities. *Bioorgan. Med. Chem.* 11, 2163–2174. doi:10.1016/S0968-0896(03)00120-2

Hajjo, R., Grulke, C. M., Golbraikh, A., Setola, V., Huang, X. P., Roth, B. L., et al. (2010). Development, validation, and use of quantitative structure-activity relationship models of 5-hydroxytryptamine (2B) receptor ligands to identify novel receptor binders and putative valvulopathic compounds among common drugs. *J. Med. Chem.* 53, 7573–7586. doi: 10.1021/jm100600y

Hajjo, R., Setola, V., Roth, B. L., and Tropsha, A. (2012). Chemocentric informatics approach to drug discovery: identification and experimental validation of selective estrogen receptor modulators as ligands of 5-hydroxytryptamine-6 receptors and as potential cognition enhancers. *J. Med. Chem.* 55, 5704–5719. doi: 10.1021/jm2011657

Hamacher, A., Weigt, M., Wiese, M., Hoefgen, B., Lehmann, J., and Kassack, M. U. (2006). Dibenzazecine compounds with a novel dopamine/5-HT2A receptor profile and 3D-QSAR analysis. *BMC Pharmacol.* 15, 6–11. doi: 10.1186/1471-2210-6-11

Hansch, C., Maloney, P. P., Fujita, T., and Muir, R. M. (1962). Correlation of biological activity of phenoxyacetic acids with hammett substituent constants and partition coefficients. *Nature* 194, 178–180. doi:10.1038/194178b0

Hansch, C., Unger, S. H., and Forsythe, A. B. (1973). Strategy in drug design. Cluster analysis as an aid in the selection of substituents. *J. Med. Chem.* 16, 1217–1222.

Hein, M., Zilian, D., and Sotriffer, C. A. (2010). Docking compared to 3D pharmacophores: the scoring function challenge. *Drug Discov. Today* 7, e229–e239. doi:10.1016/j.ddtec.2010.12.003

Hitchcock, S. A. (2012). Structural modifications that alter the P-glycoprotein efflux properties of compounds. *J. Med. Chem.* 55, 4877–4895. doi: 10.1021/jm201136z

Hitchcock, S. A., and Pennington, L. D. (2006). Structure-brain exposure relationships. *J. Med. Chem.* 49, 7559–7583. doi: 10.1021/jm060642i

Hopkins, A. L. (2008). Network pharmacology: the next paradigm in drug discovery. *Nat. Chem. Biol.* 4, 682–690. doi: 10.1038/nchembio.118

Hu, B., and Lill, M. A. (2014). PharmDock: a pharmacophore -based docking program. *J. Cheminform.* 6:14. doi: 10.1186/1758-2946-6-14

Humbert-Claude, M., Morisset, S., Gbahou, F., and Arrang, J. M. (2007). Histamine H3 and dopamine D2 receptor-mediated [35S]GTPγ[S] binding in rat striatum: evidence for additive effects but lack of interactions. *Biochem. Pharmacol.* 73, 1172–1181. doi:10.1016/j.bcp.2007.01.006

Jiang, X., Kumar, K., Hu, X., Wallqvist, A., and Reifman, J. (2008). DOVIS 2.0: an efficient and easy to use parallel virtual screening tool based on AutoDock 4.0. *Chem. Cent. J* 2, 18. doi: 10.1186/1752-153X-2-18

Johnson, D. S., Choi, C., Fay, L. K., Favor, D. A., Repine, J. T., White, A. D., et al. (2011). Discovery of PF-00217830: aryl piperazine napthyridinones as D2 agonists for schizophrenia and bipolar disorder. *Bioorg. Med. Chem. Lett.* 21, 2621–2625. doi: 10.1016/j.bmcl.2011.01.059

Jones, G., Willett, P., and Glen, R. C. (1995). Molecular recognition of receptor sites using a genetic algorithm with a description of desolvation. *J. Mol. Biol.* 245, 43–53.

Karaman, B., and Sippl, W. (2015). Docking and binding free energy calculations of sirtuin inhibitors. *Eur. J. Med. Chem.* 93, 584–598. doi: 10.1016/j.ejmech.2015.02.045

Khan, K. M., Wadood, A., Ali, M., Zia-Ullah, Ul-Haq, Z., Lodhi, M. A., et al. (2010). Identification of potent urease inhibitors via ligand- and structure-based virtual screening and *in vitro* assay. *J. Mol. Graph. Model.* 28, 792–798. doi: 10.1016/j.jmgm.2010.02.004

Kinnings, S. L., Liu, N., Tonge, P. J., Jackson, R. M., Xie, L., and Bourne, P. E. (2011). A machine learning-based method to improve docking scoring functions and its application to drug repurposing. *J. Chem. Inf. Model.* 51, 408–419. doi: 10.1021/ci100369f

Kiss, B., Horváth, A., Némethy, Z., Schmidt, E., Laszlovszky, I., Bugovics, G., et al. (2010). Cariprazine (RGH-188), a dopamine D(3) receptor-preferring, D(3)/D(2) *J. Pharmacol. Exp. Ther.* 333, 328–340. doi: 10.1124/jpet.109.160432

Kitchen, D. B., Decornez, H., Furr, J. R., and Bajorath, J. (2004). Docking and scoring in virual screening for drug discovery: methods and applications. *Nat. Rev. Drug Discov.* 3, 935–949. doi:10.1038/nrd1549

Klebe, G., Abraham, U., and Mietzner, T. (1994). Molecular similarity indexes in a comparative-analysis (CoMSIA) of drug molecules to correlate and predict their biological-activity. *J. Med. Chem.* 37, 4130–4146.

Knox, C., Law, V., Jewison, T., Liu, P., Ly, S., Frolkis, A., et al. (2011). DrugBank 3.0: a comprehensive resource for 'omics' research on drugs. *Nucleic Acids Res.* 39, D1035–D1041. doi: 10.1093/nar/gkq1126

Koeppen, H., Kriegl, J., Lessel, U., Tautermann, C. S., and Wellenzohn, B. (2011). "Ligand-based virtual screening," in *Virtual Screening*, ed C. Sotriffer (Weinheim: Wiley-VCH Verlag GmbH & Co. KGaA), 61–85.

Kupershmidt, L., Amit, T., Bar-Am, O., Youdim, M. B., and Weinreb, O. (2012). The Novel multi-target iron chelating-radical scavenging compound M30 possesses beneficial effects on major hallmarks of Alzheimer's disease. *Antiox. Redox Sign.* 17, 860–877. doi: 10.1089/ars.2011.4279

Lakshmi, V., Kannan, V. S., and Boopathy, R. (2013). Identification of potential bivalent inhibitors from natural compounds for acetylcholinesterase through *in silico* screening using multiple pharmacophores. *J. Mol. Graph. Model.* 40, 72–79. doi:10.1016/j.jmgm.2012.12.008

Laskowski, R. A., Watson, J. D., and Thornton, J. M. (2005). ProFunc: a server for predicting protein function from 3D structure. *Nucleic Acids Res.* 33, W89–W93. doi: 0.1093/nar/gki414

Leach, A. R., Gillet, V. J., Lewis, R. A., and Taylor, R. (2010). Three-dimensional pharmacophore methods in drug discovery. *J. Med. Chem.* 53, 539–558. doi: 10.1021/jm900817u

Leeson, P. D., and Davis, A. M. (2004). Time-related differences in the physical property profiles of oral drugs. *J. Med. Chem.* 47, 6338–6348. doi: 10.1021/jm049717d

Leeson, P. D., and Springthorpe, B. (2007). The influence of drug-like concepts on decision-making in medicinal chemistry. *Nat. Rev. Drug Discov.* 6, 881–890. doi:10.1038/nrd2445

Lengauer, T., and Rarey, M. (1996). Computational methods for biomolecular docking. *Curr. Opin. Struct. Biol.* 6, 402–406.

León, R., Garcia, A. G., and Marco-Contelles, J. (2013). Recent advances in the multitarget-directed ligands approach for the treatment of Alzheimer's disease. *Med. Res. Rev.* 33, 139–189. doi: 10.1002/med.20248

Lepailleur, A., Freret, T., Lemaître, S., Boulouard, M., Dauphin, F., Hinschberger, A., et al. (2014). Dual histamine H3R/serotonin 5-HT4R ligands with antiamnesic properties: pharmacophore-based virtual screening and polypharmacology. *J. Chem. Inf. Model.* 54, 1773–1784. doi: 10.1021/ci500157n

Lešnik, S., Štular, T., Brus, B., Knez, D., Gobec, S., Janežič, D., et al. (2015). LiSiCA: a software for ligand-based virtual screening and its application for the discovery of butyrylcholinesterase inhibitors. *J. Chem. Inf. Model.* 55, 1521–1528. doi: 10.1021/acs.jcim.5b00136

Li, Y. P., Weng, X., Ning, F. X., Ou, J. B., Hou, J. Q., Luo, H. B., et al. (2013). 3D-QSAR studies of azaoxoisoaporphine, oxoaporphine, and oxoisoaporphine derivatives as anti-AChE and anti-AD agents by the CoMFA method. *J. Mol. Graph. Model.* 41, 61–67. doi: 10.1016/j.jmgm.2013.02.003

Ligneau, X., Lin, J., Vanni-Mercier, G., Jouvet, M., Muir, J. L., Ganellin, C. R., et al. (1998). Neurochemical and behavioural effects of ciproxifan, a potent histamine H3-receptor antagonist. *J. Pharmacol. Exp. Ther.* 287, 658–666.

Ligneau, X., Morisset, S., Tardivel-Lacombe, J., Gbahou, F., Ganellin, C. R., Stark, H., et al. (2000). Distinct pharmacology of rat and human histamine H(3) receptors: role of two amino acids in the third transmembrane domain. *Br. J. Pharmacol.* 131, 1247–1250. doi: 10.1038/sj.bjp.0703712

Lipina, T. V., Palomo, V., Gil, C., Martinez, A., and Roder, J. C. (2013). Dual Inhibitor of PDE7 and GSK-3-VP1.15 Acts as Antipsychotic and Cognitive Enhancer in C57BL/6J Mice. *Neuropharmacology* 64, 205–214. doi: 10.1016/j.neuropharm.2012.06.032

Lipina, T. V., Wang, M., Liu, F., and Roder, J. C. (2012). Synergistic Interactions between PDE4B and GSK-3: DISC1 Mutant Mice. *Neuropharmacology* 62, 1252–1262. doi: 10.1016/j.neuropharm.2011.02.020

Lounkine, E., Keiser, M. J., Whitebread, S., Mikhailov, D., Hamon, J., Jenkins, J. L., et al. (2012). Large-scale prediction and testing of drug activity on side-effect targets. *Nature* 486, 361–367. doi: 10.1038/nature11159

Lu, J. J., Pan, W., Hu, Y. J., and Wang, Y. T. (2012). Multi-target drugs: the trend of drug research and development. *PLoS ONE* 7:e40262. doi: 10.1371/journal.pone.0040262

Lu, S. H., Wu, J. W., Liu, H. L., Zhao, J. H., Liu, K. T., Chuang, C. K., et al. (2011). The discovery of potential acetylcholinesterase inhibitors: a combination of pharmacophore modeling, virtual screening, and molecular docking studies. *J. Biomed. Sci.* 18:8. doi: 10.1186/1423-0127-18-8

Marco-Contelles, J., León, R., de Los Ríos, C., Guglietta, A., Terencio, J., López, M. G., et al. (2006). Novel multipotent tacrine-dihydropyridine hybrids with improved acetylcholinesterase inhibitory and neuroprotective activities as potential drugs for the treatment of Alzheimer's disease. *J. Med. Chem.* 49, 7607–7610. doi: 10.1021/jm061047j

Marco-Contelles, J., León, R., de los Ríos, C., Samadi, A., Bartolini, M., Andrisano, V., et al. (2009). Tacripyrines, the first tacrine-dihydropyridine hybrids, as multitarget-directed ligands for the treatment of Alzheimer's disease. *J. Med. Chem.* 52, 2724–2732. doi: 10.1021/jm801292b

Mavridis, L., and Mitchell, J. B. O. (2013). Predicting the protein targets for athletic performance-enhancing substances. *J. Cheminformatics* 5:31. doi: 10.1186/1758-2946-5-31

Mavridis, L., Nath, N., and Mitchell, J. B. O. (2013). PFClust: a novel parameter free clustering algorithm. *BMC Bioinformatics* 14:213. doi: 10.1186/1471-2105-14-213

Meltzer, H. Y., Massey, B. W., and Horiguchi, M. (2012). Serotonin receptors as targets for drugs useful to treat psychosis and cognitive impairment in schizophrenia. *Curr. Pharm. Biotechnol.* 13, 1572–1586. doi: 10.2174/138920112800784880

Mestres, J., and Gregori-Puigjané, E. (2009). Conciliating binding efficiency and polypharmacology. *Trends Pharmacol. Sci.* 30, 470–474. doi: 10.1016/j.tips.2009.07.004

Millan, M. J. (2005). N-Methyl-d-aspartate receptors as a target for improved antipsychotic agents: novel insights and clinical perspectives. *Psychopharmacology* 179, 30–53. doi: 10.1007/s00213-005-2199-1

Millan, M. J. (2006). Multi-target strategies for the improved treatment of depressive states: conceptual foundation and neuronal substrates, drug discovery and therapeutic application. *Pharmacol. Therapeut.* 110, 135–370. doi: 10.1016/j.pharmthera.2005.11.006

Millan, M. J. (2014). On 'polypharmacy' and multi-target agents, complementary strategies for improving the treatment of depression: a comparative appraisal. *Int. J. Neuropsychopharmacol.* 17, 1009–1037. doi: 10.1017/S1461145712001496

Mitchell, J. B. O., Laskowski, R. A., Alex, A., and Thornton, J. M. (1999). BLEEP - potential of mean force describing protein-ligand interactions: I. Generating potential. *J. Comput. Chem.* 20, 1165–1176.

Morphy, R., and Rankovic, Z. (2005). Designed multiple ligands. An emerging drug discovery paradigm. *J. Med. Chem.* 48, 6523–6543. doi: 10.1021/jm058225d

Morris, G. M., Goodsell, D. S., Halliday, R. S., Huey, R., Hart, W. E., Belew, R. K., et al. (1998). Automated docking using a Lamarckian genetic algorithm and empirical binding free energy function. *J. Comput. Chem.* 19, 1639–1662.

Morris, G. M., Huey, R., Lindstrom, W., Sanner, M. F., Belew, R. K., Goodsell, D. S., et al. (2009). Autodock4 and AutoDockTools4: automated docking with selective receptor flexiblity. *J. Comput. Chem.* 30, 2785–2791. doi: 10.1002/jcc.21256

Napolitano, F., Zhao, Y., Moreira, V., Tagliaferri, R., Kere, J., D'Amato, M., et al. (2013). Drug repositioning: a machine-learning approach through data integration. *J. Cheminformatics* 5:30. doi: 10.1186/1758-2946-5-30

Nikolic, K., Agbaba, D., and Stark, H. (2015a). Pharmacophore modeling, drug design and virtual screening on multi-targeting procognitive agents approaching histaminergic pathways. *J. Taiwan Inst. Chem. E.* 46, 15–29. doi:10.1016/j.jtice.2014.09.017

Nikolic, K., Mavridis, L., Bautista-Aguilera, O. M., Marco-Contelles, J., Stark, H., do Carmo Carreiras, M., et al. (2015b). Predicting targets of compounds against neurological diseases using cheminformatic methodology. *J. Comput. Aided Mol. Des.* 29, 183–198. doi: 10.1007/s10822-014-9816-1

Ning, X., Rangwala, H., and Karypis, G. (2009). Multi-Assay-based structure-activity relationship models: improving structure-activity relationship models by incorporating activity information from related targets. *J. Chem. Inform. Mod.* 49, 2444–2456. doi: 10.1021/ci900182q

Pajouhesh, H., and Lenz, G. R. (2005). Medicinal chemical properties of successful central nervous system drugs. *NeuroRx* 2, 541–553. doi: 10.1602/neurorx.2.4.541

Pal, D., and Eisenberg, D. (2005). Inference of protein function from protein structure. *Structure* 13, 121–130. doi:10.1016/j.str.2004.10.015

Panjkovich, A., and Daura, X. (2012). Exploiting protein flexibility to predict the location of allosteric sites. *BMC Bioinformatics* 13:273. doi: 10.1186/1471-2105-13-273

Pardridge, W. M. (2005). The blood-brain barrier: bottleneck in brain drug development. *NeuroRx* 2, 3–14. doi: 10.1602/neurorx.2.1.3

Park, H., Eom, J. W., and Kim, Y. H. (2014). Consensus scoring approach to identify the inhibitors of AMPA activated protein kinase α2 with virtual screening. *J. Chem. Inf. Model.* 54, 2139–2146. doi: 10.1021/ci500214e

Parzen, E. (1962). On estimation of a probability density function and mode. *Ann. Math. Statist.* 33, 1065–1076.

Pastor, M., Cruciani, G., McLay, I., Pickett, S., and Clementi, S. (2000). GRid-INdependent descriptors (GRIND): a novel class of alignment- independent three-dimensional molecular descriptors. *J. Med. Chem.* 43, 3233–3243. doi: 10.1021/jm000941m

Patel, H., Lucas, X., Bendik, I., Günther, S., and Merfort, I. (2015). Target fishing by cross-docking to explain polypharmacological effects. *ChemMedChem.* 10, 1209–1217. doi: 10.1002/cmdc.201500123

Pérez, V., Marco, J. L., Fernández-Alvarez, E., and Unzeta, M. (1999). Relevance of benzyloxy group in 2-indolyl methylamines in the selective MAO-B inhibition. *Brit. J. Pharmacol.* 127, 869–876. doi: 10.1038/sj.bjp.0702600

Peters, J. U. (2013). Polypharmacology-foe or friend? *J. Med. Chem.* 56, 8955–8971. doi: 10.1021/jm400856t

Petroianu, G., Arafat, K., Sasse, B. C., and Stark, H. (2006). Multiple enzyme inhibitions by histamine H3 receptor antagonists as potential procognitive agents. *Pharmazie* 61, 179–182.

Planesas, J. M., Claramunt, R. M., Teixidó, J., Borrell, J. I., and Pérez-Nueno, V. I. (2011). Improving VEGFR-2 docking-based screening by pharmacophore postfiltering and similarity search postprocessing. *J. Chem. Inf. Model.* 51, 777–787. doi: 10.1021/ci1002763

Postigo, M. P., Guido, R. V., Oliva, G., Castilho, M. S., da R Pitta, I., de Albuquerque, J. F., et al. (2010). Discovery of new inhibitors of Schistosoma mansoni PNP by pharmacophore-based virtual screening. *J. Chem. Inf. Model.* 50, 1693–1705. doi: 10.1021/ci100128k

Prado-Prado, F., García-Mera, X., Escobar, M., Alonso, N., Caamaño, O., Yañez, M., et al. (2012). 3D MI-DRAGON: new model for the reconstruction of US FDA drug- target network and theoretical-experimental studies of inhibitors of rasagiline derivatives for AChE. *Curr. Top. Med. Chem.* 12, 1843–1865. doi: 10.2174/156802661120906184

Quesseveur, G., Nguyen, H. T., Gardier, A. M., and Guiard, B. P. (2012). 5-HT2 ligands in the treatment of anxiety and depression. *Expert Opin. Inv. Drug.* 21, 1701–1725. doi: 10.1517/13543784.2012.719872

Rajagopalan, R., Bandyopadhyaya, A., Rajagopalan, D. R., and Rajagopalan, P. (2014). The synthesis and comparative receptor binding affinities of novel, isomeric pyridoindolobenzazepine scaffolds. *Bioorg. Med. Chem. Lett.* 24, 576–579. doi: 10.1016/j.bmcl.2013.12.024

Rankovic, Z. (2015a). "Designing CNS drugs for optimal brain exposure" in *Blood-Brain Barrier in Drug Discovery: Optimizing Brain Exposure of CNS Drugs and Minimizing Brain Side Effects, 1st Edn.*, eds L. Di and E. H. Kerns (New York, NY: Wiley), 385–425.

Rankovic, Z. (2015b). CNS drug design: balancing physicochemical properties for optimal brain exposure. *J. Med. Chem.* 58, 2584–2608. doi: 10.1021/jm501535r

Rankovic, Z., and Bingham, M. (2013). "Medicinal chemistry challenges in CNS drug discovery," in *Drug Discovery for Psychiatric Disorders, 1st Edn.*, eds Z. Rankovic, M. Bingham, E. Nestler, and R. Hargreaves (London: Royal Society of Chemistry), 465–509.

Raub, T. J., Lutzke, B. S., Andrus, P. K., Sawada, G. A., and Staton, B. A. (2006). "Early preclinical evaluation of brain exposure in support of hit identification and lead optimization," in *Optimizing the 'Drug-Like' Properties of Leads in Drug Discovery*, eds R. T. Borchardt, E. H. Kerns, M. J. Hageman, D. R. Thakker, and J. L. Stevens (New York, NY: Springer), 355–410.

Reinikainen, K. J., Soininen, H., and Riekkinen, P. J. (1990). Neurotransmitter changes in Alzheimer's disease: implications to diagnostics and therapy. *J. Neurosci. Res.* 27, 576–586.

Remington, G. (2003). Understanding antipsychotic "atypicality": a clinical and pharmacological moving target. *J. Psychiatr. Neurosci.* 28, 275–284.

Reynolds, G. P. (2004). Receptor mechanisms in the treatment of schizophrenia. *J. Psychopharmacol.* 18, 340–345. doi: 10.1177/0269881104044562

Ripphausen, P., Nisius, B., Peltason, L., and Bajorath, J. (2010). Quo vadis, virtual screening? A comprehensive survey of prospective applications. *J. Med. Chem.* 53, 8461–8467. doi: 10.1021/jm101020z

Rosenblatt, M. (1956). Remarks on some nonparametric estimates of a density function. *Ann. Math. Statist.* 27, 832–837.

Roth, B. L., Sheffler, D. J., and Kroeze, W. K. (2004). Magic shotguns versus magic bullets: selectively non-selective drugs for mood disorders and schizophrenia. *Nat. Rev. Drug Discov.* 3, 353–359. doi: 10.1038/nrd1346

Roy, S., Kumar, A., Baig, M. H., MasaÁŽík, M., and Provazník, I. (2015). Virtual screening, ADMET profiling, molecular docking and dynamics approaches to search for potent selective natural molecules based inhibitors against metallothionein-III to study Alzheimer's disease. *Methods* 83, 105–110. doi: 10.1016/j.ymeth.2015.04.021

Sander, K., Kottke, T., and Stark, H. (2008). Histamine H3 receptor antagonists go to clinics. *Biol. Pharm. Bull.* 31, 2163–2181. doi: 10.1248/bpb.31.2163

Schmitt, K. C., Mamidyala, S., Biswas, S., Dutta, A. K., and Reith, M. E. (2010). Bivalent phenethylamines as novel dopamine transporter inhibitors: evidence for multiple substrate-binding sites in a single transporter. *J. Neurochem.* 112, 1605–1618. doi: 10.1111/j.1471-4159.2010.06583.x

Schuster, D. (2010). 3D pharmacophores as tools for activity profiling. *Drug Discov. Today Technol.* 7, e203–e270. doi: 10.1016/j.ddtec.2010.11.006

Sedvall, G. C., and Karlsson, P. (2006). Pharmacological manipulation of D1-dopamine receptor function in schizophrenia. *Neuropsychopharmacol.* 21, S181–S188. doi:10.1016/S0893-133X(99)00104-9

Shapiro, D. A., Renock, S., Arrington, E., Chiodo, L. A., Liu, L. X., Sibley, D. R., et al. (2003). Aripiprazole, a novel atypical antipsychotic drug with a unique and robust pharmacology. *Neuropsychopharmacology* 28, 1400–1411. doi:10.1038/sj.npp.1300203

Sirci, F., Istyastono, E. P., Vischer, H. F., Kooistra, A. J., Nijmeijer, S., Kuijer, M., et al. (2012). Virtual fragment screening: discovery of histamine H3 receptor ligands using ligand-based and protein-based molecular fingerprints. *J. Chem. Inf. Model.* 52, 3308–3324. doi: 10.1021/ci3004094

Son, S. Y., Ma, J., Kondou, Y., Yoshimura, M., Yamashita, E., and Tsukihara, T. (2008). Structure of human monoamine oxidase A at 2.2-A resolution: the control of opening the entry for substrates/inhibitors. *Proc. Natl. Acad. Sci. U.S.A.* 105, 5739–5744. doi:10.1073/pnas.0710626105

Sousa, S. F., Fernandes, P. A., and Ramos, M. J. (2006). Protein–ligand docking: current status and future challenges. *Proteins* 65, 15–26. doi: 10.1002/prot.21082

Sperandio, O., Miteva, M. A., and Villoutreix, B. O. (2008). Combining ligand- and structure-based methods in drug design projects. *Curr. Comput-Aid Drug* 4, 250–258. doi: 10.2174/157340908785747447

Spitzer, G. M., Heiss, M., Mangold, M., Markt, P., Kirchmair, J., Wolber, G., et al. (2010). One concept, three implementations of 3D pharmacophore-based virtual screening: distinct coverage of chemical search space. *J. Chem. Inf. Model.* 50, 1241–1247. doi: 10.1021/ci100136b

Steinbeck, C., Han, Y., Kuhn, S., Horlacher, O., Luttmann, E., and Willighagen, E. (2003). The chemistry development kit (CDK): an open-source java library for chemo- and bioinformatics. *J. Chem. Inf. Comput. Sci.* 43, 493–500. doi: 10.1021/ci025584y

Svensson, F., Karlén, A., and Sköld, C. (2012). Virtual screening data fusion using both structure- and ligand-based methods. *J. Chem. Inf. Model.* 52, 225–232. doi: 10.1021/ci2004835

Swann, S. L., Brown, S. P., Muchmore, S. W., Patel, H., Merta, P., and Locklear, J. (2011). A unified, probabilistic framework for structure- and ligand-based virtual screening. *J. Med. Chem.* 54, 1223–1232. doi: 10.1021/jm1013677

Tan, L., Geppert, H., Sisay, M. T., Gütschow, M., and Bajorath, J. (2008). Integrating structure- and ligand-based virtual screening: comparison of individual, parallel, and fused molecular docking and similarity search calculations on multiple targets. *Chem. Med. Chem.* 3, 1566–1571. doi: 10.1002/cmdc.200800129

Tauscher, J., Hussain, T., Agid, O., Verhoeff, N. P., Wilson, A. A., Houle, S., et al. (2004). Equivalent occupancy of dopamine D1 and D2 receptors with clozapine: differentiation from other atypical antipsychotics. *Am. J. Psychiatr.* 161, 1620–1625. doi:10.1176/appi.ajp.161.9.1620

Threlfell, S., Cragg, S. J., Kalló, I., Turi, G. F., Coen, C. W., and Greenfield, S. A. (2004). Histamine H3 receptors inhibit serotonin release in substantia nigra pars reticulata. *J. Neurosci.* 24, 8704–8710. doi: 10.1523/JNEUROSCI.2690-04.2004

Topliss, J. G. (1972). Utilization of operational schemes for analog synthesis in drug design. *J. Med. Chem.* 15, 1006–1011.

van Westen, G. J. P., Gaulton, A., and Overington, J. P. (2014). Chemical, target, and bioactive properties of allosteric modulation. *PLoS Comput. Biol.* 10:e1003559. doi: 10.1371/journal.pcbi.1003559

Varela, R., Walters, W. P., Goldman, B. B., and Jain, A. N. (2012). Iterative refinement of a binding pocket model: active computational steering of lead optimization. *J. Med. Chem.* 55, 8926–8942. doi: 10.1021/jm301210j

Venkatraman, V., Pérez-Nueno, V. I., Mavridis, L., and Ritchie, D. W. (2010). Comprehensive comparison of ligand-based virtual screening tools against the DUD data set reveals limitations of current 3D methods. *J. Chem. Inf. Model.* 50, 2079–2093. doi: 10.1021/ci100263p

Verloop, A., Hoogenstraaten, W., and Tipker, J. (1976). "Development and application of new steric substituent parameters in drug design," in *Drug Design*, ed E. J. Ariens (New York, NY: Academic Press), 165–207.

Vijayan, R. S., Prabu, M., Mascarenhas, N. M., and Ghoshal, N. (2009). Hybrid structure-based virtual screening protocol for the identification of novel BACE1 inhibitors. *J. Chem. Inf. Model.* 49, 647–657. doi: 10.1021/ci800386v

Warren, G. L., Andrews, C. W., Capelli, A. M., Clarke, B., LaLonde, J., Lambert, M. H., et al. (2006). A critical assessment of docking programs and scoring functions. *J. Med. Chem.* 49, 5912–5931. doi: 10.1021/jm050362n

Weidlich, I. E., Dexheimer, T., Marchand, C., Antony, S., Pommier, Y., and Nicklaus, M.C. (2010). Inhibitors of human tyrosyl-DNA phosphodiesterase (hTdp1) developed by virtual screening using ligand-based pharmacophores. *Bioorg. Med. Chem.* 18, 182–189. doi: 10.1016/j.bmc.2009.11.008

Weiss, M. M., Williamson, T., Babu-Khan, S., Bartberger, M. D., Brown, J., Chen, K., et al. (2012). Design and preparation of a potent series of hydroxyethylamine containing β-secretase inhibitors that demonstrate robust reduction of central β-amyloid. *J. Med. Chem.* 55, 9009–9024. doi: 10.1021/jm300119p

Wilson, G. I., and Lill, M. A. (2011). Integrating structure-based and ligand-based approaches for computational drug design. *Future Med. Chem.* 3, 735–750. doi: 10.4155/fmc.11.18

Witkin, J. M., and Nelson, D. L. (2004). Selective histamine H3 receptor antagonists for treatment of cognitive deficiencies and other disorders of the central nervous system. *Pharmacol. Therapeut.* 103, 1–20. doi:10.1016/j.pharmthera.2004.05.001

Wold, S., Ruhe, A., Wold, H., and Dunn, W. J. (1984). The collinearity problem in linear regression. The partial least squares (PLS) approach to generalized inverses. *SIAM J. Sci. Stat. Comput.* 5, 735–743. doi: 10.1137/0905052

Wu, G. S., Robertson, D. H., Brooks, C. L. III., and Vieth, M. (2003). Detailed analysis of grid-based molecular docking: a case study of CDOCKER—A CHARMm-based MD docking algorithm. *J. Comput. Chem.* 24, 1549–1562. doi: 10.1002/jcc.10306

Wu, W. L., Burnett, D. A., Spring, R., Greenlee, W. J., Smith, M., Favreau, L., et al. (2005). Dopamine D1/D5 receptor antagonists with improved pharmacokinetics: design, synthesis, and biological evaluation of phenol bioisosteric analogues of benzazepine D1/D5 antagonists. *J. Med. Chem.* 48, 680–693. doi: 10.1021/jm030614p

Ye, N., Song, Z., and Zhang, A. (2014). Dual ligands targeting dopamine D2 and serotonin 5-HT1A receptors as new antipsychotical on anti-parkinsonian agents. *Curr. Med. Chem.* 21, 437–457. doi: 10.2174/0929867311320660300

Yelekci, K., Büyüktürk, B., and Kayrak, N. (2013). *In silico* identification of novel and selective monoamine oxidase B inhibitors. *J. Neural. Transm.* 120, 853–858. doi: 10.1007/s00702-012-0954-0

Youdim, M. B., Edmondson, D., and Tipton, K. F. (2006). The therapeutic potential of monoamine oxidase inhibitors. *Nat. Rev. Neurosci.* 7, 295–309. doi:10.1038/nrn1883

Youdim, M. B. H., and Buccafusco, J. J. (2005). Multi-functional drugs for various CNS targets in the treatment of neurodegenerative disorders. *Trends Pharmacol. Sci.* 26, 27–35. doi:10.1016/j.tips.2004.11.007

Zhang, L., Fourches, D., Sedykh, A., Zhu, H., Golbraikh, A., Ekins, S., et al. (2013). Discovery of novel antimalarial compounds enabled by QSAR-based virtual screening. *J. Chem. Inf. Model.* 53, 475–492. doi: 10.1021/ci300421n

Zheng, H., Fridkin, M., and Youdim, M. B. (2010). Site-activated chelators derived from anti-parkinson drug rasagiline as a potential safer and more effective approach to the treatment of Alzheimer's disease. *Neurochem. Res.* 35, 2117–2123. doi: 10.1007/s11064-010-0293-1

Conflict of Interest Statement: The authors declare that the research was conducted in the absence of any commercial or financial relationships that could be construed as a potential conflict of interest.

The handling Editor declared a shared affiliation with one of the authors [JM] and states that the process nevertheless met the standards of a fair and objective review.

8

Dopamine D3 Receptor Antagonists as Potential Therapeutics for the Treatment of Neurological Diseases

Samuele Maramai[1], Sandra Gemma[1], Simone Brogi[1], Giuseppe Campiani[1], Stefania Butini[1]*, Holger Stark[2] and Margherita Brindisi[1]

[1] European Research Centre for Drug Discovery and Development and Department of Biotechnology, Chemistry and Pharmacy, University of Siena, Siena, Italy, [2] Institut fuer Pharmazeutische und Medizinische Chemie, Heinrich-Heine-Universitaet Duesseldorf, Duesseldorf, Germany

D3 receptors represent a major focus of current drug design and development of therapeutics for dopamine-related pathological states. Their close homology with the D2 receptor subtype makes the development of D3 selective antagonists a challenging task. In this review, we explore the relevance and therapeutic utility of D3 antagonists or partial agonists endowed with multireceptor affinity profile in the field of central nervous system disorders such as schizophrenia and drug abuse. In fact, the peculiar distribution and low brain abundance of D3 receptors make them a valuable target for the development of drugs devoid of motor side effects classically elicited by D2 antagonists. Recent research efforts were devoted to the conception of chemical templates possibly endowed with a multi-target profile, especially with regards to other G-protein-coupled receptors (GPCRs). A comprehensive overview of the recent literature in the field is herein provided. In particular, the evolution of the chemical templates has been tracked, according to the growing advancements in both the structural information and the refinement of the key pharmacophoric elements. The receptor/multireceptor affinity and functional profiles for the examined compounds have been covered, together with their most significant pharmacological applications.

Keywords: GPCR, dopamine, drug optimization, receptor antagonists, selectivity, multi-targeting approach

Edited by:
Rona R. Ramsay,
University of St. Andrews, UK

Reviewed by:
Dasiel Oscar Borroto-Escuela,
Karolinska Institutet, Sweden
György M. Keseru,
RCNS - Hungarian Academy of
Sciences, Hungary

*Correspondence:
Stefania Butini
butini3@unisi.it

INTRODUCTION

By the last midcentury, it was claimed that dopamine (DA) plays a pivotal role as neurotransmitter in the central nervous system (CNS). Due to its peculiar distribution in the brain DA controls, by interacting with its receptors, a variety of functions including locomotor activity, learning (Beninger, 1983), reward (Wise and Rompre, 1989), motivation, emotion, cognition (Nieoullon, 2002; Cools, 2008), food intake (Volkow et al., 2011), and endocrine regulation (Beaulieu and Gainetdinov, 2011). Later on, the dopaminergic system has been the focus of intense study and research, following the evidence that dysfunction of the dopaminergic system could be associated to a number of pathological conditions such as Parkinson's disease (Brooks, 2000), schizophrenia (Brisch et al., 2014), drug abuse and dependence (Volkow et al., 2007). The disclosure of specific sites of action for DA led to the identification of more than one kind of DA receptors in the brain (Sibley and Monsma, 1992). Originally, the DA receptors were classified into two subtypes, D1 and D2, owning different biochemical and pharmacological properties, and mediating distinct physiological functions. Both the D1 and D2 subtypes are G protein-coupled receptors (GPCRs) where diverse G proteins (classified in Gs, Gi, and Gq) and effectors are involved in mediating their effects on different signaling pathways (Beninger, 1983).

Subsequent biochemical studies, while suggesting the heterogeneity for the originally described D1 and D2 receptors, revealed the presence of 5 distinct receptor subtypes (Sibley and Monsma, 1992). These subtypes, based on sequence homology, were in turn clustered into two subfamilies, the so called D1-like receptors (D1 and D5) and the D2-like receptors (D2, D3, and D4). Typically, D1-like receptors are positively coupled to adenylyl cyclase (AC) and lead to intracellular cyclic 3,5-adenine monophosphate (cAMP) accumulation and activation of the protein kinase A (PKA). In contrast, D2-like receptors are negatively coupled to AC and negatively modulate the activity of PKA and its effectors (Rangel-Barajas et al., 2015). Over the past decades, a large number of agonists and antagonists for both D1-like and D2-like subfamilies have been developed and characterized (Butini et al., 2016). Although the design of ligands characterized by overall selectivity for the D1-like vs. the D2-like receptors is quite an easy task to be achieved, the development of specific ligands for a single receptor subtype has proven to be a tough challenge especially within the same receptor subfamily. Each receptor possesses an extracellular amino terminus and seven membrane spanning-helices linked by intracellular and extracellular protein loops. The carboxyl terminus is located in the intracellular space and may form a further link to the membrane. Structurally the D1-like receptors have a short third intracellular loop and a long carboxyl terminal tail, whereas the D2-like receptors display opposite features showing long third loops and short carboxyl terminus (**Figure 1**).

These differences provided the structural basis for the clustering of these receptors into the two mentioned subfamilies; moreover, they could also be linked to their functional outcome and significance and to specific receptor/G protein interaction potentially exploitable for the development of subtype selective ligands.

Detailed information about the structure of DA receptors, also provided by crystallographic studies for D3 subtypes (Chien et al., 2010), has greatly facilitated, in the last years, the development of subtype selective ligands.

In this review, we discuss the development of compounds behaving as D3 receptor antagonists by focusing our attention on the literature of the last 10 years. Besides a general discussion on their structure, affinity and functional profile on DA and other receptor subtypes, we also provide an overview of their application in the field of DA-related pathological states, with a particular focus on schizophrenia and drug addiction models.

D3 RECEPTORS AS MEMBERS OF THE D2-LIKE FAMILY OF DOPAMINE RECEPTORS

The D2-like receptor family represented by D2, D3, and D4 receptors exhibits pharmacological properties similar to those of the originally defined D2 receptor (Missale et al., 1998). Post-synaptic D2 receptors are present in dopaminergic projection areas such as the striatum (50%), limbic areas (nucleus accumbens, olfactory tubercle), hypothalamus and pituitary gland. D2 receptors are also located pre-synaptically in the substantia nigra pars compacta, ventral tegmental area and striatum, where they modulate the release of DA (De Mei et al., 2009). Activation of the striatal D2 receptor subfamily in rats results in a behavioral syndrome known as stereotypy (repetitive sniffing and gnawing, accompanied by hyperactivity). The repetitive behaviors observed in humans following amphetamine ingestion may have a similar neurochemical basis. By contrast, blockade of the striatal D2 receptor subfamily produces marked increase in muscle rigidity in rats and a Parkinson-like syndrome in humans. Administration of a D2 antagonist in humans results in a rapid and large increase in prolactin release from the anterior pituitary gland, since the physiological DA inhibition of prolactin release is blocked.

The D3 and D4 subtypes are much less abundant than the D2 subtype and have different and more restricted tissue localization. D3 receptors are predominantly located in areas considered important for psychotic symptoms such as ventral striatum including nucleus accumbens, thalamus, hippocampus, and cortex (Hall et al., 1996; Suzuki et al., 1998; Gurevich and Joyce, 1999). Some D3 receptors are also found in regions associated with motor function such as the putamen, whereas D4 receptors are found in the frontal cortex, amygdala, mid-brain and medulla.

Notably, D3 receptors possess a high affinity for DA (420-fold higher than that of D2 receptors) and, unlike D2 receptors, small changes in their number or function may lead to dramatic effects on synaptic transmission, suggesting that D3 receptors could be critical modulators of normal dopaminergic function and, despite their localization, also of cognition.

Recently, the resolution of the crystal structure of the human D3 receptor in complex with eticlopride, a potent D2/D3 antagonist (Chien et al., 2010) provided essential hints for rational drug design aiming at the development of D3 selective ligands. The crystal structure, in fact, highlighted useful structural differences between closely related GPCRs that can be exploited for drug design. In particular, the structural observation of the extracellular binding pocket, which may interact with bitopic or allosteric ligands, shed light on the role of the extracellular loops as relevant for defining a specific region for ligand binding not only at the orthosteric site (Brogi et al., 2014).

In the last decade, several evidences pointed out the dimerization phenomena of GPCRs as a pivotal issue for modulating their biological function paving the way to the future development of innovative drugs. In particular, many GPCRs have been described to form homodimers, heteromers, or oligomers (Borroto-Escuela et al., 2014). DA receptors are the most promiscuous proteins able to form dimers among the rhodopsin-like GPCRs. Dimerization can occur through their extracellular loops, transmembrane helices and intracellular loops. The dimers can be stabilized by covalent (disulphide bonds) or non-covalent (hydrophobic interactions between transmembrane helices or coiled coil structures) bonds or a

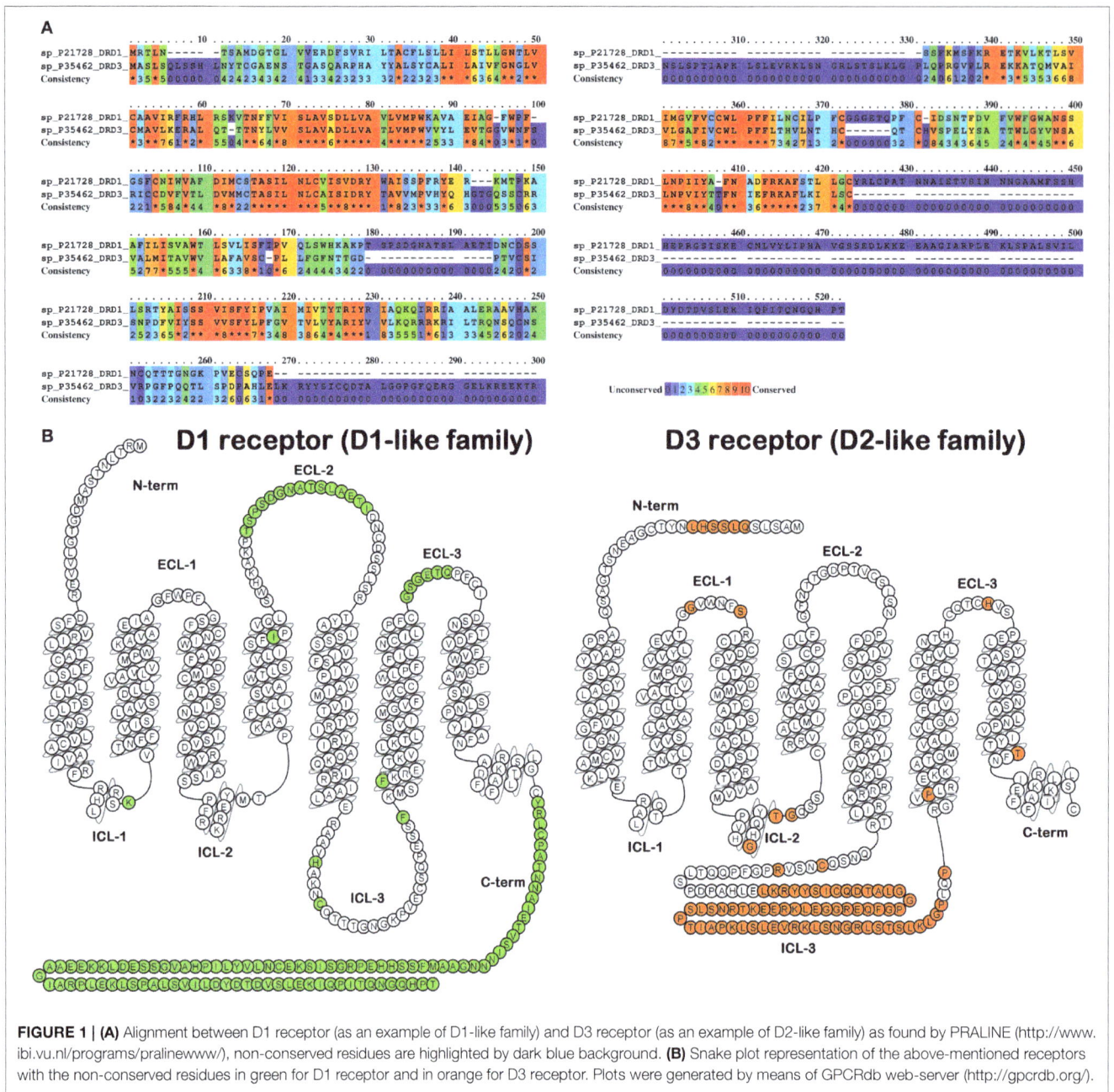

FIGURE 1 | (A) Alignment between D1 receptor (as an example of D1-like family) and D3 receptor (as an example of D2-like family) as found by PRALINE (http://www.ibi.vu.nl/programs/pralinewww/), non-conserved residues are highlighted by dark blue background. **(B)** Snake plot representation of the above-mentioned receptors with the non-conserved residues in green for D1 receptor and in orange for D3 receptor. Plots were generated by means of GPCRdb web-server (http://gpcrdb.org/).

combination of both. Although their physiological function is not completely understood yet, receptor dimers or oligomers have major consequences on ligand binding, activation of signaling pathways and cellular trafficking. These complexes, showing properties different from those found for each single monomer, may modify the action of DA itself and of different agonists and antagonists (Maggio et al., 2015). Therefore, targeting specific GPCR dimers may provide drugs with enhanced potency, selectivity, and therapeutic index, representing a promising alternative to conventional drug development approaches for CNS disorders.

In particular, D3 receptors can form homodimers or heteromers with D1 or D2 receptors (Agnati et al., 2016).

D1-D3 receptor heterodimers have been described possessing different D3 receptor-mediated activation levels on D1 receptors, and this would make interesting to investigate the differences in the pharmacological profile of various D1 agonists. D1-D3 heteromers represent an important functional unit in the brain and are considered promising targets for neuropsychiatric disorders including Parkinson's disease and drug addiction (Guitart et al., 2014; Agnati et al., 2016). Additionally, heterodimerization was also described for D3 receptors with other GPCRs such as A2A and neurotensin receptors. Recently heteromultimers were also reported involving D3 or D2 receptors with adenosine A2A and cannabinoid CB1 receptors (Maggio et al., 2015).

PHARMACOLOGICAL IMPLICATIONS OF D3 ANTAGONISM

D3 receptors have attracted interest as pharmacological targets since their peculiar anatomical distribution in the limbic areas suggests that they may play a role in cognitive and emotional functions. Accordingly, they hold a valuable potential for the treatment of neurological and psychiatric disorders being potentially devoid of the classical D2 receptor subtype side effects (Hackling and Stark, 2002; Luedtkea and Mach, 2003; Joyce and Millan, 2005; Newman et al., 2005; Kassel et al., 2015). This hypothesis has prompted many research groups to develop D3 receptor selective ligands. In this context, there is increasingly strong evidence that D3 receptor antagonists could be effective antipsychotic agents and could also be involved in behavioral sensitization, with potential efficacy in the treatment of drug abuse.

The most considerable number of reports concerns the development of D3 antagonists for the treatment of schizophrenia (Joyce and Millan, 2005) and this approach is substantiated by a series of evidences. It is well known that the inhibition of D2 receptors, which is essential for obtaining antipsychotic efficacy, is accompanied by detrimental effects on motor functions, causes extrapyramidal side effects, and increases prolactin release. In this frame, DA receptor antagonists characterized by D3 selectivity (over D2 receptors) are not expected to elicit such marked side effects (Millan et al., 2000). This lack of side effects liability is paralleled by the encouraging evidence that selective blockade of D3 receptors enhances social interaction and novel object recognition in rats (Watson et al., 2012). These rodent models efficiently mimic the negative symptoms of schizophrenia, which are poorly treated by conventional antipsychotics thus supporting D3 antagonism as a valuable approach for the treatment of this cluster of symptoms. Further, D3 receptor antagonists might also improve cognitive deficits in schizophrenic patients which are also poorly treated by currently available agents, including clozapine (Meltzer, 2004). Indeed, blockade of D2 receptors may compromise cognitive performance, while D3 antagonism was suggested to improve certain cognitive spheres. This could be due to a modulation of the cholinergic system, by increasing acetylcholine release at the prefrontal cortex level, operated by the D3 receptor antagonism (Millan et al., 2008). In fact, treatment of rats with S33138, a preferential D3 vs. D2 receptor antagonist, was demonstrated to provide enhanced efficacy against cognitive dysfunction induced by several contrasting manipulations (Millan and Brocco, 2008).

Moreover, deficits in the sensorimotor gating, assessed by the prepulse inhibition (PPI) of the startle reflex, have been reported in schizophrenia, and might correlate with the positive symptoms (Meincke et al., 2004). PPI is an operational measure of sensorimotor gating, reflected as a reduced startle response when a startling stimulus is preceded by a weaker acoustic stimulus (Zhang et al., 2007). Current data indicate that although the disruption of PPI is mediated by D2 receptors, but not D3 or D4 receptor subtypes, selective D3 antagonists can reverse the PPI-disruptive effects of other substances such as apomorphine.

The selective involvement of the D3 receptors in crucial neuronal circuits controlling motivational events triggered the identification of selective D3 receptor antagonism as a feasible therapeutic strategy against addiction (Heidbreder and Newman, 2010). This perception was further substantiated by several evidences highlighting plasticity changes in drug-addicted subjects, such as the increase in D3 receptor density in cocaine addicts and metamphetamine polydrug users (Staley and Mash, 1996; Boileau et al., 2012). Cocaine addiction represents a risk factor for schizophrenia and is likewise associated with a sensitization of the mesolimbic dopaminergic pathways and increased DA release in the mesolimbic brain area (Xi et al., 2004). In analogy with this observation, schizophrenic patients show a high incidence of abuse of drugs including cocaine.

Craving is a general central trait of addictive disorders. Drug-seeking behavior can be triggered by drug withdrawal or after a "priming dose." Moreover, drug craving can follow the exposure to stimuli previously associated with consumption of the drug of abuse ("cue-induced craving").

Neuroimaging studies in humans link drug-associated visual cues with DA release in the dorsal striatum and cocaine craving (Wong et al., 2006; Volkow et al., 2006, 2008). In animals, cocaine-associated cues sustain cocaine self-administration (Ito et al., 2004), increase cocaine seeking (Ciccocioppo et al., 2004), and elevate extracellular DA levels in the nucleus accumbens (Aragona et al., 2009), dorsal striatum, and amygdala (Carelli et al., 2003). A more recent study also evidences that cue-induced incubation of cocaine craving coincides with an increase of D3 (and not D1 or D2) receptor expression in the nucleus accumbens and ventral caudate-putamen in rats after prolonged withdrawal from cocaine self-administration (Conrad et al., 2010), suggesting a possible role for increased D3 receptor signaling in incubation of cocaine craving. These evidences delineate a clear direction of intervention, based on D3 receptors antagonism or partial agonism, for the treatment of craving and drug addiction.

D3 RECEPTOR ANTAGONISTS

Based on the interest that D3 receptors raised as an intriguing therapeutic target for the treatment of different neurological disorders and drug abuse, many efforts were dedicated in the last two decades to the development of D3 receptor ligands.

As regards to D3 receptor antagonists, a pharmacophore model was proposed based on the structure of a series of antagonists characterized by a different degree of selectivity for D3 vs. the close homologous D2 receptor subtype (for more details see Butini et al., 2016). The model consists in an aryl moiety (Ar1 of **Figure 2**) linked by a H-bond acceptor function (an amide) to a spacer of appropriate length (usually four methylene units) to the basic moiety very frequently represented by an arylpiperazine system (Hackling and Stark, 2002; Löber et al., 2011).

Amongst the big variety of structures reported in the literature of the last two decades, some early ligands, which were claimed as D3 receptors selective antagonists (or partial agonists) attracted particular attention and in our opinion deserve some "historical" mention: BP897 (**1**, **Figure 3**; Pilla et al., 1999; Garcia-Ladona and Cox, 2003), NGB2904 (**2**, **Figure 3**; Yuan et al., 1998; Xi and Gardner, 2007), SB277011A (**3a**, **Figure 3**; Reavill et al., 2000; Thanos et al., 2005), and FAUC 365 (**4**, **Figure 3**; Bettinetti et al., 2002).

Compound **1** was a potent DA D3 receptor ligand ($K_i = 0.92$ nM), showing a 70-fold selectivity vs. D2 receptors and a moderate affinity for 5-HT1A receptors, ($K_i = 84$ nM), adrenergic alpha1 ($K_i = 60$ nM), and alpha2 adrenoceptors ($K_i = 83$ nM). Although **1** behaved as partial agonist for the D3 receptors, it was not endowed with intrinsic activity and potently inhibited DA agonist effects in agonist-induced acidification rate or increase of GTPγS binding. This compound raised a big interest, since it was demonstrated to reduce cocaine-seeking behavior in rats (1 mg/kg i.p.) without producing reinforcement on its own, thus highlighting and endorsing the role D3 receptor for the treatment of cocaine abuse.

By substitution of the 2-methoxyphenyl- with the 2,3-dichlorophenyl- moiety linked to the piperazine nitrogen, another series of potent and selective D3 ligands was developed. The representative compound of this series, the fluorenylcarboxamide-based derivative NGB2409 (**2**), was originally described in 1998. It showed a selective D3 antagonism profile ($K_i = 0.90$ nM), displaying high affinity for this receptor subtype with greater than 150-fold selectivity over all other DA receptor subtypes (Yuan et al., 1998). Following studies highlighted its role in animal models of addiction, by inhibiting intravenous cocaine self-administration maintained under a progressive-ratio reinforcement schedule, cocaine- or cocaine cue–induced reinstatement of cocaine-seeking behavior, and cocaine- or other addictive drug-enhanced brain stimulation reward (Xi and Gardner, 2007).

In 2005 compound **3a** (SB277011A) was described as a brain-penetrant, high-affinity, and selective D3 receptor antagonist ($pK_i = 7.95$) with 100-fold selectivity over the D2 receptor and over 60 other receptors, enzymes, and ion channels (Thanos et al., 2005). Notably a structurally related compound, SB269,652 (**3b**) able to bind D2 and D3 receptors and behaving as atypical antagonist was recently reinvestigated in light of the D3 receptor dimerization. Binding kinetic studies and crystallographic analysis pointed out that **3b** behaves as dual-steric agent targeting orthosteric and allosteric binding sites of heteromers. In fact this so called "dual-steric ligand" is long enough to bridge orthosteric and allosteric binding sites, providing an exceptional selectivity for D2-D3 dimers, with relevant clinical implications (Silvano et al., 2010; Maggio et al., 2015, see also Butini et al., 2016 for further details). Structural

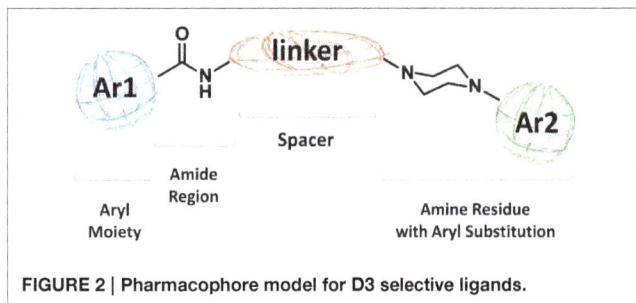

FIGURE 2 | Pharmacophore model for D3 selective ligands.

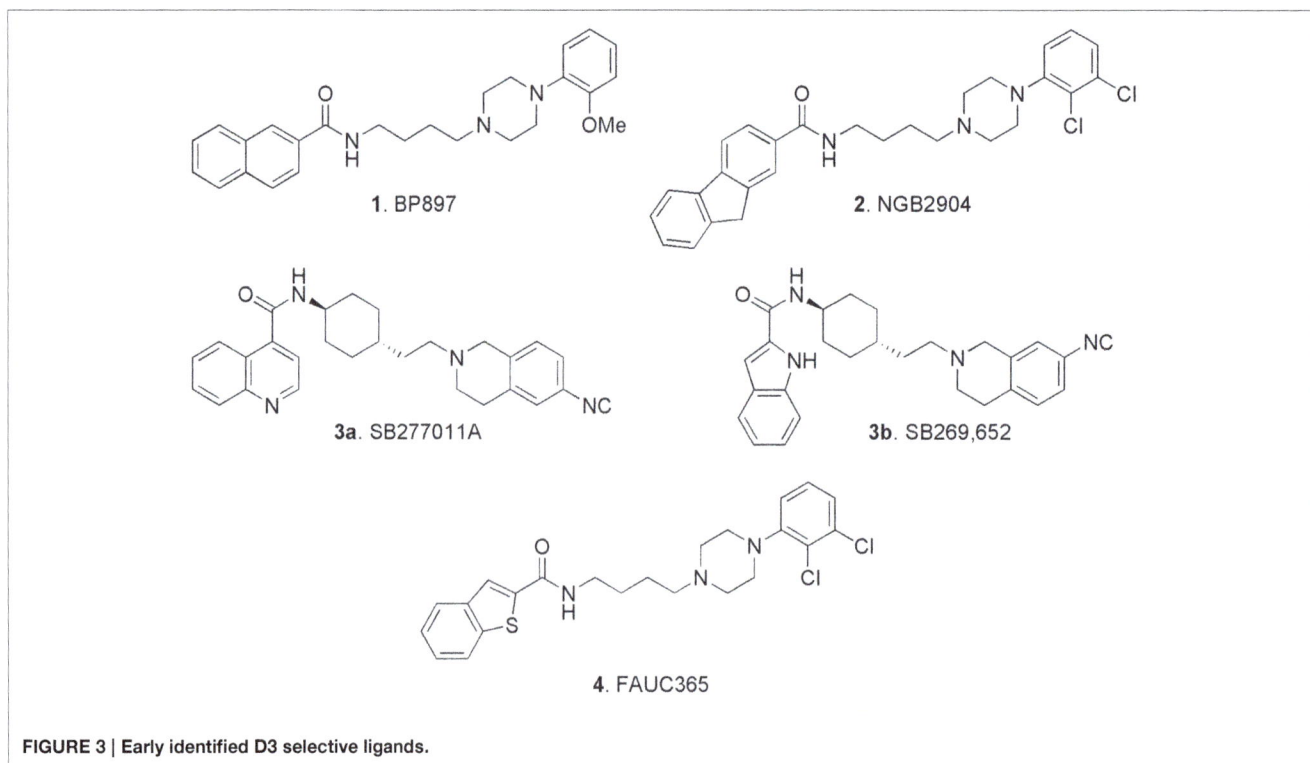

FIGURE 3 | Early identified D3 selective ligands.

elaboration of the D3 receptor pharmacophore allowed the identification of the benzothiophene-2-carboxamide FAUC365 (4) which resulted in a complete D3 receptors antagonist profile, endowed with high affinity (K_i = 0.50 nM) and selectivity (Bettinetti et al., 2002).

ARYLPIPERAZINE-BASED D3 RECEPTOR INHIBITORS

In the following years, a number of manuscripts describing the development of arylpiperazine-based compounds appeared in the literature.

Amongst the variety of retrieved compounds, KKHA-761 (5, Figure 4) was interesting since it was described as a potent D3 receptor antagonist with high 5-HT1A receptor affinity, exhibiting antipsychotic properties in animal models of schizophrenia (Park et al., 2005). In particular, it behaved as a D2-like receptor antagonist with a high affinity for human D3 receptor (K_i = 3.85 nM) with 70-fold selectivity over the D2 receptor (K_i = 270 nM) and it also displayed high affinity for human 5-HT1A receptor (K_i = 6.4 nM). Compound 5

was characterized by a pharmacological profile tracing out that of atypical antipsychotics, like clozapine. In fact 5, among other behavioral effects indicative of antipsychotic activity, could significantly reverse the apomorphine-induced disruption of PPI in mice thus suggesting a therapeutic potential for the treatment of anxiety, psychotic depression, and other related disorders (Park et al., 2005).

In this context, also Campiani et al. reported the synthesis of highly selective D3 receptor ligands (compounds 6a-c and 7a,b, Figure 4) characterized by antagonist or partial agonist activity at D3 receptors and with a D3 vs. D2 selectivity higher than 100-fold combined with 5-HT1A and 5-HT2A receptor occupancy. This represented a novel paradigm for the development of innovative and effective antipsychotics. In particular, compound 6c emerged as interesting hit displaying high affinity for D3, 5-HT1A and 5-HT2A receptors, coupled with a low affinity for D2 receptors (to minimize extrapyramidal side liabilities), 5-HT2C receptors (to decrease the risk of obesity under chronic treatment), and for ether-a-go-go related gene (hERG) channels (to reduce cardiotoxicity). Moreover, c-fos expression in mesocorticolimbic areas, confirmed the atypical antipsychotic profile of 6c in vivo, flanked by the absence of

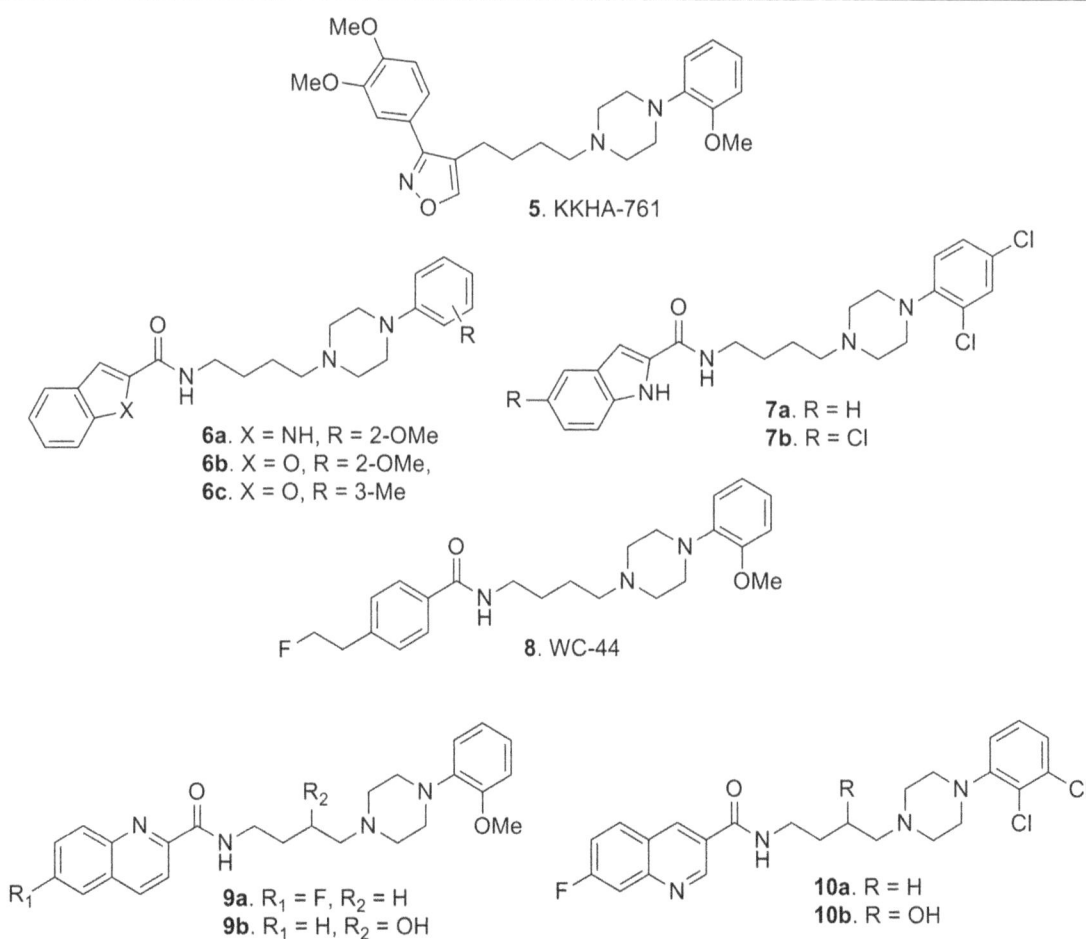

FIGURE 4 | Arylpiperazine-based derivatives 5-10.

catalepsy at antipsychotic dose (Campiani et al., 2003; Butini et al., 2009).

In 2009 Weber and colleagues demonstrated that some derivatives such as WC-44 (**8**, **Figure 4**), initially identified as a selective D3 receptor agonist (K_i = 2.4 ± 0.5 nM), showed instead functional D3 receptor antagonism and possibly an innovative antipsychotic profile. Indeed, in apomorfine- and pramipexole-induced PPI deficits studies, it did not significantly oppose to PPI deficits in apomorfine experiments while it opposed to that of pramipexole-induced analysis, thus suggesting

a novel antipsychotic profile for **8** linked to functional D3 receptor antagonism (Weber et al., 2009).

To the same end, Newman and co-workers prepared some 2-methoxyphenylpiperazine compounds bearing a quinoline heterocycle and explored whether the position of the quinoline nitrogen (2-, 3-, or 7-position) had any effect on binding affinity and/or selectivity. Also they inserted a 3-hydroxy substituent in the linker between the arylamide terminus and the 4-phenylpiperazine moiety. The best results, in terms of D3 affinity and selectivity, were obtained with derivatives

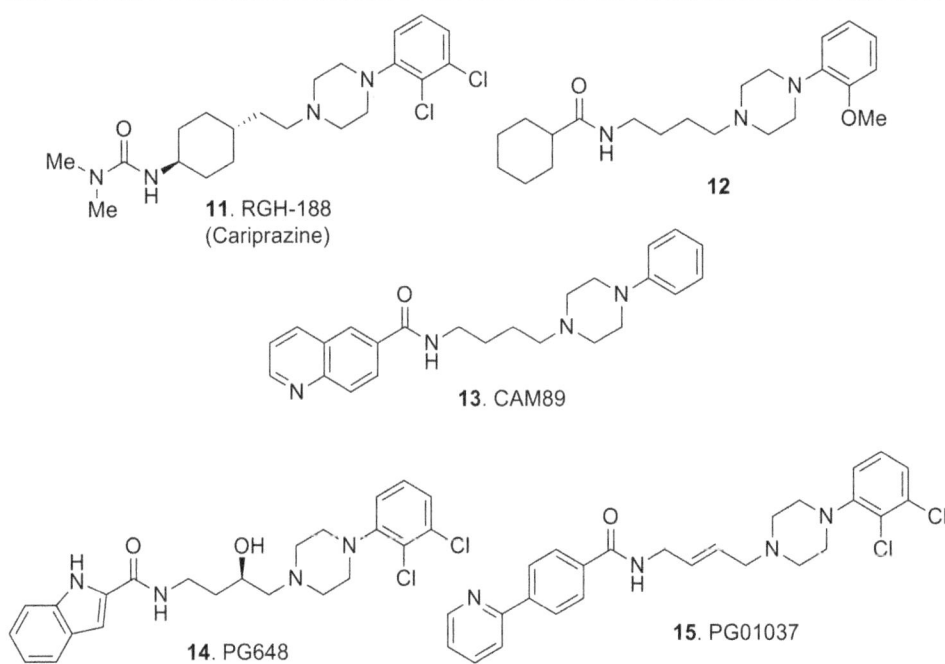

FIGURE 5 | Arylpiperazine-based derivatives 11-15.

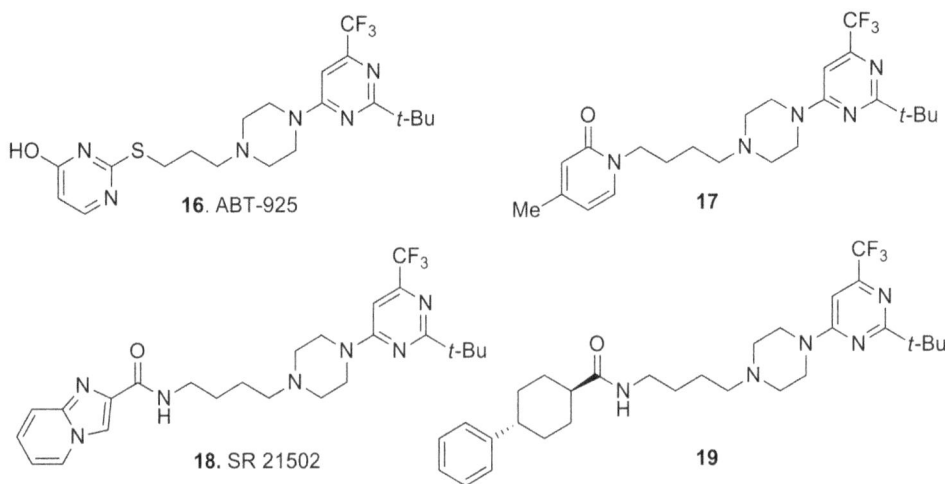

FIGURE 6 | Pyrimidinylpiperazine-based compounds 16–19.

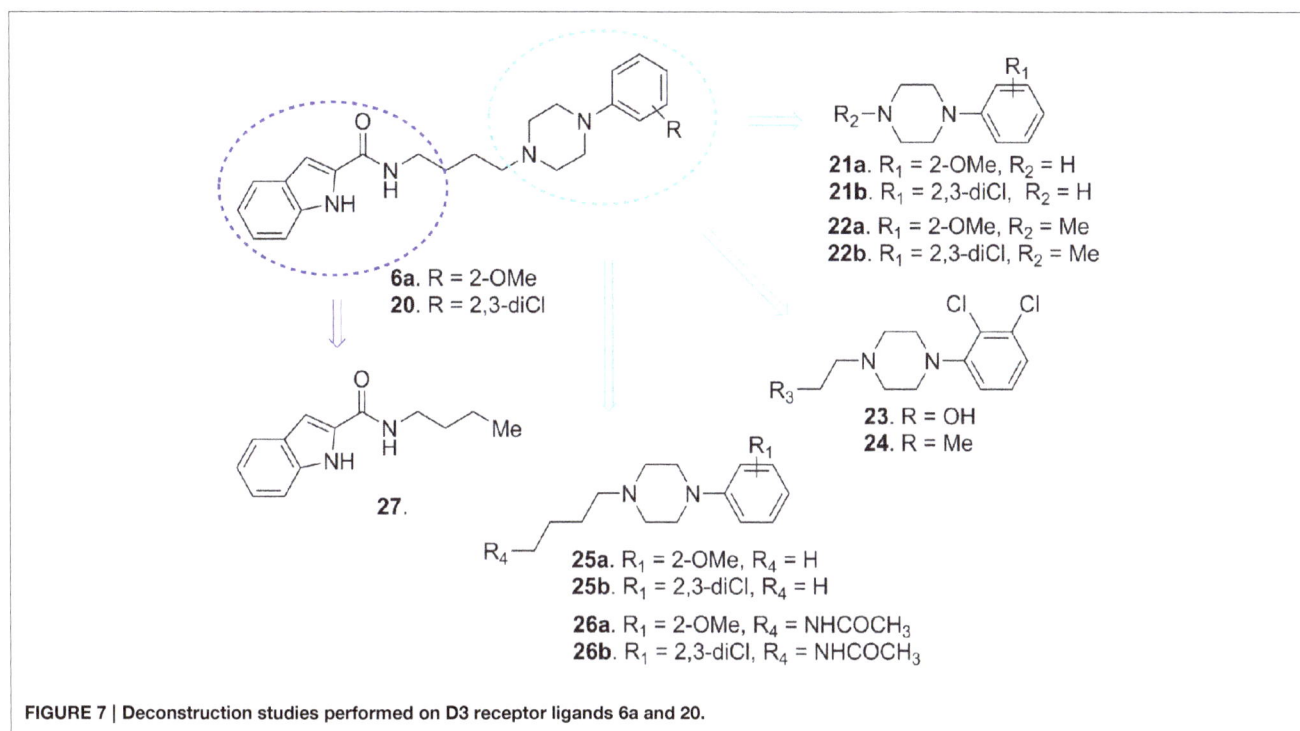

FIGURE 7 | Deconstruction studies performed on D3 receptor ligands 6a and 20.

9a,b (Figure 4), even though the hydroxy group at the 3-position brought a small drop of activity (K_i = 2.51 nM and 33.8 nM, respectively). The connection point of the amide functionality to the quinoline ring did not appear to strongly influence binding affinity and/or selectivity at D3 receptors, as well as the presence of an electron-withdrawing group on the quinoline ring. These compounds resulted in moderately potent antagonists, expressing weak partial agonist profiles at higher concentrations. This report further confirmed that the quinoline system represents a good scaffold for the development of D3 antagonists in terms of selectivity over D2 receptors. In fact, also derivatives **10a,b (Figure 4)**, in line with their 2-methoxyphenylpiperazine counterparts **9a,b**, behaved as potent and selective D3 antagonists displaying ability in reducing heroin self-administration. The same effect was not encountered in D3 knockout mice thus clearly demonstrating the involvement of D3 receptors (Boateng et al., 2015). The data regarding intrinsic affinity described in this paper essentially match with previous findings by Campiani et al. (2003), described by the development of compounds **7a,b** which were tested in cocaine craving.

Substantial elaboration of the pharmacophore model of **Figure 2** allowed the identification of RGH-188 (**11, Figure 5**), also known as cariprazine, a compound demonstrating subnanomolar affinity for D3 receptors and nanomolar affinity for D2 receptors (Kiss et al., 2010). This compound was developed in a medicinal chemistry approach (Agai-Csongor et al., 2012) aiming at the optimization of an impurity originally isolated during the scale-up process of a pyridylsulfonamide-based lead which behaved as D3/D2 antagonist. Cariprazine, was approved in 2015 in the USA for the treatment of schizophrenia and bipolar disorders under the trade name of Vraylar. The

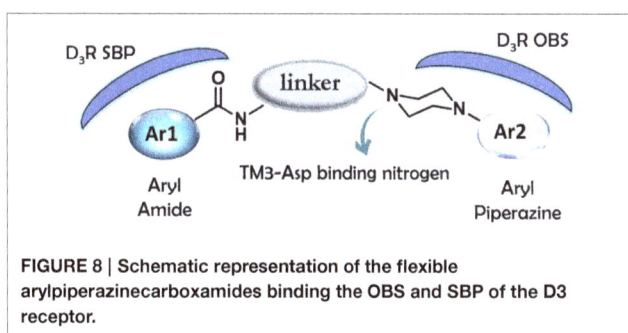

FIGURE 8 | Schematic representation of the flexible arylpiperazinecarboxamides binding the OBS and SBP of the D3 receptor.

structural innovation that this compound brought to the pharmacophoric model of **Figure 2** resided in the absence of one aromatic moiety which was efficiently replaced by a hydrophobic cyclohexyl ring system. Also the lack of the amide function connected to Ar1 of **Figure 2** was replaced by an ureido moiety on the west end of the molecule. Cariprazine was demonstrated to have antagonist–partial agonist activity at both D2 and D3 receptors and animal studies highlighted its efficacy for the treatment of schizophrenia and bipolar mania (Kiss et al., 2010). Further studies demonstrated that compound **11** was able to parallel the effect of the atypical antipsychotic aripiprazole in reducing the rewarding effect of cocaine and attenuated relapse to cocaine seeking (Román et al., 2013). In adult male rats, **11** dose-dependently reversed delay-induced impairment in novel object recognition. Further, acute administration (0.1 and 0.3 mg/kg orally) to animal models of phencyclidine-induced social isolation (in neonatal rats) reduced the symptoms and induced locomotor hyperactivity (Watson et al., 2016). Seminal clinical trials allowed to confirm the therapeutic potential of **11** in patients with acute exacerbation of schizophrenia (Durgam et al., 2015, 2016). Efficacy, safety, and tolerability of **11** were assessed in patients with acute mania associated with bipolar I disorders (Calabrese et al., 2015).

Notably, some studies also evidenced the efficacy of the compound in the treatment of the negative symptoms of schizophrenia (Debelle et al., 2015). The clinical efficacy of this D3 preferring ligand further confirms the role of D3 receptors in the management of the symptoms of schizophrenia (Citrome, 2016). Learning from **11** that the aromatic group such as Ar1 of **Figure 2** is not mandatory for attaining potent and selective D3 antagonism, Capet and colleagues synthesized a series of aliphatic amides and some ureidic analogs. Structure-activity relationship studies on this set of compounds showed that, as far as these products were lipophilic enough, they behaved as potent ligands (partial agonists) for human D3 receptors and the cyclohexyl amide analog **12** (**Figure 5**) was characterized as the best performing compound of the series (Capet et al., 2016).

One of the major drawbacks shared by many centrally active molecules, particularly those active at monoaminergic receptors, is the detection of high affinity at hERG potassium channels. Channel inhibition is associated to drug-induced torsades de pointes arrhythmia which is a major safety concern in the process of drug design and development. In fact hERG affinity is hard to be reduced in a drug design approach while retaining high receptor affinity. Unfortunately, compound **12** potently interacted with the hERG channels (82% inhibition of dofetilide binding when tested at 1 μM; Capet et al., 2016).

In a recent report describing the development of a series of arylpiperazines as potential atypical antipsychotics endowed with a multireceptor affinity profile, Brindisi and colleagues provided evidence that for compound **13** (**Figure 5**) they could achieve to lower hERG affinity up to 10 μM while retaining subnanomolar affinity for D3 receptors and nanomolar potency at 5-HT1A and 5-HT2A receptors [K_i (D3) = 0.6 nM, K_i (5-HT1A) = 99 nM, K_i (5-HT2A) = 66 nM; Brindisi et al., 2014]. This analog is endowed with a unique *in vitro* multireceptor pharmacological profile characterized by pronounced selectivity over the D2 (K_i (D2) > 1000 nM) and 5-HT2C receptors (K_i (5- HT2C) > 1000 nM). To further complement the significant efficacy profile of compound **13**, assessed in behavioral tests predictive of antipsychotic efficacy (e.g., MK801-induced hyperactivity and phencyclidine–induced PPI in mice) a promising therapeutic window was also ascertained by the absence of catalepsy at the antipsychotic effective dose and also in passive avoidance tests. Lack of cardiotoxicity in isolated Langendorff heart was also verified for this compound (Brindisi et al., 2014).

Newman and colleagues identified the first enantioselective D3 antagonists PG648 (*R*-**14**, **Figure 5**), bearing an indole system as suitable substructure for D3 ligand affinity, in which enantioselectivity was more pronounced at D3 than at D2 receptors and could represent a valuable characteristic for D3 receptor selectivity (K_i = 1.12 nM, 400-fold selective

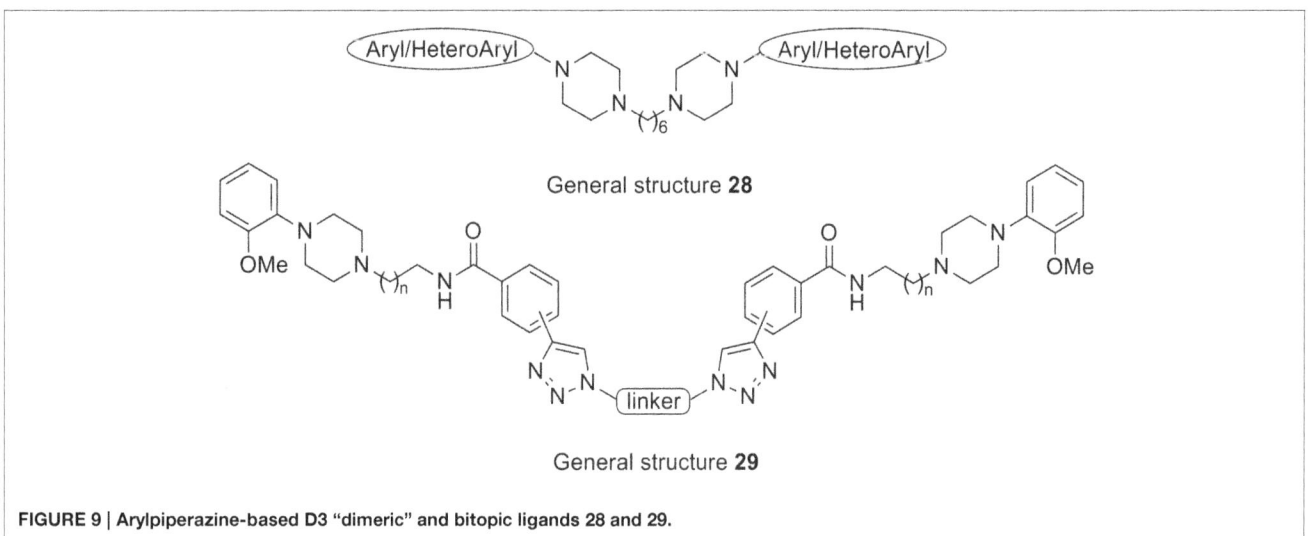

FIGURE 9 | Arylpiperazine-based D3 "dimeric" and bitopic ligands 28 and 29.

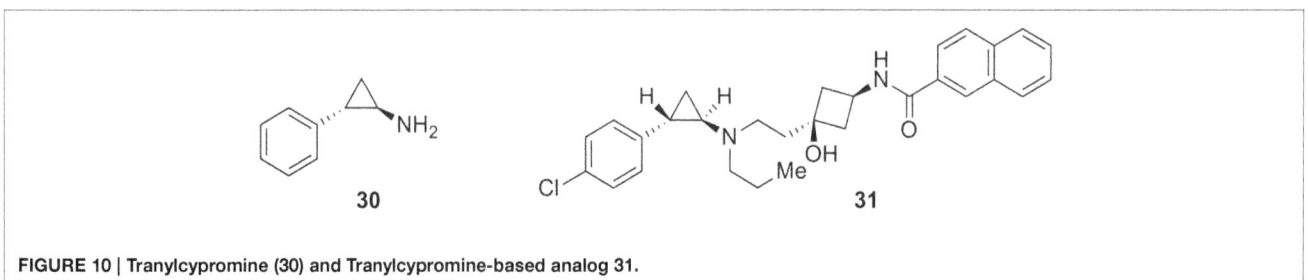

FIGURE 10 | Tranylcypromine (30) and Tranylcypromine-based analog 31.

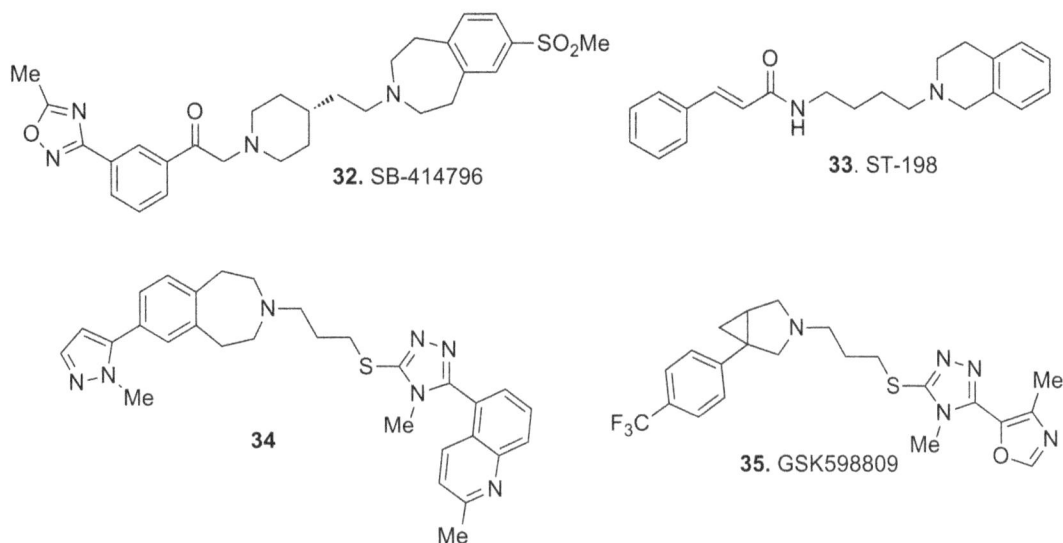

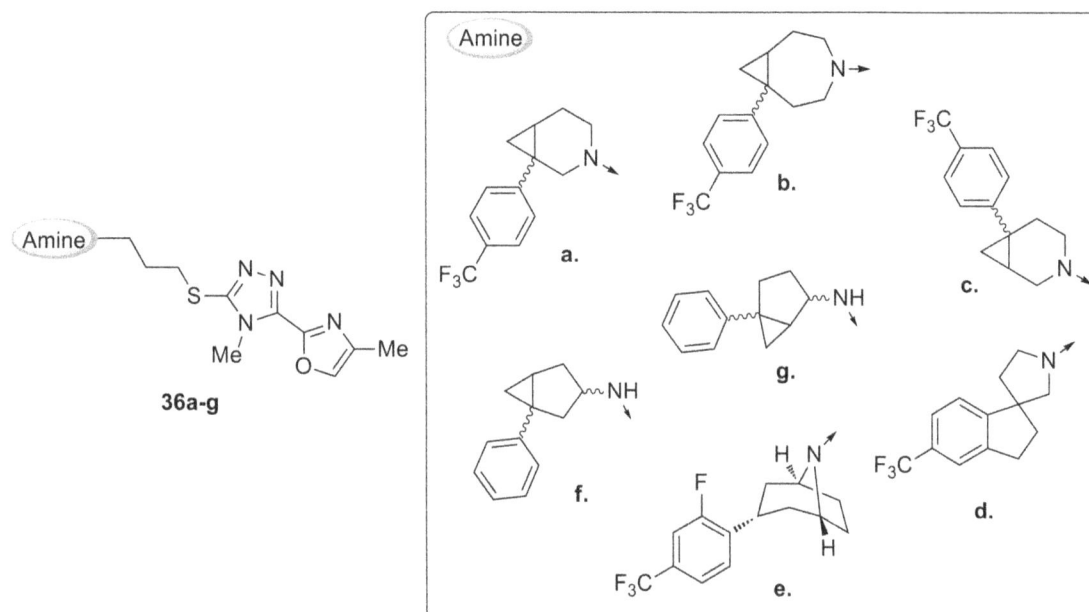

FIGURE 11 | Compounds 32 and 33 and structurally related triazole-based D3 antagonists 34–36.

D2/D3). Interestingly, this compound also exhibited balanced physico-chemical characteristics, useful for an appropriate *in vivo* exploration and determination of intrinsic activity at D3 receptors in animal models of addiction and other neuropsychiatric disorders (Newman et al., 2009).

The 2-pyridylphenyl analog **15** (**Figure 5**) with a $K_i = 0.7$ nM for D3 receptors and a D2/D3 selectivity ratio of 133, originally described in 2005 and after evaluation in animal models of cocaine abuse, served as an important pharmacological tool for highlighting the contribution of D3 receptors in drug reinforcement *in vivo* (Grundt et al., 2005). A more recent investigation of the same compound reported its useful application on methamphetamine self-administration,

methamphetamine-associated cue-induced reinstatement of drug seeking and methamphetamine-enhanced brain stimulation reward, thus highlighting the possible role of D3 antagonists also in the treatment of methamphetamine addiction (Higley et al., 2011).

A series of interesting compounds displayed a *tert*-butyl-trifluoromethylpyrimidine moiety connected to the piperazine. An early lead of this series was compound ABT-925 (**16**, **Figure 6**), which showed high affinity for the human D3 receptor ($K_i = 2.9$ nM), with at least 100-fold selectivity over the human D2 and other receptors, enzymes, and ion channels. This compound was a potent antagonist of D3 receptors, it could easily cross the blood–brain barrier and exerted efficacy in different animal models predictive of antipsychotic activity without inducing catalepsy or raising plasma prolactin levels (Geneste et al., 2006). The same report also described the methylpyridin-2-one analog **17** (**Figure 6**) which retained a good activity and selectivity for D3 vs. D2 receptors ($K_i = 0.8$ nM, with >80-fold selectivity vs. D2 receptors). However, within this class of compounds the best performances were achieved with the disclosure of SR21502 (**18**, **Figure 6**) which displayed a $K_i = 4.2$ nM at the D3 receptors with >120-fold of selectivity over the D2 receptors. Although, **18** behaved as weak partial agonist at the D3 receptors, in the agonist-stimulated mitogenesis assay, it behaved as an antagonist at D3 receptors (Ananthan et al., 2014). Compound **18** was recently employed as a pharmacological tool for evaluating its *in vivo* activity against cocaine reward and cocaine-seeking behaviors. Experimental data demonstrated efficacy of **18** against these behaviors which was not accompanied by effect on food reward or spontaneous locomotor activity (Galaj et al., 2014; Hachimine et al., 2014).

Among the pyrimidinylpiperazine derivatives, compound **19** (**Figure 6**) bearing a phenylcyclohexanecarboxamide moiety was recently characterized as a potent D3 vs. D2 receptors antagonist ($K_i = 9.4$ nM) with >150-fold selectivity over D2 receptors, thus fostering further investigation for these analogs as antipsychotics or in models of drug addiction (Ananthan et al., 2014).

In order to elucidate the structural features responsible both for D3 vs. D2 receptors efficacy and selectivity, in 2012 Newman and co-workers reported a deconstruction study on substituted-4-phenylpiperazines **6a** and **20** (**Figure 7**; Newman et al., 2012).

D3 receptors feature an orthosteric binding site (OBS), which binds DA, that is very similar to that of D2 receptors, and this represents a major issue in the development of D3 selective ligands. The Authors evidenced how selectivity could be managed by means of divergent interactions within a second binding pocket (SBP) which is distinct from the OBS. Notably, they also indicated that, the binding mode at SBP is highly influenced by that observed at the OBS. For reaching this conclusion the Authors studied the binding mode (by computational analysis) and affinity profile of a series of fragments (**21-27**, **Figure 7**) of compounds **6a** (Campiani et al., 2003) and **20** (Chu et al., 2005). They identified a primary pharmacophore element (the arylpiperazine moiety, **Figure 8**) which should bind the OBS, and a secondary pharmacophore element (the arylamide moiety, **Figure 8**) which should bind the SBP. Interestingly, these aspects could be translated to other GPCRs and, as a general "rule," it could be assumed that the SBP can be targeted by bitopic or allosteric ligands.

An earlier report by Butini and co-workers described the development of bishomo- or hetero-arylpiperazines (**28**, **Figure 9**) as flexible ligands for specific occupancy of D3, 5-HT1A, and 5-HT2A receptors. These compounds represent a different class of ligands when compared to the general structure of the proposed pharmacophoric model (see **Figure 2**; Butini et al., 2010). However, the same compounds may also comply with the above mentioned study of Newman and coworkers, but the nature of these homodimeric or heterodimeric ligands implies that both the primary pharmacophore element and the secondary pharmacophore element are arylpiperazines indeed.

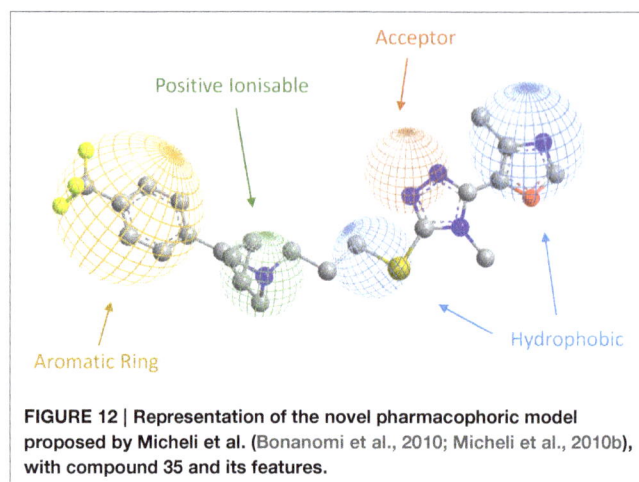

FIGURE 12 | Representation of the novel pharmacophoric model proposed by Micheli et al. (Bonanomi et al., 2010; Micheli et al., 2010b), with compound 35 and its features.

The same consideration may be true for bitopic ligands such as **29** (**Figure 9**) developed by Huber and colleagues in 2009 (Huber et al., 2009).

A further structural modification characterizes the new compound **31** (**Figure 10**), developed by Chen and co-workers, with marked differences from the classical arylpiperazine selective ligands. However, **31** still perfectly fitted the arlypiperazine–based pharmacophore of **Figure 2**. Compound **31** was a potent and selective D3 receptor antagonist based upon tranylcypromine (**30**, **Figure 10**) which effectively replaced the arylpiperazine moiety (Chen et al., 2014).

Although **30** had a low affinity for rat D3 receptors ($K_i = 12.8$ μM), derivative **31** showed K_i values of 2.7 and 2.8 nM at the rat and human D3 receptors, respectively, and displayed a high selectivity over the rat and human D2 receptors (>10,000-fold and 223-fold respectively). These features of compound **31** complemented by a good pharmacokinetic profile and brain permeability made it a promising candidate for the potential treatment of drug abuse.

1,2,4-TRIAZOLE-BASED D3 RECEPTOR LIGANDS

The arylpiperazine system proved to be an exceptionally valuable option for the design and development of selective D3 ligands, endowing the new compounds with different *in vitro* outcomes as both partial agonists and antagonists. However, in the last years, alternative scaffolds emerged such as 1,2,4-triazole-based derivatives which have been characterized as optimal alternative to the more conventional arylpiperazine-based pharmacophore of **Figure 2**. These studies led to the discovery of interesting structures potentially useful for the treatment of schizophrenia and related disorders.

An early series of triazole-based D3 antagonists was developed by drawing inspiration from the structure of compound **32** (**Figure 11**), a tetrahydro-1H-3-benzazepine which was described as a potent and selective D3 receptors antagonist with high oral bioavailability and blood-brain barrier permeability (Macdonald et al., 2003).

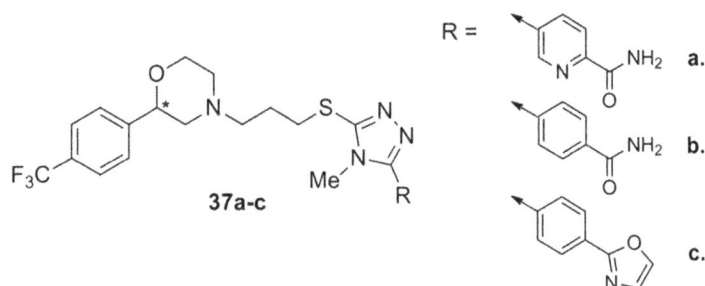

FIGURE 13 | Morpholino/triazole analogs 37a–c.

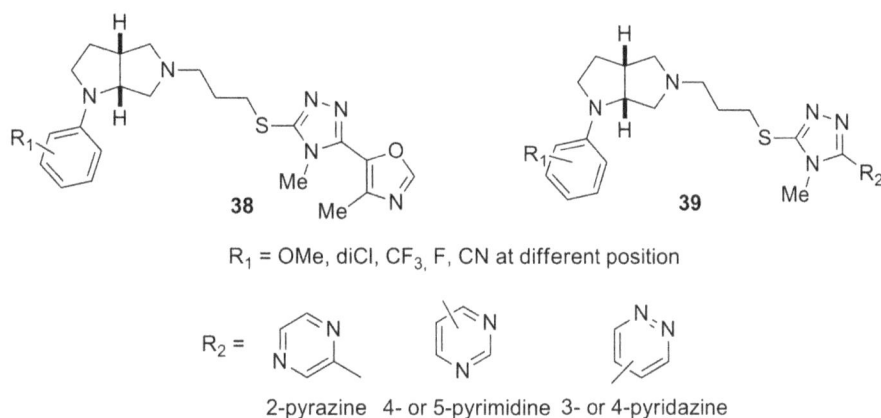

R_1 = OMe, diCl, CF_3, F, CN at different position

R_2 =   2-pyrazine   4- or 5-pyrimidine   3- or 4-pyridazine

FIGURE 14 | General structure of octahydropyrrolo[2,3-*b*]pyrrole-based D3 antagonists 38 and 39.

Also compound ST-198 (**33, Figure 11**), developed by Bézard and colleagues, bearing a tetrahydroisoquinoline moiety, resulted in a selective D3 antagonist over a wide panel of receptors (Bézard et al., 2003).

Subsequently, with the development of compound **34** (**Figure 11**) Micheli and co-workers highlighted that the thiotriazole scaffold coupled to a pyrazolyl moiety represented a promising combination for the design of D3 antagonists. In particular, **34** (**Figure 11**) showed good oral bioavailability and brain penetration associated with high potency and selectivity for D3 receptors *in vitro* (functional pK_i obtained from the GTPγS functional assay = 8.8). An in depth *in vivo* characterization of **34** showed its ability to prevent nicotine-induced conditioned place preference behavior in rats and to reduce alcohol self-administration. Moreover, it retained a low interaction with hERG channels and no QTc interval prolongation was observed in electrocardiograms, thus indicating a favorable potential for **34** to turn into an optimal candidate for the treatment of drug addiction, psychosis, and schizophrenia (Micheli et al., 2007).

More recently Micheli and collaborators reported an ample series of 1,2,4-triazolyl azabicyclo[3.1.0]hexanes as selective D3 receptors antagonists in which the oxazolyl derivative **35** (**Figure 11**) showed good affinity and selectivity coupled with optimal pharmacokinetic properties (Bonanomi et al., 2010; Micheli et al., 2010b). Successively, compound **35** was used

in studies regarding food cues in a human addict population, where it showed a lack of attentional bias toward food if compared with the placebo (Nathan et al., 2012). These data provided additional support that antagonism for D3 receptors may attenuate attentional processing of salient or rewarding cues. On the basis of the abovementioned results, the same Authors proposed a new pharmacophore model useful for the rationalization of the activity and selectivity profiles of this new series of compounds (**Figure 12**).

This also allowed the identification of alternative scaffolds to the azabicyclo[3.1.0]hexane, by the analysis of differently decorated amines that nicely fitted in the proposed pharmacophore model and prompted the synthesis of derivatives (**36a-g, Figure 11**; Micheli et al., 2010a).

Very recently, Micheli and colleagues reported the development of D3 ligands by means of a "scaffold hopping" strategy that resulted in the identification of a variety of original basic moieties and, more specifically, a morpholine system, to be spaced from the thiotriazole by a three-methylene tether (Micheli et al., 2016b). Derivative **37a** (**Figure 13**), one of the most active and selective D3 ligand of this interesting series, displayed a very high D3/D2 selectivity (800-fold) accompanied by a 60-fold selectivity vs. the hERG channel. Structure-activity relationship studies demonstrated that shift of the position of pyridine nitrogen reduced the affinity at D3 receptors, while its removal (benzamide **37b**, **Figure 13**) still allowed to maintain high D3 receptors affinity and D3/D2 selectivity accompanied by a notable 150-fold selectivity vs. the hERG channel. The compound bearing the oxazole moiety (**37c**, **Figure 13**) surprisingly showed increased affinity at the D3 receptors with 300-fold selectivity vs. D2 and 200-fold vs. hERG channel. These compounds, bearing a chiral center at the morpholino system level, were described and tested as racemates, although some of the pure enantiomers were tested showing different selectivity profile, highlighting a stereoselective interaction with DA receptors.

Another interesting and very wide series of ligands was reported by the same Authors (Micheli et al., 2016a) bearing an octahydropyrrolo[2,3-*b*]pyrrole scaffold characterized by high affinity and selectivity at D3 receptors (general structures **38** and **39**, **Figure 14**). Substituents at R1 position were -OMe, 2,3-dichloro, -CF$_3$ groups or fluorine atoms in general structure **38**, while R2, when different from the oxazole ring, could be a pyridine, pyrazine, pyrimidine, or pyridazine moiety, combined with the above listed R1 substituents (general structure **39**). Many of these derivatives proved to have ideal *in vitro* pharmacokinetic developability and, for some selected analogs, a large selectivity panel assessment campaign was performed including hERG channels.

CONCLUSION

In this review, an overview of the literature of the last 10 years in the field of D3 antagonists was provided. The

careful examination and clustering of the most significant compounds taken into consideration allowed delivering an overall picture of their structural variability. At the same time, the proposed analysis highlighted the substantial structural commonalities, despite the efforts of different research groups for providing pharmacophore refinements aiming at the discovery of innovative scaffolds for attaining high D3 receptor affinity and selectivity over the D2 receptors. The description of the pharmacodynamic (multi)receptor affinity profile and the most significant pharmacological applications for the examined compounds in the field of DA-related brain disorders were also covered, in order to provide clear-cut hints for their therapeutic potential.

AUTHOR CONTRIBUTIONS

SM wrote the paper. SG collected and clustered the literature data. SiBr collaborated in writing the introduction section and prepared the figures. GC collaborated in literature selection with particular reference to D3 antagonists as antipsychotics. SB collaborated to paper writing, supervised the overall work and revised the paper. HS collaborated in the reference literature selection and revised the paper. MB wrote the paper.

ACKNOWLEDGMENTS

The EU COST Action CM1103 is kindly acknowledged for financial support.

REFERENCES

Agai-Csongor, E., Domány, G., Nogradi, K., Galambos, J., Vago, I., Keseru, G. M., et al. (2012). Discovery of cariprazine (RGH-188): a novel antipsychotic acting on dopamine D3/D2 receptors. *Bioorg. Med. Chem. Lett.* 22, 3437–3440. doi: 10.1016/j.bmcl.2012.03.104

Agnati, L. F., Guidolin, D., Cervetto, C., Borroto-Escuela, D. O., and Fuxe, K. (2016). Role of iso-receptors in receptor-receptor interactions with a focus on dopamine iso-receptor complexes. *Rev. Neurosci.* 27, 1–25. doi: 10.1515/revneuro-2015-0024

Ananthan, S., Saini, S. K., Zhou, G., Hobrath, J. V., Padmalayam, I., Zhai, L., et al. (2014). Design, synthesis, and structure-activity relationship studies of a series of [4-(4-carboxamidobutyl)]-1-arylpiperazines: insights into structural features contributing to dopamine D3 versus D2 receptor subtype selectivity. *J. Med. Chem.* 57, 7042–7060. doi: 10.1021/jm500801r

Aragona, B. J., Day, J. J., Roitman, M. F., Cleaveland, N. A., Wightman, R. M., and Carelli, R. M. (2009). Regional specificity in the real-time development of phasic dopamine transmission patterns during acquisition of a cue-cocaine association in rats. *Eur. J. Neurosci.* 30, 1889–1899. doi: 10.1111/j.1460-9568.2009.07027.x

Beaulieu, J. M., and Gainetdinov, R. R. (2011). The physiology, signaling, and pharmacology of dopamine receptors. *Pharmacol. Rev.* 63, 182–217. doi: 10.1124/pr.110.002642

Beninger, R. J. (1983). The role of dopamine in locomotor activity and learning. *Brain Res.* 287, 173–196.

Bettinetti, L., Schlotter, K., Hübner, H., and Gmeiner, P. (2002). Interactive SAR studies: rational discovery of super-potent and highly selective dopamine D3 receptor antagonists and partial agonists. *J. Med. Chem.* 45, 4594–4597. doi: 10.1021/jm025558r

Bézard, E., Ferry, S., Mach, U., Stark, H., Leriche, L., Boraud, T., et al. (2003). Attenuation of levodopa-induced dyskinesia by normalizing dopamine D3 receptor function. *Nat. Med.* 9, 762–767. doi: 10.1038/nm875

Boateng, C. A., Bakare, O. M., Zhan, J., Banala, A. K., Burzynski, C., Pommier, E., et al. (2015). High affinity Dopamine D3 Receptor (D3R)-Selective Antagonists Attenuate Heroin Self-Administration in Wild-Type but not D3R Knockout Mice. *J. Med. Chem.* 58, 6195–6213. doi: 10.1021/acs.jmedchem.5b00776

Boileau, I., Payer, D., Houle, S., Behzadi, A., Rusjan, P. M., Tong, J., et al. (2012). Higher binding of the dopamine D3 receptor-preferring ligand [11C]-(+)-propyl-hexahydro-naphtho-oxazin in methamphetamine polydrug users: a positron emission tomography study. *J. Neurosci.* 32, 1353–1359. doi: 10.1523/JNEUROSCI.4371-11.2012

Bonanomi, G., Braggio, S., Capelli, A. M., Checchia, A., Di Fabio, R., Marchioro, C., et al. (2010). Triazolyl azabicyclo[3.1.0]hexanes: a class of potent and selective dopamine D(3) receptor antagonists. *ChemMedChem* 5, 705–715. doi: 10.1002/cmdc.201000026

Borroto-Escuela, D. O., Brito, I., Romero-Fernandez, W., Di Palma, M., Oflijan, J., Skieterska, K., et al. (2014). The G protein-coupled receptor heterodimer network (GPCR-HetNet) and its hub components. *Int. J. Mol. Sci.* 15, 8570–8590. doi: 10.3390/ijms15058570

Brindisi, M., Butini, S., Franceschini, S., Brogi, S., Trotta, F., Ros, S., et al. (2014). Targeting dopamine D3 and serotonin 5-HT1A and 5-HT2A receptors for developing effective antipsychotics: synthesis, biological characterization, and behavioral studies. *J. Med. Chem.* 57, 9578–9597. doi: 10.1021/jm501119j

Brisch, R., Saniotis, A., Wolf, R., Bielau, H., Bernstein, H. G., Steiner, J., et al. (2014). The role of dopamine in schizophrenia from a neurobiological and evolutionary perspective: old fashioned, but still in vogue. *Front. Psychiatry* 5:47. doi: 10.3389/fpsyt.2014.00047

Brogi, S., Tafi, A., Désaubry, L., and Nebigil, C. G. (2014). Discovery of GPCR ligands for probing signal transduction pathways. *Front. Pharmacol.* 5:255. doi: 10.3389/fphar.2014.00255

Brooks, D. J. (2000). Dopamine agonists: their role in the treatment of Parkinson's disease. *J. Neurol. Neurosurg. Psychiatr.* 68, 685–689. doi: 10.1136/jnnp.68.6.685

Butini, S., Campiani, G., Franceschini, S., Trotta, F., Kumar, V., Guarino, E., et al. (2010). Discovery of bishomo(hetero)arylpiperazines as novel multifunctional ligands targeting dopamine D(3) and serotonin 5-HT(1A) and 5-HT(2A) receptors. *J. Med. Chem.* 53, 4803–4807. doi: 10.1021/jm100294b

Butini, S., Gemma, S., Campiani, G., Franceschini, S., Trotta, F., Borriello, M., et al. (2009). Discovery of a new class of potential multifunctional atypical antipsychotic agents targeting dopamine D3 and serotonin 5-HT1A and 5-HT2A receptors: design, synthesis, and effects on behavior. *J. Med. Chem.* 52, 151–169. doi: 10.1021/jm800689g

Butini, S., Nikolic, K., Kassel, S., Brückmann, H., Filipic, S., Agbaba, D., et al. (2016). Polypharmacology of dopamine receptor ligands. *Prog. Neurobiol.* 142, 68–103. doi: 10.1016/j.pneurobio.2016.03.011

Calabrese, J. R., Keck, P. E. Jr., Starace, A., Lu, K., Ruth, A., Laszlovszky, I., et al. (2015). Efficacy and safety of low- and high-dose cariprazine in acute and mixed mania associated with bipolar I disorder: a double-blind, placebo-controlled study. *J. Clin. Psychiatry* 76, 284–292. doi: 10.4088/JCP.14m09081

Campiani, G., Butini, S., Trotta, F., Fattorusso, C., Catalanotti, B., Aiello, F., et al. (2003). Synthesis and pharmacological evaluation of potent and highly selective D3 receptor ligands: inhibition of cocaine-seeking behavior and the role of dopamine D3/D2 receptors. *J. Med. Chem.* 46, 3822–3839. doi: 10.1021/jm0211220

Capet, M., Calmels, T., Levoin, N., Danvy, D., Berrebi-Bertrand, I., Stark, H., et al. (2016). Improving selectivity of dopamine D3 receptor ligands. *Bioorg. Med. Chem. Lett.* 26, 885–888. doi: 10.1016/j.bmcl.2015.12.068

Carelli, R. M., Williams, J. G., and Hollander, J. A. (2003). Basolateral amygdala neurons encode cocaine self-administration and cocaine-associated cues. *J. Neurosci.* 23, 8204–8211.

Chen, J., Levant, B., Jiang, C., Keck, T. M., Newman, A. H., and Wang, S. (2014). Tranylcypromine substituted cis-hydroxycyclobutylnaphthamides as potent and selective dopamine D(3) receptor antagonists. *J. Med. Chem.* 57, 4962–4968. doi: 10.1021/jm401798r

Chien, E. Y., Liu, W., Zhao, Q., Katritch, V., Han, G. W., Hanson, M. A., et al. (2010). Structure of the human dopamine D3 receptor in complex with a D2/D3 selective antagonist. *Science* 330, 1091–1095. doi: 10.1126/science.1197410

Chu, W., Tu, Z., Mcelveen, E., Xu, J., Taylor, M., Luedtke, R. R., et al. (2005). Synthesis and *in vitro* binding of N-phenyl piperazine analogs as potential dopamine D3 receptor ligands. *Bioorg. Med. Chem.* 13, 77–87. doi: 10.1016/j.bmc.2004.09.054

Ciccocioppo, R., Martin-Fardon, R., and Weiss, F. (2004). Stimuli associated with a single cocaine experience elicit long-lasting cocaine-seeking. *Nat. Neurosci.* 7, 495–496. doi: 10.1038/nn1219

Citrome, L. (2016). Cariprazine for the treatment of Schizophrenia: a review of this Dopamine D3-Preferring D3/D2 receptor partial agonist. *Clin. Schizophr. Relat. Psychoses* 10, 109–119. doi: 10.3371/1935-1232-10.2.109

Conrad, K. L., Ford, K., Marinelli, M., and Wolf, M. E. (2010). Dopamine receptor expression and distribution dynamically change in the rat nucleus accumbens after withdrawal from cocaine self-administration. *Neuroscience* 169, 182–194. doi: 10.1016/j.neuroscience.2010.04.056

Cools, R. (2008). Role of dopamine in the motivational and cognitive control of behavior. *Neuroscientist* 14, 381–395. doi: 10.1177/1073858408317009

Debelle, M., Németh, G., Szalai, E., Szatmári, B., Harsányi, J., Barabassy, A., et al. (2015). P.3.d.053 Cariprazine as monotherapy for the treatment of schizophrenia patients with predominant negative symptoms: a double-blind, active controlled trial. *Eur. Neuropsychopharmacol.* 25(Suppl. 2), S510. doi: 10.1016/S0924-977X(15)30701-X

De Mei, C., Ramos, M., Iitaka, C., and Borrelli, E. (2009). Getting specialized: presynaptic and postsynaptic dopamine D2 receptors. *Curr. Opin. Pharmacol.* 9, 53–58. doi: 10.1016/j.coph.2008.12.002

Durgam, S., Cutler, A. J., Lu, K., Migliore, R., Ruth, A., Laszlovszky, I., et al. (2015). Cariprazine in acute exacerbation of schizophrenia: a fixed-dose, phase 3, randomized, double-blind, placebo- and active-controlled trial. *J. Clin. Psychiatry* 76, e1574–e1582. doi: 10.4088/JCP.15m09997

Durgam, S., Litman, R. E., Papadakis, K., Li, D., Nemeth, G., and Laszlovszky, I. (2016). Cariprazine in the treatment of schizophrenia: a proof-of-concept trial. *Int. Clin. Psychopharmacol.* 31, 61–68. doi: 10.1097/YIC.00000000 00000110

Galaj, E., Ananthan, S., Saliba, M., and Ranaldi, R. (2014). The effects of the novel DA D3 receptor antagonist SR 21502 on cocaine reward, cocaine seeking and

cocaine-induced locomotor activity in rats. *Psychopharmacology (Berl).* 231, 501–510. doi: 10.1007/s00213-013-3254-y

Garcia-Ladona, F. J., and Cox, B. F. (2003). BP 897, a selective dopamine D3 receptor ligand with therapeutic potential for the treatment of cocaine-addiction. *CNS Drug Rev.* 9, 141–158. doi: 10.1111/j.1527-3458.2003. tb00246.x

Geneste, H., Amberg, W., Backfisch, G., Beyerbach, A., Braje, W. M., Delzer, J., et al. (2006). Synthesis and SAR of highly potent and selective dopamine D3-receptor antagonists: variations on the 1H-pyrimidin-2-one theme. *Bioorg. Med. Chem. Lett.* 16, 1934–1937. doi: 10.1016/j.bmcl.2005.12.079

Grundt, P., Carlson, E. E., Cao, J., Bennett, C. J., Mcelveen, E., Taylor, M., et al. (2005). Novel heterocyclic trans olefin analogues of N-{4-[4-(2,3-dichlorophenyl)piperazin-1-yl]butyl}arylcarboxamides as selective probes with high affinity for the dopamine D3 receptor. *J. Med. Chem.* 48, 839–848. doi: 10.1021/jm049465g

Guitart, X., Navarro, G., Moreno, E., Yano, H., Cai, N. S., Sánchez-Soto, M., et al. (2014). Functional selectivity of allosteric interactions within G protein-coupled receptor oligomers: the dopamine D1-D3 receptor heterotetramer. *Mol. Pharmacol.* 86, 417–429. doi: 10.1124/mol.114. 093096

Gurevich, E. V., and Joyce, J. N. (1999). Distribution of dopamine D3 receptor expressing neurons in the human forebrain: comparison with D2 receptor expressing neurons. *Neuropsychopharmacology* 20, 60–80. doi: 10.1016/S0893-133X(98)00066-9

Hachimine, P., Seepersad, N., Ananthan, S., and Ranaldi, R. (2014). The novel dopamine D3 receptor antagonist, SR 21502, reduces cocaine conditioned place preference in rats. *Neurosci. Lett.* 569, 137–141. doi: 10.1016/j.neulet.2014.03.055

Hackling, A. E., and Stark, H. (2002). Dopamine D3 receptor ligands with antagonist properties. *Chembiochem* 3, 946–961. doi: 10.1002/1439-7633(20021004)3:10<946::AID-CBIC946>3.0.CO;2-5

Hall, H., Halldin, C., Dijkstra, D., Wikström, H., Wise, L. D., Pugsley, T. A., et al. (1996). Autoradiographic localisation of D3-dopamine receptors in the human brain using the selective D3-dopamine receptor agonist (+)-[3H]PD 128907. *Psychopharmacology (Berl).* 128, 240–247.

Heidbreder, C. A., and Newman, A. H. (2010). Current perspectives on selective dopamine D(3) receptor antagonists as pharmacotherapeutics for addictions and related disorders. *Ann. N.Y. Acad. Sci.* 1187, 4–34. doi: 10.1111/j.1749-6632.2009.05149.x

Higley, A. E., Spiller, K., Grundt, P., Newman, A. H., Kiefer, S. W., Xi, Z. X., et al. (2011). PG01037, a novel dopamine D3 receptor antagonist, inhibits the effects of methamphetamine in rats. *J. Psychopharmacol. (Oxford).* 25, 263–273. doi: 10.1177/0269881109358201

Huber, D., Hübner, H., and Gmeiner, P. (2009). 1,1′-Disubstituted ferrocenes as molecular hinges in mono- and bivalent dopamine receptor ligands. *J. Med. Chem.* 52, 6860–6870. doi: 10.1021/jm901120h

Ito, R., Robbins, T. W., and Everitt, B. J. (2004). Differential control over cocaine-seeking behavior by nucleus accumbens core and shell. *Nat. Neurosci.* 7, 389–397. doi: 10.1038/nn1217

Joyce, J. N., and Millan, M. J. (2005). Dopamine D3 receptor antagonists as therapeutic agents. *Drug Discov. Today* 10, 917–925. doi: 10.1016/S1359-6446(05)03491-4

Kassel, S., Schwed, J. S., and Stark, H. (2015). Dopamine D3 receptor agonists as pharmacological tools. *Eur. Neuropsychopharmacol.* 25, 1480–1499. doi: 10.1016/j.euroneuro.2014.11.005

Kiss, B., Horváth, A., Némethy, Z., Schmidt, E., Laszlovszky, I., Bugovics, G., et al. (2010). Cariprazine (RGH-188), a dopamine D(3) receptor-preferring, D(3)/D(2) dopamine receptor antagonist-partial agonist antipsychotic candidate: *in vitro* and neurochemical profile. *J. Pharmacol. Exp. Ther.* 333, 328–340. doi: 10.1124/jpet.109.160432

Löber, S., Hübner, H., Tschammer, N., and Gmeiner, P. (2011). Recent advances in the search for D3- and D4-selective drugs: probes, models and candidates. *Trends Pharmacol. Sci.* 32, 148–157. doi: 10.1016/j.tips.20 10.12.003

Luedtkea, R. R., and Mach, R. H. (2003). Progress in developing D3 dopamine receptor ligands as potential therapeutic agents for neurological and neuropsychiatric disorders. *Curr. Pharm. Des.* 9, 643–671. doi: 10.2174/1381612033391199

Macdonald, G. J., Branch, C. L., Hadley, M. S., Johnson, C. N., Nash, D. J., Smith, A. B., et al. (2003). Design and synthesis of trans-3-(2-(4-((3-(3-(5-methyl-1,2,4-oxadiazolyl))- phenyl)carboxamido)cyclohexyl)ethyl)-7-methylsulfonyl-2,3,4,5-tetrahydro-1H-3-ben zazepine (SB-414796): a potent and selective dopamine D3 receptor antagonist. *J. Med. Chem.* 46, 4952–4964. doi: 10.1021/jm030817d

Maggio, R., Scarselli, M., Capannolo, M., and Millan, M. J. (2015). Novel dimensions of D3 receptor function: focus on heterodimerisation, transactivation and allosteric modulation. *Eur. Neuropsychopharmacol.* 25, 1470–1479. doi: 10.1016/j.euroneuro.2014.09.016

Meincke, U., Mörth, D., Voss, T., Thelen, B., Geyer, M. A., and Gouzoulis-Mayfrank, E. (2004). Prepulse inhibition of the acoustically evoked startle reflex in patients with an acute schizophrenic psychosis–a longitudinal study. *Eur. Arch. Psychiatry Clin. Neurosci.* 254, 415–421. doi: 10.1007/s00406-004-0523-0

Meltzer, H. Y. (2004). Cognitive factors in schizophrenia: causes, impact, and treatment. *CNS Spectr.* 9, 15–24. doi: 10.1017/S1092852900025098

Micheli, F., Arista, L., Bertani, B., Braggio, S., Capelli, A. M., Cremonesi, S., et al. (2010a). Exploration of the amine terminus in a novel series of 1,2,4-triazolo-3-yl-azabicyclo[3.1.0]hexanes as selective dopamine D3 receptor antagonists. *J. Med. Chem.* 53, 7129–7139. doi: 10.1021/jm100832d

Micheli, F., Arista, L., Bonanomi, G., Blaney, F. E., Braggio, S., Capelli, A. M., et al. (2010b). 1,2,4-Triazolyl azabicyclo[3.1.0]hexanes: a new series of potent and selective dopamine D(3) receptor antagonists. *J. Med. Chem.* 53, 374–391. doi: 10.1021/jm901319p

Micheli, F., Bernardelli, A., Bianchi, F., Braggio, S., Castelletti, L., Cavallini, P., et al. (2016a). 1,2,4-Triazolyl octahydropyrrolo[2,3-b]pyrroles: a new series of potent and selective dopamine D3 receptor antagonists. *Bioorg. Med. Chem.* 24, 1619–1636. doi: 10.1016/j.bmc.2016.02.031

Micheli, F., Bonanomi, G., Blaney, F. E., Braggio, S., Capelli, A. M., Checchia, A., et al. (2007). 1,2,4-triazol-3-yl-thiopropyl-tetrahydrobenzazepines: a series of potent and selective dopamine D(3) receptor antagonists. *J. Med. Chem.* 50, 5076–5089. doi: 10.1021/jm0705612

Micheli, F., Cremonesi, S., Semeraro, T., Tarsi, L., Tomelleri, S., Cavanni, P., et al. (2016b). Novel morpholine scaffolds as selective dopamine (DA) D3 receptor antagonists. *Bioorg. Med. Chem. Lett.* 26, 1329–1332. doi: 10.1016/j.bmcl.2015.12.081

Millan, M. J., and Brocco, M. (2008). Cognitive impairment in schizophrenia: a review of developmental and genetic models, and pro-cognitive profile of the optimised D(3) > D(2) antagonist, S33138. *Therapie* 63, 187–229. doi: 10.2515/therapie:2008041

Millan, M. J., Dekeyne, A., Rivet, J. M., Dubuffet, T., Lavielle, G., and Brocco, M. (2000). S33084, a novel, potent, selective, and competitive antagonist at dopamine D(3)-receptors: II. Functional and behavioral profile compared with GR218,231 and L741,626. *J. Pharmacol. Exp. Ther.* 293, 1063–1073.

Millan, M. J., Loiseau, F., Dekeyne, A., Gobert, A., Flik, G., Cremers, T. I., et al. (2008). S33138 (N-[4-[2-[(3aS,9bR)-8-cyano-1,3a,4,9b-tetrahydro[1] benzopyrano[3,4-c]pyrrol-2(3H)-yl]-ethyl]phenyl-acetamide], a preferential dopamine D3 versus D2 receptor antagonist and potential antipsychotic agent: III. Actions in models of therapeutic activity and induction of side effects. *J. Pharmacol. Exp. Ther.* 324, 1212–1226. doi: 10.1124/jpet.107.134536

Missale, C., Nash, S. R., Robinson, S. W., Jaber, M., and Caron, M. G. (1998). Dopamine receptors: from structure to function. *Physiol. Rev.* 78, 189–225.

Nathan, P. J., O'Neill, B. V., Mogg, K., Bradley, B. P., Beaver, J., Bani, M., et al. (2012). The effects of the dopamine D(3) receptor antagonist GSK598809 on attentional bias to palatable food cues in overweight and obese subjects. *Int. J. Neuropsychopharmacol.* 15, 149–161. doi: 10.1017/S1461145711001052

Newman, A. H., Beuming, T., Banala, A. K., Donthamsetti, P., Pongetti, K., Labounty, A., et al. (2012). Molecular determinants of selectivity and efficacy at the dopamine D3 receptor. *J. Med. Chem.* 55, 6689–6699. doi: 10.1021/jm300482h

Newman, A. H., Grundt, P., Cyriac, G., Deschamps, J. R., Taylor, M., Kumar, R., et al. (2009). N-(4-(4-(2,3-dichloro- or 2-methoxyphenyl)piperazin-1-yl)butyl)heterobiarylcarboxamides with functionalized linking chains as high affinity and enantioselective D3 receptor antagonists. *J. Med. Chem.* 52, 2559–2570. doi: 10.1021/jm900095y

Newman, A. H., Grundt, P., and Nader, M. A. (2005). Dopamine D3 receptor partial agonists and antagonists as potential drug abuse therapeutic agents. *J. Med. Chem.* 48, 3663–3679. doi: 10.1021/jm040190e

Nieoullon, A. (2002). Dopamine and the regulation of cognition and attention. *Prog. Neurobiol.* 67, 53–83. doi: 10.1016/S0301-0082(02)00011-4

Park, W. K., Jeong, D., Cho, H., Lee, S. J., Cha, M. Y., Pae, A. N., et al. (2005). KKHA-761, a potent D3 receptor antagonist with high 5-HT1A receptor affinity, exhibits antipsychotic properties in animal models of schizophrenia. *Pharmacol. Biochem. Behav.* 82, 361–372. doi: 10.1016/j.pbb.2005.09.006

Pilla, M., Perachon, S., Sautel, F., Garrido, F., Mann, A., Wermuth, C. G., et al. (1999). Selective inhibition of cocaine-seeking behaviour by a partial dopamine D3 receptor agonist. *Nature* 400, 371–375. doi: 10.1038/22560

Rangel-Barajas, C., Coronel, I., and Florán, B. (2015). Dopamine Receptors and Neurodegeneration. *Aging Dis.* 6, 349–368. doi: 10.14336/AD.2015.0330

Reavill, C., Taylor, S. G., Wood, M. D., Ashmeade, T., Austin, N. E., Avenell, K. Y., et al. (2000). Pharmacological actions of a novel, high-affinity, and selective human dopamine D(3) receptor antagonist, SB-277011-A. *J. Pharmacol. Exp. Ther.* 294, 1154–1165.

Román, V., Gyertyán, I., Sághy, K., Kiss, B., and Szombathelyi, Z. (2013). Cariprazine (RGH-188), a D(3)-preferring dopamine D(3)/D(2) receptor partial agonist antipsychotic candidate demonstrates anti-abuse potential in rats. *Psychopharmacology (Berl).* 226, 285–293. doi: 10.1007/s00213-012-2906-7

Sibley, D. R., and Monsma, F. J. Jr. (1992). Molecular biology of dopamine receptors. *Trends Pharmacol. Sci.* 13, 61–69.

Silvano, E., Millan, M. J., Mannoury La Cour, C., Han, Y., Duan, L., Griffin, S. A., et al. (2010). The tetrahydroisoquinoline derivative SB269,652 is an allosteric antagonist at dopamine D3 and D2 receptors. *Mol. Pharmacol.* 78, 925–934. doi: 10.1124/mol.110.065755

Staley, J. K., and Mash, D. C. (1996). Adaptive increase in D3 dopamine receptors in the brain reward circuits of human cocaine fatalities. *J. Neurosci.* 16, 6100–6106.

Suzuki, M., Hurd, Y. L., Sokoloff, P., Schwartz, J. C., and Sedvall, G. (1998). D3 dopamine receptor mRNA is widely expressed in the human brain. *Brain Res.* 779, 58–74.

Thanos, P. K., Katana, J. M., Ashby, C. R. Jr., Michaelides, M., Gardner, E. L., Heidbreder, C. A., et al. (2005). The selective dopamine D3 receptor antagonist SB-277011-A attenuates ethanol consumption in ethanol preferring (P) and non-preferring (NP) rats. *Pharmacol. Biochem. Behav.* 81, 190–197. doi: 10.1016/j.pbb.2005.03.013

Volkow, N. D., Fowler, J. S., Wang, G. J., Swanson, J. M., and Telang, F. (2007). Dopamine in drug abuse and addiction: results of imaging studies and treatment implications. *Arch. Neurol.* 64, 1575–1579. doi: 10.1001/archneur.64.11.1575

Volkow, N. D., Wang, G. J., and Baler, R. D. (2011). Reward, dopamine and the control of food intake: implications for obesity. *Trends Cogn. Sci.* 15, 37–46. doi: 10.1016/j.tics.2010.11.001

Volkow, N. D., Wang, G. J., Telang, F., Fowler, J. S., Logan, J., Childress, A. R., et al. (2006). Cocaine cues and dopamine in dorsal striatum: mechanism of craving in cocaine addiction. *J. Neurosci.* 26, 6583–6588. doi: 10.1523/JNEUROSCI.1544-06.2006

Volkow, N. D., Wang, G. J., Telang, F., Fowler, J. S., Logan, J., Childress, A. R., et al. (2008). Dopamine increases in striatum do not elicit craving in cocaine abusers unless they are coupled with cocaine cues. *Neuroimage* 39, 1266–1273. doi: 10.1016/j.neuroimage.2007.09.059

Watson, D. J., King, M. V., Gyertyán, I., Kiss, B., Adham, N., and Fone, K. C. (2016). The dopamine D(3)-preferring D(2)/D(3) dopamine receptor partial agonist, cariprazine, reverses behavioural changes in a rat neurodevelopmental model for schizophrenia. *Eur. Neuropsychopharmacol.* 26, 208–224. doi: 10.1016/j.euroneuro.2015.12.020

Watson, D. J., Loiseau, F., Ingallinesi, M., Millan, M. J., Marsden, C. A., and Fone, K. C. (2012). Selective blockade of dopamine D3 receptors enhances while D2 receptor antagonism impairs social novelty discrimination and novel object recognition in rats: a key role for the prefrontal cortex. *Neuropsychopharmacology* 37, 770–786. doi: 10.1038/npp.2011.254

Weber, M., Chang, W. L., Durbin, J. P., Park, P. E., Luedtke, R. R., Mach, R. H., et al. (2009). Using prepulse inhibition to detect functional D3 receptor antagonism: effects of WC10 and WC44. *Pharmacol. Biochem. Behav.* 93, 141–147. doi: 10.1016/j.pbb.2009.04.022

Wise, R. A., and Rompre, P. P. (1989). Brain dopamine and reward. *Annu. Rev. Psychol.* 40, 191–225. doi: 10.1146/annurev.ps.40.020189.001203

Wong, D. F., Kuwabara, H., Schretlen, D. J., Bonson, K. R., Zhou, Y., Nandi, A., et al. (2006). Increased occupancy of dopamine receptors in human striatum during cue-elicited cocaine craving. *Neuropsychopharmacology* 31, 2716–2727. doi: 10.1038/sj.npp.1301194

Xi, Z. X., and Gardner, E. L. (2007). Pharmacological actions of NGB 2904, a selective dopamine D3 receptor antagonist, in animal models of drug addiction. *CNS Drug Rev.* 13, 240–259. doi: 10.1111/j.1527-3458.2007.00013.x

Xi, Z. X., Gilbert, J., Campos, A. C., Kline, N., Ashby, C. R. Jr., Hagan, J. J., et al. (2004). Blockade of mesolimbic dopamine D3 receptors inhibits stress-induced reinstatement of cocaine-seeking in rats. *Psychopharmacology (Berl).* 176, 57–65. doi: 10.1007/s00213-004-1858-y

Yuan, J., Chen, X., Brodbeck, R., Primus, R., Braun, J., Wasley, J. W., et al. (1998). NGB 2904 and NGB 2849: two highly selective dopamine D3 receptor antagonists. *Bioorg. Med. Chem. Lett.* 8, 2715–2718.

Zhang, M., Ballard, M. E., Unger, L. V., Haupt, A., Gross, G., Decker, M. W., et al. (2007). Effects of antipsychotics and selective D3 antagonists on PPI deficits induced by PD 128907 and apomorphine. *Behav. Brain Res.* 182, 1–11. doi: 10.1016/j.bbr.2007.04.021

Conflict of Interest Statement: The authors declare that the research was conducted in the absence of any commercial or financial relationships that could be construed as a potential conflict of interest.

9

The Use of Multiscale Molecular Simulations in Understanding a Relationship between the Structure and Function of Biological Systems of the Brain: The Application to Monoamine Oxidase Enzymes

Robert Vianello[1]*, Carmen Domene[2, 3] and Janez Mavri[4]

[1] *Computational Organic Chemistry and Biochemistry Group, Ruđer Bošković Institute, Zagreb, Croatia,* [2] *Department of Chemistry, King's College London, London, UK,* [3] *Chemistry Research Laboratory, University of Oxford, Oxford, UK,* [4] *Department of Computational Biochemistry and Drug Design, National Institute of Chemistry, Ljubljana, Slovenia*

Edited by:
Rona R. Ramsay,
University of St. Andrews, UK

Reviewed by:
Sulev Kõks,
University of Tartu, Estonia
Kemal Yelekci,
Kadir Has University, Turkey

*Correspondence:
Robert Vianello
robert.vianello@irb.hr

HIGHLIGHTS

- Computational techniques provide accurate descriptions of the structure and dynamics of biological systems, contributing to their understanding at an atomic level.
- Classical MD simulations are a precious computational tool for the processes where no chemical reactions take place.
- QM calculations provide valuable information about the enzyme activity, being able to distinguish among several mechanistic pathways, provided a carefully selected cluster model of the enzyme is considered.
- Multiscale QM/MM simulation is the method of choice for the computational treatment of enzyme reactions offering quantitative agreement with experimentally determined reaction parameters.
- Molecular simulation provide insight into the mechanism of both the catalytic activity and inhibition of monoamine oxidases, thus aiding in the rational design of their inhibitors that are all employed and antidepressants and antiparkinsonian drugs.

Aging society and therewith associated neurodegenerative and neuropsychiatric diseases, including depression, Alzheimer's disease, obsessive disorders, and Parkinson's disease, urgently require novel drug candidates. Targets include monoamine oxidases A and B (MAOs), acetylcholinesterase (AChE), butyrylcholinesterase (BChE), and various receptors and transporters. For rational drug design it is particularly important to combine experimental synthetic, kinetic, toxicological, and pharmacological information with structural and computational work. This paper describes the application of various modern computational biochemistry methods in order to improve the understanding of a relationship between the structure and function of large biological systems including ion channels, transporters, receptors, and metabolic enzymes. The methods covered stem from classical molecular dynamics simulations to understand the physical basis and the time evolution of the structures, to combined QM, and

QM/MM approaches to probe the chemical mechanisms of enzymatic activities and their inhibition. As an illustrative example, the later will focus on the monoamine oxidase family of enzymes, which catalyze the degradation of amine neurotransmitters in various parts of the brain, the imbalance of which is associated with the development and progression of a range of neurodegenerative disorders. Inhibitors that act mainly on MAO A are used in the treatment of depression, due to their ability to raise serotonin concentrations, while MAO B inhibitors decrease dopamine degradation and improve motor control in patients with Parkinson disease. Our results give strong support that both MAO isoforms, A and B, operate through the hydride transfer mechanism. Relevance of MAO catalyzed reactions and MAO inhibition in the context of neurodegeneration will be discussed.

Keywords: computational enzymology, molecular dynamics simulation, central nervous system, neural signal transduction, drug design, hydride transfer reaction, neurotransmitter metabolism, multiscale simulations

INTRODUCTION

Neurodegenerative disorder, such as Alzheimer's disease, Parkinson's disease, and Huntington's disease, is an umbrella term for a range of incurable and debilitating conditions which primarily affect the neurons in the human brain and result in their progressive degeneration and/or death, causing problems with movement (ataxias) or mental functioning (dementias). Although perceived as the diseases of the elderly, these disorders can have a much earlier onset, starting even before the age of 40, leading to long-term treatment and substantial financial burden for the public healthcare systems. Two recent landmark reports (Gustavsson et al., 2011; Wittchen et al., 2011), conducted within EU–27 countries plus three allied countries (Norway, Iceland, Switzerland), providing the most complete picture ever of these disorders in Europe, estimated that the societal burden of brain disorders is immense: over 160 million people are affected, more than 36% of the total population, while the costs are equally disturbing amounting to a total of €798 billion per year in 2010—one third of all health related expenses—higher than for heart diseases, cancer, and diabetes combined. A breakdown of the nature of the costs shows that just over one third are direct healthcare costs, a quarter direct non-medical costs and the remaining 40% indirect costs associated with loss of productivity. In spite of this, there is at present no effective treatment able to slow down or stop the deterioration of brain

---

Abbreviations: MAO, monoamine oxidase; GPCR, G-protein coupled receptors; QM, quantum mechanics; MM, molecular mechanics; MD, molecular dynamics; QM/MM, quantum mechanical/molecular mechanical; EVB, empirical valence bond; VB, valence bond; AChE, acetylcholinesterase; BChE, butyrylcholinesterase; WT, wild type; QCP, quantum classical path; KIE, kinetic isotope effect; DFT, density functional theory; FEP, free-energy perturbation; US, umbrella sampling; CCM, cholesterol consensus motif; CRAC, cholesterol recognition/interaction amino acid; TRP, transient receptor potential; FAD, flavin adenine dinucleotide; RMSD, root-mean-square deviation; PDLP/S–LRA, semimacroscopic protein dipole/Langevin dipole approach in its linear response approximation version; DAAO, D–amino acid oxidases; TMO, tryptophan-2-monooxygenase; MTOX, N-methyltryptophan oxidase; CPCM, conductor-like polarizable continuum model; NBO, natural bond orbitals; SCAAS, surface-constrained all atom solvent model; FEP/US, free energy perturbation/umbrella sampling; IRC, intrinsic reaction coordinate; ROS, reactive oxygen species; αSyn, α–synuclein; ET, electron transfer; CNS, central nervous system; GSH, Glutathione; NSAID, non-steroidal anti-inflammatory drugs.

function. Early diagnosis is close to impossible, and because it often occurs too late, treatment to mitigate the effects of the illness remains limited. It is, therefore, highly desirable to understand those complex processes at the molecular level in order to pave way toward prevention, diagnosis, and treatment.

Biogenic amines are a large group of naturally occurring biologically active compounds, most of which act as neurotransmitters—endogenous chemicals that allow the transmission of signals from a neuron to target cells across synapses. Neurotransmitters can be excitatory, where there is a direct communication between the presynaptic neuron and postsynaptic neuron through the synaptic gap, or neuromodulators, where the mode of transmission includes diffusion transport over large distances in the central nervous system. There are five established amine neurotransmitters: the three catecholamines (dopamine, noradrenaline, and adrenaline), histamine, and serotonin. These substances are active in regulating many centrally mediated body functions, including behavioral, cognitive, motor and endocrine processes, and can cause adverse symptoms when they are out of balance (Di Giovanni et al., 2008). Despite immense functional importance, we are currently far from understanding the complex cellular and molecular actions of biogenic amines, the timing of their release and the full spectrum of processes that are influenced by them. An important prerequisite to fully realize the actions of biogenic amines is to study, at the molecular level, the mechanisms of both the catalytic activity and inhibition of their metabolic enzymes, and the way these small molecules interact with larger systems such as transporters and receptors, which all represent the starting points for development of tools to diagnose and drugs to treat specific clusters of symptoms of neurodegenerative disorders.

Brain monoaminergic systems have been extensively implicated in the etiology and course of various neurodegenerative disorders, causing problems with movement (ataxias) or mental functioning (dementias; Di Giovanni et al., 2008; Ramsay, 2012). In spite of this, there is, at present, no effective treatment able to substantially slow down or even stop the deterioration of neurons resulting in impaired brain function. All drugs employed nowadays exhibit a range of adverse effects, and drugs tend to address only symptoms rather than the causes of the dysfunction. Early diagnosis is close to impossible and, because it often occurs too late, treatment to mitigate the effects of the illness remains limited. In view of this background, the development of novel compounds for psychiatric manifestations in neurodegenerative disorders is not only of scientific interest to advance understanding of the brain at a systems level, but also fundamental to improving the management of symptoms, the therapeutic compliance and the quality of life of patients.

The present paper focuses on the use of modern molecular dynamics and multi-scale methods of computational biochemistry—from classical molecular dynamics simulations to quantum mechanical (QM) and combined quantum mechanical/molecular mechanical (QM/MM) approaches within the Empirical Valence Bond framework—in order to aid in understanding of a close relationship between the structure and function of some biological systems of the brain with particular focus on a common metabolic enzyme, monoamine oxidase (MAO), responsible for regulating the concentration of biogenic, and dietary amines in various parts of the body. Elucidating the precise atomistic details about the catalytic activity of MAO enzymes is of paramount importance for understanding the chemistry of neurodegeneration on molecular level. The knowledge gained in this area would facilitate research on other members of the large family of flavoenzymes and would, in addition to general biochemistry and physiology, be of significant value for designing and preparing novel effective MAO inhibitors as transition state analogs, which are potential clinical drugs for the treatment of depression, Parkinson, and Alzheimer diseases (Youdim et al., 2006).

CLASSICAL MOLECULAR DYNAMICS OF PROTEINS

Molecular dynamics simulation (MD) is a powerful computational technique that provides accurate descriptions of the structure and dynamics of biological systems, contributing to their understanding at an atomic level. In MD simulations, the motion of interacting particles is calculated by integrating Newton's equations of motion. The potential energy of the system and the forces, derived from the negative gradient of the potential with respect to displacements in a specified direction, are used to forecast the time evolution of the system in the form of a trajectory. Equilibrium quantities are then calculated using statistical mechanics by averaging over trajectories of sufficient length which would have sampled a representative ensemble of the state of the system. The potential energies can be obtained by either classical or quantum mechanical methods, with the former predominant due to reduced computational expense of utilizing empirical force fields. A force field refers to the functional form and parameter sets used to calculate the potential energy of a system of particles classically. A wide variety of force fields for biological molecules are available including, but not limited to, CHARMM (Chemistry at Harvard Molecular Mechanics; Brooks et al., 1983), AMBER (Assisted Model Building with Energy Requirement; Cornell et al., 1995), and OPLS (Optimized Potentials for Liquid Simulations; Jorgensen and Tirado-Rives,

1988). Each varies in their functional form and parameters therein, which are generally obtained to provide a suitable reproduction of experimental and/or quantum mechanical data. In classical potentials, atoms are considered as spheres with a particular mass and associated charge interlinked by springs that model the bonds. Atomic motions are evaluated using classical mechanics under the Born-Oppenheimer approximation where it is assumed that the motion of atomic nuclei and electrons in a molecule can be separated as a result of the vast difference in mass between electrons and nuclei. Electrons are said to adjust "instantaneously" to changes in the nuclear positions, and they can be ignored when solving the equations of motion. For this reason, the analytic expression that represents the energy of a system described by classical potentials is composed solely by inter- and intra-molecular contributions to the energy function. The most time-consuming part of the simulation is the calculation of the non-bonded interactions. A general functional form includes bond stretching, angle bending, bond rotations, and non-bonded terms. In general, all these interactions are calculated between pairs of atoms neglecting the many-body nature of some of the interactions. This many-body nature refers to the fact that the motion of every single particle influences and depends on the motion of the surrounding particles which would require coupled equations to describe the dynamics of the system. Classical force fields typically consider effective values of electronic polarization which is a significant limitation inherent to all additive force fields, although significant efforts to develop polarizable force fields for biological molecules have resulted in several schemes including the fluctuating charge model, the induced dipole model, and the Drude oscillator approach (Lamoureux et al., 2003; Patel and Brooks, 2004; Patel et al., 2004; Shi et al., 2013). A large majority of biomolecular simulation is currently performed by effectively polarized force fields. In addition, in order to describe chemical reactions, bond breaking or forming, nuclear effects, etc., a quantum formulation is required such as the one described. In systems with a few atoms, solutions of the aforementioned equation of motions can be achieved analytically. However, in larger systems, the subsistence of a continuous potential instigates a many body problem for force evaluations, rendering analytic solutions unattainable. Under these circumstances, finite difference methods are employed and forces are assessed at discrete intervals.

Although the basic idea behind classical molecular dynamics appears to be rather simple, in practice there are many complications and one has to be careful at setting the initial conditions, analyzing in a systematic way the influence of simulation protocols to ensure reliability, choosing appropriate algorithms or storing, and analyzing the huge amount of data generated. Among many applications, classical MD has become an established tool to identify putative binding sites, and consequentially establish how drugs function on a molecular level, to study transport in proteins, to rationalize conformational changes or to study aggregation and recognition. Nonetheless, the high computational expense of atomistic MD simulations for large biological systems remains a significant limitation. Many biological phenomena occur on extended timescales which are generally unattainable by classical MD and alternative approaches to accelerate sampling have been developed. Coarse-grained or reduced representations of molecules where a group of atoms is treated as a single entity or a "bead" are one of such approaches. By employing classical MD simulations using coarse-grained models, larger systems, and longer timescales can be achieved. In addition, several algorithms also exist to accelerate sampling along a pre-defined set of reaction coordinates and estimate the potential of mean force of a process. Enhanced sampling algorithms are crucial to investigate processes that involve overcoming an energetic barrier or exceeding the microsecond timescale, whilst maintaining full atomic detail or when a substantial system size is required even when considering a coarse-grained representation. Among these techniques are thermodynamic integration, umbrella sampling, metadynamics, adaptive biasing force, steered MD, and many other variants.

With the relentless development of computational algorithms together with progress in the experimental determination of three-dimensional structures of membrane proteins and the increasing speed and availability of supercomputers, it is now possible to investigate an immense range of biological phenomenon using MD simulations.

QUANTUM MECHANICAL TREATMENT OF THE CHEMICAL REACTIVITY

The past century has seen substantial advances, both in computational techniques and in our understanding of how enzymes really work. The use of quantum chemical methods to address enzymatic reaction mechanisms has become a booming area in enzymology (Ramos and Fernandes, 2008; Lonsdale et al., 2010; Shaik et al., 2010; Carvalho et al., 2014). Nevertheless, studying an enzyme at atomic resolution is a computationally demanding task. In this case, the complexity of the system prevents resorting to pure quantum-mechanical (QM) methods to treat the entire system, while the phenomena under study cannot be accurately represented by molecular-mechanical (MM) methods (since MM methods are in their traditional functional form unable to describe chemical reactions). Currently, there are two popular approaches to describe enzymatic processes: the quantum mechanics-only (QM-only) (Himo, 2006; Siegbahn and Borowski, 2006; Siegbahn and Himo, 2011), which uses a small but carefully selected cluster model of the active site, and the multiscale quantum mechanics/molecular mechanics (QM/MM) method (Senn and Thiel, 2009; van der Kamp and Mulholland, 2013), which employs a layer-based approach using the entire protein. Both methods have been successfully applied to the study of various classes of enzymes, and in many cases similar results and conclusions have been obtained (Ramos and Fernandes, 2008; Shaik et al., 2010).

In the QM-only approach, commonly also called the cluster approach (Siegbahn and Borowski, 2006), a model of the active site is designed on the basis of available crystal structures. The basic idea of this approach for modeling enzyme active sites and reaction mechanisms is to cut out a relatively small but well-chosen part of the enzyme and treat it with as accurate quantum chemical methods as possible. The model should be a good representation of the whole enzyme, and should behave and react like the real system. Hybrid density functional theory (DFT) methods are most frequently used for the calculation of the geometries and energies of all stationary points along the reaction pathways. The missing steric and electrostatic effects from the remaining part of the protein are considered by two simple procedures. The steric effects imposed by the protein matrix are taken into account by applying position constraints to certain key atoms at the periphery of the cluster model, while electrostatic effects are modeled by the dielectric cavity method, usually with a dielectric constant of four. In this respect the experimental structure is included in the calculation. Recent work even demonstrated that the solvation effects saturate with increasing the size of a cluster and that the particular choice of dielectric constant is then no longer of much concern (Liao et al., 2011).

The first application of the cluster model on an enzyme reaction mechanism using a high accuracy electronic structure method was done for methane monooxygenase in 1997 (Siegbahn and Crabtree, 1997). In the past 20 years, the cluster approach has gradually developed to become more robust and accurate, a work that is still continuing. For example, different models of the amino acids were tested (Siegbahn, 2001), and also how second-shell amino acids should be handled (Pelmenschikov et al., 2002). As a result of the accelerating computer power, active site models have become increasingly larger, which has enabled the modeling of evermore complex problems. At present, models with up to 200 atoms are often used, which should yield higher accuracy but has also introduced several new problems in the modeling, for example, a large number of local geometric minima. These problems are minimized by trying to limit the size of the model and include only those residues that are found to have significant effects. When this is successful, the approach is extremely powerful and yields a wealth of new information. On the basis of extensive calculations for a large number of enzymes, the error of the cluster approach for modeling metalloenzymes has been assessed by Siegbahn and co-workers to be <5 kcal/mol (Siegbahn, 2006).

MULTISCALE SIMULATION ON THE QM/MM LEVEL

Despite a tremendous increase in computer power, including the availability of tailor-made massively parallelized computer architectures, together with specialized and more efficient computer algorithms, it is still impossible to rigorously treat chemical reactivity in enzymes and solution describing the entire system at the quantum chemical level. Two key underlying issues for a correct description of reactions and processes with chemical character are: (i) an accurate and computationally efficient description of the bond breaking/forming processes, and (ii) proper modeling of the complex environment of the reaction, which involves efficient thermal averaging of the energy landscape. For converged calculations of free energy profiles for a typical enzyme reaction with applied position restraints for reactive species, it is necessary to perform at least a nanosecond trajectory, what requires evaluation of forces and energies for a million configurations. The use of molecular mechanics (MM) approaches, which are based on classical potentials, is extremely helpful, as they allow inclusion of environmental effects (either solvent molecules or enzymes) in a cost-efficient way. However, traditional MM force field functional forms are unable to describe changes in the electronic structure associated with making and breaking chemical bonds of a system undergoing a chemical reaction.

A solution to these challenges is the use of multiscale approaches, in which the interesting part of the system (usually the reactive atoms plus some additional environment) is described at the electronic level by high-level QM models, while the rest of the system is represented by empirical force fields (or by a lower-level QM method). Multiscale approaches have now become established *state-of-the-art* computational techniques for the modeling of chemical reactions in the condensed phase, including complex processes in organic chemistry, biochemistry, and heterogeneous catalysis, among others. Over the past decade, a number of so-called combined quantum mechanical and molecular mechanical (QM/MM) methods have been implemented, using different approximations and interaction schemes. The award of the 2013 Nobel Prize in Chemistry to Martin Karplus, Michael Levitt, and Arieh Warshel for "the development of multiscale models for complex chemical systems" has demonstrated how mature and highly important multiscale simulations for enzymology and drug design are.

Ab initio or DFT QM/MM methods are still computationally very demanding since they do not allow for well-converged reaction free energy profiles. The Empirical Valence Bond (EVB) approach introduced by Warshel and Levitt (1976) was the first QM/MM method, and after nearly four decades it remains the most practical approach in computational enzymology and the computational treatment of chemical reactivity in polar solutions in general. In their seminal work *Theoretical Study of Enzymatic Reactions: Dielectric, Electrostatic, and Steric Stabilization of the Carbonium Ion in the Reaction of Lysozyme* (Warshel and Levitt, 1976), Warshel and Levitt introduced all of the basic concepts of the QM/MM methodology, including the partitioning of the system, the form of the potential energy function, and the interactions between the QM and MM parts. The rest of this section will be devoted to the description of EVB that provides a powerful way to connect classical concepts of physical organic chemistry to the study of chemical reactions. On purpose, most of the mathematical formulation is not shown, and the interested reader is referred to review articles describing progress in EVB theory and implementation (Olsson et al., 2006; Kamerlin and Warshel, 2011a,b).

As within a standard Valence Bonds (VB) framework, EVB uses a set of VB configurations, which can involve covalent, ionic, or a mixture of bonding types, to describe the reactive system participating in the chemical reaction. However, in this case, each VB state corresponds to different bonding patterns of key essential energy minima (reactants, products, and any intermediates) along the postulated reaction coordinate. Energy of covalent bonds is described by Morse functions that allow for bond breaking and making, while bond angle and dihedral

angle terms are functionally identical to other force fields. For molecular simulation of a simple S_N2 reaction with the EVB method with graphical interface visit http://www.ki.si/L01/EVB.

Most enzymatic reactions involve high barriers that cannot be sampled directly by molecular dynamics. In order to calculate reaction energy profiles in terms of free energy, it is necessary to proceed with biased sampling in conjunction with a special method for the free energy calculation. The strategy for this involves the free-energy perturbation (FEP) approach and the so-called umbrella sampling (US) procedure. The FEP approach is based on gradual transformation between the reactant and the product state using the coupling parameter, λ. At each step, a molecular dynamics (MD) simulation is performed with fixed λ. This technique ensures that the system explores areas of the phase space that would not be accessible otherwise in real time, due to the high potential energy (i.e., around the transition state).

The reaction barrier, $\Delta G^\ddagger$, extracted from the computed free energy profile is directly related to the rate constant k as $k = \frac{K_B T}{h} \exp\left(-\frac{\Delta G^\ddagger}{K_B T}\right)$, where T is the absolute temperature while h and k_B are Planck and Boltzmann constant, respectively. Therefore, once the free energy profiles are computed, they can be trivially converted into reaction rates. The applied procedure proved to be computationally robust and allows for practical calculation of the reaction rates. Currently, many research groups are actively developing and applying different approaches based on the EVB philosophy. These recent developments, which include new methodologies and program packages, have greatly expanded the scope of problems that can be studied with EVB, enabling applications from small to large-scale molecular systems. Still, computational enzymology remains the most important field where EVB is applied.

EXAMPLES OF CLASSICAL MOLECULAR DYNAMICS OF MEMBRANE PROTEINS

Neurotransmitters such as dopamine and serotonin play a central role in the pathophysiology of major neuropsychiatric illnesses, such as anxiety and mood disorders, schizophrenia, autism spectrum disorders, Parkinson's disease, epilepsy, and dementias. Neurotransmitter-binding proteins such as receptors, transporters, and common metabolic enzymes are the starting points for development of tools to diagnose and drugs to treat specific clusters of symptoms. How these proteins function on a molecular level, remains largely unresolved. A fuller understanding is steadily emerging due to the increasing availability of three-dimensional structures of membrane proteins, in combination with computational methodologies, such as molecular dynamics simulations. In this context, computational labs have focused their efforts in studying at atomistic level how membrane proteins work probing events such as selectivity, permeation, gating, or the conformational changes associated with these processes, and more recently, on studies illustrating protein-lipid interactions (Domene, 2007; Domene and Furini, 2009; Illingworth and Domene, 2009; Furini and Domene, 2013; Ingolfsson et al., 2014). For instance, the composition of biological cell membranes is integral in controlling the structure, and subsequently function, of membrane proteins. Cholesterol is an essential component of the plasma membrane, with concentrations of over 30% in some tissues (Lange, 1991). It has been identified to be extremely influential in the functioning of G-protein couple receptors (GPCR's) such as the serotonin$_{1A}$ receptor, β2-adrenergic receptor and the rhodopsin receptor (Burger et al., 2000; Pucadyil and Chattopadhyay, 2006; Paila and Chattopadhyay, 2010; Oates and Watts, 2011; Jafurulla and Chattopadhyay, 2013). However, the mechanism by which cholesterol modulates protein structure and function is largely unknown. Various theories have been proposed throughout the literature suggesting that cholesterol acts by either varying the physical properties of the membrane, binding directly to specific sites on the protein surface, or facilitating interactions with a third party which biases the activation state. Indeed, these effects may not be mutually exclusive but act cooperatively. Crystallographic data of GPCR's in complex with cholesterol molecules, such as the β2-adrenergic receptor (Cherezov et al., 2007; Hanson et al., 2008), β1-adrenergic receptor (Warne et al., 2011), A$_{2A}$-adenosine receptor (Liu et al., 2012), 5-HT$_{2B}$-receptor (Wang et al., 2013), and metabotropic glutamate type 1 receptor (Wu et al., 2014), has led to the identification of specific cholesterol interaction sites. Elucidation of the β2-adrenergic receptor (Hanson et al., 2008) structure established the cholesterol consensus motif (CCM), a groove region between helices II and VII constituted of highly conserved residues and sequence analysis of several GPCR's identified additional putative binding sites (Jafurulla et al., 2011), the cholesterol recognition/interaction amino acid consensus (CRAC) motif (Li and Papadopoulos, 1998) and the inverted form of the CRAC motif (Baier et al., 2011), termed the CARC motif. However, the affinity of cholesterol for these sites and the influence on the functional state of GPCR's has not been widely categorized and thus MD simulations are underway to investigate the interactions of GPCR's and cholesterol.

Likewise, ion channels are a large and bio-medically important family of membrane proteins that constitute significant drug targets. They govern the electrical properties of the membranes of excitable cells such as neurons or myocytes by allowing thousands of millions of ions to diffuse down their electrochemical gradient across the membrane. Channels do not stay open all of the time but they are "gated" by changes in voltage across the membrane, changes in the pH, the binding of small molecules, etc. This process is called "gating" and it operates via conformational changes. One of the keys to rationalize the way drugs modulate ion channels is to understand the ability of such small molecules to access their respective binding sites, from which they can exert an activating or inhibitory effect. Drug access depends both on the target conformational state as well as on the real-time dynamics of the residues lining the fenestrations and entry tunnels of the target. Although many computational studies have probed the mechanisms of selectivity and gating as well as the energetics of ion permeation, few have focused on investigating the existence and characteristics of cavities in ion channels through which drugs can exert their action. For example, a recent study in our lab explored the presence, structure and conformational dynamics of transmembrane fenestrations accessible by drugs in potassium channels (Jorgensen et al.,

2015). Molecular dynamics simulation trajectories were analyzed from three potassium channels one from a different family, a voltage-gated channel, an inward rectifying channel, and a two-pore domain one. Four lateral fenestrations across the range of potassium channels studied were identified and using structural and sequence alignment and analysis was carried out to characterize the similarities and differences among the K$^+$-channel subtypes considered. The study rendered a framework for rationalizing the differential response of potassium channels to drugs targeting the transmembrane domain of these proteins and provided insight about the potential role of lateral fenestrations in K$^+$-channels for drug delivery and for designing single and multi-target drugs with improved selectivity.

Another example where MD simulations have recently contributed to the atomistic understanding of a membrane protein is that of the transient receptor potential (TRP) ion channels. The three-dimensional structure of the vanilloid receptor 1 or TRPV1, and TRPV2 were recently determined by single particle electron cryo-microscopy, providing the opportunity to explore ionic conduction in TRP channels at atomic detail (Liao et al., 2013; Zubcevic et al., 2016). They constitute an extensive family of cation channels involved in the ability of organisms to detect noxious mechanical, thermal, and chemical stimuli that give rise to the perception of pain. TRPV1 is the main representative of a subfamily of thermosensitive TRP channels that enable a sensation of scalding heat and pain. Additionally, tissue damage and inflammation products modulate the channel by decreasing its thermal activation threshold (~43°C). This feature makes the TRPV1 channel an essential player in the molecular mechanisms responsible for injury-related hyperalgesia and pain (Brederson et al., 2013; Julius, 2013). In addition to temperature greater than 43°C and acidic conditions, TRPV1 is also activated by capsaicin and allyl isothiocyanate, the irritating chemical in hot chili peppers and the pungent compound in mustard and wasabi, respectively (Everaerts et al., 2011; Julius, 2013). MD simulations using the TRPV1 channel revealed the presence of three main binding sites for cations in the transmembrane domain that were not appreciable in the cryo-EM structure (Darre et al., 2015). Two rings of acidic residues are disposed at the extracellular side of the conduction path generating an electrostatic attraction to cations and a delineating the first binding site. A second binding site was found at the intracellular side of the selectivity filter, and a further site in the central water-filled cavity analogous to those observed in other ion channels. Simulations evidenced the flexibility of the selectivity filter, the area of the protein that discriminates the type of ions that permeates the pore that responds to the type of permeating ions by adjusting the global symmetry of this area. A comprehensive picture of the thermodynamics governing the binding of capsaicin to the TRPV1 channel was also accomplished (Darre and Domene, 2015) by combining molecular docking, unbiased MD simulations, and free energy methods in good agreement with earlier experimental reports. These exploratory calculations have provided an early glimpse of the amino acids engaged in favorable capsaicin–channel interactions defining the key structural determinants of the TRPV1 vanilloid binding site.

Ion channels modulate electrical signals across cell membranes and therefore are key in a myriad of physiological processes. Establishing the mechanisms of selectivity, conduction, and gating is central in biomedical sciences studies in order to establish the connection between structure and function. For many years, molecular dynamics simulations have been used to explore these relationships, and it is likely that they will continue to do so in the future, where the challenges lie initially in tackling systems where the realism of the biological environment is improved and subsequently in simulating higher and more complex levels of organization in living systems.

PHARMACOLOGY OF MONOAMINE OXIDASES

Monoamine oxidases are mitochondrial outer membrane-bound enzymes that catalyze the oxidative deamination of a broad range of biogenic and dietary amines into their corresponding imines, thus playing a critical role in the degradation of monoamine neurotransmitters in the central and peripheral nervous systems. They contain the covalently bound cofactor flavin adenine dinucleotide (FAD) and are, thus, classified as flavoproteins. Formed imines leave the active site and are then non-enzymatically hydrolyzed to the final carbonyl compounds and ammonia. The enzyme itself is regenerated to its active form by molecular oxygen, O_2, which is in turn reduced to hydrogen peroxide, H_2O_2, according to the overall equation (**Scheme 1**):

The aldehyde intermediate is rapidly metabolized, usually by oxidation via the enzyme aldehyde dehydrogenase to the corresponding carboxylic acid, or is reduced in some circumstances to the alcohol or glycol by the enzyme aldehyde reductase. MAOs operate using the FAD cofactor, which is, in contrast to the majority of other flavoenzymes, covalently bound to a cysteine through an 8α-thioether linkage (Miller and Edmondson, 1999a). During the catalytic reaction, FAD is reduced to $FADH_2$ by accepting two protons and two electrons from the substrate. Although having around 70% sequence identity and a conserved pentapeptidic sequence (Ser-Gly-Gly-Cys-Tyr) that binds the identical FAD cofactor (Klinman, 2007), both the A and the B isoforms of MAO differ on the basis of their substrate affinities and inhibitor sensitivities. However, it is assumed that they act by the same mechanism. In humans, MAO A predominates in the gastrointestinal tract, placenta, and heart, whereas MAO B predominates in platelets and glial cells in the brain. Both are found in liver where biogenic amines are rapidly metabolized and excreted. The primary role of MAO in the gastrointestinal tract is removal of monoamines absorbed by food in order to prevent their uncontrolled interaction with the receptors. It is interesting to mention that the required time for MAO synthesis in the gastrointestinal tract is 2–3 days, while in the central nervous system it is about 2–3 weeks. Under normal physiologic conditions, noradrenalin and serotonin are the preferred substrates of MAO A, while dopamine and β-phenylethylamine are the preferred substrates of MAO B, while both isoforms metabolize dopamine, albeit with differing kinetic parameters. Inhibitors that mainly act on MAO A are used in the treatment of depression, due to their ability to raise serotonin concentrations. In contrast, MAO B inhibitors decrease dopamine degradation and improve motor control in patients with Parkinson disease. Inhibition of MAOs has a notable neuroprotective effect, since MAO catalyzed reactions yield neurotoxic products such as hydrogen peroxide and aldehydes (Gadda, 2012; Edmondson, 2014; Pavlin et al., 2016). The cloning of two separate cDNAs encoding two isoforms of MAO by Shih and co-workers (Bach et al., 1988) provided the basis for a range of important discoveries, thereby allowing the elucidation of their biological roles and development of inhibitors. However, despite tremendous research efforts devoted to MAOs over several decades, neither the catalytic nor the inhibition mechanisms of MAO have been unambiguously established.

STRUCTURES OF MAO A AND MAO B ISOFORMS

Structures of MAO A and MAO B appeared relatively late and the main obstacle was the protein crystallization. They are trans-membrane proteins and their crystallization represents a very demanding task. After successful heterologous over-expression and purification of recombinant human MAO in yeast or *P. Pastoris* (Newton-Vinson et al., 2000; Li et al., 2002), the three-dimensional structures of human MAO A (Binda et al., 2002; De Colibus et al., 2005) and MAO B (Son et al., 2008) have been solved at a resolution of 2.2 Å and 1.65 Å, respectively. The X–ray structures of both human MAO, A and B, showed that the active-site cavities extend from the flavin-binding site at the core to the surface of the protein. The FAD cofactor binding site is highly conserved between the two enzymes, but several details in the substrate-binding site show major differences. It was hypothesized that substrate preferences and inhibitor specificities are attributed to differences between Phe208–Ile335 in MAO A and Ile199–Tyr326 in MAO B (Li et al., 2006). The covalently-bound FAD lies at the end of a long tunnel leading from the outside of the protein close to the membrane surface. The tunnel is generally considered to be hydrophobic, ending in an aromatic

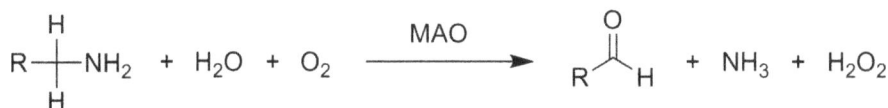

SCHEME 1 | Overall oxidative deamination of biogenic and dietary amines catalyzed by the MAO enzyme. Amines are enzymatically converted to the corresponding imines, which leave the MAO active site and are non-enzymatically hydrolyzed to aldehydes.

cage near the flavin where two tyrosines align the substrate toward the C4–N5 region of the flavin (Li et al., 2006; Akyuz et al., 2007). The influence of the catalytic site tyrosines (Tyr398 and Tyr435 in MAO B) has been investigated in careful kinetic investigation of several mutants. Although neither is essential to catalysis in terms of complete loss of activity, the affinity for and turnover of substrates is altered in the mutant enzymes. For example, the K_m for benzylamine increases by more than 10-fold in the Tyr435Phe mutant (Li et al., 2006). The evidence reveals a clear role for these tyrosines in aligning the substrate correctly for catalysis, perpendicular to the N5 and on the *re* face of the isoalloxazine ring. These tyrosines also exert a dipole effect on the substrate that can make the amine more susceptible to oxidation. The key features of substrate position in the active site are proximity and orientation relative to the N5–C4a region of the flavin ring. All these features result in changed activation free energy and therewith associated rate constants on the point mutations.

At this point it is worth to emphasize that availability of the high-resolution MAO structures represents crucial information for the multiscale simulation of the reactive step and rational design of both irreversible and reversible inhibitors.

MAO PREORGANIZED ELECTROSTATICS IS REFLECTED IN THE pK_a VALUES

Computational studies gave clear evidence that the enzyme active sites provide specific polar environments that do not resemble the gas phase or simple solvent. The enzyme environment is designed for the electrostatic stabilization of transition states, enabling solvation higher than in water. Therefore, the bulk of the enzyme catalytic power originates from the electrostatic preorganization of its active sites. Essentially, solvent molecules must reorient during the reaction due to polarization induced by a changing charge distribution, while this energetic penalty is much smaller in enzymes, as they provide an electrostatic environment that has evolved to require much less reorganization. A change in the protonation states of ionizable residues results in an altered electrostatic potential pattern in the enzyme, which gives rise to altered activation free energies and manifests as pH dependence of the reaction rate. Electrostatic potential of the enzyme active site is, by definition, a fluctuating scalar field and cannot be directly measured experimentally. However, there are few experimentally accessible quantities that are closely related to the electrostatic potential. Recent studies by the vibrational Stark effect spectroscopy applied to carbonyl group stretching give some insight into the preorganized electrostatics. The authors calibrated the sensitivity of these vibrations to electric fields and used this calibration to quantitatively interpret the electric field environment experienced by a probe. The approach was pioneered by Boxer's group and applied to quantify the contribution of electric fields to the catalytic rate enhancement by the enzyme ketosteroid isomerase (Sigala et al., 2007; Fried et al., 2014). Much more practical, established and abundant approach is the measurement and calculation of the corresponding pK_a values.

The pK_a values of ionizable residues in the enzyme active site are an excellent probe for the electrostatic environment, since pK_a is very sensitive to any structural change and the associated alteration in the electrostatic potential. Since MAO A and MAO B isozymes are 70% homologous and the overall geometric matching is high (RMSD between the X-ray structures is only 0.66 Å), it is reasonable to expect that their electrostatic potential pattern in the active site will be quite similar and accompanied by a similarity in the pK_a values of the corresponding residues. It is worth to stress that, in contrast to the point-wise electrostatic potential comparison, pK_a values can also be determined experimentally. Change of the pK_a value is also a measure of hydrophobicity: hydrophobic environment does not favor presence of charged species giving rise to significant shifts in the pK_a values. Despite the fact that monoamines are predominantly monocations at a physiological pH of 7.4, a hydrophobic active site in MAOs has been proposed to favor unprotonated substrates. Furthermore, every catalytic proposal to date has agreed that the substrate must be neutral for the reaction to take place. Active site pK_a values are difficult to determine experimentally and, similarly, while experimental pH rate profiles can provide tremendous insight, it can be hard to conclusively determine the identity of residues whose protonation state is being affected. For MAO some attempts were performed to determine pK_a values of some surface residues (Dunn et al., 2008; Repić et al., 2014a). The work of Scrutton and co-workers addressed the pK_a values of the enzyme active site and the substrates (Dunn et al., 2008). The authors studied pH dependence of MAO A kinetic parameters by stopped-flow and steady state methodology and H/D isotope substitution. The authors came to a conclusion that substrates such as benzylamine, kynuramine, and phenylethyl amine bind in the protonated form, while deprotonation is required for chemical step. Moreover, the authors have demonstrated that the pH dependence of the kinetic isotope effect decreases from ~13 to 8 with increasing pH, leading to the assignment of this catalytically important deprotonation of the amine substrate. The strong H/D kinetic isotope effect dependence gives evidence that at low pH values the substrate deprotonation interferes with the rate-limiting step. Moreover, Scrutton and co-workers suggested that the pK_a values of the studies substrates are decreased for about 2 pK_a units when transferring the substrate from aqueous solution to the enzyme. To get an insight into the nature of the MAO active sites, the pK_a values of a few ionisable residues were calculated in order to compare the electrostatic potential pattern in the active sites of both isoforms (Dunn et al., 2008). Well-converged free energy calculations of the pK_a values were performed using the MOLARIS program package together with an all-atom representation of the solvated enzymes. In line with the general consensus that dopamine enters the chemical step in a neutral form, a neutral dopamine molecule was manually docked in the active site in a way suitable for the catalytic step. We chose only one substrate on purpose in order to avoid the effects associated with ligands of different sizes on the pK_a values. pK_a calculations were performed using the semimacroscopic protein dipole/Langevin dipole approach of Warshel and co-workers in its linear response approximation version (PDLD/S–LRA), allowing for converged free energy calculations (Lee et al., 1993; Schutz and Warshel, 2001).

The calculated pK_a values are sensitive to the applied external dielectric constant during simulations. The choice of the correct dielectric constant to describe the protein interior is a very complex issue and has been the subject of heated debates over the years (Schutz and Warshel, 2001). In our work, we employed $\varepsilon = 10\text{–}16$, still, due to the focus on the relative difference between pK_a values in MAO A and MAO B, the choice would not change the qualitative picture and is thus of lesser importance. Specifically, we have examined the pK_a values of four tyrosine residues that are part of the so-called aromatic cage and a Lys residue close to the reacting atoms of FAD. Among isoforms, the average absolute differences over a dielectric constant of 10–16 in the corresponding pK_a values are assumed to be 0.05, 0.07, 0.12, 0.75, and 1.23 for MAO A/B pairs Tyr69/Tyr60, Lys305/Lys296, Tyr407/Tyr398, Tyr444/Tyr435, and Tyr197/Tyr188, respectively. These results clearly demonstrate that, for both isozymes, the pK_a values for the Tyr and Lys residues in question are not substantially different (1.23 pK_a units at maximum), thus providing strong evidence that the electrostatic potential pattern in the active sites of both isozymes is very closely matched. Since enzymes work by preorganized electrostatics, the same electrostatic environment cannot be at the same time suitable for optimal solvation of the transition state with a positive and a negative charge build-up, as would be the case in the hydride and polar nucleophilic mechanisms. Superimposition of both experimental X-ray structures also reveals a high similarity in the spatial configuration of charged groups in MAOs (**Figure 1**). It is therefore unlikely that MAO A and MAO B would work by different chemical mechanisms on the same family of substrates, thus contradicting an interesting proposal of Orru and co-workers (Orru et al., 2013). The pK_a value of the bound dopamine (8.8) is practically unchanged compared to the corresponding value in aqueous solution (8.9), as would be expected from a charged amine placed in a hydrophobic active site consisting of aromatic moieties (Li et al., 2006). The MAO active sites are in this respect not hydrophobic and practically unchanged dopamine pK_a relative to aqueous solution may be attributed to favorable cation–π interactions between the dopamine $-NH_3^+$ group and aromatic moieties, which provide a stabilizing effect to the charged fragment. Our results can be contrasted with the study of Scrutton and co-workers reporting the pK_a shift of the substrates for about 2 pK_a units. The discrepancy can be, among other factors, explained by the sizes of different substrates.

MECHANISTIC STUDIES OF MONOAMINE OXIDASE BY QUANTUM MECHANICAL CLUSTER MODEL

The general reaction of flavin amine oxidases, including MAO, can be divided into two half-reactions. In the reductive half-reaction, a hydride equivalent is transferred from the substrate to the flavin, thus reducing it to $FADH_2$, while the oxidative half-reaction involves the oxidation of the reduced flavin back to FAD by molecular oxygen, producing H_2O_2 (**Scheme 1**).

The chemical mechanism of the reductive half-reaction in MAO has been the source of controversy and debate (MacMillar et al., 2011). Oxidation of an amine substrate necessarily involves the removal of two protons and two electrons as the carbon–nitrogen single bond is converted to a double bond. Three-dimensional structures of MAO A and MAO B isoforms (Binda et al., 2002; De Colibus et al., 2005; Son et al., 2008), together with extensive kinetic and spectroscopic studies on mutant enzymes (Binda et al., 2002; De Colibus et al., 2005; Li et al., 2006), have led researchers to propose three possible catalytic scenarios for MAO (MacMillar et al., 2011): (a) the direct hydride mechanism, (b) the radical mechanism, and (c) the polar nucleophilic mechanism. Studies on deuterated substrate analogs have suggested that the rate-limiting step is the cleavage of a carbon-hydrogen bond vicinal to the amino group (Klinman and Matthews, 1985) and, hence, the catalytic proposals differ in the nature of the hydrogen being transferred, namely a hydride (H^-) in (a), a hydrogen atom ($H^\bullet$) in (b), and a proton (H^+) in (c) (Walker and Edmondson, 1994; Wang and Edmondson, 2011), commonly by the flavin N5 atom. In contrast, the other hydrogen from the amino N–H moiety is generally proposed to be abstracted as a proton (Harris et al., 2001). Thus, establishing the MAO catalytic mechanism necessarily requires the knowledge of the timing of the removal of hydrogens from both the carbon and nitrogen atoms.

The possibility of the hydride mechanism for MAOs was based on their structural similarities to flavoprotein D-amino acid oxidases (DAAO), for which both kinetic measurements (Kurtz et al., 2000; Ralph et al., 2007) and related calculations (Ralph et al., 2007) suggested a hydride or a single electron transfer. Additionally, deuterium and ^{15}N kinetic isotope effect studies of flavin amine oxidases including DAAO (Kurtz et al., 2000), tryptophan-2-monooxygenase (TMO; Ralph et al., 2006), and N-methyltryptophan oxidase (MTOX; Ralph et al., 2007), are most consistent with a hydride transfer mechanism. However, Erdem et al. (2006) assumed that a hydride mechanism was unlikely, and concluded that in MAO it would be associated with a barrier too high to be readily crossed. In addition, a combined ^{15}N and deuterium isotope effects demonstrated that the C–H bond cleavage is not concerted with the rehybridization of the substrate amino group (MacMillar et al., 2011), which seem to rule out the feasibility of a concerted hydride transfer mechanism.

According to Silverman and co-workers (Silverman, 1995) the radical mechanism is initiated by a single-electron transfer from the substrate to the flavin, producing an aminium radical cation and a flavin semiquinone as transient intermediates. The lowered pK_a of the α–CH bond of the aminium radical cation can result in either a stepwise (Silverman, 1995) or concerted (Vintém et al., 2005) deprotonation and a second electron transfer producing reduced flavin and the iminium ion. The main supporting evidence for the radical mechanism is the observation that both MAOs are inactivated by cyclopropylamine analogs with subsequent ring opening, a process characteristic of radical reactions (Silverman, 1983). An argument against the radical mechanism has been the failure of any laboratory to detect semiquinone radical species during turnover in a

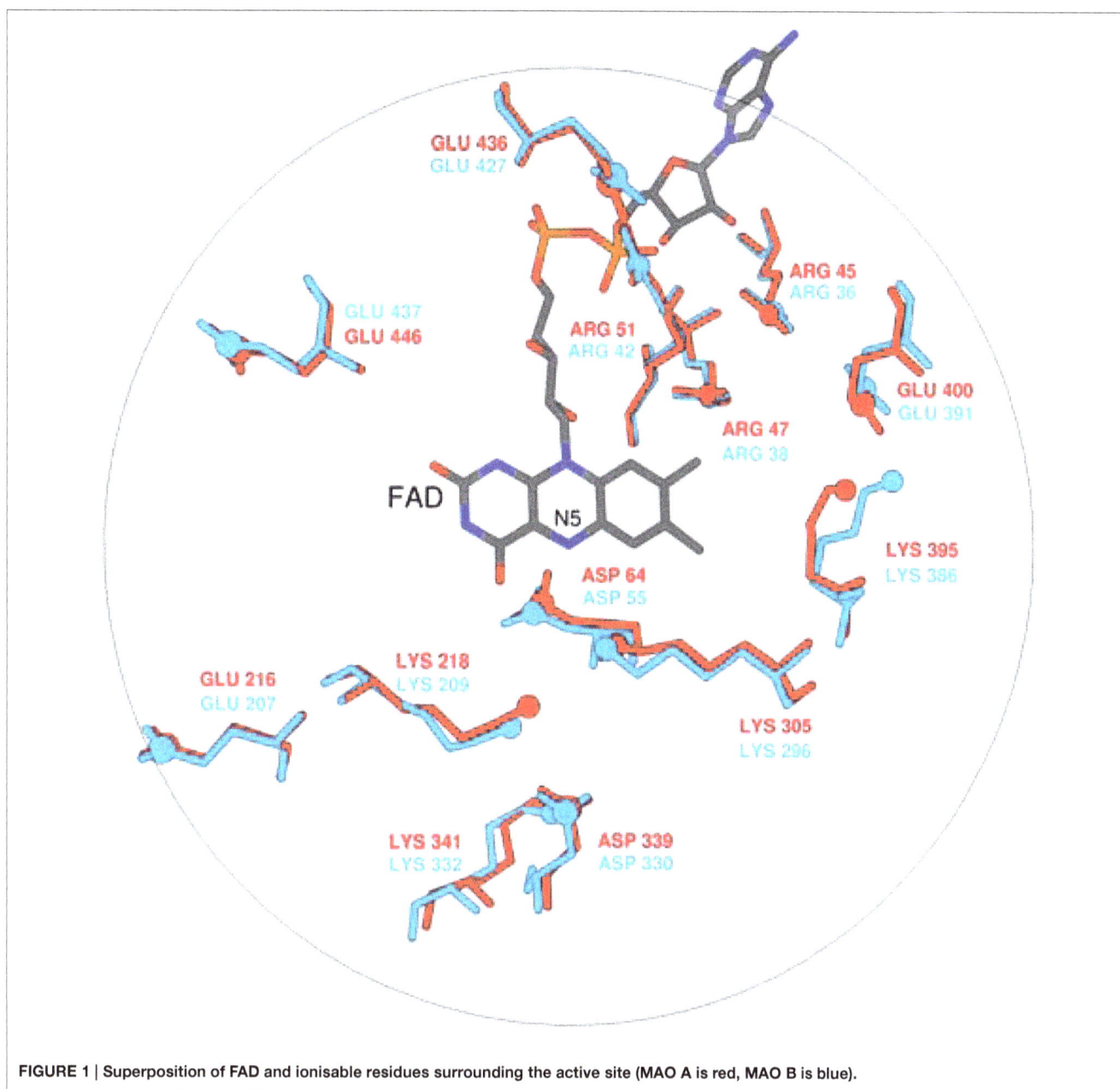

FIGURE 1 | Superposition of FAD and ionisable residues surrounding the active site (MAO A is red, MAO B is blue).

stopped-flow monitored reduction or using radical traps (see later). The chemistry of the cyclopropylamine probes and resulting products supported the view that single electron transfer is possible at least with these compounds, but the lack of inactivation by, and a ring-opened product from trans-2-phenyl(aminomethyl)cyclopropane suggested that other mechanisms must be possible (Fitzpatrick, 2010). In a modified single electron transfer mechanism, the involvement of protein-based radicals has also been proposed but questioned (Rigby et al., 2005; Kay et al., 2007). Mutation of the substrate-orienting tyrosines and isotopic labeling of the tyrosines in MAO A, and the fungal counterpart MAO B, provide evidence for radicals delocalized away from the active site (Dunn et al., 2010).

The experiments by Edmondson and co-workers (Walker and Edmondson, 1994), as well as related electron paramagnetic resonance studies (Tan et al., 1983; Miller et al., 1995; Nandigama and Edmondson, 2000) and stopped-flow kinetic determinations (Nandigama and Edmondson, 2000), failed to provide any evidence for radical intermediates, and no influence of the magnetic field on the kinetics of enzyme reduction was observed (Miller et al., 1995). In addition, Taft correlation studies of Miller and Edmondson with benzylamines showed that attaching the electron-withdrawing groups to the substrate para-position increases the rate of the reaction in both human (Miller and Edmondson, 1999a) and rat (Wang and Edmondson, 2011) MAO A, implying negative charge build-up on the substrate α–carbon atom, thus suggesting that proton transfer is an integral part of the rate limiting step. This led authors to propose the polar nucleophilic mechanism for MAO A (Miller and Edmondson, 1999b), originally formulated by Hamilton (Hamilton, 1971). This mechanism involves the creation of a highly energetic substrate–flavin adduct which then decomposes to the protonated imine, with proton abstraction concerted with either the adduct formation or the product formation. The crucial issue related to this mechanism is what moiety on the enzyme would be strong enough base to perform this task, since the pK_a of a benzyl proton is expected to be around 25 (Smith and March, 2001). Structural analysis of both MAO isoforms showed there are no active site basic residues that could act as proton acceptors. Also, no direct evidence for a stable amine–flavin adduct has been found experimentally. A study on human MAO B, however, showed an inverse Taft correlation (Orru et al., 2013), supporting the hydride transfer mechanism, which led the authors to propose different mechanisms for two isozymes: H^+ transfer in MAO A and H^- transfer in MAO B, although, the same authors had previously ruled out H^- transfer in human MAO B, based on the nitrogen secondary kinetic isotope effects (MacMillar et al., 2011). Based on the similarities in the continuous wave electronic paramagnetic resonance spectrum between MAO and D-amino acid oxidase, determined to operate by the H^- transfer mechanism (Umhau et al., 2000), Kay and co-workers suggested a hydride transfer mechanism should be re-examined for MAO (Kay et al., 2007). Therefore, it is clear that, despite the widespread use of MAO inhibitors, the mechanism of MAO catalysis is not unambiguously determined which calls for its rationalization using advanced computational techniques.

The first computational study on the complete mechanism of MAO catalysis was performed by our groups (Vianello et al., 2012), employing DFT methodology within the cluster model of the enzyme. The starting point for our calculations was the high-resolution (1.6 Å) X-ray structure of MAO B complexed with 2-(2-benzofuranyl)-2-imidazoline (accession code 2XFN; De Colibus et al., 2005). We truncated the enzyme to the flavin moiety (isoalloxazine group 2, Figure 2) and three tyrosine side-chains (p-hydroxytoluenes of Tyr188, Tyr398, and Tyr435), which all form the mentioned hydrophobic "aromatic cage" (Li et al., 2006; Akyuz et al., 2007). Previously, we calculated the pK_a values of the Tyr residues with bound dopamine (Borštnar et al., 2012), and obtained an upward shift to 13.0–14.7 (pK_a for Tyr in aqueous solution is 10.1). This clearly confirmed the hydrophobic nature of the active site, which indicates that gas-phase calculations on truncated MAOs are reliable. Also, we showed that the pK_a value of bound dopamine changes to only 8.8 (8.9 in aqueous solution), a result of stabilizing cation–π interactions with the tyrosine side-chains (Borštnar et al., 2012). This implies that dopamine binds to the MAO active site as a protonated monocation, but the free-energy cost to deprotonate it to the bulk, being as low as 1.9 kcal mol^{-1}, allows it to enter the chemical step either as an ionized or neutral molecule, which led us to consider both alternatives. Based on crystal structures (Binda et al., 2002; De Colibus et al., 2005; Son et al., 2008) and our MD simulations (Borštnar et al., 2012) that both indicate the presence of few

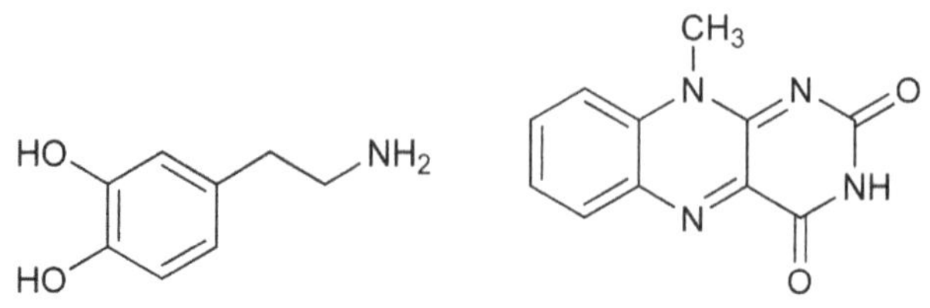

FIGURE 2 | Structures of dopamine (1) and isoalloxazine moiety (2) of the FAD cofactor used in the cluster model of the MAO active site.

water molecules in the active site, our model also included four crystal water molecules (HOH$_{2157}$, HOH$_{2181}$, HOH$_{2329}$, and HOH$_{2372}$). It turned out that two of those are chemically involved in catalysis. We manually placed dopamine 1 within the cluster, resulting in the initial stationary-point (SP) complexes (Figure 3). The system was modeled at the (CPCM)/M06–2X/6–311++G(2df,2pd)//(CPCM)/M06–2X/6–31+G(d) level of theory employing the M06–2X functional designed by Zhao and Truhlar to accurately reproduce thermodynamic and kinetic parameters (Zhao and Truhlar, 2008, 2011; Bell and Head-Gordon, 2011; Cheong et al., 2011; Picek et al., 2015; Saftić et al., 2015), being particularly successful in treating non-bonding interactions. To account for the polarization effects caused by the rest of the enzyme, we included a conductor-like polarizable continuum model (CPCM) (Cossi et al., 2003) with a dielectric constant of ε = 4, taking the rest of the parameters for pure water, as employed in many studies by Siegbahn, Himo and their co-workers in elucidating the catalytic mechanism of a large variety of enzymes (Himo, 2006; Siegbahn and Borowski, 2006; Siegbahn and Himo, 2011).

For 1$_{SP1}$ (Figure 3) we first considered the single-electron radical mechanism, which would initially create a biradical either in the singlet or triplet electronic states. (CPCM)/UM06–2X/6–31+G(d) calculations for the triplet state produced the system 54.2 kcal mol^{-1} higher in energy than 1$_{SP1}$. For the singlet state, we employed "symmetry-broken" open-shell calculations, defining dopamine and the rest of the system as two different fragments each having an unpaired electron of opposite spin, which resulted in a stable wave-function with both the energy and electron distribution identical to that in 1$_{SP1}$. Overall, this suggests that the singlet-state biradical is non-existent, whereas the free-energy cost to generate the triplet is too high for an efficient catalysis. This agrees well with the experimentally observed mismatch between the oxidation/reduction potentials of the FAD cofactor, which is too low (−0.2 V; Newton-Vinson and Edmondson, 1999) for it to be an effective oxidant of the neutral amine (around +1.0–1.5 V) (Hull et al., 1969). On top of the fact that there is no experimental evidence for a radical intermediate, our results suggest that it is very unlikely that a radical pathway is feasible and we did not consider it further.

The polar nucleophilic mechanism is another alternative for the amine oxidation and involves proton abstraction from the α–carbon atom as the rate-limiting step (Miller and Edmondson, 1999b). The crucial issue relating to this mechanism is what

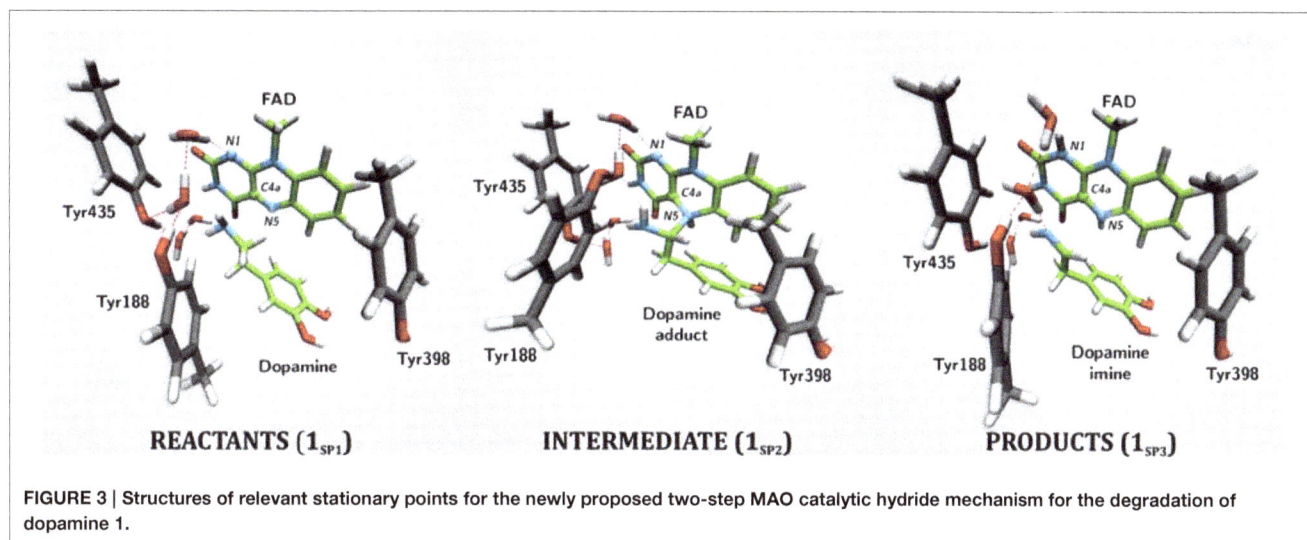

FIGURE 3 | Structures of relevant stationary points for the newly proposed two-step MAO catalytic hydride mechanism for the degradation of dopamine 1.

moiety on the enzyme would be a strong enough base to perform this task, because the pK_a of a benzyl proton is expected to be around 25 (Smith and March, 2001). Structural analysis of both MAO isoforms shows there are no basic active-site residues that could act as proton acceptors (Binda et al., 2003). Edmondson and coworkers upheld their arguments by stating that in MAOs the flavin is bent by around 30° from planarity about the N5–N10 axis (Binda et al., 2003), which enhances the basicity of the N5 atom and depletes the electron density on the C4a atom, thus facilitating substrate–flavin complex formation with the former flavin site making subsequent proton abstraction possible. We feel that, even if all of these effects are operational, it would still be insufficient to downshift the substrate pK_a value by around 10–15 units in order to make the α–CH bond acidic enough for an efficient catalysis. Furthermore, a relaxed-geometry scan of the latter bond, by compressing it with 0.1 Å increments, showed no indication of the formation of a stable complex. In addition, NBO charges on the flavin C4a and N5 sites and the substrate N atom in 1_{SP1} are 0.13, −0.35, and −0.97|e|, respectively, which demonstrate that they do not change much from the values found in isolated flavin **2** and dopamine **1** (0.10, −0.34, and −0.93|e|; **Table 1**), and that there is no charge transfer already in the Michaellis complex, as proposed by some authors in favor of the polar nucleophilic mechanism (Abad et al., 2013). This all indicates that neutral amines do not exhibit the necessary nucleophilicity to readily add to the flavin C4a position, in agreement with the fact that no direct evidence for a stable amine–flavin adduct has been found experimentally. Taken all together, these results also led us to rule out this mechanism as feasible.

The geometry of stationary structure 1_{SP1} (**Figure 3**) suggests that the following two pathways are possible. The substrate amino group is connected through two active-site water molecules to the flavin N1 atom, which is the most basic position within the isoalloxazine moiety (Vianello et al., 2012). This implies that the substrate could be first activated by amino deprotonation to the flavin N1 site. Also, the α–C(substrate) · · ·N5 bond

length in 1_{SP1} is 3.198 Å, being sufficiently short to suggest that the substrate is properly oriented for a direct α–CH abstraction.

Deprotonation of the neutral substrate amino group is feasible, but the process is associated with a large barrier of 37.3 kcal mol^{-1} (**Figure 4**; Vianello et al., 2012). The transition-state structure 1_{TS1} has one imaginary frequency of 270i cm^{-1} and the corresponding eigenvector represents a proton transfer to the flavin N1 atom assisted by two water molecules by the de Grotthuss mechanism (de Grotthuss, 1806). Such a high energy requirement is rationalized by the large difference in the pK_a values between proton donor and acceptor sites. For the flavin N1–H deprotonation pK_a was measured to be around 7.0 (Macheroux et al., 2005), whereas amine deprotonation typically has a pK_a of around 35 (Smith and March, 2001). Upon proton removal, the anionic substrate turns nucleophilic and covalently binds to the flavin C4a atom. The formed complex facilitates subsequent H$^-$ abstraction from the α–CH group, requiring only 13.2 kcal mol^{-1} to arrive at the transition-state structure 1_{TS2} ($v_{imag} = 871i$ cm^{-1}). Abstraction of the H$^-$ is concerted with the loosening of the N(substrate) · · ·C4a bond from 2.439 Å in 2_{TS2-N} to 3.505 Å in the final products 1_{SP3}, being reduced flavin FADH$_2$ and neutral imine. This pathway is associated with collective activation energy of 44.6 kcal mol^{-1}, which is too high to be feasible. In an analogous pathway, only starting from the substrate with the protonated amino group, the flavin N1 deprotonation of the –NH$_3^+$ group becomes easier requiring only 20.7 kcal mol^{-1} ($v_{imag} = 980i$ cm^{-1}) The subsequent α–hydride abstraction by the flavin N5 atom costs an additional 24.4 kcal mol^{-1} to add up to an overall reaction free-energy barrier of 43.1 kcal mol^{-1}, yielding protonated imine, R–CH$_2$CH$_2$ = NH$_2^+$. Although the collective activation barrier for this process is slightly lower than with the unionized substrate, it is still too high for this mechanism to be plausible.

Traditional notion of the hydride abstraction should generate positive charge on the substrate α–carbon atom, which would

TABLE 1 | Evolution of atomic charges during the C(α)–H hydride abstraction reaction from dopamine to flavin as obtained with the NBO approach at the (CPCM)/M06–2X/6–31G(d) level of theory.

System	Atom/group	Isolated	Reactants (1_{SP1})	TS (2_{TS1})	Intermediate (2_{SP2})
	N(amino)	−0.93	−0.97	−0.79	−0.90
	α–C	−0.26	−0.25	−0.11	0.16
	β–C	−0.50	−0.49	−0.50	−0.52
	C1(phenyl)	−0.06	−0.04	−0.06	−0.07
	dopamine	0.00	−0.03	0.31	0.43
	N5(flavin)	−0.34	−0.35	−0.50	−0.50
	N1(flavin)	−0.63	−0.68	−0.71	−0.70
	flavin	0.00	0.01	−0.29	−0.35

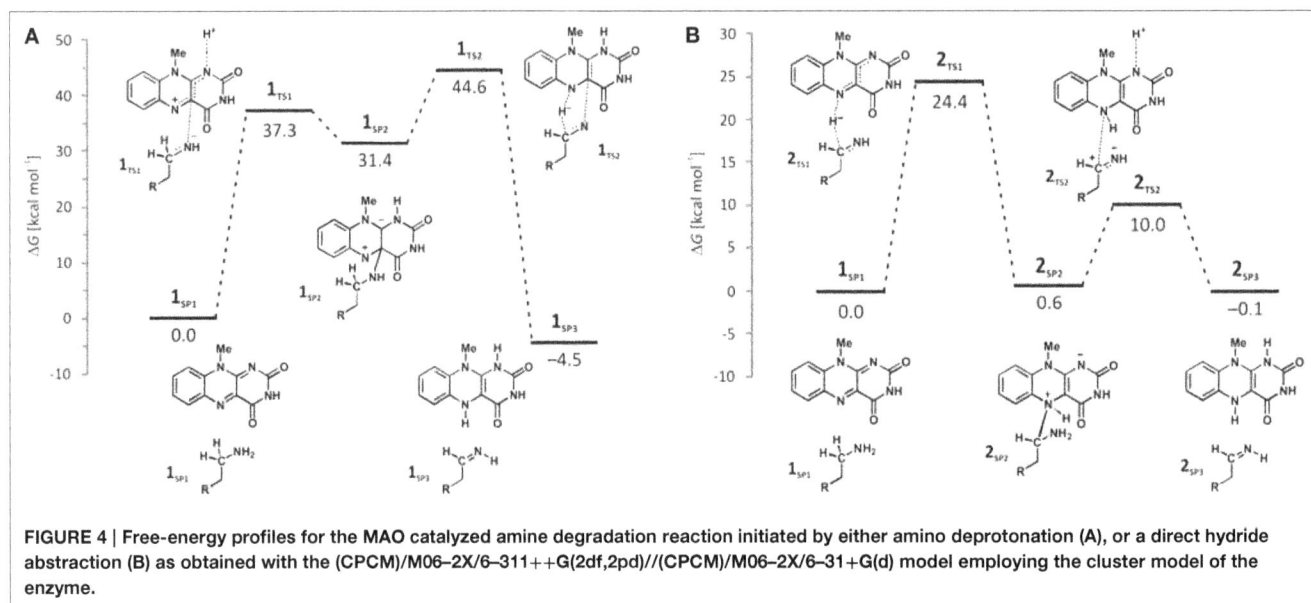

FIGURE 4 | Free-energy profiles for the MAO catalyzed amine degradation reaction initiated by either amino deprotonation (A), or a direct hydride abstraction (B) as obtained with the (CPCM)/M06–2X/6–311++G(2df,2pd)//(CPCM)/M06–2X/6–31+G(d) model employing the cluster model of the enzyme.

seem to contrast the aforementioned positive Taft correlation (Miller and Edmondson, 1999a) that suggested negative charge development on the stated carbon atom. However, due to H$^-$ abstraction, the depletion of electron density on the α–carbon atom is completely outperformed by the strong electron-donating ability of the vicinal amino group, as evidenced by a decrease in both the corresponding N(amino)-C(α) bond length and the nitrogen atomic charge from 1.466 Å and 0.97|e| in 1_{SP1} to 1.354 Å and −0.79|e| in 2_{TS1}. As a result, the charge on the α–carbon atom changes from −0.25|e| in 1_{SP1} to −0.11|e| in 2_{TS1}, surprisingly preserving a significant portion of the negative charge (**Table 1**). More importantly, the charge on the dopamine β–carbon atom, which is in terms of *para*-substituent effects analogous to the benzylamine α–carbon atom, even increases from −0.49|e| (1_{SP1}) to −0.50|e| (2_{TS1}), which, taken all together, gives strong evidence to why this reaction is facilitated by the electron-withdrawing *para*-substituents on the aromatic ring, thus putting our results in firm agreement with the work of Miller and Edmondson (1999a,b). After the flavin accommodates H$^-$, its N5 atom becomes sp^3-hybridized with excess negative charge, having enough nucleophilicity to

form a covalent bond with the thus formed cationic substrate (**Figures 3, 4**). Macheroux et al. (2005) measured the pK_a value of the fully hydrogenated flavin N(5)–H$_2$ moiety to be pK_a = 4, which indicates that the N(5)–H$^-$ group possesses sufficient basicity to act as a base. The calculated substrate-flavin interaction free energy in 2_{SP2} is as high as 27.7 kcal mol^{-1}, which, together with the corresponding N5-C(α) bond length of only 1.703 Å, suggests that the formed complex is rather strong. With the complex formation, the necessity for another step in this process becomes apparent, which represents an important advantage over other mechanistic proposals that all advise protonated imine as the final product. We disagree with the latter for two reasons. First, it would be difficult for a protonated imine to leave the active site, because on its way out it would relatively strongly bind to the "aromatic cage" through favorable cation–π interactions (Borštnar et al., 2012). Secondly, it is well-established that the final imine hydrolysis to aldehydes occurs non-enzymatically outside the MAO (Edmondson et al., 1993; Woo and Silverman, 1995). However, the protonated product would immediately be hydrolyzed by the nearest water molecule within the enzyme, because in organic chemistry this reaction readily proceeds with the protonated imine under acidic conditions (Smith and March, 2001).

The next step involves amino group deprotonation by the flavin N1 atom with an activation free energy of 9.4 kcal mol^{-1} (**Figure 4**), being concerted with the weakening of the adduct N5(flavin) $\cdots$ Cα(dopamine) bond. The transition-state 2_{TS2} ($\upsilon_{imag} = 933i$ cm^{-1}) again describes a de Grotthuss-type proton transfer proceeding with the two active-site water molecules. Upon deprotonation, the system is stabilized by 10.1 kcal mol^{-1} to 2_{SP3}, making the whole reaction energetically feasible and yielding the neutral trans-imine and the fully reduced flavin (FADH$_2$) as final products (**Figures 3, 4**). It has to be strongly emphasized that the presence of the acidic N–H bond enables the completion of MAO turnover and explains why many alkyl- and arylamines change from being MAO substrates to MAO inhibitors upon *N,N*-dimethylation (Ding et al., 1993). The fact that dopamine is converted into a neutral imine is significant, because this suggests it will predominantly remain unprotonated in the hydrophobic active site, based on consideration of the pK_a values of similar unconjugated imines, which are, as a rule, found to be below the physiological value of 7.4 (for example, the pK_a value of Me$_2$C$=$N$-$Me is 5.5) (Smith and March, 2001), ensuring that the neutral product could go past the "aromatic cage" on its release from the active site. This, however, does not rule out the possibility that, when it is finally liberated from the enzyme, the imine formed could be readily protonated, because, during its departure, changes in the environment could make the protonation feasible. It is also possible that the protonation occurs already close to the active site since hydrated enzyme represents proton rich environment. This would then fully agree with Edmondson et al. (1993), who showed that the protonated *p*-(dimethylamino) benzylimine is released from the enzyme. Also, the fact that flavin is fully reduced to FADH$_2$ enables an important prerequisite for MAO regeneration by molecular oxygen to revert flavin into its oxidized form (FAD) by creating hydrogen peroxide (H$_2$O$_2$), a reaction for which two hydrogen atoms are required (**Scheme 1**). Please note that hydrogen peroxide further reacts and produces reactive oxygen species that are responsible for the oxidative stress and neurodegeneration (*vide infra*).

In concluding this section, let us emphasize that presented results have convincingly demonstrated the prevailing feasibility of the two-step hydride transfer mechanism (**Figure 5**). In recent years, there have been several additional computational studies showing its prevailing feasibility in MAO (Akyüz and Erdem, 2013; Atalay and Erdem, 2013; Zapata-Torres et al., 2015), or some other flavoenzymes (Kopacz et al., 2014; Karasulu and Thiel, 2015). Furthermore, in what follows, we will demonstrate that when we moved from the QM-only cluster model toward including the full enzyme structure, *via* the Empirical Valence Bond QM/MM approach, the calculated activation free energy for the MAO B catalyzed degradation of dopamine drops down to $\Delta G^{\ddagger} = 16.1$ kcal/mol (Repić et al., 2014b), being in excellent agreement with the available experimental value of 16.5 kcal/mol (Walker and Edmondson, 1994; Wang and Edmondson, 2011), thus providing a strong support for our mechanistic picture.

MULTISCALE SIMULATION OF MAO CATALYZED CHEMICAL STEP FOR DIFFERENT SUBSTRATES

In this section, we focus to the extension of the static cluster model study of the rate-limiting step in MAO B to a full enzyme dimensionality using multiscale EVB approach with extensive thermal averaging allowing for a direct evaluation of the enzyme catalytic effect compared to the reference reaction in the gas phase or aqueous solution (Warshel, 2014).

For enzyme reactions and reactions in polar solutions, transition state theory is practically always valid. To calculate the rate constant for the reaction it is, therefore, necessary to know the barrier height in terms of free energy. Faster reaction has lower barrier than the slower one. Catalysis is the reaction rate enhancement relative to the reference reaction and catalyzed reaction has, therefore, lower free energy of activation than the uncatalyzed reaction. The natural reference state for an enzymatic reaction is the corresponding uncatalyzed reaction in aqueous solution, since biology occurs in this medium. However, considering the lack of direct experimental kinetic data in aqueous solution, our calculated reference state for the MAO B catalyzed reaction is the corresponding hydride transfer in the gas phase, as this is the state for which one is most likely to obtain reliable estimates of the activation barrier using quantum chemical approaches. For the gas phase reference reaction between lumiflavin **2** and dopamine **1** we used the optimized geometries of the reactants and transition state from the cluster study. The gas phase energetics of the reaction were calculated using the M06–2X density functional in conjunction with the 6–31+G(d,p) basis set as described in previous section. For simulation using full dimensionality of the enzyme with included water molecules, atomic coordinates were obtained from the high-resolution (1.6 Å) crystal structure of MAO B obtained from the Protein Data Bank (accession code 2XFN). The charges of all relevant structures were fitted to the electrostatic potential and calculated with inclusion of the solvent reaction field at the (CPCM)/B3LYP/6–311G(d,p) level. The dopamine substrate was manually docked into the MAO B active site. EVB calculations were performed *in vacuo* representing the reference state, aqueous solution as well as full dimensionality of the MAO B enzyme, to examine the effect of different environments on the reaction barrier. For all EVB calculations the same EVB region was used, consisting of lumiflavin moiety and dopamine for a total simulation time of 15.3 ns, while for other technical details the reader is referred to the original publication (Repić et al., 2014b). All EVB calculations were performed using the standard EVB free energy perturbation/umbrella sampling (EVB–FEP/US) procedure (Kamerlin and Warshel, 2011b) and the MOLARIS simulation package in combination with the ENZYMIX force field (Schutz and Warshel, 2001).

In order to study enzyme catalysis, it is highly desirable to have the experimental kinetic data for the reference reaction in aqueous solution. To our best knowledge experimental kinetic data for the reaction between flavin and dopamine in aqueous solution are not available. There are also no available data

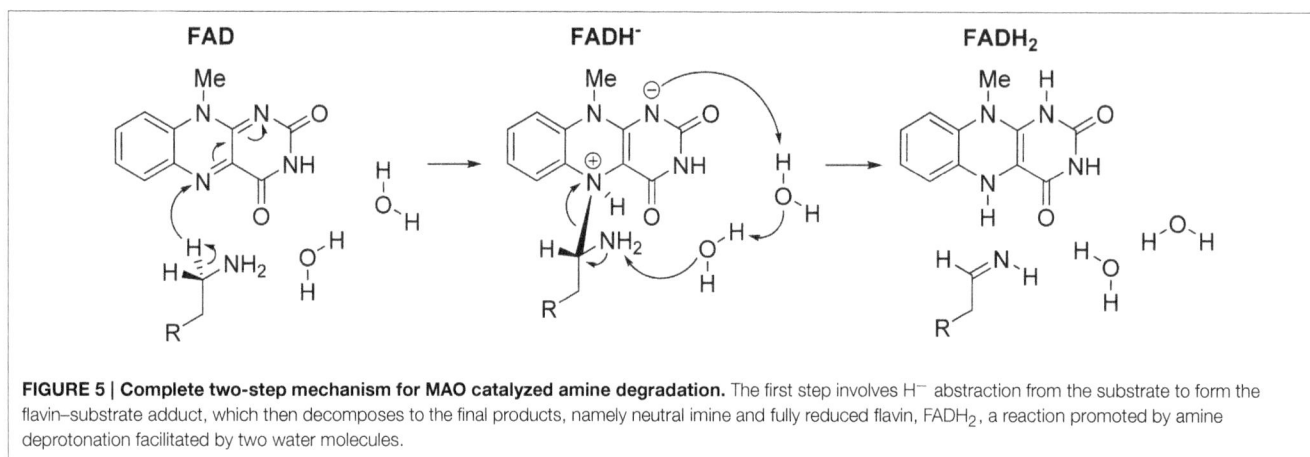

FIGURE 5 | Complete two-step mechanism for MAO catalyzed amine degradation. The first step involves H$^-$ abstraction from the substrate to form the flavin–substrate adduct, which then decomposes to the final products, namely neutral imine and fully reduced flavin, FADH$_2$, a reaction promoted by amine deprotonation facilitated by two water molecules.

about the kinetics of uncatalyzed reactions between flavins and phenethylamines or some suitable model compounds. Some studies has shown that flavins react with amines and alcohols in aqueous solution on a timescale of days, but no further kinetic data were provided and, therefore, experimental value for activation free energy of the reference reaction cannot be deduced (Brown and Hamilton, 1970; Kim et al., 1993). Therefore, we parameterized our EVB Hamiltonian to reproduce reliable M06–2X/6–31+G(d,p) energetics *in vacuo* ($\Delta G^{\ddagger}_{gas}$ and ΔG^{0}_{gas}). The system was subsequently moved to aqueous solution and to the MAO B active site using the same parameter set (EVB off-diagonal term plus the gas phase shift). This is a valid approximation, due to the demonstrated phase-independence of the EVB off-diagonal (H_{ij}) coupling term (Hong et al., 2006).

To model the hydride transfer step using EVB, the activation free energy ($\Delta G^{\ddagger}_{gas}$) and the free energy ($\Delta G^{0}_{gas}$) of the reference reaction need to be known. While it is straightforward to obtain $\Delta G^{\ddagger}_{gas}$, the calculation of ΔG^{0}_{gas} is complicated by the fact that, in the gas phase, the resulting FADH$_2$ anion and dopamine cation form a bound adduct immediately upon hydride transfer. In order to circumvent this issue we selected the point in the Intrinsic Reaction Coordinate (IRC) profile where the structure of FADH$^-$ moiety matches the geometry of the gas-phase optimized FADH$^-$. In addition, the IRC profile shows a shoulder in the potential energy surface around the same point, thus suggesting a transient intermediate. Full geometrical optimization of the reactant, the transition state, and the adduct, including the thermal correction to Gibbs free energy, shows that the transition state and adduct are 32.8 and 10.0 kcal mol^{-1} higher in energy than the reactants, respectively. Taking into account the thermal correction, the product is 24.9 kcal mol^{-1} higher in energy than the reactants. The EVB gas-phase shift and coupling parameter were thus parameterized to reproduce these $\Delta G^{\ddagger}_{gas}$ and ΔG^{0}_{gas} values. Using the same parameters as in the gas-phase EVB simulation the reaction in aqueous solution and in the enzyme was simulated. In aqueous solution the activation free energy is still high, 26.5 kcal mol^{-1}, it is lowered by 6.3 kcal mol^{-1} relative to the gas phase. Even more pronounced is the effect of the aqueous environment to the free energy of reaction, which is lowered to 4.2 kcal mol^{-1}. By inclusion of

the full dimensionality of the enzyme environment, reduction of the barrier to 14.2 kcal mol^{-1} is observed and the reaction becomes exergonic with a reaction free energy of −0.6 kcal mol^{-1} (Repić et al., 2014b). The reduction in the activation barrier compared to the aqueous solution is 12.3 kcal mol^{-1}, which corresponds to a rate-enhancement of more than nine orders of magnitude. The reaction is not excessively exergonic, allowing for the reverse reaction in the case of product overproduction. Experimental studies revealed that the substrates are bound to the MAO B active site in the protonated form, while they enter the reaction only if they are neutral. We calculated the pK_a value for dopamine placed at the MAO B active site and we have shown that it is not significantly changed relative to its value in water. The reversible work necessary for dopamine deprotonation can be calculated then analytically and its value is 1.9 kcal mol^{-1}. When this correction is added to the calculated barrier of 14.2 kcal mol^{-1}, it gives an activation free energy of 16.1 kcal mol^{-1}. The latter is in excellent agreement with the experimental value of 16.5 kcal mol^{-1} (Edmondson et al., 2009) thus strongly supporting the proposed hydride transfer mechanism. A snapshot from the simulation of MAO B active site with the reactive dopamine molecule is shown in **Figure 6**.

The Lys296 residue is a part of the FAD–H$_2$O–Lys296 motif conserved in many flavin-dependent oxidases and we speculated that it might be important in the MAO catalysis. We have performed our calculations with both the neutral and protonated form of Lys296 to quantify the effect of the ionization state of this residue on the hydride transfer reaction. Our results show that the protonation state of Lys296 does not affect the reductive half-reaction of MAO B and that the barrier for the reaction is virtually unchanged at 14.0 kcal mol^{-1}. One may speculate that the protonation state of Lys296 may be relevant for the oxidative half-reaction, what is in accordance with the conclusion for mouse polyamine oxidase (Henderson Pozzi and Fitzpatrick, 2010).

Following the same methodology, we also addressed the catalytic step of MAO A catalyzed decomposition of noradrenaline (Poberžnik et al., unpublished data). We showed that MAO A lowers the activation barrier by 14.3 kcal mol^{-1} relative to the same reaction in aqueous solution. Taking

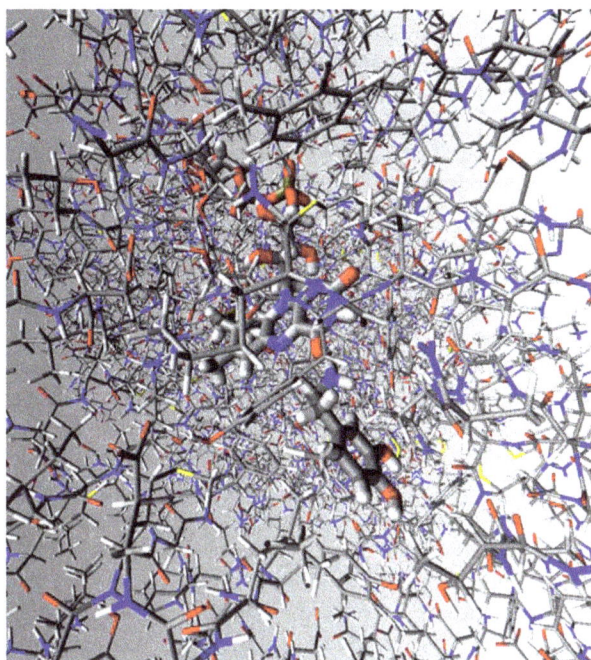

FIGURE 6 | Structure of the MAO B active site with the reactive neutral dopamine. The FAD prosthetic group is shown in orange, dopamine in light blue, and Lys296 in violet.

into account the deprotonation of noradrenaline prior to the hydride transfer reaction, the activation barrier in the enzyme is calculated to be 20.3 ± 1.6 kcal mol^{-1}, being in reasonably good agreement with the correlated experimental value of 16.3 kcal mol^{-1} (O'Carroll et al., 1986). The results presented here offer a strong support that both MAO A and MAO B isoforms function by the same hydride transfer mechanism.

In this study we also calculated the effects of point mutations on the activation free energy. The choice of investigated systems was prompted by the experimental work of Edmondson and co-workers (Husain et al., 1982; Li et al., 2006). Our results show that the pK_a uncorrected values for the activation free energies are as follows (in kcal mol^{-1}): WT MAO A 18.7, Tyr444Phe 18.2, Tyr444Leu 19.3, Tyr444Trp, and Tyr444His 25.7. For the last mutant, it is essential that His444 is neutral, otherwise in monoprotonated His444 the barrier raises for additional 5 kcal mol^{-1}. Taken all together, our analysis confirmed the functional importance of the probed tyrosine residue, since mutations to Leu, Trp, and His produced enzymes which are less efficient, culminating with the Tyr444His mutant that is five orders of magnitude a slower enzyme than WT. Interestingly, Tyr444Phe mutation even slightly lowered the activation free-energy, which strongly suggests that the role of the probed Tyr44 residue is predominantly exerted through its aromatic moiety, rather than through the hydroxyl –OH group, which is a significant observation. It follows that the efficiency of the wild-type MAO A enzyme and its Tyr444 mutants is WT = Tyr444Phe > Tyr444Leu > Tyr444Trp > Tyr444His, and it could be qualitatively related to the mentioned experimental

results in MAO B (Husain et al., 1982; Li et al., 2006), which read WT > Tyr444Phe > Tyr444His≈Tyr444Leu > Tyr444Trp. Another very interesting aspect is provided with His and Glu mutants regarding their protonation forms. It turns out that Tyr444His(0) mutant, where His residue is neutral, gives an enzyme with 7 kcal mol^{-1} higher activation free-energy than WT, which is even further increased by another 9 kcal mol^{-1} to $\Delta G^{\ddagger} = 34.9$ kcal mol^{-1} in Tyr444His(+) upon protonating the histidine residue, thus even exceeding the value for the aqueous solution. This observation is consistent with the idea of a positive charge build-up on the substrate in the transition state, thus strongly confirming the anionic nature of the abstracted hydride H$^-$. Therefore, positively charged species near the active site have an anti-catalytic effect as clearly indicated by our results. To further test this concept, we investigated two additional Tyr444Glu mutants corresponding to unionized and negatively charged glutamic acid residues. For the neutral form, Tyr444Glu(0), the barrier is higher than for the WT, assuming $\Delta G^{\ddagger} = 23.8$ kcal mol^{-1}, but is significantly reduced to $\Delta G^{\ddagger} = 21.7$ kcal mol^{-1}, when Glu residue is deprotonated to – CH$_2$–CH$_2$–COO$^-$. The induced negative charge in this active site residue stabilizes the cationic transition state, which lowers the barrier. Taken all together, the results obtained for both Tyr444His and Tyr444Glu mutants and their protonation forms provide a straightforward confirmation that MAO enzymes operate through the hydride transfer mechanism (Poberžnik et al., unpublished data).

HOW IMPORTANT IS NUCLEAR TUNNELING FOR THE MAO CATALYTIC STEP?

The rate limiting step of MAO catalyzed reaction involves a hydride transfer and, as a light particle, its motion obeys the laws of quantum mechanics rather than the laws of classical mechanics. Nuclear quantum effect contributes to enzyme kinetics by vibrational zero point energy that elevates the reactant well and by tunneling through the barrier. Both effects have no classical analog and often they are refereed in the literature as "tunneling." Both contributions give rise to the effective lowering of the barrier reflected in enlarged rate constant. Since nuclear quantum effects are mass dependent they are therefore different for H and D.

Experimentally the quantum-mechanical nature of nuclei motion in the reaction process is reflected as kinetic isotope effect (KIE) that is, by definition, the ratio of the rate constants for the species involving various isotopomers. The most pronounced are always the KIE values involving H/D isotopes, because of the large relative mass ratio of the isotopomers. Tunneling reflected in H/D KIE for MAO catalyzed reactions was addressed by several experimental studies. Husain et al. (1982) studied bovine liver MAO B catalyzed decomposition of benzylamine. The kinetic parameters were deduced from UV/VIS detection of an aldehyde signal as a function of time at 25°C. The H/D KIE was dependent on the oxygen level. For the oxygen and benzylamine saturation case the observed H/D KIE was 6.4–6.7, while at low oxygen levels the value increased to 8.7. In a detailed study of Walker and Edmondson (Walker and Edmondson, 1994) the authors applied advanced data processing techniques to address a series of *para* and *meta* substituted benzylamine analogs. The H/D KIE value for unsubstituted benzylamine was between 8.2 and 10.1, depending on the level of oxygen. For the other substituted benzylamine species the H/D KIE values were between 6.5 for *p*-Br substitution and 14.1 for *m*-Cl substitution. Tunneling in recombinant human liver MAO A catalyzed decomposition of *para*-substituted benzylamines was studied by Miller and Edmondson (1999a) and the reported values range between 6 and 13. Scrutton and co-workers studied pH dependence of KIE in recombinant human liver MAO A catalyzed decomposition of benzylamine and the value decreases from ~13 to 8 with increasing pH value (Dunn et al., 2008). Wang and Edmondson addressed tunneling in a rat MAO A for a series of *p*-substituted benzylamines (Walker and Edmondson, 1994; Wang and Edmondson, 2011), concluding that H/D KIE values are pH–independent and range from 7 to 14, demonstrating a rate-limiting α–CH bond cleavage step in catalysis.

Interesting proposals were given for the role of tunneling and dynamical effects in enzyme catalysis. These proposals were mainly based on experimental detection and careful quantization of hydrogen (radical, proton, and hydride) tunneling in enzymatic reactions. Several independent groups gathered evidence that room temperature nuclear tunneling occurs in several enzymatic reaction, especially those involving C–H bond activation (Hay et al., 2009; Klinman, 2009, 2013; Klinman and Kohen, 2013). The donor-acceptor distance played a special role in these proposals on which depends the shape of the potential for hydrogen transfer. It was long ago proposed that steric strain and compression can help catalysis (Jencks, 1987). The rationale behind assigning special relevance for catalysis to the modes involving donor-acceptor distance is that the authors suggest that for the compressed case the barrier for hydrogen transfer just gets narrower at the preserved height, which is a prerequisite for tunneling. The experimental results were interpreted by the vibronic formula approach (Klinman, 2013; Klinman and Kohen, 2013) and by a theory of electron transfer-coupled hydrogen transfer (Hammes-Schiffer, 2010). In particular, recent studies argued that the promoting mode proposal is consistent with pressure effects on enzymatic reactions, and that the observed pressure effects support the idea of vibrationally enhanced catalysis. By critical recompilation of the experimental and multiscale simulation data we have demonstrated that serious inconsistencies exist in the evidence to support these hypotheses (Kamerlin et al., 2010). Tunneling reflected in H/D KIE decreases upon compression, and external pressure does not lead to the applicable compression of the free energy surface. Moreover, pressure experiments do not provide actual evidence for vibrationally enhanced catalysis (Hay et al., 2007). Finally, the temperature dependence of the entropy change in hydrogen transfer reactions is shown to reflect simple electrostatic effects (Liu and Warshel, 2007). Hydrogen transfer reactions in enzymology can be explained by the transition state theory and the concept of promoting modes is not necessary. It is

enough to know the probability density for the reactive system at the transition state and at the equilibrium. Speaking about the computational methods to calculate the KIE, the method of choice is path integration, where each quantum atoms is represented by a necklace of beads. The method yields correct ensemble averages and probability densities are different for H and D giving rise to different activation free energies. Tunneling is not a dynamical phenomenon and technically speaking KIE can be calculated also by Monte Carlo method.

In this section we report the results of the path integration calculated H/D KIE of the rate-limiting step of dopamine decomposition catalyzed by MAO B (Mavri et al., 2016). We would like to reiterate that the experimental data for dopamine are not available, but for structurally closely related substituted benzylamines and MAO B the values are between 6.5 and 14.1 indicating sensitivity of tunneling to all atomic details of the reactive system. We decided to proceed with dopamine, because of its immense importance in neuroscience and because we have developed simulation protocol for this reaction for classical treatment of nuclear motion (Repić et al., 2014b). In our study, we considered the full dimensionality of the enzyme. Path integration was implemented in the form of quantum classical path (QCP) method with an EVB potential energy surface. We obtained classical EVB reaction profile of the reacting system and its surrounding protein with water molecules by the procedure described above. The QCP approach is based on the isomorphism between the nuclear wavefunction involving all the vibrational levels and the ring of quasiparticles. As the temperatures are approaching zero, the quantum correction to free energy reduces to the contribution of the zeroth vibrational level and matches the zero point energy. At the finite temperature values contribution from all the excited states are included. Please note that the harmonic force constants connection quasiparticles are larger for D than for H and the H necklace is, therefore, more delocalized.

In order to evaluate the QCP correction to the activation free energy, it is necessary to perform simulation for the transition state and the reactant minimum. Both simulations are performed for H and D, respectively. Since the wave function is more delocalized for hydrogen than for deuterium, the corresponding probability densities and therewith associated free energy values are different. The procedure was as follows. Initially, we used exactly the same protocol as for calculation of the reaction profile with the classical treatment of nuclear motion. Equilibration of 600 ps proved to be sufficient and was performed for the system constrained with reaction coordinate corresponding to the reactant well and to the transition state. We quantized nuclear motion for the dopamine methylene group next to the amino group and the N5 atom of the flavin moiety using 18 beads. In this way, the motion of four atoms was quantized corresponding to 12 degrees of freedom. 100 ps of QCP simulations followed for both H and D. When performing calculations for the D isotopomer, both hydrogen atoms of the methylene group were replaced by D in order to facilitate comparison with the experiment. The error was estimated by using 8 different starting points that were 1 ps apart. Our computational strategy evaluated the relevant nuclear quantum corrections and gave the observed kinetic isotope effect of 12.8 ± 0.3 what is in agreement with the available experimental values in the range 6.5–14.1 for MAO B catalyzed decomposition of substituted benzylamines. The latter represent structurally the closest analogs of dopamine for which H/D KIE was determined. The calculated H/D KIE gives additional piece of evidence that the proposed hydride mechanism is valid. The H/D KIE values for the enzymes where the contribution to the rate constant comes only from the zero point energy of the reactant well are between 3 and 8. The elevated value for MAO B indicates that non-negligible contribution comes from tunneling through the barrier in the reaction coordinate region around the transition state. The calculated H/D KIE can be compared with the work of Kästner and co-workers for benzylamine decomposition catalyzed by MAO B (Zenn et al., 2015), who calculated H/D KIE by diagonalizing mass weighted Hessian for reactant well and transition state, respectively, by considering DFT described reactive QM part of the system. Zero point energy corrections were calculated for both isotopomers. The "through the barriers" contribution to tunneling was calculated by one-dimensional Eckart model allowing for the analytical solution. For the lowest barrier conformation the authors obtained a H/D KIE value of 3.5, while for three others conformations the values 2.4, 2.7, and 3.7 were reported. We feel that these H/D KIE values cluster around the lower limit, since they do not include anharmonicities of all other vibrational modes but the CH stretching.

Our calculations once more demonstrated that the applied rigorous QCP approach is a reliable computational tool and it allows for quantum mechanical contributions to activation free energies even in the case when significant tunneling contributions to the rate constant are present. It is worth to comment about the meaning of the H/D kinetic isotope effect for the catalytic decomposition of dopamine. The fact is that H isotopomer is decomposed over twelve times faster than the corresponding D isotopomer. Since very much the same effect is expected in the corresponding reaction in aqueous solution the contribution to catalytic effect is highly probable expected to be zero. This phenomenon was observed for lypoxygenase with a spectacular H/D KIE of 81. It remains a challenge to perform the isotope resolved kinetic experiments for the reaction between dopamine and lumiflavin in aqueous solution. Because of very low reaction rate this is a very demanding task.

Studies of H/D KIE have, beside insight to the enzyme mechanism, relevance in the field of deuterated drugs. For drug design and pharmacokinetics H/D KIE are highly relevant in the context of advent of D substituted drug D isotopomers (Katsnelson, 2013). In the present case treatment of patients with deuterated L-dopa would result in a prolonged clearance time.

MAO, REACTIVE OXYGEN SPECIES, AND NEURODEGENERATION

Neurodegenerative diseases are mainly caused by oxidative stress. Among other sources, MAO catalyzed oxidative deamination reactions produce hydrogen peroxide as a by-product giving rise to several reactive oxygen species (ROS) that are responsible for oxidative stress. For example, H_2O_2 molecules easily undergo Fenton-type chemistry to give OH$^\bullet$ radicals. A gross scheme

of neurodegeneration on the molecular level is based on two pathways. Firstly, reactive species oxidize heavy atom ions, which enhances the interaction with α–synuclein (αSyn), thus promoting its folding to the beta form and giving rise to insoluble amyloid plaques. The latter prevents the function of vesicular transport leading to gradual neuronal death. In the second pathway, radical species, OH$^\bullet$ in particular, react with the methylene groups of the apolar part of the lipid bilayer of either the cell or mitochondrial wall, resulting in membrane leakage followed by dyshomeostasis, loss of resting potential and neuron death. Inflammation that follows is additional rich source of ROS. Epidemiological data show that the incidence of neurodegenerative diseases rapidly increases with the age. MAO inhibition is an important strategy for the prevention and treatment of neurodegenerative diseases. MAO is not the only source of ROS, electron transfer (ET) chain is even a richer source. It is worth to stress that ET cannot be inhibited, while MAO inhibition is possible. ROS originating from inflammation can be avoided to significant extents by COX–2 inhibition. In this section we will give an overview of the processes associated with these reactions that can be employed in developing strategies for the prevention and treatment of neurodegeneration. For a very recent review the reader should refer to reference (Pavlin et al., 2016).

The central nervous system (CNS) is vulnerable to oxidative stress and neurodegeneration is its direct consequence. An important reason why central nervous system is so prone to oxidative stress is that human brain consumes about 10 times more oxygen than is the average over all other tissues, which is directly linked to the high-energy consumption of neural signal transduction. Human brain represents about 2% of the body weight and consumes 20% of the oxygen. In addition, neurons have large surface to volume ratio and therefore there is higher probability for the cellular membrane damage than for other cells. In contrast to other cells, neurons are non-replicating and the brain is, despite massive redundancy, sensitive to the loss of function if too many neurons die. Neurodegeneration is a very complex pathological process. We are still very far from understanding all the details, particularly on a molecular level. Nevertheless, ROS, arising from several sources, including the non-enzymatic oxidation of dopamine, electron transfer chain, molecular oxygen, MAO catalyzed metabolism of biogenic and dietary amines, and inflammatory processes, are largely responsible for the damage to neurons. Additional complication is that initial damage of neurons triggers inflammatory process response that produces even more ROS resulting in perpetual damages of the neurons. ROS can harm the membranes of either neurons or mitochondria, thus inducing spillage of the contents, depolarization and loss of function, followed by fast neuronal death. Possibly more important than the toxic mechanism of ROS, is the heavy metal ion mediated one, in which the metal ions, especially copper and iron are oxidized, enhancing their binding to αSyn that then folds to a significantly less soluble beta form, which further aggregates into amyloid plaques. Keeping reasonably low levels of ROS is essential for homeostasis, while complete removal of ROS would have deleterious effect on the immune system. Glutathione (GSH), present at milimolar concentrations in most cell types, is a major intracellular reducing agent owing to its cysteine thiol group. Heavy metal ions form stable complexes with GSH, thus significantly decreasing its scavenging potential, and are involved in the Fenton and Haber–Weiss reactions producing $OH^\bullet$. On the other hand, H_2O_2 production from the non-enzymatic metal ions mediated oxidative deamination of dopamine and noradrenaline seems to be particularly problematic, since it is not restricted to the mitochondrial membrane, where H_2O_2 decomposing enzymes, such as catalase and glutathione peroxidase are located in significant quantities. These are possible explanations for the involvement of dopaminergic neurons in the initial stages of Parkinson's disease, while, at the same time, the loss of olfactory neurons, which are mainly glutaminergic, gives strong evidence for the essential role of either the electron transfer chain or inflammatory processes in neurodegeneration.

There are many dietary components that can not only scavenge ROS but also influence some of the biochemical events (signal transduction, stress protein synthesis, glycation, and toxin generation) associated with neurodegenerative pathologies, thereby either ameliorating the risks or slowing down the progression of the disease. In general, food containing sulfur rich compounds, such as garlic, onion, and avocados, are also good options. Bilirubin is a very efficient ROS scavenger (Joshi et al., 1995), which provides a possible explanation for a low incidence of cardiovascular diseases and, to a certain extent, neurodegeneration in patients with Gilbert–Meulengracht syndrome. A promising strategy for the prevention and, to a certain extent, treatment of neurodegeneration is the administration of curcumin, an essential ingredient of curry, which has recently been demonstrated to have significant neuroprotective potential (Trujillo et al., 2014). Interestingly, the prevalence of Alzheimer's disease in India among adults aged between 70 and 79 years is 4.4 times lower than in the USA (Mishra and Palanivelu, 2008). Green tea and coffee drinking seems to have neuroprotective potential. Catechins found in green tea can penetrate the hematoencephalic barrier and they act as metal chelating agents and ROS scavengers.

The ROS production originating from inflammatory processes in the central neural system can be blocked at the level of the arachidonic acid cascade with one of the COX–2 selective non-steroidal anti-inflammatory drugs (NSAID). Ibuprofen seems to be a first-choice, because of its low ulceration potential (Gao et al., 2011). However, it remains a challenge to balance the benefit of NSAID administration with its unwanted side effects and to give recommendations for administering NSAID in the context of neuroprotection. It is probably not recommendable to administer NSAID to patients with no signs of neurodegenerative diseases, particularly as long-term therapies.

One can lower ROS production through the MAO pathway by inhibiting MAO with one of the irreversible MAO B inhibitors, such as selegiline and rasagiline. We suggested chemical mechanism of the inhibition reaction (Borštnar et al., 2011). MAO A inhibitors, such as clorgyline, seem to be less appropriate because of their psychoactive properties (Pavlin et al., 2013). An unknown substance(s) in tobacco smoke also irreversibly inhibit MAO by up to 60%, suggesting that sporadic smoking in low quantities, e.g., one cigar per week, could be beneficial for the prevention of neurodegeneration (Fowler et al., 1996), while balancing its potential in the development of neoplasia and cardiovascular diseases. Interestingly, nicotine *per se* is a reversible inhibitor of MAO (Pavlin and Sket, 1993), while its metabolite nornicotine binds to the arginine side chain in αSyn, thus preventing conformational change to its β–form (Dickerson and Janda, 2003). Novel, promising strategies for design of drugs used in treatment of neurodegeneration are appearing. An interesting strategy is development of multi-target drugs possessing both cholinesterase and MAO-inhibitory activity like Ladostygil (Weinstock et al., 2000).

We have presented a few known chemical mechanisms of neurodegeneration on the molecular level. One can view neurodegeneration as the interplay of several chemical reactions with complex kinetics. It is still plenty of work ahead to get insight into the features of molecular events linked to neurodegeneration, paving the way toward new strategies for the prevention of and protection from these debilitating diseases.

CONCLUSION AND PERSPECTIVES

In this article, an overview of computational methods relevant for molecular modeling of the processes relevant for central nervous system was given with a focus on simulations of enzymes, receptors, transporters, and reactions relevant for central nervous system. We reviewed our work concerning monomine oxidases, enzymes that catalyze the oxidative deamination of biogenic neurotransmitters and cardio- and vasoactive amines. We demonstrated by using quantum chemical methods on the cluster model level that the rate-limiting first step for monoamine oxidases represents a hydride transfer from the methylene group next to the amino moiety to the flavin N5 atom. This is followed by the substrate amino group deprotonation to the flavin N1 site, which creates a fully reduced flavin, $FADH_2$, and neutral imine. Comparison between the structure and pK_a values of the ionisable groups of the active centers of MAO A and MAO B enzymes gives strong evidence that both enzymes operate by the same chemical mechanism. By using the empirical valence bond QM/MM approach, we showed that MAO B lowers the barrier of the hydride transfer reaction by 12.3 kcal mol^{-1} relative to the reference reaction in aqueous solution, corresponding to a rate-enhancement of more than 9 orders of magnitude. The barrier for the enzymatic reaction starting from the deprotonated substrate is 14.2 kcal mol^{-1}. Taking into account the free energy cost of dopamine deprotonation in the active site prior to the enzymatic reaction, the reaction barrier becomes 16.1 kcal mol^{-1}, being in excellent agreement with the available experimental value of 16.5 kcal mol^{-1}. Assuming hydride transfer, we calculated H/D kinetic isotope effect for MAO B catalyzed decomposition of dopamine that is also in agreement with the experimental value. In conjunction with additional experimental and computational work, the data presented here improve the understanding of the mechanism of the catalytic activity of MAO, as well as a large family of flavoenzymes, which can allow for the design of novel and improved MAO B inhibitors for antiparkinsonian and neuroprotective use. Understanding and treating depression on the level of MAO A polymorphism and serotonin transporter (SERT) polymorphism is a challenge for future. Very recently published structure of SERT (Coleman et al., 2016), along with the experimental genomic data and molecular simulation of mutants represents a step forward toward the precision medicine.

AUTHOR CONTRIBUTIONS

All authors listed, have made substantial, direct and intellectual contribution to the work, and approved it for publication.

FUNDING

RV gratefully acknowledges the European Commission for an individual FP7 Marie Curie Career Integration Grant (contract number PCIG12–GA–2012–334493). CD's lab is funded by grants from The Royal Society, the Engineering and Physical Sciences Research Council (EPSRC) and the Biotechnology and Biological Sciences Research Council (BBSRC). JM thanks the Slovenian Research Agency for the financial support in the framework of Programme Group P1-0012. The authors thank COST Action CM1103 for the productive collaborations that inspired this work and for open access funding.

ACKNOWLEDGMENTS

RV wishes to thank the Zagreb University Computing Centre (SRCE) for generously granting computational resources on the ISABELLA cluster (isabella.srce.hr) and the CRO—NGI infrastructure (www.cro-ngi.hr). CD acknowledges use of the infrastructure in the Hartree Centre, the EPSRC UK National Service for Computational Chemistry Software (NSCCS), and ARCHER, the UK National Supercomputing Service (http://www.archer.ac.uk). The authors thank the participants in COST Action CM1103 "Structure-based drug design for diagnosis and treatment of neurological diseases: dissecting and modulating complex function in the monoaminergic systems of the brain" for productive collaborations. We would like to thank Urška Jug for critical reading of the manuscript.

REFERENCES

Abad, E., Zenn, R. K., and Kästner, J. (2013). Reaction mechanism of monoamine oxidase from QM/MM calculations. *J. Phys. Chem. B* 117, 14238–14246. doi: 10.1021/jp4061522

Akyüz, M. A., and Erdem, S. S. (2013). Computational modeling of the direct hydride transfer mechanism for the MAO catalyzed oxidation of phenethylamine and benzylamine: ONIOM (QM/QM) calculations. *J. Neural Transm.* 120, 937–945. doi: 10.1007/s00702-013-1027-8

Akyuz, M. A., Erdem, S. S., and Edmondson, D. E. (2007). The aromatic cage in the active site of monoamine oxidase B: effect on the structural and electronic properties of bound benzylamine and p-nitrobenzylamine. *J. Neural Transm.* 114, 693–698. doi: 10.1007/s00702-007-0670-3

Atalay, V. E., and Erdem, S. S. (2013). A comparative computational investigation on the proton and hydride transfer mechanisms of monoamine oxidase using model molecules. *Comp. Biol. Chem.* 47, 181. doi: 10.1016/j.compbiolchem.2013.08.007

Bach, A. W., Lan, N. C., Johnson, D. L., Abell, C. W., Bembenek, M. E., Kwan, S. W., et al. (1988). cDNA cloning of human liver monoamine oxidase A and B: molecular basis of differences in enzymatic properties. *Proc. Natl. Acad. Sci. U.S.A.* 85, 4934–4938. doi: 10.1073/pnas.85.13.4934

Baier, C. J., Fantini, J., and Barrantes, F. J. (2011). Disclosure of cholesterol recognition motifs in transmembrane domains of the human nicotinic acetylcholine receptor. *Sci. Rep.* 1:69. doi: 10.1038/srep00069

Bell, A. T., and Head-Gordon, M. (2011). Quantum mechanical modeling of catalytic processes. *Annu. Rev. Chem. Biomol. Eng.* 2, 453–477. doi: 10.1146/annurev-chembioeng-061010-114108

Binda, C., Li, M., Hubalek, F., Restelli, N., Edmondson, D. E., and Mattevi, A. (2003). Insights into the mode of inhibition of human mitochondrial monoamine oxidase B from high-resolution crystal structures. *Proc. Natl. Acad. Sci. U.S.A.* 100, 9750–9755. doi: 10.1073/pnas.1633804100

Binda, C., Newton-Vinson, P., Hubalek, F., Edmondson, D. E., and Mattevi, A. (2002). Structure of human monoamine oxidase B, a drug target for the treatment of neurological disorders. *Nat. Struct. Biol.* 9, 22–26. doi: 10.1038/nsb732

Borštnar, R., Repič, M., Kamerlin, S. C. L., Vianello, R., and Mavri, J. (2012). Computational study of the pK_a values of potential catalytic residues in the active site of monoamine oxidase B. *J. Chem. Theory Comput.* 8, 3864–3870. doi: 10.1021/ct300119u

Borštnar, R., Repič, M., Kržan, M., Mavri, J., and Vianello, R. (2011). Irreversible inhibition of monoamine oxidase B by the antiparkinsonian medicines rasagiline and selegiline: a computational study. *Eur. J. Org. Chem.* 32, 6419–6433. doi: 10.1002/ejoc.201100873

Brederson, J.-D., Kym, P. R., and Szallasi, A. (2013). Targeting TRP channels for pain relief. *Eur. J. Pharm.* 716, 61–76. doi: 10.1016/j.ejphar.2013.03.003

Brooks, B. R., Bruccoleri, R. E., Olafson, B. D., States, D. J., Swaminathan, S., and Karplus, M. (1983). CHARMM: A program for macromolecular energy, minimization, and dynamics calculations. *J. Comp. Chem.* 4, 187–217. doi: 10.1002/jcc.540040211

Brown, L. E., and Hamilton, G. A. (1970). Model reactions and a general mechanism for flavoenzyme-catalyzed dehydrogenations. *J. Am. Chem. Soc.* 92, 7225–7227. doi: 10.1021/ja00727a049

Burger, K., Gimpl, G., and Fahrenholz, F. (2000). Regulation of receptor function by cholesterol. *Cell. Mol. Life Sci.* 57, 1577–1592. doi: 10.1007/PL00000643

Carvalho, A. T. P., Barrozo, A., Doron, D., Kilshtain, A. V., Major, D. T., and Kamerlin, S. C. L. (2014). Challenges in computational studies of enzyme structure, function and dynamics. *J. Mol. Graph. Model.* 54, 62–79. doi: 10.1016/j.jmgm.2014.09.003

Cheong, P. H.-Y., Legault, C. Y., Um, J. M., Çelebi-Ölçüm, N., and Houk, K. N. (2011). Quantum mechanical investigations of organocatalysis: mechanisms, reactivities, and selectivities. *Chem. Rev.* 111, 5042–5137. doi: 10.1021/cr100212h

Cherezov, V., Rosenbaum, D. M., Hanson, M. A., Rasmussen, S. G. F., Thian, F. S., Kobilka, T. S., et al. (2007). High Resolution Crystal Structure of an Engineered Human β(2)-Adrenergic G protein-Coupled Receptor. *Science* 318, 1258–1265. doi: 10.1126/science.1150577

Coleman, J. A., Green, E. M., and Gouaux, E. (2016). X-ray structures and mechanism of the human serotonin transporter. *Nature* 532, 334–339. doi: 10.1038/nature17629

Cornell, W. D., Cieplak, P., Bayly, C. I., Gould, I. R., Merz, K. M., Ferguson, D. M., et al. (1995). A Second Generation Force Field for the Simulation of Proteins, Nucleic Acids, and Organic Molecules. *J. Am. Chem. Soc.* 117, 5179–5197. doi: 10.1021/ja00124a002

Cossi, M., Rega, N., Scalmani, G., and Barone, V. (2003). Energies, structures, and electronic properties of molecules in solution with the C-PCM solvation model. *J. Comp. Chem.* 24, 669–681. doi: 10.1002/jcc.10189

Darre, L., and Domene, C. (2015). Binding of Capsaicin to the TRPV1 Ion Channel. *Mol. Pharm.* 12, 4454–4465. doi: 10.1021/acs.molpharmaceut.5b00641

Darre, L., Furini, S., and Domene, C. (2015). Permeation and dynamics of an open-activated TRPV1 channel. *J. Mol. Biol.* 427, 537–549. doi: 10.1016/j.jmb.2014.11.016

De Colibus, L., Li, M., Binda, C., Lustig, A., Edmondson, D. E., and Mattevi, A. (2005). Three-dimensional structure of human monoamine oxidase A (MAO A): relation to the structures of rat MAO A and human MAO B. *Proc. Natl. Acad. Sci. U.S.A.* 102, 12684–12689. doi: 10.1073/pnas.0505975102

de Grotthuss, C. J. T. (1806). Sur la décomposition de l'eau et des corps qu'elle tient en dissolution À l'aide de l'électricité galvanique. *Ann. Chim. Rome* 58, 54–73.

Dickerson, T. J., and Janda, K. D. (2003). Glycation of the amyloid β–protein by a nicotine metabolite: a fortuitous chemical dynamic between smoking and Alzheimer's disease. *Proc. Natl. Acad. Sci. U.S.A.* 100, 8182–8187. doi: 10.1073/pnas.1332847100

Di Giovanni, G., Di Matteo, V., and Esposito, E. (2008). *Serotonin-Dopamine Interaction: Experimental Evidence and Therapeutic Relevance.* Amsterdam: Elsevier.

Ding, C. Z., Lu, X., Nishimura, K., and Silverman, R. B. (1993). Transformation of monoamine oxidase-B primary amine substrates into time-dependent inhibitors. Tertiary amine homologs of primary amine substrates. *J. Med. Chem.* 36, 1711–1715. doi: 10.1021/jm00064a004

Domene, C. (2007). Molecular dynamics simulations of potassium channels. *Cent. Eur. J. Chem.* 5, 635–671. doi: 10.2478/s11532-007-0028-6

Domene, C., and Furini, S. (2009). Examining ion channel properties using free-energy methods. *Methods Enzymol.* 466, 155–177. doi: 10.1016/s0076-6879(09)66007-9

Dunn, R. V., Marshall, K. R., Munro, A. W., and Scrutton, N. S. (2008). The pH dependence of kinetic isotope effects in monoamine oxidase A indicates stabilization of the neutral amine in the enzyme–substrate complex. *FEBS J.* 275, 3850–3858. doi: 10.1111/j.1742-4658.2008.06532.x

Dunn, R. V., Munro, A. W., Turner, N. J., Rigby, S. E. J., and Scrutton, N. S. (2010). Tyrosyl radical formation and propagation in flavin dependent monoamine oxidases. *ChemBioChem* 11, 1228–1231. doi: 10.1002/cbic.201000184

Edmondson, D. E. (2014). Hydrogen peroxide produced by mitochondrial monoamine oxidase catalysis: biological implications. *Curr. Pharm. Des.* 20, 155–160. doi: 10.2174/13816128113190990406

Edmondson, D. E., Bhattacharyya, A. K., and Walker, M. C. (1993). Spectral and kinetic studies of imine product formation in the oxidation of p (N,N-dimethylamino)benzylamine analogs by monoamine oxidase B. *Biochemistry* 32, 5196–5202. doi: 10.1021/bi00070a031

Edmondson, D. E., Binda, C., Wang, J., Upadhyay, A. K., and Mattevi, A. (2009). Molecular and mechanistic properties of the membrane-bound mitochondrial monoamine oxidases. *Biochemistry* 48, 4220–4230. doi: 10.1021/bi900413g

Erdem, S. S., Karahan, O., Yildiz, I., and Yelekci, K. (2006). A computational study on the amine-oxidation mechanism of monoamine oxidase: Insight into the polar nucleophilic mechanism. *Org. Biomol. Chem.* 4, 646–658. doi: 10.1039/b511350d

Everaerts, W., Gees, M., Alpizar, Y. A., Farre, R., Leten, C., Apetrei, A., et al. (2011). The capsaicin receptor TRPV1 Is a crucial mediator of the noxious effects of mustard oil. *Curr. Biol.* 21, 316–321. doi: 10.1016/j.cub.2011.01.031

Fitzpatrick, P. F. (2010). Oxidation of amines by flavoproteins. *Arch. Biochem. Biophys.* 493, 13–25. doi: 10.1016/j.abb.2009.07.019

Fowler, J. S., Volkow, N. D., Wang, G.-J., Pappas, N., Logan, J., Shea, C., et al. (1996). Brain monoamine oxidase A inhibition in cigarette smokers. *Proc. Natl. Acad. Sci. U.S.A.* 93, 14065–14069. doi: 10.1073/pnas.93.24.14065

Fried, S. D., Bagchi, S., and Boxer, S. G. (2014). Extreme electric fields power catalysis in the active site of ketosteroid isomerase. *Science* 346, 1510–1514. doi: 10.1126/science.1259802

Furini, S., and Domene, C. (2013). K+ and Na+ conduction in selective and nonselective ion channels via molecular dynamics simulations. *Biophys. J.* 105, 1737–1745. doi: 10.1016/j.bpj.2013.08.049

Gadda, G. (2012). Oxygen activation in flavoprotein oxidases: the importance of being positive. *Biochemistry* 51, 2662–2669. doi: 10.1021/bi300227d

Gao, X., Chen, H., Schwarzschild, M. A., and Ascherio, A. (2011). Use of ibuprofen and risk of Parkinson disease. *Neurology* 76, 863–869. doi: 10.1212/WNL.0b013e31820f2d79

Gustavsson, A., Svensson, M., Jacobi, F., Allgulander, C., Alonso, J., Beghi, E., et al. (2011). Cost of disorders of the brain in Europe 2010. *Eur. Neuropsychopharm.* 21, 718–779. doi: 10.1016/j.euroneuro.2011.08.008

Hamilton, G. A. (1971). Proton in biological redox reactions. *Prog. Bioorg. Chem.* 1, 83–157.

Hammes-Schiffer, S. (2010). Introduction: Proton-coupled electron transfer, *Chem. Rev.* 110, 6937–6938. doi: 10.1021/cr100367q

Hanson, M. A., Cherezov, V., Roth, C. B., Griffith, M. T., Jaakola, V.-P., Chien, E. Y. T., et al. (2008). A specific cholesterol binding site is established by the 2.8 Å structure of the human β(2)-adrenergic receptor in an alternate crystal form. *Structure* 16, 897–905. doi: 10.1016/j.str.2008.05.001

Harris, C. M., Pollegioni, L., and Ghisla, S. (2001). pH and kinetic isotope effects in D-amino acid oxidase catalysis: Evidence for a concerted mechanism in substrate dehydrogenation via hydride transfer. *Eur. J. Biochem.* 268, 5504–5520. doi: 10.1046/j.1432-1033.2001.02462.x

Hay, S., Pudney, C. R., McGrory, T. A., Pang, J., Sutcliffe, M. J., and Scrutton, N. S. (2009). Barrier compression enhances an enzymatic hydrogen-transfer reaction. *Angew. Chem. Int. Ed.* 121, 1480–1482. doi: 10.1002/ange.200805502

Hay, S., Sutcliffe, M. J., and Scrutton, N. S. (2007). Promoting motions in enzyme catalysis probed by pressure studies of kinetic isotope effects. *Proc. Natl. Acad. Sci. U.S.A.* 104, 507–512. doi: 10.1073/pnas.0608408104

Henderson Pozzi, M., and Fitzpatrick, P. F. (2010). A lysine conserved in the monoamine oxidase family is involved in oxidation of the reduced flavin in mouse polyamine oxidase. *Arch. Biochem. Biophys.* 498, 83–88. doi: 10.1016/j.abb.2010.04.015

Himo, F. (2006). Quantum chemical modeling of enzyme active sites and reaction mechanisms. *Theor. Chem. Acc.* 116, 232–240. doi: 10.1007/s00214-005-0012-1

Hong, G., Rosta, E., and Warshel, A. (2006). Using the constrained DFT approach in generating diabatic surfaces and off diagonal empirical valence bond terms for modeling reactions in condensed phases. *J. Phys. Chem. B* 110, 19570–19574. doi: 10.1021/jp0625199

Hull, L. A., Davis, G. T., Rosenblatt, D. H., and Mann, C. K. (1969). Oxidations of amines. VII. Chemical and electrochemical correlations. *J. Phys. Chem.* 73, 2142–2146. doi: 10.1021/j100727a007

Husain, M., Edmondson, D. E., and Singer, T. P. (1982). Kinetic studies on the catalytic mechanism of liver monoamine oxidase. *Biochemistry* 21, 595–600. doi: 10.1021/bi00532a028

Illingworth, C. J., and Domene, C. (2009). Many-body effects and simulations of potassium channels. *Proc. R. Soc. A* 465, 1701–1716. doi: 10.1098/rspa.2009.0014

Ingolfsson, H. I., Lopez, C. A., Uusitalo, J. J., de Jong, D. H., Gopal, S. M., Periole, X., et al. (2014). The power of coarse graining in biomolecular simulations. *Wiley Interdiscip. Rev. Comp. Mol. Sci.* 4, 225–248. doi: 10.1002/wcms.1169

Jafurulla, M., and Chattopadhyay, A. (2013). Membrane lipids in the function of serotonin and adrenergic receptors. *Curr. Med. Chem.* 20, 47–55. doi: 10.2174/0929867311302010006

Jafurulla, M., Tiwari, S., and Chattopadhyay, A. (2011). Identification of cholesterol recognition amino acid consensus (CRAC) motif in G-protein coupled receptors. *Biochem. Biophys. Res. Commun.* 404, 569–573. doi: 10.1016/j.bbrc.2010.12.031

Jencks, W. P. (1987). *Catalysis in Chemistry and Enzymology.* New York, NY: Dover Publications.

Jorgensen, C., Darre, L., Vanommeslaeghe, K., Omoto, K., Pryde, D., and Domene, C. (2015). In silico identification of PAP-1 binding sites in the Kv1.2 potassium channel. *Mol. Pharm.* 12, 1299–1307. doi: 10.1021/acs.molpharmaceut.5b00023

Jorgensen, W. L., and Tirado-Rives, J. (1988). The OPLS potential functions for proteins, energy minimizations for crystals of cyclic peptides and crambin. *J. Am. Chem. Soc.* 110, 1657–1666. doi: 10.1021/ja00214a001

Joshi, M., Billing, B. H., and Hallinan, T. (1995). Investigation of the role of reactive oxygen species in bilirubin metabolism in the Gunn rat. *Biochim. Biophys. Acta* 1243, 244–250. doi: 10.1016/0304-4165(94)00135-K

Julius, D. (2013). TRP channels and pain. *Annu. Rev. Cell Dev. Biol.* 29, 355–384. doi: 10.1146/annurev-cellbio-101011-155833

Kamerlin, S. C. L., Mavri, J., and Warshel, A. (2010). Examining the case for the effect of barrier compression on tunneling, vibrationally enhanced catalysis, catalytic entropy and related issues. *FEBS Lett.* 584, 2759–2766. doi: 10.1016/j.febslet.2010.04.062

Kamerlin, S. C. L., and Warshel, A. (2011a). Multiscale Modeling of Biological Functions. *Phys. Chem. Chem. Phys.* 13, 10401–10411. doi: 10.1039/c0cp02823a

Kamerlin, S. C. L., and Warshel, A. (2011b). The empirical valence bond model: theory and applications. *Wiley Interdiscip. Rev. Comp. Mol. Sci.* 1, 30–45. doi: 10.1002/wcms.10

Karasulu, B., and Thiel, W. (2015). Amine oxidation mediated by *N*-methyltryptophan oxidase: computational insights into the mechanism, role of active-site residues, and covalent flavin binding. *ACS Catal.* 5, 1227–1239. doi: 10.1021/cs501694q

Katsnelson, A. (2013). Heavy drugs draw heavy interest from pharma backers. *Nat. Med.* 19:656. doi: 10.1038/nm0613-656

Kay, C. W. M., El Mkami, H., Molla, G., Pollegioni, L., and Ramsay, R. R. (2007). Characterization of the covalently bound anionic flavin radical in monoamine oxidase a by electron paramagnetic resonance. *J. Am. Chem. Soc.* 129, 16091–16097. doi: 10.1021/ja076090q

Kim, J. M., Bogdan, M. A., and Mariano, P. S. (1993). Mechanistic analysis of the 3-methyllumiflavin-promoted oxidative deamination of benzylamine. A potential model for monoamine oxidase catalysis. *J. Am. Chem. Soc.* 115, 10591–10595. doi: 10.1021/ja00076a017

Klinman, J. P. (2007). How do enzymes activate oxygen without inactivating themselves? *Acc. Chem. Res.* 40, 325–333. doi: 10.1021/ar6000507

Klinman, J. P. (2009). An integrated model for enzyme catalysis emerges from studies of hydrogen tunneling. *Chem. Phys. Lett.* 471, 179–193. doi: 10.1016/j.cplett.2009.01.038

Klinman, J. P. (2013). Importance of protein dynamics during enzymatic C–H bond cleavage. *Biochemistry* 52, 2068–2077. doi: 10.1021/bi301504m

Klinman, J. P., and Kohen, A. (2013). Hydrogen tunneling links protein dynamics to enzyme catalysis. *Ann. Rev. Biochem.* 82, 471–496. doi: 10.1146/annurev-biochem-051710-133623

Klinman, J. P., and Matthews, R. G. (1985). Calculation of substrate dissociation constants from steady-state isotope effects in enzyme-catalyzed reactions. *J. Am. Chem. Soc.* 107, 1058–1060. doi: 10.1021/ja00290a052

Kopacz, M. M., Heuts, D. P. H. M., and Fraaije, M. W. (2014). Kinetic mechanism of putrescine oxidase from *Rhodococcus erythropolis*. *FEBS J.* 281, 4384–4393. doi: 10.1111/febs.12945

Kurtz, K. A., Rishavy, M. A., Cleland, W. W., and Fitzpatrick, P. F. (2000). Nitrogen isotope effects as probes of the mechanism of D-amino acid oxidase. *J. Am. Chem. Soc.* 122, 12896–12897. doi: 10.1021/ja002528+

Lamoureux, G., MacKerell, A. D., and Roux, B. T. (2003). A simple polarizable model of water based on classical Drude oscillators. *J. Chem. Phys.* 119, 5185–5197. doi: 10.1063/1.1598191

Lange, Y. (1991). Disposition of intracellular cholesterol in human fibroblasts. *J. Lipid Res.* 32, 329–339.

Lee, F. S., Chu, Z. T., and Warshel, A. (1993). Microscopic and semimicroscopic calculations of electrostatic energies in proteins by the POLARIS and ENZYMIX programs. *J. Comp. Chem.* 14, 161–185. doi: 10.1002/jcc.540140205

Li, H., and Papadopoulos, V. (1998). Peripheral-type benzodiazepine receptor function in cholesterol transport. Identification of a putative cholesterol recognition/interaction amino acid sequence and consensus pattern. *Endocrinology* 139, 4991–4997. doi: 10.1210/en.139.12.4991

Li, M., Binda, C., Mattevi, A., and Edmondson, D. E. (2006). Functional role of the "aromatic cage" in human monoamine oxidase B: Structures and catalytic properties of Tyr435 mutant proteins. *Biochemistry* 45, 4775–4784. doi: 10.1021/bi051847g

Li, M., Hubálek, F., Newton-Vinson, P., and Edmondson, D. E. (2002). High-level expression of human liver monoamine oxidase A in Pichia pastoris: comparison with the enzyme expressed in *Saccharomyces cerevisiae*. *Protein Expr. Purif.* 24, 152–162. doi: 10.1006/prep.2001.1546

Liao, M., Cao, E., Julius, D., and Cheng, Y. (2013). Structure of the TRPV1 ion channel determined by electron cryo-microscopy. *Nature* 504, 107. doi: 10.1038/nature12822

Liao, R.-Z., Yu, J.-G., and Himo, F. (2011). Quantum chemical modeling of enzymatic reactions: the case of decarboxylation. *J. Chem. Theory Comput.* 7, 1494–1501. doi: 10.1021/ct200031t

Liu, H., and Warshel, A. (2007). Origin of the temperature dependence of isotope effects in enzymatic reactions: the case of dihydrofolate reductase. *J. Phys. Chem. B* 111, 7852–7861. doi: 10.1021/jp070938f

Liu, W., Chun, E., Thompson, A. A., Chubukov, P., Xu, F., Katritch, V., et al. (2012). Structural basis for allosteric regulation of GPCRs by sodium ions. *Science* 337, 232–236. doi: 10.1126/science.1219218

Lonsdale, R., Ranaghan, K. E., and Mulholland, A. J. (2010). Computational enzymology. *Chem. Commun.* 46, 2354–2372. doi: 10.1039/b925647d

Macheroux, P., Ghisla, S., Sanner, C., Ruterjans, H., and Muller, F. (2005). Reduced flavin: NMR investigation of N(5)-H exchange mechanism, estimation of ionisation constants and assessment of properties as biological catalyst. *BMC Biochem.* 6:26. doi: 10.1186/1471-2091-6-26

MacMillar, S., Edmondson, D. E., and Matsson, O. (2011). Nitrogen kinetic isotope effects for the Monoamine Oxidase B-catalyzed oxidation of benzylamine and (1,1-^{2}H$_2$)benzylamine: nitrogen rehybridization and C–H bond cleavage are not concerted. *J. Am. Chem. Soc.* 133, 12319–12321. doi: 10.1021/ja205629b

Mavri, J., Matute, R., Chu, Z. T., and Vianello, R. (2016). Path integral simulation of the H/D kinetic isotope effect in monoamine oxidase b catalyzed decomposition of dopamine. *J. Phys. Chem. B* 120, 3488–3492. doi: 10.1021/acs.jpcb.6b00894

Miller, J. R., and Edmondson, D. E. (1999a). Structure–activity relationships in the oxidation of para-substituted benzylamine analogues by recombinant human liver monoamine oxidase A. *Biochemistry* 38, 13670–13683.

Miller, J. R., and Edmondson, D. E. (1999b). Influence of flavin analogue structure on the catalytic activities and flavinylation reactions of recombinant human liver monoamine oxidases A and B. *J. Biol. Chem.* 274, 23515–23525.

Miller, J. R., Edmondson, D. E., and Grissom, C. B. (1995). Mechanistic probes of monoamine oxidase B catalysis: rapid-scan stopped flow and magnetic field independence of the reductive half-reaction. *J. Am. Chem. Soc.* 117, 7830–7831. doi: 10.1021/ja00134a038

Mishra, S., and Palanivelu, K. (2008). The effect of curcumin (turmeric) on Alzheimer's disease: an overview. *Ann. Indian Acad. Neurol.* 11, 13–19. doi: 10.4103/0972-2327.40220

Nandigama, R. K., and Edmondson, D. E. (2000). Structure–activity relations in the oxidation of phenethylamine analogues by recombinant human liver monoamine oxidase A. *Biochemistry* 39, 15258–15265. doi: 10.1021/bi001957h

Newton-Vinson, P., and Edmondson, D. E. (1999). "High-level expression, structural, kinetic, and redox characterization of recombinant human liver monoamine oxidase B," in *Flavins and Flavoproteins*, eds S. Ghisla, P. Kroneck, P. Macheroux, and H. Sund (Berlin: Agency for Scientific Publications), 431–434.

Newton-Vinson, P., Hubálek, F., and Edmondson, D. E. (2000). High-level expression of human liver monoamine oxidase B in Pichia pastoris. *Protein Expr. Purif.* 20, 334–345. doi: 10.1006/prep.2000.1309

Oates, J., and Watts, A. (2011). Uncovering the intimate relationship between lipids, cholesterol and GPCR activation. *Curr. Opin. Struct. Biol.* 21, 802–807. doi: 10.1016/j.sbi.2011.09.007

O'Carroll, A. M., Bardsley, M. E., and Tipton, K. F. (1986). The oxidation of adrenaline and noradrenaline by the two forms of monoamine oxidase from human and rat brain. *Neurochem. Int.* 8, 493–500. doi: 10.1016/0197-0186(86)90182-8

Olsson, M. H. M., Parson, W. W., and Warshel, A. (2006). Dynamical Contributions to Enzyme Catalysis: Critical Tests of a Popular Hypothesis. *Chem. Rev.* 106, 1737–1756. doi: 10.1021/cr040427e

Orru, R., Aldeco, M., and Edmondson, D. E. (2013). Do MAO A and MAO B utilize the same mechanism for the C–H bond cleavage step in catalysis? Evidence suggesting differing mechanisms. *J. Neural Transm.* 120, 847–851. doi: 10.1007/s00702-013-0991-3

Paila, Y. D., and Chattopadhyay, A. (2010). Membrane cholesterol in the function and organization of G-protein coupled receptors. *Subcell. Biochem.* 51, 439–466. doi: 10.1007/978-90-481-8622-8_16

Patel, S., and Brooks, C. L. (2004). CHARMM fluctuating charge force field for proteins: I parameterization and application to bulk organic liquid simulations. *J. Comp. Chem.* 25, 1–16. doi: 10.1002/jcc.10355

Patel, S., Mackerell, A. D. Jr., and Brooks, C. L. (2004). CHARMM fluctuating charge force field for proteins: II protein/solvent properties from molecular dynamics simulations using a nonadditive electrostatic model. *J. Comput. Chem.* 25, 1504–1514. doi: 10.1002/jcc.20077

Pavlin, M., Mavri, J., Repić, M., and Vianello, R. (2013). Quantum-chemical approach to determining the high potency of clorgyline as an irreversible acetylenic monoamine oxidase inhibitor. *J. Neural Transm.* 120, 875–882. doi: 10.1007/s00702-013-1016-y

Pavlin, M., Repić, M., Vianello, R., and Mavri, J. (2016). The chemistry of neurodegeneration: kinetic data and their implications. *Mol. Neurobiol.* 53, 3400–3415. doi: 10.1007/s12035-015-9284-1

Pavlin, R., and Sket, D. (1993). Effect of cigarette smoke on brain monoamine oxidase activity. *Farmacevtski Vestnik* 44, 185–192.

Pelmenschikov, V., Blomberg, M. R. A., and Siegbahn, P. E. M. (2002). A theoretical study of the mechanism for peptide hydrolysis by thermolysin. *J. Biol. Inorg. Chem.* 7, 284–298. doi: 10.1007/s007750100295

Picek, I., Vianello, R., Šket, P., Plavec, J., and Foretić, B. (2015). Tandem β-elimination/hetero-michael addition rearrangement of an N-alkylated pyridinium oxime to an O-alkylated pyridine oxime ether: an experimental and computational study. *J. Org. Chem.* 80, 2165–2173. doi: 10.1021/jo5026755

Pucadyil, T. J., and Chattopadhyay, A. (2006). Role of cholesterol in the function and organization of G-protein coupled receptors. *Prog. Lipid Res.* 45, 295–333. doi: 10.1016/j.plipres.2006.02.002

Ralph, E. C., Anderson, M. A., Cleland, W. W., and Fitzpatrick, P. F. (2006). Mechanistic studies of the flavoenzyme tryptophan 2-monooxygenase: Deuterium and ^{15}N kinetic isotope effects on alanine oxidation by an L-amino acid oxidase. *Biochemistry* 45, 15844–15852. doi: 10.1021/bi0618940

Ralph, E. C., Hirschi, J. S., Anderson, M. A., Cleland, W. W., Singleton, D. A., and Fitzpatrick, P. F. (2007). Insights into the mechanism of the flavoprotein-catalyzed amine oxidation from nitrogen isotope effects of the reaction of N-methyltryptophan oxidase. *Biochemistry* 46, 7655–7664. doi: 10.1021/bi700482h

Ramos, M. J., and Fernandes, P. A. (2008) Computational enzymatic catalysis. *Acc. Chem. Res.* 41, 689–698. doi: 10.1021/ar7001045

Ramsay, R. R. (2012). Monoamine oxidases: the biochemistry of the proteins as targets in medicinal chemistry and drug discovery. *Curr. Top. Med. Chem.* 12, 2189–2209. doi: 10.2174/156802612805219978

Repić, M., Purg, M., Vianello, R., and Mavri, J. (2014a). Examining electrostatic preorganization in monoamine oxidases A and B by structural comparison and pK$_a$ calculations. *J. Phys. Chem. B* 118, 4326–4332. doi: 10.1021/jp500795p

Repić, M., Vianello, R., Purg, M., Duarte, F., Bauer, P., Kamerlin, S. C. L., et al. (2014b). Empirical valence bond simulations of the hydride transfer step in the monoamine oxidase B catalyzed metabolism of dopamine. *Proteins* 82, 3347–3355. doi: 10.1002/prot.24690

Rigby, S. E. J., Hynson, R. M. G., Ramsay, R. R., Munro, A. W., and Scrutton, N. S. (2005). A stable tyrosyl radical in monoamine oxidase A. *J. Biol. Chem.* 280, 4627–4631. doi: 10.1074/jbc.M410596200

Saftić, D., Vianello, R., and Žinić, B. (2015). 5-Triazolyluracils and their N1-sulfonyl derivatives: intriguing reactivity differences in the sulfonation of triazole N1′-substituted and N1′-unsubstituted uracil molecules. *Eur. J. Org. Chem.* 35, 7695–7704. doi: 10.1002/ejoc.201501088

Schutz, C. N., and Warshel, A. (2001). What are the dielectric "constants" of proteins and how to validate electrostatic models? *Proteins* 44, 400–417. doi: 10.1002/prot.1106

Senn, H. M., and Thiel, W. (2009). QM/MM methods for biomolecular systems. *Angew. Chem. Int. Ed.* 48, 1198–1229. doi: 10.1002/anie.200802019

Shaik, S., Cohen, S., Wang, Y., Chen, H., Kumar, D., and Thiel, W. (2010). P450 enzymes: their structure, reactivity, and selectivity-modeled by QM/MM calculations. *Chem. Rev.* 110, 949–1017. doi: 10.1021/cr900121s

Shi, Y., Xia, Z., Zhang, J., Best, R., Wu, C., Ponder, J. W., et al. (2013). Polarizable atomic multipole-based AMOEBA force field for proteins. *J. Chem. Theory Comput.* 9, 4046–4063. doi: 10.1021/ct4003702

Siegbahn, P. E. M. (2001). Modeling aspects of mechanisms for reactions catalyzed by metalloenzymes. *J. Comp. Chem.* 22, 1634–1645. doi: 10.1002/jcc.1119

Siegbahn, P. E. M. (2006). The performance of hybrid DFT for mechanisms involving transition metal complexes in enzymes. *J. Biol. Inorg. Chem.* 11, 695–701. doi: 10.1007/s00775-006-0137-2

Siegbahn, P. E. M., and Borowski, T. (2006). Modeling enzymatic reactions involving transition metals. *Acc. Chem. Res.* 39, 729–738. doi: 10.1021/ar050123u

Siegbahn, P. E. M., and Crabtree, R. H. (1997). The mechanism of C-H activation by di-iron methane monooxygenases: quantum chemical studies. *J. Am. Chem. Soc.* 119, 3103–3113. doi: 10.1021/ja963939m

Siegbahn, P. E. M., and Himo, F. (2011). The quantum chemical cluster approach for modeling enzyme reactions. *Wiley Interdiscip. Rev. Comp. Mol. Sci.* 1, 323–336. doi: 10.1002/wcms.13

Sigala, P. A., Fafarman, A. T., Bogard, P. E., Boxer, S. G., Herschlag, D. (2007). Do ligand binding and solvent exclusion alter the electrostatic character within the oxyanion hole of an enzymatic active site? *J. Am. Chem. Soc.* 129, 12104–12105. doi: 10.1021/ja075605a

Silverman, R. B. (1983). Mechanism of inactivation of monoamine oxidase by trans-2-phenylcyclopropylamine and the structure of the enzyme-inactivator adduct. *J. Biol. Chem.* 258, 14766–14769.

Silverman, R. B. (1995). Radical ideas about monoamine oxidase. *Acc. Chem. Res.* 28, 335–342. doi: 10.1021/ar00056a003

Smith, M., and March, J. (2001). *March's Advanced Organic Chemistry: Reactions, Mechanisms and Structure, 5th Edn.* New York, NY: Wiley.

Son, S. Y., Ma, J., Kondou, Y., Yoshimura, M., Yamashita, E., and Tsukihara, T. (2008). Structure of human monoamine oxidase A at 2.2 Å resolution: the control of opening the entry for substrates/inhibitors. *Proc. Natl. Acad. Sci. U.S.A.* 105, 5739–5744. doi: 10.1073/pnas.0710626105

Tan, A., Glantz, M. D., Piette, L. H., and Yasunobu, K. T. (1983). Electron spin-resonance analysis of the FAD in bovine liver monoamine oxidase. *Biochem. Biophys. Res. Commun.* 117, 517–523. doi: 10.1016/0006-291X(83)91230-5

Trujillo, J., Granados-Castro, L. F., Zazueta, C., Andérica-Romero, A. C., Chirino, Y. I., and Pedraza-Chaverrí, J. (2014). Mitochondria as a target in the therapeutic properties of curcumin. *Arch. Pharm.* 347, 873–884. doi: 10.1002/ardp.201400266

Umhau, S., Pollegioni, L., Molla, G., Diederichs, K., Welte, W., Pilone, M. S., et al. (2000). The X-ray structure of D-amino acid oxidase at very high resolution identifies the chemical mechanism of flavin-dependent substrate dehydrogenation. *Proc. Natl. Acad. Sci. U.S.A.* 97, 12463–12468. doi: 10.1073/pnas.97.23.12463

van der Kamp, M. W., and Mulholland, A. J. (2013). Combined quantum mechanics/molecular mechanics (QM/MM) methods in computational enzymology. *Biochemistry* 52, 2708–2728. doi: 10.1021/bi400215w

Vianello, R., Repić, M., and Mavri, J. (2012). How are biogenic amines metabolized by monoamine oxidases? *Eur. J. Org. Chem.* 7057–7065. doi: 10.1002/ejoc.201201122

Vintém, A. P. B., Price, N. T., Silverman, R. B., and Ramsay, R. R. (2005). Mutation of surface cysteine 374 to alanine in monoamine oxidase A alters substrate turnover and inactivation by cyclopropylamines. *Bioorg. Med. Chem.* 13, 3487–3495. doi: 10.1016/j.bmc.2005.02.061

Walker, M. C., and Edmondson, D. E. (1994). Structure-activity relationships in the oxidation of benzylamine analogs by bovine liver mitochondrial monoamine oxidase B. *Biochemistry* 33, 7088–7098. doi: 10.1021/bi00189a011

Wang, C., Jiang, Y., Ma, J., Wu, H., Wacker, D., Katritch, V., et al. (2013). Structural basis for molecular recognition at serotonin receptors. *Science* 340, 610–614. doi: 10.1126/science.1232807

Wang, J., and Edmondson, D. E. (2011). ^{2}H kinetic isotope effects and pH dependence of catalysis as mechanistic probes of rat monoamine oxidase A: comparisons with the human enzyme. *Biochemistry* 50, 7710–7717. doi: 10.1021/bi200951z

Warne, T., Moukhametzianov, R., Baker, J. G., Nehme, R., Edwards, P. C., Leslie, A. G., et al. (2011). The structural basis for agonist and partial agonist action on a beta(1)-adrenergic receptor. *Nature* 469, 241–244. doi: 10.1038/nature09746

Warshel, A. (2014). Multiscale modeling of biological functions: from enzymes to molecular machines (Nobel lecture). *Angew. Chem.* 53, 10020–10031. doi: 10.1002/anie.201403689

Warshel, A., and Levitt, M. (1976). Theoretical study of enzymatic reactions: dielectric, electrostatic and steric stabilization of the carbonium ion in the reaction of lysozyme. *J. Mol. Biol.* 103, 227–249. doi: 10.1016/0022-2836(76)90311-9

Weinstock, M., Bejar, C., Wang, R. H., Poltyrev, T., Gross, A., Finberg, J. P., et al. (2000). TV3326, a novel neuroprotective drug with cholinesterase and monoamine oxidase inhibitory activities for the treatment of Alzheimer's disease. *J. Neural Transm. Suppl.* 60, 157–169. doi: 10.1007/978-3-7091-6301-6_10

Wittchen, H. U., Jacobi, F., Rehm, J., Gustavsson, A., Svensson, M., Jönsson, B., et al. (2011). The size and burden of mental disorders and other disorders of the brain in Europe 2010. *Eur. Neuropsychopharm.* 21, 655–679. doi: 10.1016/j.euroneuro.2011.07.018

Woo, J. C. G., and Silverman, R. B. (1995). Monoamine oxidase B catalysis in low aqueous medium. Direct evidence for an imine product. *J. Am. Chem. Soc.* 117, 1663–1664.

Wu, H., Wang, C., Gregory, K. J., Han, G. W., Cho, H. P., Xia, Y., et al. (2014). Structure of a class C GPCR metabotropic glutamate receptor 1 bound to an allosteric modulator. *Science* 344, 58–64. doi: 10.1126/science.1249489

Youdim, M. B. H., Edmondson, D. E., and Tipton, K. F. (2006). The therapeutic potential of monoamine oxidase inhibitors. *Nat. Rev. Neurosci.* 7, 295–309. doi: 10.1038/nrn1883

Zapata-Torres, G., Fierro, A., Barriga-González, G., Salgado, J. C., and Celis-Barros, C. (2015). Revealing monoamine oxidase B catalytic mechanisms by means of the quantum chemical cluster approach. *J. Chem. Inform. Model.* 55, 1349–1360. doi: 10.1021/acs.jcim.5b00140

Zenn, R. K., Abad, E., and Kästner, J. (2015). Influence of the environment on the oxidative deamination of p-substituted benzylamines in monoamine oxidase. *J. Phys. Chem. B* 119, 3678–3686. doi: 10.1021/jp512470a

Zhao, Y., and Truhlar, D. G. (2008). The M06 suite of density functionals for main group thermochemistry, thermochemical kinetics, noncovalent interactions, excited states, and transition elements: two new functionals and systematic testing of four M06-class functionals and 12 other functionals. *Theor. Chem. Acc.* 120, 215–241. doi: 10.1007/s00214-007-0310-x

Zhao, Y., and Truhlar, D. G. (2011). Density functional theory for reaction energies: test of meta and hybrid meta functionals, range-separated functionals, and other high-performance functionals. *J. Chem. Theory Comput.* 7, 669–676. doi: 10.1021/ct1006604

Zubcevic, L., Herzik, M. A. Jr., Chung, B. C., Liu, Z., Lander, G. C., Lee, S.-Y., et al. (2016). Cryo-electron microscopy structure of the TRPV2 ion channel. *Nat. Struc. Mol. Biol.* 23, 180. doi: 10.1038/nsmb.3159

Conflict of Interest Statement: The authors declare that the research was conducted in the absence of any commercial or financial relationships that could be construed as a potential conflict of interest.

10

Multi-Target Directed Donepezil-Like Ligands for Alzheimer's Disease

Mercedes Unzeta[1]*, Gerard Esteban[2], Irene Bolea[1], Wieslawa A. Fogel[3],
Rona R. Ramsay[4], Moussa B. H. Youdim[5], Keith F. Tipton[2] and José Marco-Contelles[6]

[1] Departament de Bioquímica i Biologia Molecular, Institut de Neurociències, Facultat de Medicina, Universitat Autònoma de Barcelona, Barcelona, Spain, [2] School of Biochemistry and Immunology, Trinity Biomedical Sciences Institute, Trinity College Dublin, Dublin, Ireland, [3] Department of Hormone Biochemistry, Medical University of Lodz, Lodz, Poland, [4] Biomolecular Sciences, Biomedical Sciences Research Complex, University of St Andrews, St. Andrews, UK, [5] Department of Pharmacology, Ruth and Bruce Rappaport Faculty of Medicine, Eve Topf and National Parkinson Foundation Center for Neurodegenerative Diseases Research, Haifa, Israel, [6] Laboratory of Medicinal Chemistry, Institute of General Organic Chemistry, Spanish National Research Council, Madrid, Spain

Edited by:
Francisco Lopez-Munoz,
University of Alcala, Spain

Reviewed by:
Massimo Grilli,
University of Genova, Italy
Min-Yu Sun,
Washington University in St. Louis,
USA

*Correspondence:
Mercedes Unzeta
mercedes.unzeta@uab.es

HIGHLIGHTS

- **ASS234** is a MTDL compound containing a moiety from Donepezil and the propargyl group from the PF 9601N, a potent and selective MAO B inhibitor. This compound is the most advanced anti-Alzheimer agent for preclinical studies identified in our laboratory.
- Derived from **ASS234** both multipotent donepezil-indolyl **(MTDL-1)** and donepezil-pyridyl hybrids **(MTDL-2)** were designed and evaluated as inhibitors of AChE/BuChE and both MAO isoforms. **MTDL-2** showed more high affinity toward the four enzymes than **MTDL-1**.
- **MTDL-3** and **MTDL-4,** were designed containing the N-benzylpiperidinium moiety from Donepezil, a metal- chelating 8-hydroxyquinoline group and linked to a N-propargyl core and they were pharmacologically evaluated.
- The presence of the cyano group in **MTDL-3,** enhanced binding to AChE, BuChE and MAO A. It showed antioxidant behavior and it was able to strongly complex Cu(II), Zn(II) and Fe(III).
- **MTDL-4** showed higher affinity toward AChE, BuChE.
- **MTDL-3** exhibited good brain penetration capacity (ADMET) and less toxicity than Donepezil. Memory deficits in scopolamine-lesioned animals were restored by **MTDL-3**.
- **MTDL-3** particularly emerged as a ligand showing remarkable potential benefits for its use in AD therapy.

Alzheimer's disease (AD), the most common form of adult onset dementia, is an age-related neurodegenerative disorder characterized by progressive memory loss, decline in language skills, and other cognitive impairments. Although its etiology is not completely known, several factors including deficits of acetylcholine, β-amyloid deposits, τ-protein phosphorylation, oxidative stress, and neuroinflammation are considered to play significant roles in the pathophysiology of this disease. For a long time, AD patients have been treated with acetylcholinesterase inhibitors such as donepezil (Aricept®) but with limited therapeutic success. This might be due to the complex multifactorial nature of AD, a fact that has prompted the design of new Multi-Target-Directed Ligands (MTDL) based on the "one molecule, multiple targets" paradigm. Thus, in this context, different series of novel multifunctional molecules with antioxidant, anti-amyloid, anti-inflammatory, and metal-chelating properties able to interact with multiple enzymes of therapeutic interest in AD pathology including acetylcholinesterase, butyrylcholinesterase, and monoamine oxidases A and B have been designed and assessed biologically. This review describes the multiple targets, the design rationale and an in-house MTDL library, bearing the *N*-benzylpiperidine motif present in donepezil, linked to different heterocyclic ring systems (indole, pyridine, or 8-hydroxyquinoline) with special emphasis on compound **ASS234**, an *N*-propargylindole derivative. The description of the *in vitro* biological properties of the compounds and discussion of the corresponding structure-activity-relationships allows us to highlight new issues for the identification of more efficient MTDL for use in AD therapy.

Keywords: **multi-target-directed ligands, donepezil, oxidative stress, anti-β-amyloid aggregation, Alzheimer's disease**

INTRODUCTION

Alzheimer's disease (AD) is one of the most common neurodegenerative diseases accounting for more than 80% of total dementia cases in elderly people. It is estimated that currently 47 million victims of AD exist worldwide and that number is expected to grow up to more than 130 million by 2050 as a result of life expectancy increase over the next decades (Thies and Bleiler, 2012, 2013). In 2015, the World Alzheimer Report estimated that the current annual societal and economic cost of dementia was US $818 billion worldwide and that amount is expected to rise up to 1 trillion by 2018. This study also reported that the cost associated with dementia has increased by 35% since 2010.

The clinical manifestations of AD are characterized by misfunctioning and gradual neuronal death resulting in a progressive memory deterioration and cognitive decline, related with the loss of cholinergic dysfunction. The anatomopathology of AD has been described by progressive loss of synaptic neurons triggering atrophy in the hippocampus and frontal and tempo-parietal cortex. Two distinctive hallmarks of AD include the presence of accumulated amyloid beta (Aβ) plaques around neurons (Glenner and Murphy, 1989) and hyperphosphorylated microtubules associated with tau protein in the form of intracellular neurofibrillary tangles (NFT) (Goedert et al., 2006).

The pathogenesis of this neurodegenerative disorder is not yet fully understood, but the scientific consensus is quite firm in describing it as a multifactorial disease caused by several elements. These include loss of cholinergic transmission, excessive protein misfolding and Aβ aggregation (Terry et al., 1964; Grundke-Iqbal et al., 1986), oxidative stress and free radical formation (Coyle and Puttfarcken, 1993), metal dyshomeostasis (Huang et al., 2004), excitotoxic, and neuroinflammatory

processes (Coyle and Puttfarcken, 1993). Although a large number of genes has been associated with the AD late-onset condition, these appear to affect susceptibility or rate of progression rather than being directly causative (Bertram and Tanzi, 2008; Chouraki and Seshadri, 2014; Karch and Goate, 2015).

CHOLINERGIC HYPOTHESIS

Cholinergic neurotransmission modulates cognitive function and cortical plasticity (Arendt and Bigl, 1986) and also plays key roles in the control of cerebral blood flow (Biesold et al., 1989), cortical activity (Détári et al., 1999), and the sleep-wake cycle (Lee et al., 2005). In 1971, Deutsch postulated the involvement of the cholinergic system in learning and memory (Deutsch, 1971), which was later corroborated in studies with animal models and humans (Fibiger, 1991; Schliebs, 2005).

The first physiological evidence for the involvement of the cholinergic system in AD pathology was a reduction in pre-synaptic acetylcholine (ACh) and a reduced expression of choline acetyltransferase (ChAT), the enzyme responsible for ACh synthesis. In addition, decreases in the binding parameters of both muscarinic acetylcholine receptors (mAChR) and nicotinic acetylcholine receptors (nAChR) have been reported. These findings suggest a direct link between cholinergic neurotransmission and AD, and constitute the basis for the so-called "cholinergic hypothesis of AD" (Deutsch, 1971), which the main therapeutic approach used to date to address the cognitive loss associated with AD is based on.

Cholinesterases

Cholinesterases (ChE) catalyse the hydrolysis of ACh into choline and acetic acid, an essential process in the cholinergic neurotransmission. There are two types of ChEs: acetylcholinesterase (AChE, EC 3.1.1.7) and butyrylcholinesterase (BuChE, EC 3.1.1.8). Both enzymes

Abbreviations: AD, Alzheimer's disease; Aβ, amyloid beta; NFT, neurofibrillary tangles; AChE, acetylcholinesterase; BuChE, butyrylcholinesterase; MAO, monoamine oxidase; APP, amyloid precursor protein; ROS, reactive oxygen species; MTDL, multi-target-directed ligand.

are type α/β hydrolases folded with an α-helix bound with β-sheet containing a catalytic domain (Ollis et al., 1992).

Acetylcholinesterase

AChE is expressed in cholinergic neurons and neuromuscular junctions where its primary function is the rapid breakdown of the neurotransmitter ACh released during cholinergic neurotransmission. Although AChE and BuChE are structurally similar, resembling each other by more than 50%, both their significance and location are substantially different.

The structure of AChE has been widely studied since the 1990s. The active site of the enzyme lies on a bottom of a long and narrow cavity of 20 Å deep and contains a catalytic triad with amino acid residues Ser200, His440 and Glu327 that catalyses the hydrolysis of the ester bond. The active site also includes an anionic site or α-anionic site that interacts with the quaternary ammonium atom of ACh, ensuring its correct orientation. A peripheral anionic site (PAS) or β-anionic site, located on the enzyme surface around the cavity entrance (**Figure 1**) has been described to play an important role in AD. This site was first recognized in the 1960s as a target for AChE activity modulators (see Sussman et al., 1991) such as toxins and promising drugs. Furthermore, interaction of the Aβ peptide with the PAS contributes to the formation of amyloid plaques by accelerating the aggregation process. Propidium iodide is an example of an inhibitor binding to this site (Inestrosa et al., 1996).

One of the most consistent changes associated with AD has been the degeneration of neurons from the cholinergic nuclei in the basal forebrain region and their terminals in the hippocampus (Struble et al., 1982). The neuronal atrophy has been associated with a loss of cholinergic markers, occurring specifically in the nucleus basalis of Meynert (Vogels et al., 1990). The cholinergic system function, responsible for the storage and retrieval of items in memory, is therefore highly impaired in AD pathology, which has been corroborated by some neuroimaging data (Jack et al., 2010).

Butyrylcholinesterase

BuChE is expressed in the hippocampus and temporal neocortex but at lower levels than AChE, and associated with glial cells (Mesulam et al., 2002), suggesting that these enzymes may have complementary functions. In AD brain, neuritic plaques, and NFTs contain large amounts of AChE and BuChE, the latter being present in the neuroglia (Wright et al., 1993), Moreover, these enzymes have been reported to play a role in the processing of APP (Wright et al., 1993), although it is unclear whether their inhibition could influence the pathogenic course of AD. While AChE is expressed in nerve and blood cells, hydrolysing ACh, the biological significance of BuChE still remains poorly understood, although it has been reported to partially modulate or compensate for the diminished AChE activity in deficient animals (Xie et al., 2000).

Likewise AChE, glial BuChE hydrolyses ACh into choline and acetate (Daikhin and Yudkoff, 2000; Mesulam et al., 2002) but with a different kinetic behavior. While AChE predominates in neurons and exhibits high affinity for ACh, with low K_M values, BuChE is mainly present in endothelia, glia and neuronal cells with low affinity (high K_M value) for ACh (Soreq and Seidman, 2001).

In addition to its role in the hydrolysis of ACh, non-enzymatic functions have also been attributed to BuChE. Whereas, AChE may accelerate amyloid deposition in the brain of AD patients, as previously mentioned, BuChE can associate with Aβ protein possibly delaying the onset and rate of neurotoxic Aβ fibril formation as observed *in vitro* (Diamant et al., 2006).

Activity of BuChE has been found either unaltered or increased in certain AD brain regions (Perry et al., 1978; Ciro et al., 2012). The increase has been associated with amyloid plaques and NFTs (Geula and Mesulam, 1989; Guillozet et al., 1997). In addition to changes in activity, changes in AChE and BuChE protein expression also occur during the progression of AD. An increase in the levels of glial-derived BuChE and decrease in synaptic AChE have been observed, triggering a dramatic increase in the BuChE: AChE ratio in cortical regions from 0.6, in healthy conditions, to 11 in AD pathology (Giacobini, 2003). The observed changes in BuChE activity and expression throughout the course of AD, and its relationship with cognitive function, emphasize the potential value of BuChE and AChE inhibition as therapeutic targets in AD condition.

AMYLOID HYPOTHESIS

The amyloid cascade hypothesis postulates that neurodegeneration in AD is caused by abnormal accumulation of Aβ plaques in various areas of the brain (Hardy and Higgins, 1992; Evin and Weidemann, 2002). This accumulation acts as a pathological trigger for a cascade that includes neuritic injury, formation of NFTs via tau protein to neuronal dysfunction and cell death (Hardy and Higgins, 1992; Selkoe, 1994).

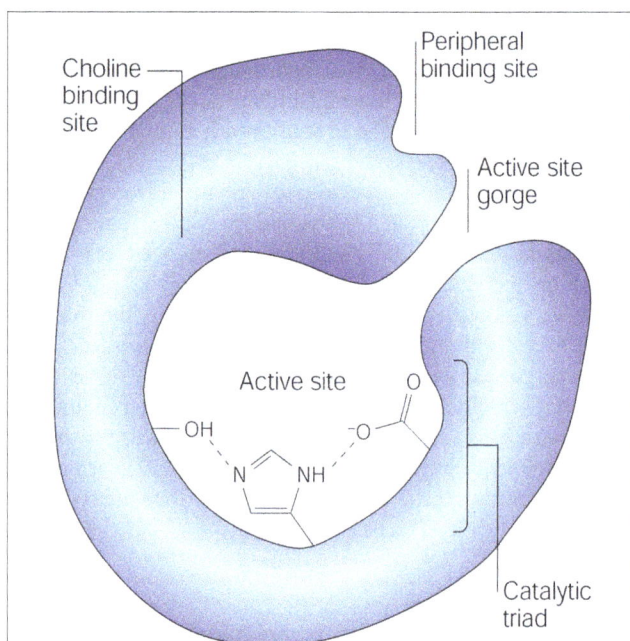

FIGURE 1 | Structure of AChE displaying the active site at the bottom of a narrow gorge, lined with hydrophobic amino-acid side chains within the catalytic triad, the choline binding site, and the peripheral binding site (Reproduced, with permission from Soreq and Seidman, 2001).

Genetic, biochemical, and pathological evidences support this hypothesis as the primary cause of AD (Kayed et al., 2003). The Aβ senile plaques are composed by Aβ peptides, which consist of 39–43 amino acid residues proteolytically derived from the sequential enzymatic action of β- and γ-secretases on transmembrane APP (Coulson et al., 2000). The length of Aβ peptides varies at the C-terminal according to the cleavage pattern of APP, with $A\beta_{1-40}$ being the most prevalent form, followed by the hydrophobic form $A\beta_{1-42}$ that aggregates faster (Perl, 2010). Within plaques, Aβ peptides and β-sheet conformation assemble and polymerise into structurally distinct forms such as fibrils, protofibers, and polymorphic oligomers (Selkoe, 1994).

The kinetics of the aggregation process of Aβ peptide follows a sigmoidal curve owing to the presence of β-sheets in its structure (LeVine, 1993), and it can be monitored *in vitro* by the use of dying molecules. The aggregating process comprises two main phases: lag phase and elongation phase. Over the lag or nucleation phase, soluble monomers or dimers with random-coil structures form a nucleus that proceeds rapidly to the formation of fibrils. At the end of this phase, low-weight soluble oligomeric species are formed, which are spherical, globular, and described as micelles or amorphous aggregates. The molecular mass of these species varies between 25 and 50 KDa (Lambert et al., 1998). Throughout the elongation phase, the oligomeric species link together to form high-molecular weight oligomers of up to 1000 KDa approximately, (Huang et al., 2000). These prefibrillar species transform into protofilaments or protofibrils, which are short, flexible, and fibrillar. The protofibrils are the precursors of full-length fibrils that are formed by simple lateral association and

structural organization. Mature fibrils are straight, unbranched, twisted and can reach up to 10 μm in length (Dobson and Batich, 2004).

The Aβ aggregation process is highly susceptible to many factors, including pH, ionic strength of the solvent, purification process or temperature. These are responsible for complications in reproducibility when experimentally assayed *in vitro*. Distinct oligomerisation and assembly processes between $A\beta_{1-40}$ and $A\beta_{1-42}$ have been described (Bitan et al., 2003). While $A\beta_{1-42}$ exhibits higher neurotoxicity and is able to form hexamers, heptamers, or octamers, $A\beta_{1-40}$ reaches equilibrium from monomers to tetramers. These variances are related to differences in the Ile-41-Ala-42 dipeptide at the C-terminus of Aβ. Until recently, it was assumed that fibrillary Aβ deposits were the responsible agents for the neuronal injury and neurodegenerative process of AD (Hardy and Higgins, 1992; Selkoe, 1994). However, later findings showed that soluble oligomeric species were able to disrupt synaptic function (Lambert et al., 1998) and recent data support the belief that soluble dimeric species are highly toxic (Jin et al., 2011). The mechanism by which Aβ induces cell damage has been reported to be caused by reactive oxygen species (ROS) production (Schubert et al., 1995), altered signaling pathways (Mattson, 1997), mitochondrial dysfunction (Shoffner, 1997), and interaction with biometals (Jin et al., 2011).

Both Aβ deposition and plaque formation also lead to local microglia activation, cytokine release, reactive astrocytosis, and multi-protein inflammatory responses (Heppner et al., 2015; **Figure 2**). The multifaceted biochemical and structural changes in surrounding axons, dendrites, and neuronal cell bodies also

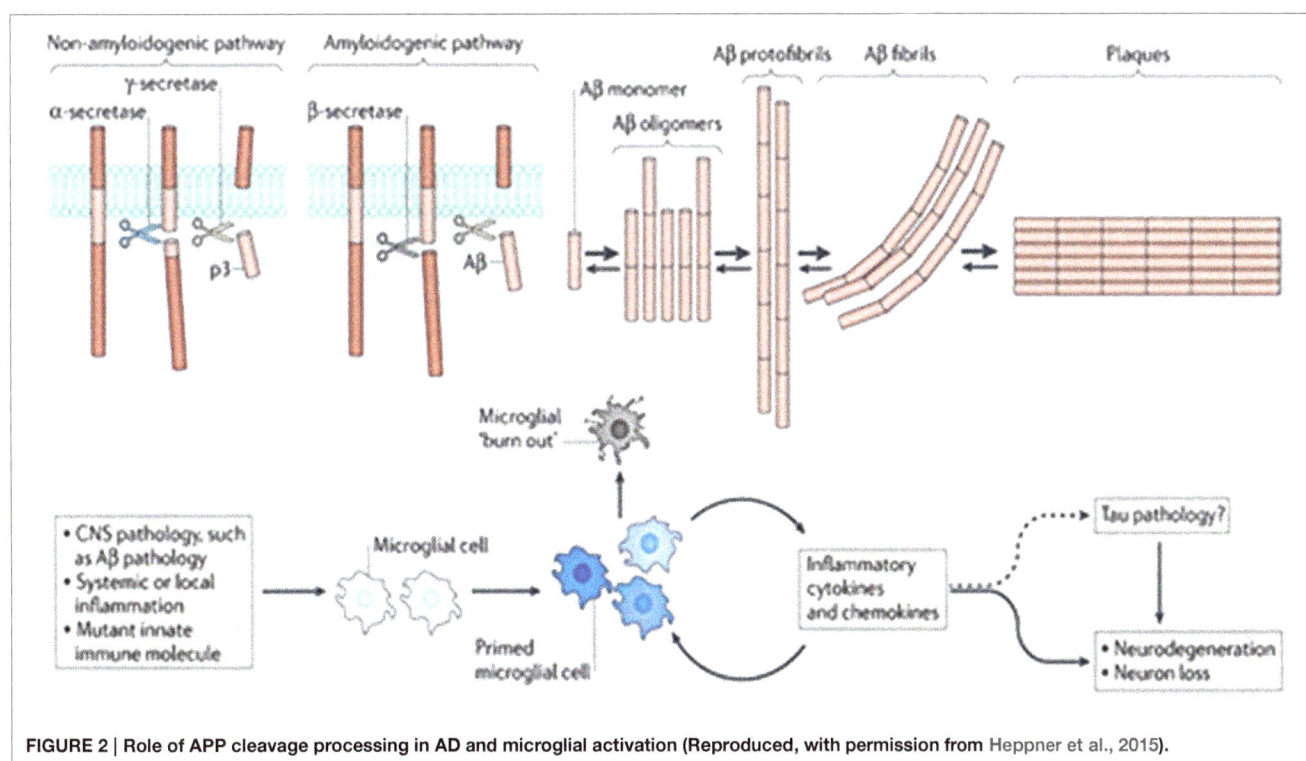

FIGURE 2 | Role of APP cleavage processing in AD and microglial activation (Reproduced, with permission from Heppner et al., 2015).

induce synapse loss as well as a remarkable cerebral atrophy in AD (Braak and Braak, 1994).

Nonetheless, to date no correlation between Aβ accumulation with extent of neuronal loss and cognitive dysfunction has been reported. In addition, direct Aβ-peptide neurotoxicity has been difficult to be identified in animal models, suggesting the existence of key intermediates between amyloidosis and neurodegeneration (Nelson et al., 2012; Serrano-Pozo et al., 2013). In addition to these studies, genetic research has suggested that neurodegenerative processes occurring in AD are the consequence of an imbalance between Aβ peptide production and clearance. Since the postulation of the amyloid hypothesis of AD, extensive but, so far unsuccessful, efforts have been undertaken in clinical research in order to develop novel therapeutics, this hypothesis has continued to gain support over the last two decades, particularly from genetic studies.

OXIDATIVE STRESS

Within any functional aerobic cell, the process involved in respiration inevitably generates ROS (Petersen et al., 2007). In particular, redox reactions are necessary for the generation of ATP and free radical intermediates are produced via the establishment of a proton gradient in oxidative phosphorylation. Multiple damaging mechanisms coexist in AD pathology, affecting each other at multiple levels (Von Bernhardi and Eugenín, 2012). In this respect, oxidative stress, which could be secondary to several other pathophysiological events, appears to be central in the progression of AD pathogenesis. Experimental evidence indicates that disturbances of the tissue redox state are important factors in early-stage AD, including the activation of multiple cell signaling pathways that contribute to the initial progression of the neurodegenerative process (Feng and Wang, 2012).

Evidence of ROS and reactive nitrogen species (RNS)-mediated injury has been reported in AD (Praticò, 2008). Increased levels of oxidative damage to biomolecules including proteins, lipids, carbohydrates, and nucleic acids have been detected in a number of studies (Moreira et al., 2008; Fukuda et al., 2009; Sultana et al., 2011). In addition, levels of antioxidant enzymes were found to be altered in specific AD brain regions (Sultana et al., 2011). Consequently, the "oxidative stress hypothesis of AD" emerged as a key factor in both the onset and progression of the disease. Oxidative stress is a widespread cellular process that currently lacks a specific treatment target such as a receptor or a single major metabolic pathway (Galasko et al., 2012). The wide variety of sources and sites of oxidative stress production paralleled by an even higher heterogeneity in the antioxidant responses. Specifically, the activity of cytochrome oxidase and pyruvate and α-ketoglutarate dehydrogenase complexes (key enzymes for the ATP supply) have been reported to be decreased as a result of oxidative damage (Aliev et al., 2011). In AD, there are established connexions between oxidative stress and other key AD events that amplify its complexity (**Figure 3**).

The presence of oxidation markers in the early stages of AD indicates that oxidative stress precedes the appearance of some other hallmarks (Rosini et al., 2014). Moreover, the accumulation of oxidative active modified products, such as 8-hydroxyguanosine (8-OHG) and nitrotyrosine in the cytoplasm of cerebral neurons from Down's syndrome patients has been reported to precede amyloid deposition (Odetti et al., 1998; Nunomura et al., 2000). This finding was also demonstrated in an APP transgenic mice model of AD (Smith et al., 1998). In post-mortem brains of myocardial infarction (MCI) patients, CSF, plasma, and urine increased levels of lipid peroxidation, nuclear acid oxidation, and diminished levels of antioxidant enzymes were found (Keller et al., 2005; Butterfield et al., 2006). Furthermore, heme oxygenase-1 (HO-1) levels were also reported to be increased in both AD and MCI post-mortem brain tissues (Schipper et al., 2006). Such findings might indicate increased oxidative stress as a general response to tissue damage in the brain, which may therefore contribute to its further progression.

Although Aβ and its aggregated senile plaques are undoubtedly involved in the neurodegenerative process of AD, the chronology of their presence has been now deemed secondary by many studies (Castellani et al., 2006; Zhu et al., 2007). Evidence suggests that secretion and deposition of Aβ within the neurons are compensatory measures taken by cells in effort to protect themselves against damage triggered by oxidative stress (Hayashi et al., 2007; Nakamura et al., 2007). Mitochondrial abnormalities, initially caused by gradual oxidative disturbances are major contributors of ROS to the cell (Bonda et al., 2010). Oxidative perturbances in mitochondrial operations result in impaired metabolic capacity (Wang et al., 2009) that would prevent the effective transfer of electrons along the respiratory chain during oxidative phosphorylation and the further generation of excessive ROS. This abnormality creates a vicious positive-feedback cycle where ROS produce oxidative stress that eventually yields more ROS along with other cellular detriments. ROS gradually accumulate in the cell and once a threshold is reached, it is no longer able to control the debilitating cycle propagation and a compensatory "steady state" is unavoidably initiated in order to regain control of its environment (Zhu et al., 2007). This hyper-defensive state, intended to prolong cell life, increases vulnerability to additional insults such as Aβ peptides. The cell therefore becomes subject to oxidative damage produced by oligomerisation and aggregation (Wang et al., 2009), that in turn, leads to neuroinflammation, mitochondrial damage, and further ROS generation.

In addition, cellular oxidative damage has also been linked to tau hyperphosphorylation and formation of NFTs (Lee et al., 2004). As a consequence of this aberrant cycle, cells succumb to neurodegeneration exhibiting the distinctive cognitive decline and dementia descriptive of AD (Zhu et al., 2007). Altogether, the primary role of oxidative stress in both AD onset and progression open the possibility of developing specific disease-modifying antioxidant approaches to confronting the disease.

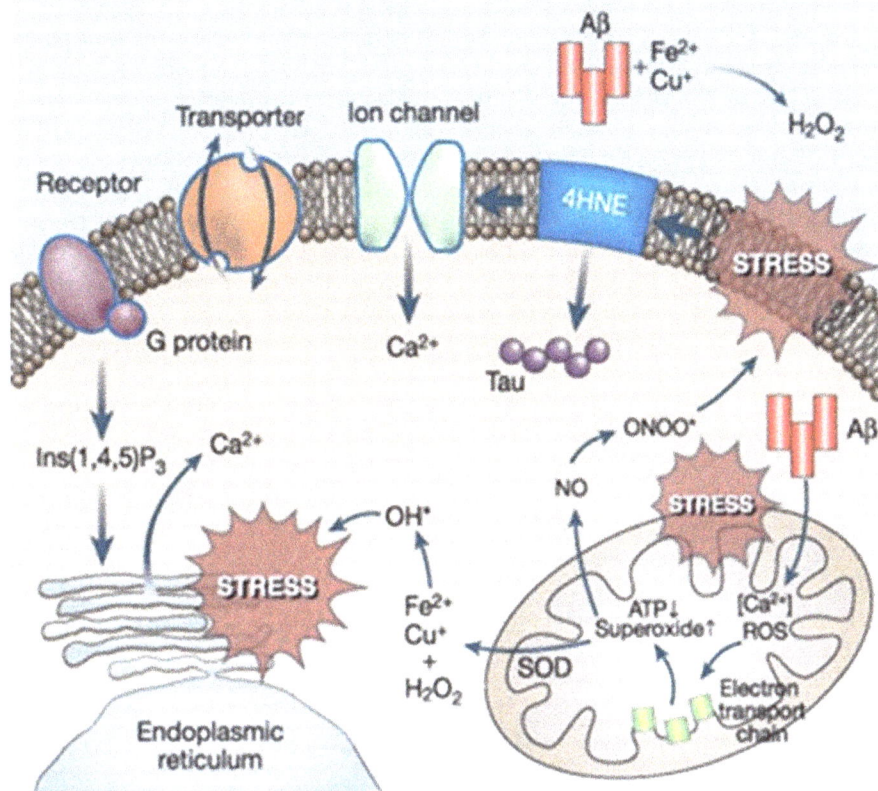

FIGURE 3 | Prevailing connections between oxidative stress and other key players in AD (Reproduced, with permission from Mattson, 2004).

BIOMETAL DYSHOMEOSTASIS

Numerous studies in AD and other neurodegenerative disorders have described an increase in the levels of oxidative stress reflected by a deregulated content of metals iron, copper, and zinc in the brain of patients. Recent findings have strongly pointed to brain oxidative stress as one of the earliest changes in AD pathogenesis that might play a central role in the disease progression (Guglielmotto et al., 2010; Lee et al., 2010). Redox-active metals, especially Fe^{2+} and Cu^{2+} are capable of stimulating free radical formation via the Fenton reaction, thereby increasing protein and DNA oxidation and enhancing lipid peroxidation (Khalil et al., 2011).

Metal ions have also been reported to mediate Aβ toxicity in AD (Duce et al., 2010). The Aβ peptide itself has been shown to be a strong redox-active catalyst able to produce hydrogen peroxide and OH^- in presence of copper or iron, which, in turn, are enriched in the amyloid cores of senile plaques (Huang et al., 1999, 2004). Metal ions can also interact with Aβ peptide enhancing its self-aggregation and oligomerisation at low physiological concentrations or under mildly acidic conditions (Huang et al., 1999). Moreover, metals can promote tau hyperphosphorylation and subsequent formation of NFTs by inducing aggregation upon tau interaction with Aβ (Yamamoto et al., 2002).

The presence of an iron-responsive element (IRE) in the 5′ untranslated regions (UTR) of AβPP mRNA was revealed as another link between iron metabolism and AD (Rogers et al., 2002; Silvestri and Camaschella, 2008). Iron closely upregulates intracellular levels of APP holo-protein by a mechanism that is similar to the translational control of ferritin L- and H- mRNAs through an IRE in their 5′ UTR (Rogers et al., 2002; Silvestri and Camaschella, 2008).

The Role of Copper in AD

Copper is an essential trace element for all living animals. Copper levels are controlled by homeostatic mechanisms to prevent an excess, or a deficiency, that may trigger a unique set of adverse health effects. Copper can undergo redox cycling between Cu^{1+} and Cu^{2+} and the activities of some copper-containing enzymes, including superoxide dismutase (SOD), cytochrome-c oxidase, ceruloplasmin, and tyrosinase, have important biological functions. However, copper is also involved in the formation of free radicals by the Fenton reaction, in which free copper catalyses the formation of toxic hydroxyl radicals from physiologically available hydrogen peroxide (Barnham et al., 2004). Two classic disorders related to copper metabolism are Menkes and Wilson diseases, in which neurodegeneration is a common complication (Kodama et al., 1999; Merle et al., 2007).

In AD pathology, copper is mislocalized in brains, where decreased levels of this metal have been reported in affected regions (Deibel et al., 1996; Magaki et al., 2007) with enrichment in amyloid plaques and tangles (Lovell et al., 1998). Copper is released into the glutamatergic synaptic cleft facilitated by the copper-transporting P-type ATPase ATP7A at concentrations of ~15 μM (Hartter and Barnea, 1988; Hopt et al., 2003). There, it causes S-nitrosylation of NMDA receptors, inhibiting their activation (Schlief et al., 2005, 2006).

Aβ toxicity has been linked to the presence of redox metals, especially the binding to copper as well as the non-redox zinc ions (Hou and Zagorski, 2006; Tougu et al., 2008), although the precise mechanisms involved are still under investigation (Syme et al., 2004; Ma et al., 2006; Minicozzi et al., 2008; Alies et al., 2011). The copper binding site to $Aβ_{1-42}$ has high affinity (K_d = 7.03 10^{-18} M; $logK_{app}$ = 17.2), as measured by competitive metal-capture analysis, whereas that of $Aβ_{1-40}$ is 10.3 (Atwood et al., 2000). The binding to copper has also been shown to modify and accelerate Aβ aggregation.

Copper also promotes dityrosine cross-linking of Aβ, which further accelerates Aβ aggregation (Atwood et al., 2000; Ali et al., 2005). The copper-induced Aβ oligomer contains a membrane-penetrating structure with histidine bridging (Curtain et al., 2001; Smith et al., 2006). This fact underlines the importance of histidine in the copper-Aβ interaction, which results in oligomers rather than the fibrils that are formed in the presence of zinc (Jiao and Yang, 2007). The copper-Aβ complex has been reported to exhibit cytotoxic properties (You et al., 2012) as this binding increases Aβ-induced cell death in cell culture (Wu et al., 2008; Perrone et al., 2010). Some hypotheses for this finding include the inhibition of cytochrome c (Crouch et al., 2005) and the increase of oxidative stress, triggered by the generation of hydrogen peroxide by Aβ and copper via a catalytic cycle (Huang et al., 1999). APP also interacts with copper by binding it between residues 142 and 166 (White et al., 1999; Barnham et al., 2003; Cappai et al., 2004) and catalytically oxidizing Cu^{1+} to Cu^{2+} (Multhaup et al., 1996). Furthermore, copper promotes APP internalization, whereas copper deficiency promotes Aβ secretion but not APP cleavage (Acevedo et al., 2011). Therefore, APP may not directly influence copper homeostasis, but inappropriate interaction with copper may be neurotoxic.

Tau phosphorylation and aggregation may also be induced by copper. Certain fragments in the four-repeat microtubule-binding domain of tau were shown to aggregate in the presence of copper *in vitro* (Ma et al., 2006; Zhou et al., 2007). Copper binding to tau induces hydrogen peroxide production *in vitro* (Su et al., 2007) and NFTs have also been shown to bind to copper in a redox-dependent manner as a source of ROS within the neuron (Sayre et al., 2000). In addition, copper exposure has been reported to induce tau hyperphosphorylation promoting tau pathology in a mouse model of AD (Kitazawa et al., 2009).

The Role of Zinc in AD

The brain is the main pool of zinc within the body (Frederickson, 1989). Zinc is an essential component for many enzymes and transcription factors. In healthy conditions, most of the zinc content is located in membrane-bound metalloproteins (MP I,

II, and III), loosely bound to zinc within the cytoplasm, and vesicular zinc, enriched in synapses. It has several functional roles in signal transmission. Synaptic transmission releases high concentrations of zinc into the synaptic cleft (Frederickson, 1989; Vogt et al., 2000; Qian and Noebels, 2005), where it acts as an antagonist of GABA (Molnar and Nadler, 2001; Ruiz et al., 2004) and NMDA receptors (Paoletti et al., 1997; Traynelis et al., 1998; Vogt et al., 2000) and activates the G-protein-coupled receptor GPR39 (Besser et al., 2009).

Inconsistent reports of zinc levels in AD have been published. Early surveys of brain tissue found no difference in zinc levels between AD and controls. Yet, later studies showed a decrease in zinc levels in neo-cortex (Danscher et al., 1997), superior frontal and parietal gyri, medial temporal gyrus and thalamus and hippocampus (Corrigan et al., 1993; Panayi et al., 2002). However, in other reports elevated zinc levels in AD-affected amygdala, hippocampus and cerebellum, (Deibel et al., 1996; Danscher et al., 1997), olfactory areas (Samudralwar et al., 1995), and superior temporal gyrus (Religa et al., 2006) were described.

The cause of this apparent zinc dysregulation remains unknown, yet it may be involved in alterations of proteins such as metallothionein III, which is found in neurons and reduced in AD brains (Uchida et al., 1991; Yu et al., 2001). In contrast, metallothionein I/II was found increased in astrocytes of post-mortem and preclinical AD brains (Adlard et al., 1998). In AD pathogenesis, enriched zinc levels have been found in amyloid plaques (Bush et al., 1994c). Studies using microparticle-induced X-ray emission tomography demonstrated a three-fold in zinc concentrations-surrounding neuropils in the amigdala (Lovell et al., 1998). These findings were later corroborated by histochemistry (Suh et al., 2000), autometallographic tracing (Stoltenberg et al., 2005) and synchrotron-based infrared and X-ray imaging (Miller et al., 2006).

Aβ binds to zinc at residues 6–28 (Bush et al., 1993, 1994a,b,c), with up to three zinc ions bound to histidines 6, 13, and 14 (Damante et al., 2009), inducing the aggregation of Aβ into soluble precipitates (Bush et al., 1994c). Therefore, zinc, like copper, accelerates Aβ-induced toxicity and zinc sequestration into amyloid deposits (Bush et al., 1994c) (Faller et al., 2013), inducing loss of functional zinc in the synapses. This loss may contribute to cognitive decline in AD due to ZnT-3 depletion (Adlard et al., 2010).

Zinc may also interfere with APP processing and function as these processes are coordinated by secretases under the zinc regulation. This metal increases the synthesis of PS-1 (Park et al., 2001); however, the γ-secretase activity is inhibited by Zn^{2+} (Hoke et al., 2007). Zinc binds directly to Aβ, hiding its proteolytic cleavage site (Bush et al., 1994b) and therefore inhibiting its degradation by matrix metalloproteases (Crouch et al., 2009). Secreted Aβ is normally degraded by proteases such as neprilysin within a short period of time. However, zinc and other metals enhance the oligomerisation and accumulation of the amyloid protein.

After being incorporated into the membrane, the conformation of Aβ changes and it aggregates on the membranes. These aggregates are able to form channels, which unlike endogenous Ca^{2+} channels, are not regulated by standard channel blockers. Thus, a continuous flow of Ca^{2+} is initiated and disruption of calcium homeostasis triggers several apoptotic pathways, including free radical formation and tau phosphorylation leading to cell death. Conversely, zinc secreted into synaptic clefts, inhibits $A\beta$-induced Ca^{2+} entry, and thus confers a protective function in AD (Kawahara et al., 2014).

In agreement with these findings, *in vivo* studies revealed that high intake of dietary zinc triggered elevated expression of APP and enhanced amyloidogenic APP cleavage and $A\beta$ deposition in APP/PS1 transgenic mice (Borchardt et al., 2000; Cuajuangco and Faget, 2003; Wang et al., 2010). Finally, zinc may also be involved in tau pathology as it is enriched in tangle-containing neurons (Suh et al., 2000). Zinc moderates translation of tau and modulates its phosphorylation by affecting the activities of GSK-3β, protein kinase B, ERK1/2, and c-Jun N-terminal kinase (An et al., 2005; Pei et al., 2006; Lei et al., 2011). Zinc can also bind to tau monomers, altering their conformation (Boom et al., 2009) and inducing both aggregation and fibrillation of this protein (Mo et al., 2009).

The Role of Iron in AD

Iron is a fundamental element in biology for oxygen transport and energy metabolism. It is a transition element that exists in oxidative states from -2 to $+8$, although in biological systems only ferrous (Fe^{2+}) and ferric (Fe^{3+}) states normally exist. The cycling between ferric to ferrous states is used in biology for various redox reactions essential to life. However, deleterious reactions with oxygen, such as Fenton reaction, which is catalyzed by the free ferrous iron and may involve bound Fe(IV) (Freinbichler et al., 2009) are a source of oxidative stress (Zigler et al., 2015).

In the brain, iron is involved in development (Beard, 2003), metabolic and neurotransmitter systems (Agarwal, 2001). It is therefore regulated by multiple proteins, reflecting its involvement in different cellular functions. In AD brains, iron is enriched in both NFTs (Smith et al., 1998) and senile plaques (Goodman, 1953) with an estimated concentration of three-fold higher that of the normal neuropil levels (Lovell et al., 1998). Iron accumulation occurs in the cortex but not in the cerebellum (Andrasi et al., 1995; Duce et al., 2010). The iron storage protein ferritin binds to most iron within the brain and its levels increase with age and in AD (Bartzokis and Tishler, 2000). Transferrin (Tf) is an extracellular iron-transporting protein expressed in the brain that exchanges iron between cells. The complex Fe-Tf is endocytosed (Eckenroth et al., 2011) and iron is reduced to its ferrous state by an unknown ferrirreductase.

Recently, AD-associated APP was identified as a neuronal ferroxidase (Duce et al., 2010). APP-knockout mice exhibit iron accumulation in the brain and peripheral tissues and loss of APP ferroxidase activity in AD brains is coincident with iron retention in the tissues (Duce et al., 2010). Recent studies reported that iron-export capability of APP requires tau protein (Lei et al., 2012), which is involved in axonal transport (Lei et al., 2010) and binds to APP (Islam and Levy, 1997). Moreover, the loss of tau in mice is reported to cause age-related iron accumulation (Lei et al., 2012). The iron-regulatory system is disturbed in AD brains and ferritin has been reported to be elevated and co-localized with senile plaques expressed in astrocytes (Connor et al., 1992) and increased in frontal cortex of AD brains (Loeffler et al., 1995). However, the amount of APP was not significantly reduced in cortex (Duce et al., 2010) but both ferroxidase activity and soluble tau protein levels were observed to be decreased (Shin et al., 1992; Khatoon et al., 1994; Zhukareva et al., 2001; Van Eersel et al., 2009; Duce et al., 2010). Genetic factors have also been linked to higher susceptibility to iron burden in AD (Blázquez et al., 2007; Bertram and Tanzi, 2008; Percy et al., 2008).

Iron burden enriches around the senile plaque region (Meadowcroft et al., 2009) and promotes $A\beta$ aggregation *in vitro* (Mantyh et al., 1993). Furthermore, iron-aggregated $A\beta$ toxicity in cell culture (Schubert and Chevion, 1995) is mediated by ROS production (Rottkamp et al., 2001) or by the activation of Bcl-2/Bax-related apoptosis pathway (Kuperstein and Yavin, 2003). As mentioned above, iron also binds to tau protein, but only Fe^{3+} has reported to induce aggregation of hyperphosphorylated tau protein, which can be reversed by reducing Fe^{3+} to Fe^{2+} (Yamamoto et al., 2002) or by the use of iron-chelators (Amit et al., 2008). In AD brain, NFTs bind iron, which acts as a source of ROS within the neurons (Sayre et al., 2000). A decrease of tau phosphorylation in hippocampal neurons treated with Fe^{3+} (Egaña et al., 2003), corresponding with a decrease in CDK5 activity. Conversely, treatment with Fe^{2+} also resulted in hyperphosphorylation (Lovell et al., 2004) without inducing aggregation, possibly resulting from upstream activation of the ERK1/2, MAPK pathway (Muñoz et al., 2006; Huang et al., 2007). Recently, oxygen tension-dependent transcriptional factor, hypoxia inducible factor-1α (HIF-1α) has emerged as a potential target in neurodegenerative diseases. This protein regulates intracellular iron by binding to HIF-responsive elements (HREs) that are located within the genes of iron-related proteins such as Tf receptor and heme oxygenase-1 (Petousi and Robbins, 2014).

Recent research and clinical trials have confirmed that HIF-1α activation may be a potent strategy for postponing the pathogenesis and ameliorating the outcomes of AD. In this context, the use of iron chelators such as M30 has been reported to increase the levels of this protein by inducing the expression of its target genes VEGF and EPO. In addition, overexpression of HIF-1α has been shown to protect cultured cortical neurons from $A\beta$-induced neurotoxicity, through activating glycolytic and hexose monophosphate shunt-related enzymes. Therefore, an additional use of iron-chelators to overexpress HIF-1α may contribute to preventing neuron death and ameliorating the symptomatology of AD by inducing the expression of neuroprotection-related genes (Benkler et al., 2010).

Thus, in the context of AD pathology, the involvement of both oxidative stress and metal ions in AD (Ayton et al., 2013), indicates the use of antioxidant-chelators as potential beneficial agents in the prevention and treatment of the disease, by scavenging free radicals and, more importantly, by blocking their production, as well as restoring normal metal balance.

Although abnormal accumulation of metals has been reported in AD for many years, it has been only recently considered as a key early factor in AD, closely related to increased levels of both oxidative stress and amyloid beta-protein toxicity in

Barone (2016). The development of metal-chelators has emerged, concurrently, as a novel pharmacological approach against this neurological disorder. In this regard Youdim and co-workers have reported a novel multifunctional molecule, M30, which combines iron-chelation with and monoamine oxidase (MAO) inhibitory properties as a possible drug for the treatment of AD (Zheng et al., 2005; Avramovich-Tirosh et al., 2007).

NEUROINFLAMMATION

Inflammation is a defensive mechanism of the body against multiple threats such as infections and injury. It is a complex event that involves both soluble factors and specialized cells (Brown et al., 2007). Similar inflammatory processes occur in the brain and peripheral tissues. In the brain, glial cells, including astrocytes and microglia, undergo activation under pro-inflammatory conditions by the increase in the production of inflammatory cytokines in the CNS, which become deleterious and leads to progressive tissue damage in degenerative diseases (Morales et al., 2014). Infiltration by peripheral macrophages may also occur (Rogers et al., 1996).

In chronic disorders such as AD pathology, inflammation plays a critical role. It has been reported that insoluble fibrillar Aβ surrounding microglia, reactive astrocytes and dystrophic neurites contributes to the process of neuronal degeneration by initiating a series of cellular events which are able to elicit an immune response. Moreover, Aβ deposition in parenchyma and blood vessels has been described to trigger microglial migration and mediation of acute and chronic inflammatory response against the aggregates, thus inducing the production of nitric oxide (NO), ROS, pro-inflammatory cytokines such as tumor necrotic factor α (TNFα) or inteleukins-1β and -6 (IL-1β, IL-6) and prostaglandin E2 (PGE2), which eventually may promote neuronal death (Kitazawa et al., 2009).

MAO AS A TARGET

One of the major observations in late AD is the loss of neuronal cells and brain shrinkage. Specific loss of dopaminergic cells has led to the use of deprenyl or selegiline as adjunctive therapy in PD to prevent removal of dopamine by metabolism (Birkmayer et al., 1977). The same principle applies in AD, where the decrease in all neurotransmitters is due mainly to a loss of neuronal connections.

Monoamine oxidases (MAO, EC 1.4.3.4) are flavin adenine dinucleotide (FAD)-containing enzymes that catalyse the oxidative deamination of primary, secondary, or tertiary amines, producing the corresponding aldehyde, hydrogen peroxide and ammonia. There are two isoforms of MAO present in mammals: MAO A and MAO B, which share ∼70% sequence identity and are encoded by separate genes located on the X chromosome. The C-terminal regions of MAOs are transmembrane α-helices that anchor the enzymes to the mitochondrial outer membrane leaving the rest of the protein exposed to the cytoplasm. The entry of a substrate or inhibitor into the active site of MAOs is predicted to occur near the intersection of the enzyme with the

surface of the membrane (De Colibus et al., 2005; Edmondson et al., 2007).

In selective MAO-knockout mice, the two MAO isoforms resulted in significantly different effects on both metabolism and behavior. Whereas, the lack of MAO A triggered aggressive phenotypes as a result of elevated levels of 5-HT and NA and lesser of DA (Chester et al., 2015), only the levels of 2-phenylethylamine were increased in MAO B-knockout mice, which exhibited traits such as sensation seeking, impulsiveness and extraversion. MAO A and MAO B were originally distinguished by their sensitivity to nanomolar concentrations of the acetylenic inhibitors clorgyline and l-deprenyl, respectively, as well as by their substrate specificities. The content of MAO varies over lifetime as MAO A appears before MAO B, the brain level of which increases dramatically after birth (Tsang et al., 1986; Strolin-Benedetti et al., 1992; Nicotra et al., 2004). MAO B levels continue to increase throughout the lifetime and in AD progression. In rat peripheral nervous system, MAO is localized in the endothelial cells of the endoneurial vessels, Schwann cells and unmyelinated axons of some neurons (Matsubayashi et al., 1986).

In human brain, MAO activity differs among regions. While the highest levels are found in basal ganglia and hippocampus, the lowest are observed in the cerebellum and neocortex (O'Carroll et al., 1983). The anatomical distribution of MAO isoforms in human brains were confirmed by positron-emission topography (PET) using intravenous ^{11}C-labeled irreversible inhibitors (Fowler et al., 1987; Saura et al., 1992). Immunohistochemical studies have revealed that serotonergic neurons and astrocytes are rich in MAO B whereas catecholaminergic neurons mainly contain MAO A (Westlund et al., 1988). Caudate dopaminergic nerve endings contain only MAO A and small amounts of this isoform are also found in the serotonergic nerve terminals (O'Carroll et al., 1987). Some differences in the dopamine metabolism have been observed between species. For instance, only MAO A isoform is involved in rat brain, whereas MAO B is primary responsible for dopamine metabolism in human brain (Fornai et al., 1999).

Inhibitors of MAO, reversible and irreversible, equipotent on both isoforms or highly selective, have been used for more than 60 years for the treatment of depression (Mendelewicz and Youdim, 1983; Youdim et al., 2006). The most successful approach has been the use of selective irreversible inhibitors as exemplified by deprenyl, now used in PD therapy. The chemical moiety of this compound includes the propargyl group, which is readily incorporated into different scaffolds to cause MAO inhibition in compounds that are designed for other targets. This finding has been identified as one of the mechanisms of various MTDL to delay the progression of neurodegeneration as it will be discussed below.

FDA-APPROVED DRUGS FOR AD

At present, only five drugs have been approved by the U.S. Food and Drug Administration (FDA, USA) for use in AD. These compounds are mainly based on the "cholinergic hypothesis" and aimed at re-establishing functional cholinergic neurotransmission. Four of these: tacrine (1), rivastigmine (2), donepezil (3), and galantamine (4) are cholinesterase inhibitors, whereas memantine (5) is a NMDA receptor antagonist (**Figure 4**).

Tacrine

Tacrine or tetrahydroaminoacridine (THA), marketed as *Cognex®*, was the first drug to be approved for use in AD by the FDA in 1993. It is a competitive AChE inhibitor with high lipid solubility (Nielsen et al., 1989) also able to interact with muscarinic receptors (Adem, 1993) and MAO A and B (Adem et al., 1989). Although it had some relatively small benefits on cognition, tacrine was withdrawn from the market in 2013 due to the high incidence of side effects, mostly related to hepatotoxicity (Qizilbash et al., 1998).

Rivastigmine

Rivastigmine, marketed under the trade name of *Exelon®* since 1998, is a non-selective pseudoreversible ChE inhibitor reported to produce enhanced benefits over AChE inhibition alone (Touchon et al., 2006; Bullock and Lane, 2007). A recent study using a transdermal patch reported a reduction in the prevalence of side effects as well as positive results after administering rivastigmine to mild-to-moderate AD patients. These studies reported better outcomes, in comparison with placebo group, for rate of cognitive function decline and daily living activities (Birks et al., 2015).

Galantamine

Galantamine (*Razadyne®*) is a well-studied drug approved in 2001 for the treatment of AD, possessing a dual mechanism of action to attenuate the symptoms of cognitive decline in AD. It is a reversible selective competitive AChE inhibitor (Greenblatt et al., 1999) that is able to simultaneously modulate nAChERs (Dajas-Bailador et al., 2003). The main mechanism of action of this molecule is the ability to increase the content of ACh, enhancing cholinergic neurotransmission and therefore improving cognition in AD patients by delay of ACh catabolism at synapse. Moreover, galantamine has also demonstrated to directly interact with the nAChER as low-affinity agonist, allosterically binding to a distinct binding site from where nicotinic agonists, such as ACh, choline, or carbachol, bind (Akk and Steinbach, 2005). Moriguchi et al. (2003) showed that galantamine also potentiates the activity of NMDARs, so that the dual mechanism of action on both cholinergic and glutamatergic systems in AD patients may elucidate the improvement in cognition, memory, and learning that have been found in clinical trials with this drug (Wilkinson and Murray, 2001).

Memantine

Memantine, marketed as *Namenda®* or *Ebixa®*, is a glutamatergic agent and the first and only NMDAR antagonist approved in 2003 for the treatment of moderate-to-severe AD and dementia. In clinical trials, memantine has shown significant benefits on cognition, function, and global status of AD patients. Moreover, it appears to be harmless and well-tolerated, with a safety profile compared to placebo (Doody et al., 2007). Memantine binds to NMDARs with a low-micromolar IC_{50} value. Furthermore, it exhibits poor selectivity among NMDARs subtypes, with under micromolar IC_{50} values for NR2A, NR2B, NR2C, and NR2D receptors expressed in *Xenopus* oocytes (Parsons et al., 1999). Although memantine was initially regarded as a poor drug candidate for AD therapy, the mechanisms by which exerts clinical benefits and its safe profile have attracted a great considerable interest in the field of medicinal chemistry (Lipton, 2006). In addition, memantine has also been reported to exhibit neuroprotective activities against Aβ toxicity (Tremblay et al., 2000; Miguel-Hidalgo et al., 2002; Hu et al., 2007), tau phosphorylation (Song et al., 2008), neuroinflammation (Willard et al., 2000), and oxidative stress (Figueiredo et al., 2013; Liu et al., 2013).

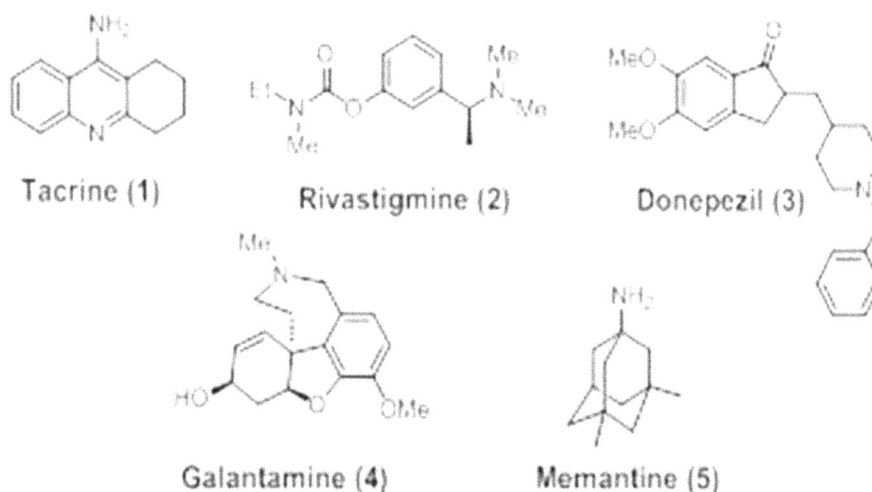

FIGURE 4 | Chemical structures of FDA-approved agents for use in AD: tacrine (1), donepezil (2), rivastigmine (3), galantamine (4), and memantine (5).

Donepezil

Donepezil, marketed under the trade name of *Aricept*® in 1996, is a brain-permeable reversible non-competitive ChE inhibitor approved for use in AD (Birks and Harvey, 2006) and currently the most widely prescribed drug for the treatment of this disease. Donepezil is highly selective for AChE over BuChE activity (405:1) (Nochi et al., 1995). Compared to other approved AChE inhibitors, donepezil is similarly effective in ameliorating cognitive and functional decline in AD with comparable safety and tolerability. Moreover, beneficial effects have been observed at lower doses (5 mg/day), which is highly valuable at minimizing adverse reactions. Although clinical trials with donepezil have been reported, modest but reproducible, improvements in cognition and global functioning in treated patients, as compared to placebo. These effects were not permanent as patients, continued to exhibit a decline in cognitive functioning over time (Doody et al., 2007).

In recent years, the consistent failure of pharmacological approaches targeting traditional AD targets such as Aβ and tau protein together with the existing number of drugs to be tested in pre-dementia stages of the disease has left no effective disease-modifying treatment of AD in sight. Thus, additional benefits of donepezil might be revealed with the use of this molecule in combination with other active moieties.

MULTI-TARGET-DIRECTED LIGANDS (MTDL)

The lack of therapeutic effectiveness of the current FDA-approved drugs based on the single-target paradigm for the treatment of cognition and memory decline, prompted to the rational design and development of a novel and improved pharmacological approach against AD: the Multi-Target-Directed Ligands (MTDL) or "dirty drugs" (Buccafusco and Terry, 2000; Youdim et al., 2005; León et al., 2013). These molecules are conceived to directly interact weakly with multiple targets associated with AD by the molecular hybridisation of different pharmacophore moieties from identified bioactive molecules. The development of MTDLs obviates the challenge of simultaneously administering multiple drugs with potentially different degrees of bioavailability, pharmacokinetics, and metabolism. Furthermore, this pharmacological approach also provides AD patients with a simplification of the therapeutic regimen (**Figure 5**).

To date, the therapeutic potential of MTDLs for the treatment of complex neurodegenerative diseases and age-related cognitive impairment has not been realized. Multifaceted diseases such as AD, mainly caused by perturbations of the complex intracellular network that links to tissue and organs systems, needs a more comprehensive pharmacological approach. Therefore, approaches relying on targeting single proteins/mechanisms are not likely to have effective outcomes. Because of the existence of feedback mechanisms in biological systems, enzyme inhibition may not be able to decrease activity in long term, but instead, may result in increased activity, as reported from the use of rapid-reversible AChE inhibitors that significantly increased both

protein activity and expression levels in the CSF of AD patients after long-term treatment (Darreh-Shori and Soininen, 2010).

Since 2005, literature has shown several promising results from applying this innovative approach to drug design. Well-known drugs such as donepezil, tacrine, or rivastigmine (Bolognesi et al., 2007; Samadi et al., 2011) as well as bioactive natural products such as curcumin (Malar and Devi, 2014), berberine (Jiang et al., 2011; Shan et al., 2011), or 8-hydroxyquinoline (Gomes et al., 2014) have been used as structural scaffolds for the development and search of new chemical entities with multiple properties or MTDLs for the treatment of AD. These new entities may be considered as simplified versions or lead drugs possessing great potential as real alternatives to the current unsuccessful pharmacological therapies for effectively fighting against AD and other complex diseases.

The next sections include an overview on the outcomes obtained from the biological assessment of several MTDLs molecules that have been lately reported by some of us. All the compounds described bear the *N*-benzylpiperidine group present in donepezil and the *N*-propargylamine motif present in **PF9601N**, a potent and selective MAO B inhibitor with neuroprotective effects *in vitro* and *in vivo* using different experimental models of neurodegenerative diseases (Cutillas et al., 2002; Pérez and Unzeta, 2003; Pérez et al., 2003; Battaglia et al., 2006; Sanz et al., 2009). Both scaffolds were linked by different heterocyclic ring systems, such as pyridine, indole or 8-hydroxyquinoline, allowing the facile synthesis of different MTDL molecules as promising drugs to be used in AD therapy (**Figure 6**). The inhibitory profile of these new MTDL molecules inhibiting ChE and MAO, their antioxidant, anti-β-aggregating, anti-inflammatory, and anti-apoptotic behavior together with their metal-chelating properties were determined and results from comparative studies were assessed. Taken together, the outcomes reported with these derivatives reveal a potential improvement of the current pharmacological therapy of AD.

ASS234

ASS234 {*N*-[5-(3-(1-benzylpiperidin-4-yl)propoxy)-1-methyl-1*H*-indol-2-ylmethyl]-*N*-methylprop-2-yn-1-amine} (**Figure 7**) was first identified by some of us as a suitable candidate for use in AD as a result of extensive screening of several series of novel derivatives. This multipotent molecule was specifically developed to combine the anti-cholinergic activity of donepezil, as an AChE inhibitor widely used in AD therapy, with a propargylamine moiety derived from selective MAO B inhibitor, **PF9601N** (**Figure 7**) with neuroprotective properties (Bolea et al., 2011).

ASS234 was revealed as a potent inhibitor of both MAO A and MAO B, with an IC_{50} values of 5.2 ± 1.1 nM and 43.1 ± 7.9 nM, respectively. It also inhibited both ChEs exhibiting IC_{50} values of 0.35 ± 0.001 and 0.46 ± 0.06 μM toward AChE and BuChE, respectively. In comparison with donepezil and **PF9601N**, analyzed under the same experimental conditions, donepezil was ineffective at inhibiting MAO activities whereas **PF9601N** potently and selectively inhibited MAO B isoform but displayed no interaction with both ChEs (Bolea et al., 2011). These data indicate that **ASS234** combines the

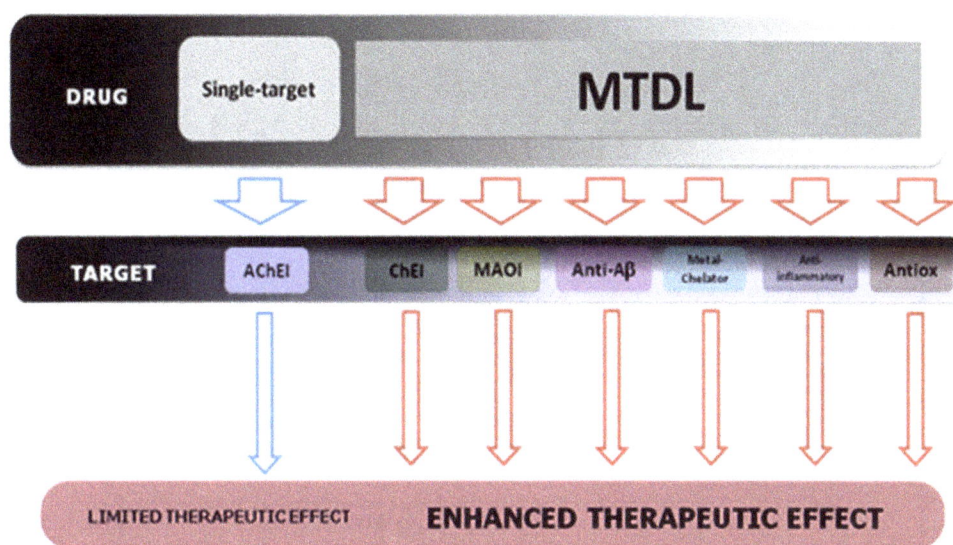

FIGURE 5 | Scheme of the therapeutic design strategy of MTDL for the treatment of the multifaceted nature of AD pathology.

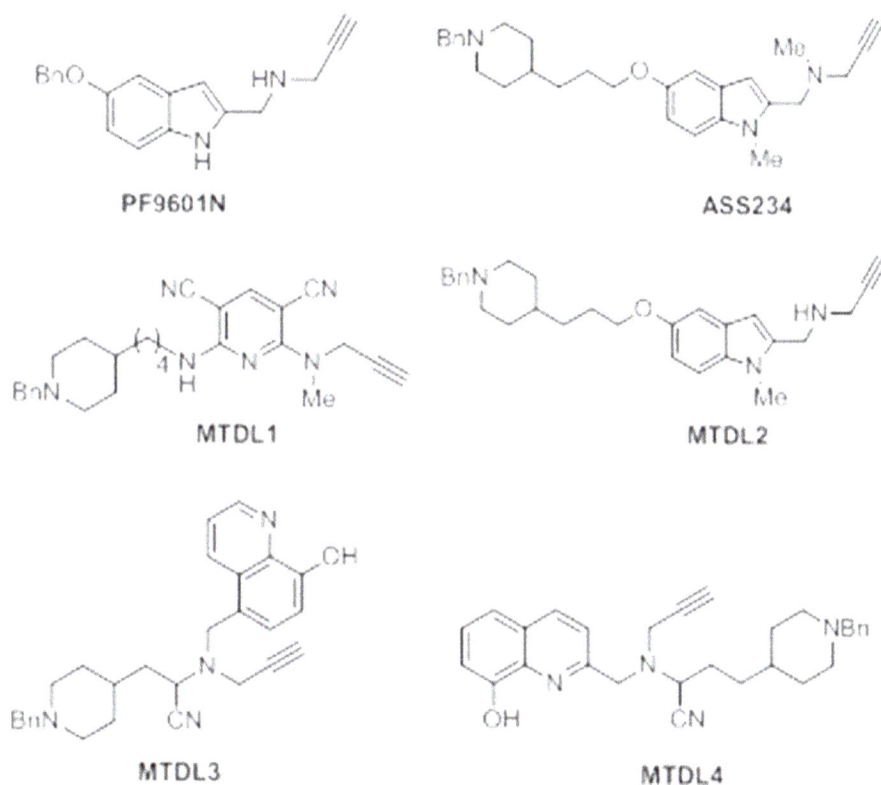

FIGURE 6 | Structure of compounds PF9601N, ASS234, and the MTDL1-4 described in this review.

desirable properties of donepezil and **PF9601N** being capable of simultaneously enhancing both cholinergic and monoaminergic transmission as well as possessing neuroprotective effects (Bolea et al., 2013a).

Kinetic studies showed that **ASS234** is a-reversible inhibitor of both ChEs, with micromolar affinity, and a highly potent irreversible MAO A inhibitor with similar behavior to clorgyline (Esteban et al., 2014). The parent propargylamine, **PF9601N**,

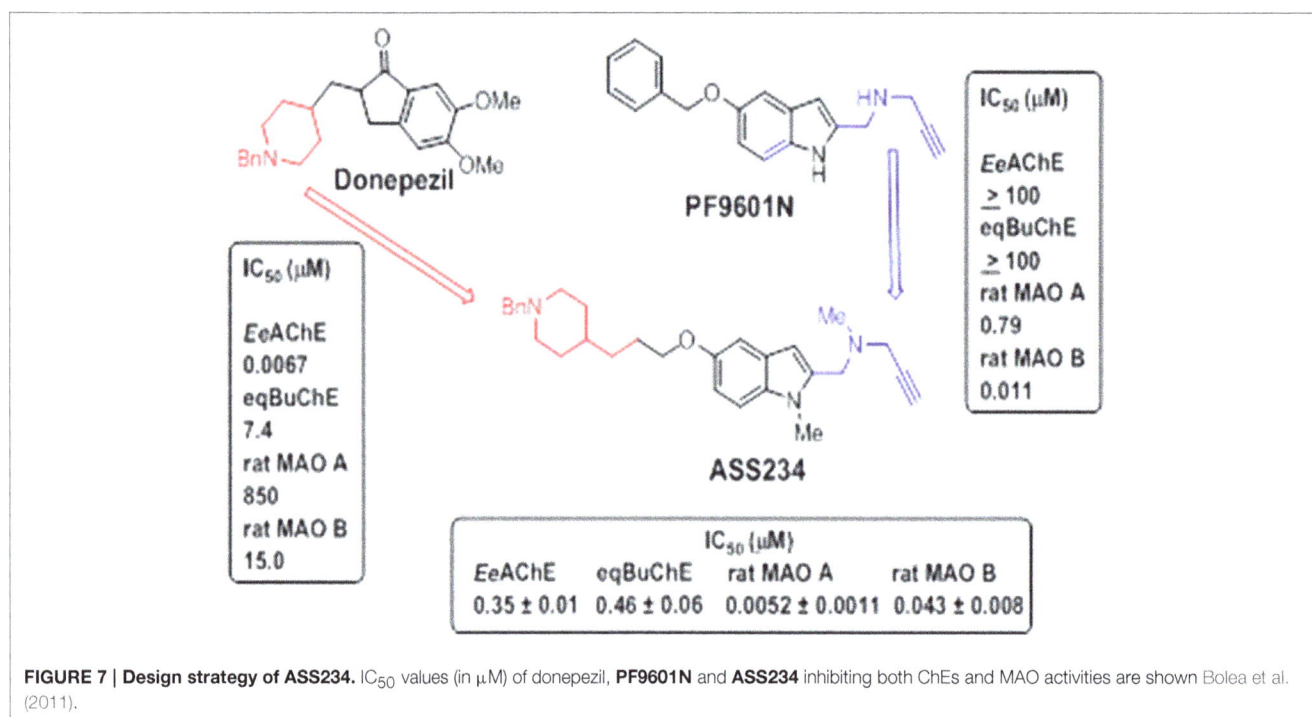

FIGURE 7 | Design strategy of ASS234. IC_{50} values (in µM) of donepezil, PF9601N and ASS234 inhibiting both ChEs and MAO activities are shown Bolea et al. (2011).

behaves similarly to *l*-deprenyl as an effective selective MAO B inhibitor. Both PF9601N and ASS234 display as mechanism-based MAO inhibitors. The selectivity of ASS234 as a MAO A inhibitor, indicated by the IC_{50} values, for both purified and membrane-bound protein samples (Pérez et al., 1999; Bolea et al., 2011), might be attributed to the shared propargylamine structure, which is larger and more hydrophobic in ASS234. The initial reversible binding parameter (K_i value of 0.2 µM) indicated that ASS234 has slightly lower affinity for MAO A than clorgyline (K_i value of 0.04 µM), and this was also reflected in higher rate constant (k_1) for the irreversible reaction.

UV-VIS spectral analyses showed an irreversible modification of the MAO flavin group by ASS234 similar to that found with other propargyl MAO inhibitors. The crystal structure of human MAO B in complex with ASS234 revealed the formation of a covalent adduct with the N5 atom of the flavin cofactor. The *N*-benzylpiperidine moiety of the compound was not able to fully bind to the intact molecule to the MAO B active site, which ruled out the possibility that the inhibitor may have undergone degradation. Thus, these outcomes demonstrated the efficacy of ASS234 as inhibitor of both the "classic" AD-targeted ChE enzymes and the MAOs (Esteban et al., 2014).

Following the search for additional activities with multi-target ASS234, the potential modulation of the monoaminergic transmission and metabolism by this molecule were also investigated both *in vitro* and *in vivo* (Van Schoors et al., unpublished results). Since some of the behavioral alterations occurring in AD such as depression are possibly caused by monoaminergic dysfunction, the therapeutic use of antidepressant drugs based on the selective inhibition of MAO A, an enzyme possessing an indispensable role in the

metabolic regulation of neurotransmitters 5-HT, NA, DA, and/or on the blockage of the corresponding reuptake systems at the pre-synaptic nerve endings, may also be considered.

In this context, a significant increase in the levels of 5-HT associated with a reduction in the levels of its metabolite 5-HIAA was observed as a result of irreversible inhibition of MAO A in SH-SY5Y cells treated with ASS234. Comparatively, similar though less pronounced effects were found with highly-selective MAO A inhibitor clorgyline under the same experimental conditions, thus revealing an active effect of this multi-target drug to in enhancing 5-HT levels. In contrast, DA levels were significantly decreased in PC12 cells that had been treated with ASS234 for 24 h. This finding may be due to a reduction of both activity and expression of the enzymes responsible for DA synthesis, tyrosine hydroxylase and aromatic L-amino acid decarboxylase as a response to initial rapid elevation of DA levels following the blockage of MAO activity. Both MAO A inhibitors ASS234 and clorgyline were able to modulate the levels of DA metabolites DOPAC and HVA, which were decreased after incubations. *In vivo* microdialysis studies of the effects upon administration of ASS234 in freely-moving rats also revealed alterations in the extracellular monoamines levels in both hippocampus and prefrontal cortex, two brain areas that are highly-impaired in AD. Interestingly, the effect of ASS234 differed from brain areas and dosage. In hippocampus, levels of 5-HT and NA were increased whereas those of DA and NA markedly augmented in prefrontal cortex.

These differences might be attributed to the presence of metabolizing enzymes in both brain areas as well as to the complexity of the monoaminergic neurochemical interactions existing in the brain. In addition, ASS234, as a multi-target compound, might be able to modulate other neurobiological systems and therefore producing a complex pharmacological outcome. The results from the *in vivo* studies revealed a time-dependent effect on extracellular levels of monoaminergic neurotransmitters after administration of a single, subcutaneous, dose of **ASS234**. This results could be used in further studies to assess both the pharmacokinetics and bioavailability of the compound in reaching its therapeutic target. Many factors, including route of administration and the existence of active metabolites may contribute to the observed delay in the *in vivo* effects observed with **ASS234**.

In AD, levels of DA and NA are diminished in cortex and hippocampus while those of 5-HT are decreased in hippocampus (Reinikainen et al., 1988), producing some distinctive behavioral symptoms including depressive-like disorder, psychosis, or memory impairment related to alterations in serotonergic, catecholaminergic, and cholinergic neurotransmissions (Vermeiren et al., 2015). Therefore, the outcomes observed *in vivo* upon the administration of **ASS234** in addition with those previously found, confirm the potential value of this compound to be used as a modulator of the monoaminergic transmission in AD, both in terms of therapy and for further elucidation of the mechanisms involved.

The therapeutic potential of **ASS234** has been also evaluated following its administration to a rat model of vascular dementia (Stasiak et al., 2014). These experiments involved the permanent bilateral occlusion of the common carotid arteries (BCCAO) with experimental vascular dementia. In this rat model, the administration of **ASS234** for five consecutive days resulted in a potent and selective inhibition of brain MAO A activity as well as a concurrent increase in the concentrations of serotonin and catecholamines dopamine and noradrenaline. BCCAO resulted in impaired time parameters and memory functions as measured by hole-board memory tests in rats. Treatment of BCCAO rats with **ASS234** showed less negative effects on cognitive parameters and exerted a significant positive effect on working memory.

Aggregation and deposition of Aβ is a key pathological hallmark of AD and there is increasing evidence suggesting that the neurotoxicity of this peptide is related to the formation of toxic oligomeric aggregates. In this regard, **ASS234** has demonstrated to possess anti-Aβ$_{1-42}$ aggregating capacity and also an ability to reduce the presence of oligomeric forms of β-amyloid, as the most toxic species in AD (Bolea et al., 2013a). Moreover, **ASS234** was able to inhibit AChE-catalyzed Aβ aggregation by binding to the PAS of the enzyme. **ASS234** also showed a protective effects on the Aβ$_{1-42}$-mediated cytotoxicity induced in human neuroblastoma cells by preventing the activation of the intrinsic mitochondrial pathway of apoptosis. Moreover, **ASS234** displayed significant antioxidant properties, arising from the increase in the expression of catalase and SOD-1 in human neuroblastoma SH-SY5Y cells. This compound also has the capacity to capture free radicals *in vitro*, as measured by the well-established ORAC-FL (Oxygen radical Absorbance Capacity) fluorescent method. It is noteworthy that in a recent *in vivo* approach using transgenic APP/PS1AE9 mice given **ASS234**, both Aβ plaques in cortex and activated glia were found decreased (Serrano et al., 2016).

These findings, summarized in **Figure 8**, allow us to conclude that **ASS234** is able to interact with multiple targets relevant to AD. They also indicate that this is an interesting MTDL molecule that should be considered for therapeutic development against AD.

Derivatives MTDL-1 and MTDL-2 (*Donepezil-Pyridyl and Indolyl-Propargyl Hybrids*) as Dual ChE/MAO Inhibitors

With the aim of searching for improved MTDLs, two series of novel structurally-derived compounds, derived from **ASS234** as multipotent donepezil-indolyl and donepezil-pyridyl hybrids were designed and pharmacologically evaluated for their potential use in AD. The synthetic strategy that was used to design these novel donepezil-pyridyl hybrids is outlined in **Figures 9, 10**.

Among all the compounds tested, the donepezil-pyridyl hybrid **MTDL-1** (**Figure 9**) was identified as a potent AChE inhibitor (IC$_{50}$ = 1.1 nM) and a moderate BuChE inhibitor (IC$_{50}$ = 0.6 μM) with total selectivity toward human MAO B (Bautista-Aguilera et al., 2014a). Interestingly, the design and development of non-selective ChE inhibitors for use in AD appears of valuable pharmacological concern, as the hydrolysis of neurotransmitter ACh may largely occur via BuChE catalysis in aged AD brains, the activity levels of which have been found elevated on late-stages of the disease as it is also the case with MAO B. Since BuChE is also found in glial cells that are recruited and activated around the plaques and tangles, the inhibition of this enzyme might provide additional benefits at reducing neuroinflammation. Suitable drug-likeness profile and ADMET properties of these two novel MTDLs were also confirmed by 3D-QSAR studies.

The donepezil-indolyl hybrid molecule **MTDL-2** (**Figure 10**), exhibited an interesting profile as potent MAO A inhibitor (IC$_{50}$ = 5.5 nM) that was moderately able to inhibit MAO B (IC$_{50}$ = 150 nM), AChE (IC$_{50}$ = 190 nM), and BuChE (IC$_{50}$ = 830 nM) (Bautista-Aguilera et al., 2014b). Moreover, this compound appeared to be a mixed-type AChE inhibitor able to span both the CAS and PAS of this enzyme, as found by molecular modeling studies. Interestingly, docking simulations revealed that the selective inhibition of MAO isoforms by propargyl-containing compounds accounts for the orientation on their propargylamine and phenyl moieties in MAO, which energetically affects the interaction with the active site.

Derivatives MTDL-3 and MTDL-4 (*Donepezil+Propargylamine+8-Hydroxyquinoline Hybrids*) As Dual ChE/MAO Inhibitors with Antioxidant Activity, Metal-Chelating Properties, and Other Pharmacological Targets

Newly-designed **MTDL-3** and **MTDL-4** derivatives containing the *N*-benzylpiperidine moiety from donepezil and a metal-chelating 8-hydroxyquinoline group (**Figures 11, 12**), were

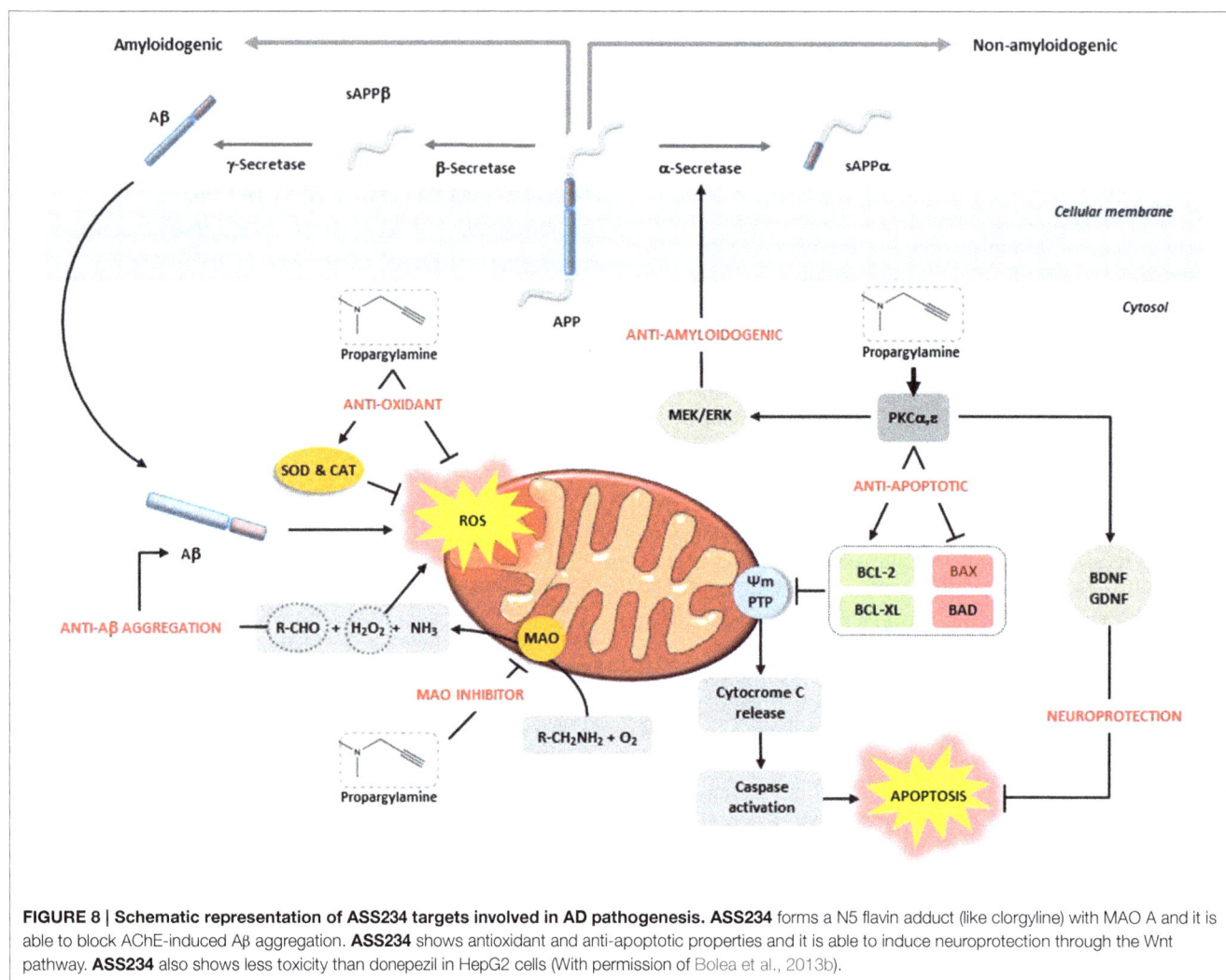

FIGURE 8 | Schematic representation of ASS234 targets involved in AD pathogenesis. ASS234 forms a N5 flavin adduct (like clorgyline) with MAO A and it is able to block AChE-induced Aβ aggregation. **ASS234** shows antioxidant and anti-apoptotic properties and it is able to induce neuroprotection through the Wnt pathway. **ASS234** also shows less toxicity than donepezil in HepG2 cells (With permission of Bolea et al., 2013b).

linked to a central N-propargylamine core and pharmacologically evaluated (Wang et al., 2014; Wu et al., 2015). This molecule contains a moiety also present in the compound M30, a brain-permeable and iron-chelating compound with antioxidant activity displaying neuroprotective activity in animal models (Salkovic-Petrisic et al., 2015). M30 modulates HIF-α-related glycolytic genes in the frontal cortex of APP/PS1 mice used as AD model (Mechlovich et al., 2014). These studies also showed M30 to have beneficial effects on several major hallmarks of AD (Kupershmidt et al., 2012), indicating the potential value of incorporating this moiety into **MTDL-3** (**Figure 11**).

MTDL-3 was revealed as an irreversible MAO inhibitor and mixed-type ChE inhibitor, in low micromolar range, able to strongly complex Cu (II), Zn (II), and Fe (III) (Wang et al., 2014). In addition, the cyano group, which was only present in some derivatives, was found to enhance the binding to AChE, BuChE, and MAO A (Wang et al., 2014). Although α-aminonitriles have seldom been investigated as ChE inhibitors, some previous

studies described nitriles as MAO inhibitors, and reported that cyanide potentiates irreversible MAO inhibition (Ramadan et al., 2007). Although cyanide is known to be a poor reversible inhibitor of the oxidation of benzylamine by MAO (Houslay and Tipton, 1973), previous studies have indicated that the inhibitory activity of several compounds against MAO is potentiated by cyanide (Davison, 1957; Ramadan and Tipton, 1998; Ramadan et al., 1999, 2007; Juárez-Jiménez et al., 2014). An earlier study by Davison (1957) on the inhibition of mitochondrial MAO by the irreversible inhibitor iproniazid revealed that, although at low concentrations, this compound alone had little effect on enzyme activity, while the inhibitory activity was significantly enhanced in the presence of cyanide ions. A similar potentiating effect was also reported for phenelzine and pheniprazine (Ramadan et al., 1999). Such studies demonstrated that, in case of pheniprazine, cyanide potentiates the inhibition by increasing the apparent binding affinity to MAO without producing significant changes in the rate of the reaction that yields the irreversibly inhibited species (Ramadan et al., 2007). This finding suggests that the

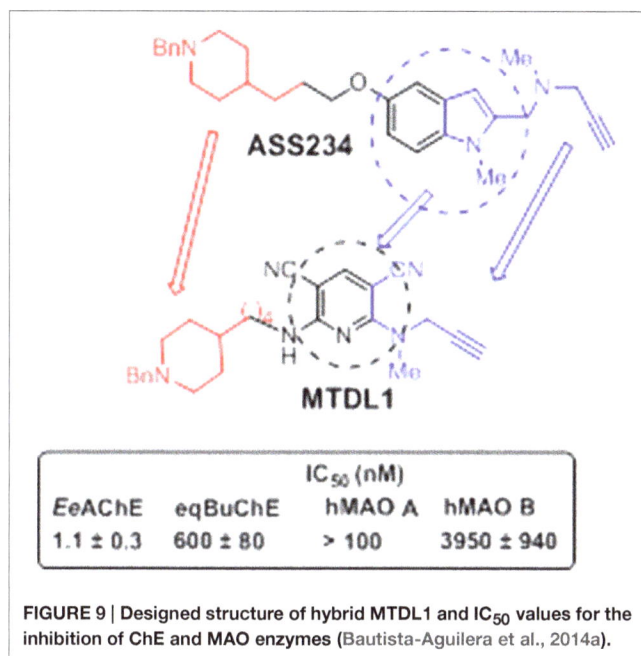

FIGURE 9 | Designed structure of hybrid MTDL1 and IC$_{50}$ values for the inhibition of ChE and MAO enzymes (Bautista-Aguilera et al., 2014a).

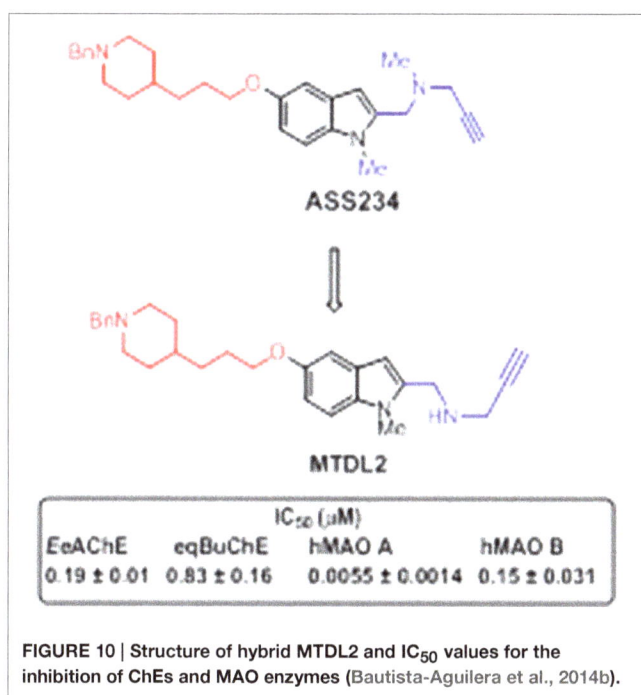

FIGURE 10 | Structure of hybrid MTDL2 and IC$_{50}$ values for the inhibition of ChEs and MAO enzymes (Bautista-Aguilera et al., 2014b).

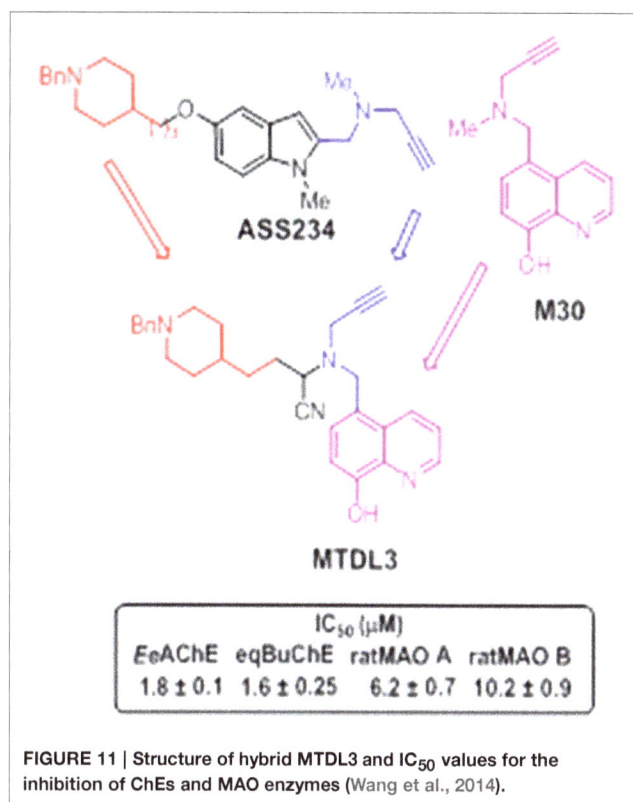

FIGURE 11 | Structure of hybrid MTDL3 and IC$_{50}$ values for the inhibition of ChEs and MAO enzymes (Wang et al., 2014).

potentiating effect of cyanide can be ascribed to an activation mechanism whereby cyanide assists the binding of the inhibitor to the enzyme.

Theoretical ADMET analyses, showed **MTDL-3** to exhibit good drug-likeness properties and brain penetration capacity for CNS activity. Moreover, less toxicity than donepezil in HepG2 cells was also revealed with these derivatives. These findings are important, of noteworthy relevance since the simultaneous administration of multiple therapeutic agents (polypharmacology) may lead to potentially lethal side effects triggered by drug-to-drug interactions. Therefore, such undesirable outcomes might be significantly reduced by the use of multi-target derivatives such as **MTDL-3**. Furthermore, these molecules also displayed good performance in terms of translational science since scopolamine-induced memory deficits were partially restored by **MTDL-3**, confirming its effective pharmacokinetics *in vivo*.

Another related molecule, **MTDL-4** (**Figure 12**), showed similar behavior as dual ChE/MAO inhibitor (Wu et al., 2015), which was identified from an initial pharmacological screening as an appropriate lead compound for further investigation. Subsequent investigations revealed further potentially valuable properties of this molecule.

CONCLUDING REMARKS

Overall, the findings presented in this review robustly reinforce the suitability of MTDLs as an appropriate pharmacological approach to target disease progression in AD therapy. Amongst all the compounds tested, multi-target **MTDL-3** particularly emerged as a ligand possessing a number of remarkable potential benefits for use in this neurological disorder including well-balanced dual AChE/MAO inhibition,

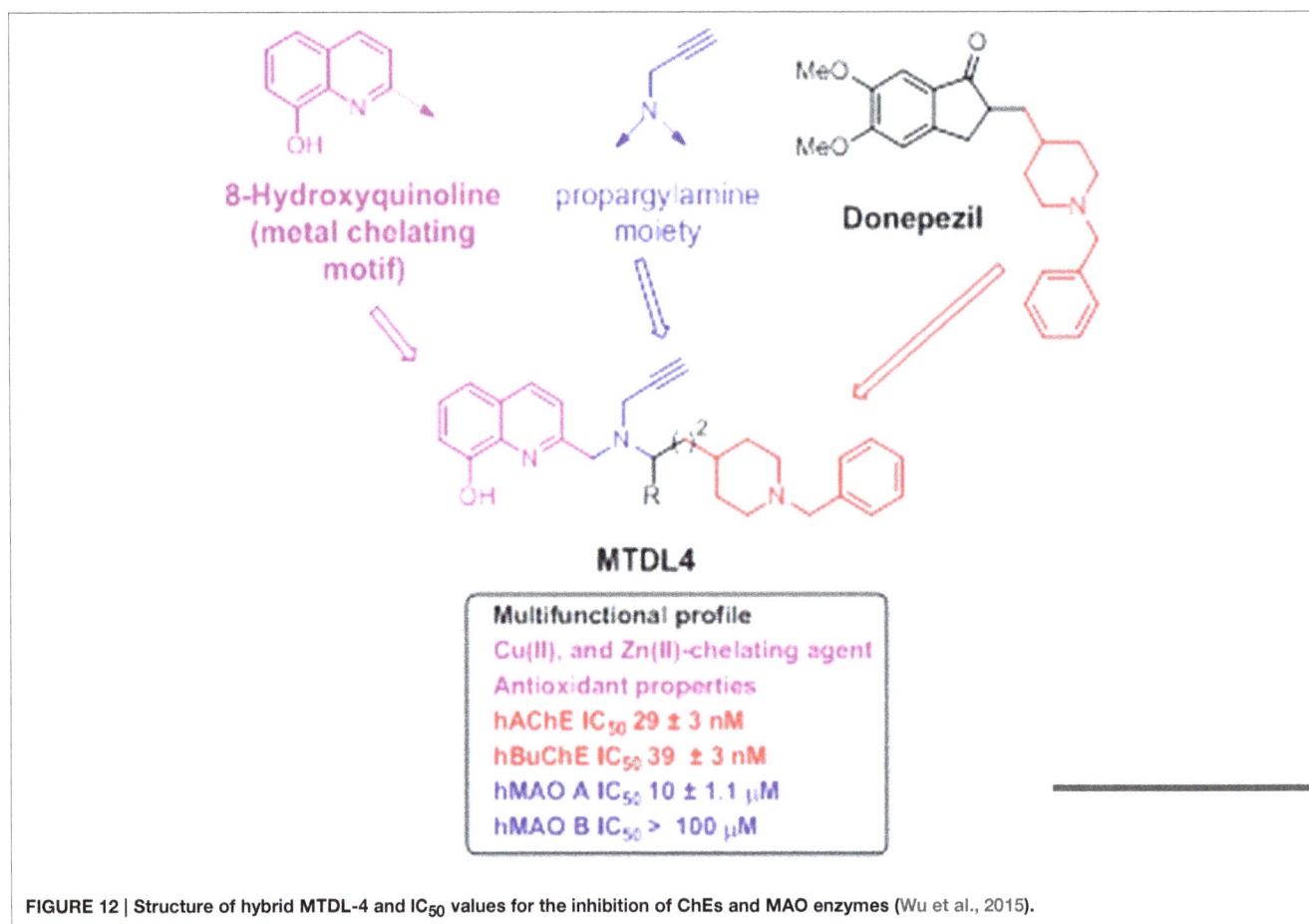

FIGURE 12 | Structure of hybrid MTDL-4 and IC$_{50}$ values for the inhibition of ChEs and MAO enzymes (Wu et al., 2015).

strong metal-chelating activity, neuroprotective and anti-apoptotic properties, potent antioxidant capacities and anti-inflammatory action. Furthermore, **MTDL-3** has effects as enhancer of cognitive functions. This prompts us to propose this molecule as the first racemic α-aminonitrile identified so far as a multifunctional chelator for biometals able to interact in two key enzymatic systems implicated in AD. We consider it as an important new lead compound that merits further investigation for the potential treatment of this disease.

AUTHOR CONTRIBUTIONS

MU, GE, JM, wrote the manuscript. RR, KT, and WF, corrected and revised the manuscript.

ACKNOWLEDGMENTS

MU, GE, JM thank to MIneco (Spain) for support Grant SAF 2012-33304, SAF 2015-65586R. All authors thank EU COST Action CM1103 for its support.

REFERENCES

Acevedo, K. M., Hung, Y. H., Dalziel, A. H., Li, Q. X., Laughton, K., Wikhe, K., et al. (2011). Copper promotes the trafficking of the amyloid precursor protein. *J. Biol. Chem.* 286, 8252–8262. doi: 10.1074/jbc.M110.128512

Adem, A. (1993). The next generation of cholinesterase inhibitors. *Acta Neurol. Scand. Suppl.* 149, 10–12. doi: 10.1111/j.1600-0404.1993.tb04246.x

Adem, A., Jossan, S. S., and Oreland, L. (1989). Tetrahydroaminoacridine inhibits human and rat brain monoamine oxidase. *Neurosci. Lett.* 107, 313–317. doi: 10.1016/0304-3940(89)90837-9

Adlard, P. A., Parncutt, J. M., Finkelstein, D. I., and Bush, A. I. (2010). Cognitive loss in zinc transporter-3 knock-out mice: a phenocopy for the synaptic and memory deficits of Alzheimer's disease? *J. Neurosci.* 30, 1631–1636. doi: 10.1523/jneurosci.5255-09.2010

Adlard, P. A., West, A. K., and Vickers, J. C. (1998). Increased density of metallothionein I/II-immunopositive cortical glial cells in the early stages of Alzheimer's disease. *Neurobiol. Dis.* 5, 349–356. doi: 10.1006/nbdi.1998.0203

Agarwal, K. N. (2001). Iron and the brain: neurotransmitter receptors and magnetic resonance spectroscopy. *Br. J. Nutr.* 85, S147–S150. doi: 10.1079/bjn2000307

Akk, G., and Steinbach, J. H. (2005). Galantamine activates muscle-type nicotinic acetylcholine receptors without binding to the acetylcholine-binding site. *J. Neurosci.* 25, 1992–2001. doi: 10.1523/JNEUROSCI.4985-04.2005

Ali, F. E., Separovic, F., Barrow, C. J., Cherny, R. A., Fraser, F., Bush, A. I., et al. (2005). Methionine regulates copper/hydrogen peroxide oxidation products of Abeta. *J. Pept. Sci.* 11, 353–360. doi: 10.1002/psc.626

Alies, B., Eury, H., Bijani, C., Rechignat, L., Faller, P., and Hureau, C. (2011). pH-dependent, Cu(II) coordination to amyloid-beta peptide: impact of sequence alterations, including the H6R and D7N familial mutations. *Inorg. Chem.* 50, 11192–11201. doi: 10.1021/ic201739n

Aliev, G., Li, Y., Palacios, H. H., and Obrenovich, M. E. (2011). Oxidative stress induced mitochondrial DNA deletion as a hallmark for the drug development in the context of the cerebrovascular diseases. *Recent Pat. Cardiovasc. Drug Discov.* 6, 222–241. doi: 10.2174/157489011797376942

Amit, T., Avramovich-Tirosh, Y., Youdim, M. B. H., and Mandel, S. (2008). Targeting multiple Alzheimer's disease etiologies with multimodal neuroprotective and neurorestorative iron chelators. *FASEB J.* 22, 1296–1305. doi: 10.1096/fj.07-8627rev

An, W. L., Bjorkdahl, C., Liu, R., Cowburn, R. F., Winblad, B., and Pei, J. J. (2005). Mechanism of zinc-induced phosphorylation of p70 S6 kinase and glycogen synthase kinase 3beta in SH-SY5Y neuroblastoma cells. *J. Neurochem.* 92, 1104–1115. doi: 10.1111/j.1471-4159.2004.02948.x

Andrasi, E., Farkas, E., Scheibler, H., Reffy, A., and Bezur, L. A. (1995). 'Zn, Cu, Mn and Fe levels in brain in Alzheimer's disease. *Arch. Gerontol. Geriatr.* 21, 89–97. doi: 10.1016/0167-4943(95)00643-Y

Arendt, T., and Bigl, V. (1986). Alzheimer plaques and cortical cholinergic innervation. *Neuroscience* 17, 277–279. doi: 10.1016/0306-4522(86)90243-5

Atwood, C. S., Scarpa, R. C., Huang, X., Moir, R. D., Jones, W. D., Fairlie, D. P., et al. (2000). Characterization of copper interactions with Alzheimer amyloid beta peptides: identification of an attomolar-affinity copper binding site on amyloid beta1-42. *J. Neurochem.* 75, 1219–1233. doi: 10.1046/j.1471-4159.2000.0751219.x

Avramovich-Tirosh, Y., Amit, T., Bar-Am, O., Zheng, H., Fridkin, M., and Youdim, B. (2007). Therapeutic targets and potential of the novel brain-permeable multifunctional iron chelator-monoamine oxidase inhibitor drug, M-30, for the treatment of Alzheimer's disease. *J. Neurochem.* 100, 490–502. doi: 10.1111/j.1471-4159.2006.04258.x

Ayton, S., Lei, P., and Bush, A. I. (2013). Metallostasis in Alzheimer's disease. *Free Radic. Biol. Med.* 62, 76–89. doi: 10.1016/j.freeradbiomed.2012.10.558

Barnham, K. J., Masters, C. L., and Bush, A. I. (2004). Neurodegenerative diseases and oxidative stress. *Nat. Rev. Drug Discov.* 3, 205–214. doi: 10.1038/nrd1330

Barnham, K. J., McKinstry, W. J., Multhaup, G., Galatis, D., Morton, C. J., Curtain, C. C., et al. (2003). Structure of the Alzheimer's disease amyloid precursor protein copper binding domain: a regulator of neuronal copper homeostasis. *J. Biol. Chem.* 278, 17401–17407. doi: 10.1074/jbc.M300629200

Barone, E. (2016). Oxidative stress and Alzheimer's Disease: Where do we stand? *Curr. Alzheimer Res.* 13, 108–111. doi: 10.2174/1567205013021601011123849

Bartzokis, G., and Tishler, T. A. (2000). MRI evaluation of basal ganglia ferritin iron and neurotoxicity in Alzheimer's and Huntingon's disease. *Cell. Mol. Biol.* 46, 821–833.

Battaglia, V., Sanz, E., Salvi, M., Unzeta, M., and Toninello, A. (2006). Protective effect of PF 9601N on mitochondrial permeability transition pore. *Cell. Mol. Life Sci.* 63, 1440–1448. doi: 10.1007/s00018-006-6105-8

Bautista-Aguilera, O. M., Esteban, G., Bolea, I., Nikolic, K., Agbaba, D., Moraleda, I., et al. (2014b). Design, synthesis, pharmacological evaluation, QSAR analysis, molecular modeling and ADMET of novel donepezil-indolyl hybrids as multipotent cholinesterase/monoamine oxidase inhibitors for the potential treatment of Alzheimer's disease. *Eur. J. Med. Chem.* 75, 82–95. doi: 10.1016/j.ejmech.2013.12.028

Bautista-Aguilera, O. M., Esteban, G., Chioua, M., Nikolic, K., Agbaba, D., Moraleda, I., et al. (2014a). Multipotent cholinesterase/monoamine oxidase inhibitors for the treatment of Alzheimer's disease: design, synthesis, biochemical evaluation, ADMET, molecular modeling, and QSAR analysis of novel donepezil-pyridyl hybrids. *Drug Des. Devel. Ther.* 8, 1893–18910. doi: 10.2147/DDDT.S69258

Beard, J. (2003). Iron deficiency alters brain development and functioning. *J. Nutr.* 133, 1468S–1472S.

Benkler, C., Offen, D., Melamed, E., Kupershmidt, L., Amit, T., Mandel, S., et al. (2010). Recent advances in amyotrophic lateral sclerosis research: Perspectives for personalized clinical application. *EPMA J.* 1, 343–361. doi: 10.1007/s13167-010-0026-1

Bertram, L., and Tanzi, R. E. (2008). Thirty years of Alzheimer's disease genetics: the implications of systematic meta-analyses. *Nat. Rev. Neurosci.* 9, 768–778. doi: 10.1038/nrn2494

Besser, L., Chorin, E., Sekler, I., Silverman, W. F., Atkin, S., Russell, J. T., et al. (2009). Synaptically released zinc triggers metabotropic signaling via a

zinc-sensing receptor in the hippocampus. *J. Neurosci.* 29, 2890–2901. doi: 10.1523/JNEUROSCI.5093-08.2009

Biesold, D., Inanami, O., Sato, A., and Sato, Y. (1989). Stimulation of the nucleus basalis of Meynert increases cerebral cortical blood flow in rats. *Neurosci. Lett.* 98, 39–44. doi: 10.1016/0304-3940(89)90370-4

Birkmayer, W., Riederer, P., Ambrozi, L., and Youdim, M. (1977). Implications of combined treatment with "Madopar" and l-Deprenyl in Prkinson's disease. *Lancet* 1, 439–443. doi: 10.1016/S0140-6736(77)91940-7

Birks, J., Grimley-Evans, J., Iakovidou, V., and Tsolaki, M. (2015). Rivastigmine for Alzheimer's disease. *Cochrane Database Syst. Rev.* 4:CD001191. doi: 10.1002/14651858.CD001191

Birks, J. S., and Harvey, R. J. (2006). Donepezil for dementia due to Alzheimer's disease. *Cochrane Database Syst. Rev.* 1:CD001190. doi: 10.1002/14651858.CD001190.pub2

Bitan, G., Kirkitadze, M. D., Lomakin, A., Vollers, S. S., Benedek, G. B., and Teplow, D. B. (2003). Amyloid beta -protein (Abeta) assembly: Abeta 40 and Abeta 42 oligomerize through distinct pathways. *Proc. Natl. Acad. Sci. U.S.A.* 100, 330–335. doi: 10.1073/pnas.222681699

Blázquez, L., De Juan, D., Ruiz-Martinez, J., Emparanza, J. I., Saenz, A., Otaegui, D., et al. (2007). Genes related to iron metabolism and susceptibility to Alzheimer's disease in Basque population. *Neurobiol. Aging* 28, 1941–1943. doi: 10.1016/j.neurobiolaging.2006.08.009

Bolea, I., Gella, A., Monjas, L., Pérez, C., Rodríguez-Franco, M. I., Marco-Contelles, J., et al. (2013a). Multipotent, permeable drug ASS234 inhibits Aβ aggregation, possesses antioxidant properties and protects from Aβ-induced apoptosis *in vitro*. *Curr. Alzheimer Res.* 10, 797–808. doi: 10.2174/15672050113109990151

Bolea, I., Gella, A., and Unzeta, M. (2013b). Propargylamine-derived multitarget-ligands: fighting Alzheimer's disease with monoamine oxidase inhibitors. *J. Neural. Trans.* 120, 893–902. doi: 10.1007/s00702-012-0948-y

Bolea, I., Juárez-Jiménez, J., de Los Ríos, C., Chioua, M., Pouplana, R., Luque, F. J., et al. (2011). Synthesis, biological evaluation, and molecular modeling of donepezil and N-[(5-(benzyloxy)-1-methyl-1H-indol-2-yl)methyl]-N-methylprop-2-yn-1-amine hybrids as new multipotent cholinesterase/monoamine oxidase inhibitors for the treatment of Alzheimer's disease. *J. Med. Chem.* 54, 8251–8270. doi: 10.1021/jm200853t

Bolognesi, M. L., Cavalli, A., Luca-Valgimigli, L., Bartolini, M., Rosini, M., Andrisano, V., et al. (2007). Multitarget-directed drug design strategy: from a dual binding site acetylcholinesterase inhibitor to a trifunctional compound against Alzheimer's disease. *J. Med. Chem.* 50, 6446–6449. doi: 10.1021/jm701225u

Bonda, D. J., Wang, X., Perry, G., Smith, M. A., and Zhu, X. (2010). Mitochondrial dynamics in Alzheimer disease: opportunities for future treatment strategies. *Drugs Aging* 27, 1–12. doi: 10.2165/11532140-000000000-00000

Boom, A., Authelet, M., Dedecker, R., Frederick, C., Van Heurck, R., Daubie, V., et al. (2009). Bimodal modulation of tau protein phosphorylation and conformation by extracellular Zn^{2+} in human-tau transfected cells. *Biochim. Biophys. Acta* 1793, 1058–1067. doi: 10.1016/j.bbamcr.2008.11.011

Borchardt, T., Schmidt, C., Camarkis, J., Cappai, R., Masters, C. L., Multhaup, G., et al. (2000). Differential effects of zinc on amyloid precursor protein (APP) processing in copper resistant variants of cultured Chinese hamster ovary cells. *Cell. Mol. Biol.* 46, 785–795.

Braak, H., and Braak, E. (1994). Morphological criteria for the recognition of Alzheimer's disease and the distribution pattern of cortical changes related to this disorder. *Neurobiol. Aging* 15, 355–356. doi: 10.1016/0197-4580(94) 90032-9

Brown, K. L., Cosseau, C., Gardy, J. L., and Hancock, R. E. (2007). Complexities of targeting innate immunity to treat infection. *Trends Immunol.* 28, 260–266. doi: 10.1016/j.it.2007.04.005

Buccafusco, J. J., Terry, A. V. Jr. (2000). Multiple central nervous system targets for elicing benefitial effects on memory and cognition. *J. Pharmacol. Exp. Ther.* 295, 438–446.

Bullock, R., and Lane, R. (2007). Executive dyscontrol in dementia, with emphasis on subcortical pathology and the role of butyrylcholinesterase. *Curr. Alzheimer Res.* 4, 277–293. doi: 10.2174/156720507781077313

Bush, A. I., Multhaup, G., Moir, R. D., Williamson, T. G., Small, D. H., Rumble, B., et al. (1993). A novel zinc (II) binding site modulates the function of the beta A4 amyloid protein precursor of Alzheimer's disease. *J. Biol. Chem.* 268, 16109–16112.

Bush, A. I., Pettingell, W. H. Jr., de Paradis, M. D., and Tanzi, R. E. (1994b). Modulation of A beta adhesiveness and secretase site cleavage by zinc. *J. Biol. Chem.* 269, 12152–12158.

Bush, A. I., Pettingell, W. H. Jr., de Paradis, M. D., Tanzi, R. E., and Wasco, W. (1994a). The amyloid beta-protein precursor and its mammalian homologues: evidence for a zinc-modulated heparin-binding superfamily. *J. Biol. Chem.* 269, 26618–26621.

Bush, A. I., Pettingell, W. H., Multhaup, G., de Paradis, M., Vonsattel, J. P., Gusella, J. F., et al. (1994c). Rapid induction of Alzheimer Abeta amyloid formation by zinc. *Science* 265, 1464–1467. doi: 10.1126/science.8073293

Butterfield, D. A., Reed, T., Perluigi, M., De Marco, C., Coccia, R., Cini, C., et al. (2006). Elevated protein-bound levels of the lipid peroxidation product, 4-hydroxy-2-nonenal, in brain from persons with mild cognitive impairment. *Neurosci. Lett.* 397, 170–173. doi: 10.1016/j.neulet.2005.12.017

Cappai, R., Kong, G., McKinstry, W., Galatis, D., Adams, J., Bellingham, S., et al. (2004). Structural and functional analysis of the Alzheimer's disease amyloid precursor protein copper binding domain. *Neurobiol. Aging* 25, s60. doi: 10.1016/s0197-4580(04)80203-3

Castellani, R. J., Lee, H. G., Zhu, X., Nunomura, A., Perry, G., and Smith, M. A. (2006). Neuropathology of Alzheimer disease: pathognomonic but not pathogenic. *Acta Neuropathol.* 111, 503–509. doi: 10.1007/s00401-006-0071-y

Chester, D. S., DeWall, C. N., Derefinko, K. J., Estus, S., Peters, J. R., Lynam, D. R., et al. (2015). Monoamine oxidase A (MAO A) genotype predicts greater aggression through impulsive reactivity to negative affect. *Behav. Brain Res.* 283, 97–101. doi: 10.1016/j.bbr.2015.01.034

Chouraki, V., and Seshadri, S. (2014). Genetics of Alzheimer's disease. *Adv. Genet.* 87, 245–294. doi: 10.1016/B978-0-12-800149-3.00005-6

Ciro, A., Park, J., Burkhard, G., Yan, N., and Geula, C. (2012). Biochemical differentiation of cholinesterases from normal and Alzheimer's disease cortex. *Curr. Alzheimer Res.* 9, 138–143. doi: 10.2174/156720512799015127

Connor, J. R., Menzies, S. L., St Martin, S. M., and Mufson, E. J. (1992). A histochemical study of iron, transferrin, and ferritin in Alzheimer's diseased brains. *J. Neurosci. Res.* 31, 75–83. doi: 10.1002/jnr.490310111

Corrigan, F. M., Reynolds, G. P., and Ward, N. I. (1993). Hippocampal tin, aluminum and zinc in Alzheimer's disease. *Biometals* 6, 149–154. doi: 10.1007/BF00205853

Coulson, E. J., Paliga, K., Beyreuther, K., and Masters, C. L. (2000). What the evolution of the amyloid protein precursor supergene family tells us about its function. *Neurochemistry* 36, 175–184. doi: 10.1016/S0197-0186(99)00125-4

Coyle, J. T., and Puttfarcken, P. (1993). Oxidative stress, glutamate and neurodegenerative dosorders. *Science* 262, 689–695. doi: 10.1126/science.7901908

Crouch, P. J., Blake, R., Duce, J. A., Ciccotosto, G. D., Li, Q. X., Barnham, K. J., et al. (2005). Copper-dependent inhibition of human cytochrome c oxidase by a dimeric conformer of amyloid-beta (1-42). *J. Neurosci.* 25, 672–679. doi: 10.1523/JNEUROSCI.4276-04.2005

Crouch, P. J., Tew, D. J., Du, T., Nguyen, D. N., Caragounis, A., Filiz, G., et al. (2009). Restored degradation of the Alzheimer's amyloid-beta peptide by targeting amyloid formation. *J. Neurochem.* 108, 1198–1207. doi: 10.1111/j.1471-4159.2009.05870.x

Cuajuangco, M. P., and Faget, K. Y. (2003). Zinc takes the center stage: Its paradoxical role in Alzheimer's disease. *Brain Res. Brain Res. Rev.* 41, 44–56. doi: 10.1016/S0165-0173(02)00219-9

Curtain, C. C., Ali, F. E., Volitaskis, I., Cherny, R. A., Norton, R. S., Beyreuther, K., et al. (2001). Alzheimer's disease amyloid-beta binds copper and zinc to generate an allosterically ordered membrane-penetrating structure containing superoxide dismutase-like subunits. *J. Biol. Chem.* 276, 20466–22047. doi: 10.1074/jbc.M100175200

Cutillas, B., Ambrosio, S., and Unzeta, M. (2002). Neuroprotective effect of the monoamin oxidase inhibitor PF 9601N on rat nigral neurons after 6-OH-Dopamine striatal lesion. *Neurosci. Lett.* 329, 165–168. doi: 10.1016/S0304-3940(02)00614-6

Daikhin, Y., and Yudkoff, M. (2000). Compartmentation of brain glutamate metabolism in neurons and glia. *J. Nutr.* 130, 1026S–1031S.

Dajas-Bailador, F. A., Heimala, K., and Wonnacott, S. (2003). The allosteric potentiation of nicotinic acetylcholine receptors by galantamine is transduced into cellular responses in neurons: Ca^{2+} signals and neurotransmitter release. *Mol. Pharmacol.* 64, 1217–1226. doi: 10.1124/mol.64.5.1217

Damante, C. A., Osz, K., Nagy, Z., Pappalardo, G., Grasso, G., Impellizzeri, G., et al. (2009). Metal loading capacity of Abeta N-terminus: a combined potentiometric and spectroscopic study of zinc (II) complexes with Abeta (1-16), its short or mutated peptide fragments and its polyethylene glycolylated analogue. *Inorg. Chem.* 48, 10405–10415. doi: 10.1021/ic9012334

Danscher, G., Jensen, K. B., Frederickson, C. J., Kemp, K., Andreasen, A., Ravid, S., et al. (1997). Increased amount of zinc in the hippocampus and amygdala of Alzheimer's diseased brains: a proton-induced X-ray emission spectroscopic analysis of cryostat sections from autopsy material. *J. Neurosci. Methods* 76, 53–59. doi: 10.1016/S0165-0270(97)00079-4

Darreh-Shori, T., and Soininen, H. (2010). Effects of cholinesterase inhibitors on the activities and protein levels of cholinesterases in the cerebrospinal fluid of patients with Alzheimer's disease: A review of recent clinical studies. *Curr. Alzheimer Res.* 7, 67–73. doi: 10.2174/156720510790274455

Davison, A. N. (1957). The mechanism of the irreversible inhibition of rat-liver monomine oxidase by iproniazid. *Biochem. J.* 67, 316–322. doi: 10.1042/bj0670316

De Colibus, C. L., Li, M., Binda, C., Lustig, A., Edmondson, D. E., and Mattevi, A. (2005). Three-dimensional structure of human monoamine oxidase A (MAO A): relation to the structures of rat MAO A and human MAO B. *Proc. Natl. Acad. Sci. U.S.A.* 102, 12684–12689. doi: 10.1073/pnas.0505975102

Deibel, M. A., Ehmann, W. D., and Markesbery, W. R. (1996). Copper, iron, and zinc imbalances in severely degenerated brain regions in Alzheimer's disease: possible relation to oxidative stress. *J. Neurol. Sci.* 143, 137–142. doi: 10.1016/S0022-510X(96)00203-1

Détári, L., Rasmusson, D. D., and Semba, K. (1999). The role of basal forebrain neurons in tonic and phasic activation of the cerebral cortex. *Prog. Neurobiol.* 58, 249–277. doi: 10.1016/S0301-0082(98)00084-7

Deutsch, J. A. (1971). The cholinergic synapse and the site of memory. *Science* 174, 788–794. doi: 10.1126/science.174.4011.788

Diamant, S., Podoly, E., Friedler, A., Ligumsky, H., Livnah, O., and Soreq, H. (2006). Butyrylcholinesterase attenuates amyloid fibril formation *in vitro*. *Proc. Natl. Acad. Sci. U.S.A.* 103, 8628–8633. doi: 10.1073/pnas.0602922103

Dobson, J., and Batich, C. (2004). A potential iron-based mechanism for enhanced deposition of amyloid plaques due to cognitive stimulation in Alzheimer disease. *J. Neuropathol. Exp. Neurol.* 63, 674–675. doi: 10.1093/jnen/63.6.674

Doody, R. S., Tariot, P. N., Pfeiffer, E., Olin, J. T., and Graham, S. M. (2007). Meta-analysis of six-month memantine trials in Alzheimer's disease. *Alzheimers Dement.* 1, 7–17. doi: 10.1016/j.jalz.2006.10.004

Duce, J. A., Tsatsanis, A., Cater, M. A., James, S. A., Robb, E., Wikhe, K., et al. (2010). Iron-export ferroxidase activity of beta-amyloid precursor protein is inhibited by zinc in Alzheimer's disease. *Cell* 142, 857–867. doi: 10.1016/j.cell.2010.08.014

Eckenroth, B. E., Steere, A. N., Chasteen, N. D., Everse, S. J., and Mason, A. B. (2011). How the binding of human transferrin primes the transferrin receptor potentiating iron release at endosomal pH. *Proc. Natl. Acad. Sci. U.S.A.* 108, 13089–13094. doi: 10.1073/pnas.1105786108

Edmondson, D. E., Binda, C., and Mattevi, A. (2007). Structural insights into the mechanism of amine oxidation by monoamine oxidases A and B. *Arch. Biochem. Biophys.* 464, 269–276. doi: 10.1016/j.abb.2007.05.006

Egaña, J. T., Zambrano, C., Núñez, M. T., González-Billault, C., and Maccioni, R. B. (2003). Iron-induced oxidative stress modifies tau phosphorylation patterns in hippocampal cell cultures. *Biometals* 16, 215–223.

Esteban, G., Allan, J., Samadi, A., Mattevi, A., Unzeta, M., Marco-Contelles, J., et al. (2014). Kinetic and structural analysis of irreversible inhibition of human monoamine oxidases by ASS234, a multi-target compound designed for use in Alzheimer's disease. *Biochim. Biophys. Acta* 1844, 1104–1110. doi: 10.1016/j.bbapap.2014.03.006

Evin, G., and Weidemann, A. (2002). Biogenesis and metabolism of Alzheimer's disease Abeta amyloid peptides. *Peptides* 23, 1285–1297. doi: 10.1016/S0196-9781(02)00063-3

Faller, P., Hureau, C., and Berthoumieu, O. (2013). Role of metal ions in the self-assembly of the Alzheimer's amyloid-beta peptide. *Inorg. Chem.* 52, 12193–12206. doi: 10.1021/ic4003059

Feng, Y., and Wang, X. (2012). Antioxidant therapies for Alzheimer's disease. *Oxid. Med. Cell. Longev.* 2012:472932. doi: 10.1155/2012/472932

Fibiger, H. C. (1991). Cholinergic mechanisms in learning, memory and dementia: a review of recent evidence. *Trends Neurosci.* 14, 220–223. doi: 10.1016/0166-2236(91)90117-D

Figueiredo, C. P., Clarke, J. R., Ledo, J. H., Ribeiro, F. C., Costa, C. V., Melo, H. M., et al. (2013). Memantine rescues transient cognitive impairment caused by high-molecular-weight aβ oligomers but not the persistent impairment induced by low-molecular-weight oligomers. *J. Neurosci.* 33, 9626–9634. doi: 10.1523/JNEUROSCI.0482-13.2013

Fornai, F., Chen, K., Giorgi, F. S., Gesi, M., Alessandri, M. C., and Shih, J. C. (1999). Striatal dopamine metabolism in monoamine oxidase B-deficient mice: a brain dialysis study. *J. Neurochem.* 73, 2434–2440. doi: 10.1046/j.1471-4159.1999.0732434.x

Fowler, J. S., Mac Gregor, R. R., Wolf, A. P., Arnett, C. D., Devey, S. L., Schlyer, D., et al (1987). Mapping human brain monoamine oxidase A and B with 11C-labeled suicide inactivators and PET. *Science* 235, 481–485. doi: 10.1126/science.3099392

Frederickson, C. J. (1989). Neurobiology of zinc and zinc-containing neuron. *Int. Rev. Neurobiol.* 31, 145–238. doi: 10.1016/s0074-7742(08)60279-2

Freinbichler, W., Tipton, K. F., Della Corte, L., and Linert, W. (2009). Mechanistic aspects of the Fenton reaction under conditions approximated to the extracellular fluid. *J. Inorg. Biochem.* 103, 28–34. doi: 10.1016/j.jinorgbio.2008.08.014

Fukuda, M., Kanou, F., Shimada, N., Sawabe, M., Saito, Y., Murayama, S., et al. (2009). Elevated levels of 4-hydroxynonenal-histidine Michael adduct in the hippocampi of patients with Alzheimer's disease. *Biomed. Res.* 30, 229–233. doi: 10.2220/biomedres.30.227

Galasko, D. R., Peskind, E., Clark, C. M., Quinn, J. F., Ringman, J. M., Jicha, G. A., et al. (2012). Antioxidants for Alzheimer disease: A randomized clinical trial with cerebrospinal fluid biomarker measures. *Arch. Neurol.* 69, 836–841. doi: 10.1001/archneurol.2012.85

Geula, C., and Mesulam, M. (1989). Special properties of cholinesterases in the cerebral cortex of Alzheimer's disease. *Brain Res.* 498, 185–189. doi: 10.1016/0006-8993(89)90419-8

Giacobini, E. (2003). Cholinesterases: new roles in brain function and in Alzheimer's disease. *Neurochem. Res.* 28, 515–522. doi: 10.1023/A:1022869222652

Glenner, G. G., and Murphy, M. A. (1989). Amyloidosis of the nervous system. *J. Neurol. Sci.* 94, 1–28. doi: 10.1016/0022-510X(89)90214-1

Goedert, M., Klug, A., and Crowther, R. A. (2006). Tau protein, the paired helical filament and Alzheimer's disease. *J. Alzheimers Dis.* 9, 195–207.

Gomes, L. M., Vieira, R. P., Jones, M. R., Wang, M. C., Dyrager, C., Souza-Fagundes, E. M., et al. (2014). 8-Hydroxyquinoline Schiff-base compounds as antioxidants and modulators of copper-mediated Aβ peptide aggregation. *J. Inorg. Biochem.* 139, 106–116. doi: 10.1016/j.jinorgbio.2014.04.011

Goodman, L. (1953). Alzheimer's disease; a clinico-pathologic analysis of twenty three cases with a theory on pathogenesis. *J. Nerv. Mental Dis.* 118, 97–130. doi: 10.1097/00005053-195308000-00001

Greenblatt, H. M., Kryger, G., Lewis, T., Silman, I., and Sussman, J. L. (1999). Structure of acetylcholinesterase complexed with (-)-galanthamine at 2.3 A resolution. *FEBS Lett.* 463, 321–326. doi: 10.1016/S0014-5793(99)01637-3

Grundke-Iqbal, I., Iqbal, K., Tung, Y. C., Quinlan, M., Wisniewski, H., and M., Binder, L. I. (1986). Abnormal phosphorilation of the microtubule-associated protein tau in Alzheimer cytoskeletal pathology. *Proc. Natl. Acad. Sci. U.S.A.* 93, 4913–4917. doi: 10.1073/pnas.83.13.4913

Guglielmotto, M., Giliberto, L., Tamagno, E., and Tabaton, M. (2010). Oxidative stress mediates the pathogenic effect of different Alzheimer's disease risk factors. *Front. Aging Neurosci.* 2:3. doi: 10.3389/neuro.24.003.2010

Guillozet, A. L., Smiley, J. F., Mash, D. C., and Mesulam, M. M. (1997). Butyrylcholinesterase in the life cycle of amyloid plaques. *Ann Neurol.* 42, 909–918. doi: 10.1002/ana.410420613

Hardy, J. A., and Higgins, G. A. (1992). Alzheimer's disease: The amyloid cascade hypothesis. *Science* 256, 184–185. doi: 10.1126/science.1566067

Hartter, D. E., and Barnea, A. (1988). Evidence for release of copper in the brain: Depolarization-induced release of newly taken-up 67 copper. *Synapse* 2, 412–415. doi: 10.1002/syn.890020408

Hayashi, T., Shishido, N., Nakayama, K., Nunomura, A., Smith, M. A., Perry, G., et al. (2007). Lipid peroxidation and 4-hydroxy-2-nonenal formation by copper

ion bound to amyloid-beta peptide. *Free Rad. Biol. Med.* 43, 1552–1559. doi: 10.1016/j.freeradbiomed.2007.08.013

Heppner, F. L., Ransohoff, R. M., and Becher, B. (2015). Immune attack: the role of inflammation in Alzheimer disease. *Nat. Rev. Neurosci.* 16, 358–372. doi: 10.1038/nrn3880

Hoke, D. E., Tan, J. L., Ilaya, N. T., Culvenor, J. G., Smith, S. J., White, A. R., et al. (2007). *In vitro* gamma-secretase cleavage of the Alzheimer's amyloid precursor protein correlates to a subset of presenilin complexes and is inhibited by zinc. *FEBS J.* 272, 5544–5557. doi: 10.1111/j.1742-4658.2005.04950.x

Hopt, A., Korte, S., Fink, H., Panne, U., Niessner, R., Jahn, R., et al. (2003). Methods for studying synaptosomal copper release. *J. Neurosci. Methods* 128, 159–172. doi: 10.1016/S0165-0270(03)00173-0

Hou, L., and Zagorski, M. G. (2006). NMR reveals anomalous copper (II) binding to the amyloid Abeta peptide of Alzheimer's disease. *J. Am. Chem. Soc.* 128, 9260–9261. doi: 10.1021/ja046032u

Houslay, M. D., and Tipton, K. F. (1973). The reaction pathway of rat liver monoamine oxidase. *Biochem. J.* 135, 173–186. doi: 10.1042/bj1350173

Hu, M., Schurdak, M. E., Puttfarcken, P. S., El Kouhen, R., Gopalakrishnan, M., and Li, J. (2007). High content screen microscopy analysis of amyloid beta 1-42-induced neurite outgrowth reduction in rat primary cortical neurons: neuroprotective effects of alpha 7 neuronal nicotinic acetylcholine receptor ligands. *Brain Res.* 1151, 227–235. doi: 10.1016/j.brainres.2007.03.051

Huang, T. H., Yang, D. S., Fraser, P. E., and Chakrabartty, A. (2000). Alternate aggregation pathways of the Alzheimer beta-amyloid peptide. An *in vitro* model of preamyloid. *J. Biol. Chem.* 275, 36436–36440. doi: 10.1074/jbc.M005698200

Huang, X., Cuajungco, M. P., Atwood, C. S., Hartshorn, M. A., Tyndall, G. R., Hanson, J. D., et al. (1999). Cu (II) potentiation of Alzheimer A-β neurotoxicity. Correlation with cell-free hydrogen peroxide production and metal reduction. *J. Biol. Chem.* 274, 37111–37116. doi: 10.1074/jbc.274.52.37111

Huang, X., Dai, J., Huang, C., Zhang, Q., Bhanot, O., and Pelle, E. (2007). Deferoxamine synergistically enhances iron-mediated AP-1 activation: a showcase of the interplay between extracellular-signal-regulated kinase and tyrosine phosphatase. *Free Rad. Res.* 41, 1135–1142. doi: 10.1080/10715760701609061

Huang, X., Moir, R. D., Tanzi, R. E., Bush, A. I., and Rogers, J. T. (2004). Redox-active metals, oxidative stress and Alzheimer's disease pathology. *Ann. N.Y. Acad. Sci.* 1012, 153–163. doi: 10.1196/annals.1306.012

Inestrosa, N. C., Alvarez, A., Perez, C. A., Moreno, R. D., Vicente, M., Linker, C., et al. (1996). Acetylcholinesterase accelerates assembly of amyloid-β-peptides into Alzheimer's Fibrils: possible role of the peripheral site of the enzyme. *Neuron* 16, 881–891.

Islam, K., and Levy, E. (1997). Carboxyl-terminal fragments of beta-amyloid precursor protein bind to microtubules and the associated protein tau. *Am. J. Pathol.* 151, 265–271.

Jack, C. R. Jr., Wiste, H. J., Vemuri, P., Weigand, S. D., Senjem, M. L., Zeng, G., et al. (2010). Brain beta-amyloid measures and magnetic resonance imaging atrophy both predict time-to-progression from mild cognitive impairment to Alzheimer's disease Neuroimaging Initiative. *Brain* 133, 3336–3348. doi: 10.1093/brain/awq277

Jiang, H., Wang, X., Huang, L., Luo, Z., Su, T., Ding, K., et al. (2011). Benzenediol-berberine hybrids: Multifunctional agents for Alzheimer's disease. *Bioorg. Med. Chem.* 19, 7228–7235. doi: 10.1016/j.bmc.2011.09.040

Jiao, Y., and Yang, P. (2007). Mechanism of copper (II) inhibiting Alzheimer's amyloid beta-peptide from aggregation: a molecular dynamics investigation. *J. Phys. Chem.* 111, 7646–7655. doi: 10.1021/jp0673359

Jin, M., Shepardson, N., Yang, T., Chen, G., Walsh, D., and Selkoe, D. J. (2011). Soluble amyloid beta-protein dimers isolated from Alzheimer cortex directly induce Tau hyperphosphorylation and neuritic degeneration. *Proc. Natl. Acad. Sci. U.S.A.* 108, 5819–5824. doi: 10.1073/pnas.1017033108

Juárez-Jiménez, J., Mendes, E., Galdeano, C., Martins, C., Silva, D. B., Marco-Contelles, J., et al. (2014). Exploring the structural basis of the selective inhibition of monoamine oxidase A by dicarbonitrile aminoheterocyles: Role of Asn181 and Ile335 validated by spectroscopic and computational studies. *Biochim. Biophys. Acta* 1844, 389–397. doi: 10.1016/j.bbapap.2013.11.003

Karch, C. M., and Goate, A. M. (2015). Alzheimer's disease risk genes and mechanisms of disease pathogenesis. *Biol. Psychiatry* 77, 43–51. doi: 10.1016/j.biopsych.2014.05.006

Kawahara, M., Mizuno, D., Koyama, H., Konora, K., Ohkawa, S., and Sadakane, Y. (2014). Disruption of Zinc homeostasis at the pathogenesis of senile dementia. *Metallomics* 6, 209–216. doi: 10.1039/C3MT00257H

Kayed, R., Head, E., Thompson, J. L., McIntire, T. M., Milton, S. C., Cotman, C. W., et al. (2003). Common structure of soluble amyloid oligomers implies common mechanism of pathogenesis. *Science* 300, 486–489. doi: 10.1126/science.1079469

Keller, J. N., Schmitt, F. A., Scheff, S. W., Ding, Q., Chen, Q., Butterfield, D. A., et al. (2005). Evidence of increased oxidative damage in subjects with mild cognitive impairment. *Neurology* 64, 1152–1156. doi: 10.1212/01.WNL.0000156156.13641.BA

Khalil, M., Teunissen, C., and Langkammer, C. (2011). Iron and neurodegeneration in multiple sclerosis. *Mult. Scler. Int.* 2011:606807. doi: 10.1155/2011/606807

Khatoon, S., Grundke-Iqbal, I., and Iqbal, K. (1994). Levels of normal and abnormally phosphorylated tau in different cellular and regional compartments of Alzheimer disease and control brains. *FEBS Lett.* 351, 80–84. doi: 10.1016/0014-5793(94)00829-9

Kitazawa, M., Cheng, D., and Laferla, F. M. (2009). Chronic copper exposure exacerbates both amyloid and tau pathology and selectively deregulates CDK5 in a mouse model of AD. *J. Neurochem.* 108, 1550–1560. doi: 10.1111/j.1471-4159.2009.05901.x

Kodama, H., Murata, Y., and Kobayashi, M. (1999). Clinical manifestations and treatment of Menkes disease and its variants. *Pediatr. Int.* 41, 423–429. doi: 10.1046/j.1442-200x.1999.01095.x

Kupershmidt, L., Amit, T., Bar-Am, O., Youdim, M. B., and Weinreb, O. (2012). The novel multi-target iron chelating-radical scavenging compound M30 possesses beneficial effects on major hallmarks of Alzheimer's disease. *Antioxid. Redox Signal.* 17, 860–877. doi: 10.1089/ars.2011.4279

Kuperstein, F., and Yavin, E. (2003). Pro-apoptotic signaling in neuronal cells following iron and amyloid beta peptide neurotoxicity. *J. Neurochem.* 86, 114–125. doi: 10.1046/j.1471-4159.2003.01831.x

Lambert, M. P., Barlow, A. K., Chromy, B. A., Edwards, C., Freed, R., Liosatos, M., et al. (1998). Diffusible, nonfibrillar ligands derived from Abeta1-42 are potent central nervous system neurotoxins. *Proc. Natl. Acad. Sci. U.S.A.* 95, 6448–6453. doi: 10.1073/pnas.95.11.6448

Lee, H. P., Zhu, X., Casadesus, G., Castellani, R. J., Nunomura, A., Smith, M. A., et al. (2010). Antioxidant approaches for the treatment of Alzheimer's disease. *Expert Rev. Neurother.* 10, 1201–1208. doi: 10.1586/ern.10.74

Lee, M. G., Hassani, O. K., Alonso, A., and Jones, B. E. (2005). Cholinergic basal forebrain neurons burst with theta during waking and paradoxical sleep. *J. Neurosci.* 25, 4365–4369. doi: 10.1523/JNEUROSCI.0178-05.2005

Lee, Y. J., Jeong, S. Y., Karbowski, M., Smith, C. L., and Youle, R. J. (2004). Roles of the mammalian mitochondrial fission and fusion mediators Fis1, Drp1, and Opa1 in apoptosis. *Mol. Bio. Cell.* 15, 5001–5011. doi: 10.1091/mbc.E04-04-0294

Lei, P., Ayton, S., Bush, A. I., and Adlard, P. A. (2011). GSK-3 in neurodegenerative diseases. *Int. J. Alzheimers Dis.* 2011:189246. doi: 10.4061/2011/189246

Lei, P., Ayton, S., Finkelstein, D. I., Adlard, P. A., Masters, C. L., and Bush, A. I. (2010). Tau protein: Relevance to Parkinson's disease. *Int. J. Biochem. Cell Biol.* 42, 1775–1778. doi: 10.1016/j.biocel.2010.07.016

Lei, P., Ayton, S., Finkelstein, D. I., Spoerri, L., Ciccotosto, G. D., Wright, D. K., et al. (2012). Tau deficiency induces parkinsonism with dementia by impairing APP-mediated iron export. *Nat. Med.* 18, 291–295. doi: 10.1038/nm.2613

León, R., García, A. G., and Marco-Contelles, J. (2013). Recent advances in the multitaret-directed ligands approach for the treatment of Alzheimer's disease. *Med. Res. Rev.* 33, 139–189. doi: 10.1002/med.20248

LeVine, H. (1993). Thioflavine T interaction with synthetic Alzheimer's disease beta-amyloid peptides: detection of amyloid aggregation in solution. *Protein Sci.* 2, 404–410. doi: 10.1002/pro.5560020312

Lipton, S. A. (2006). Paradigm shift in neuroprotection by NMDA receptor blockade: memantine and beyond. *Nat. Rev. Drug Discov.* 5, 160–170. doi: 10.1038/nrd1958

Liu, W., Xu, Z., Deng, Y., Xu, B., Wei, Y., and Yang, T. (2013). Protective effects of memantine against methylmercury-induced glutamate dyshomeostasis and oxidative stress in rat cerebral cortex. *Neurotox. Res.* 24, 320–337. doi: 10.1007/s12640-013-9386-3

Loeffler, D. A., Connor, J. R., Juneau, P. L., Snyder, B. S., Kanaley, L., DeMaggio, A. J., et al. (1995). Transferrin and iron in normal, Alzheimer's disease, and Parkinson's disease brain regions. *J. Neurochem.* 65, 710–724. doi: 10.1046/j.1471-4159.1995.65020710.x

Lovell, M. A., Robertson, J. D., Teesdale, W. J., Campbell, J. L., and Markesbery, W. R. (1998). Copper, iron and zinc in Alzheimer's disease senile plaques. *J. Neurol. Sci.* 58, 47–52. doi: 10.1016/S0022-510X(98)00092-6

Lovell, M. A., Xiong, S., Xie, C., Davies, P. L., and Markesbery, W. R. (2004). Induction of hyperphosphorylated tau in primary rat cortical neuron cultures mediated by oxidative stress and glycogen synthase kinase-3. *J. Alzheimers Dis.* 5, 659–671.

Ma, Q. F., Hu, J., Wu, W. H., Liu, H. D., Du, J. T., Fu, Y., et al. (2006). Characterization of copper binding to the peptide amyloid-beta (1-16) associated with Alzheimer's disease. *Biopolymers* 83, 20–31. doi: 10.1002/bip.20523

Magaki, S., Raghavan, R., Mueller, C., Oberg, K. C., Vinters, H. V., and Kirsch, W. M. (2007). Iron, copper, and iron regulatory protein 2 in Alzheimer's disease and related dementias. *Neurosci. Lett.* 418, 72–76. doi: 10.1016/j.neulet.2007.02.077

Malar, D. S., and Devi, K. P. (2014). Dietary polyphenols for treatment of Alzheimer's disease: future research and development. *Curr. Pharm. Biotechnol.* 15, 330–342. doi: 10.2174/1389201015666140813122703

Mantyh, P. W., Ghilardi, J. R., Rogers, S., DeMaster, E., Allen, C. J., Stimson, E. R., et al. (1993). Aluminum, iron, and zinc ions promote aggregation of physiological concentrations of beta-amyloid peptide. *J. Neurochem.* 61, 1171–1174. doi: 10.1111/j.1471-4159.1993.tb03639.x

Matsubayashi, K., Fukuyama, H., Akiguchi, I., Kameyama, M., Imai, H., and Maeda, T. (1986). Localization of monoamine oxidase (MAO) in the rat peripheral nervous system existence of MAO-containing unmyelinated axons. *Brain Res.* 368, 30–35. doi: 10.1016/0006-8993(86)91039-5

Mattson, M. P. (1997). Cellular actions of beta-amyloid precursor protein and its soluble and fibrillogenic derivatives. *Physiol. Rev.* 77, 1081–1132.

Mattson, M. P. (2004). Pathways towards and away from Alzheimer's disease. *Nature* 430, 631–639. doi: 10.1038/nature02621

Meadowcroft, M. D., Connor, J. R., Smith, M. B., and Yang, Q. X. (2009). MRI and histological analysis of beta-amyloid plaques in both human Alzheimer's disease and APP/PS1 transgenic mice. *J. Magn. Reson. Imaging.* 29, 997–1007. doi: 10.1002/jmri.21731

Mechlovich, D., Amit, T., Bar-Am, O., Mandel, S., Youdim, M. B., and Weinreb, O. (2014). The novel multi-target iron chelator, M30 modulates HIF-1α-related glycolytic genes and insulin signaling pathway in the frontal cortex of APP/PS1 Alzheimer's disease mice. *Curr. Alzheimer Res.* 2, 119–127. doi: 10.2174/1567205010666131212112529

Mendelewicz, J., and Youdim, M. B. H. (1983). L-Deprenyl: a selective monoamine oxidase type B inhibitor in the treatment of depression: a double-bind evaluation. *Br. J. Psychiatry* 142, 508–511. doi: 10.1192/bjp.142.5.508

Merle, U., Schaefer, M., Ferenci, P., and Stremmel, W. (2007). Clinical presentation, diagnosis and long-term outcome of Wilson's disease: A cohort study. *Gut* 56, 115–120. doi: 10.1136/gut.2005.087262

Mesulam, M., Guillozet, A., Shaw, P., and Quinn, B. (2002). Widely spread butyrylcholinesterase can hydrolyze acetylcholine in the normal and Alzheimer brain. *Neurobiol. Dis.* 9, 88–93. doi: 10.1006/nbdi.2001.0462

Miguel-Hidalgo, J. J., Álvarez, X. A., Cacabelos, R., and Quack, G. (2002). Neuroprotection by memantine against neurodegeneration induced by beta-amyloid (1-40). *Brain Res.* 958, 210–221. doi: 10.1016/S0006-8993(02)03731-9

Miller, L. M., Wang, Q., Telivala, T. P., Smith, R. J., Lanzirotti, A., and Miklossy, J. (2006). Synchrotron-based infrared and X-ray imaging shows focalized accumulation of Cu and Zn co-localized with beta-amyloid deposits in Alzheimer's disease. *J. Struct. Biol.* 155, 30–37. doi: 10.1016/j.jsb.2005.09.004

Minicozzi, V., Stellato, F., Comai, M., Serra, M. D., Potrich, C., Meyer-Klaucke, W., et al. (2008). Identifying the minimal copper- and zinc-binding site sequence in amyloid-beta peptides. *J. Biol. Chem.* 283, 10784–10792. doi: 10.1074/jbc.M707109200

Mo, Z. Y., Zhu, Y. Z., Zhu, H. L., Fan, J. B., Chen, J., and Liang, Y. (2009). Low micromolar zinc accelerates the fibrillization of human tau via bridging of Cys-291 and Cys-322. *J. Biol. Chem.* 284, 34648–34657. doi: 10.1074/jbc.M109.058883

Molnar, P., and Nadler, J. V. (2001). Lack of effect of mossy fiber-released zinc on granule cell GABA (A) receptors in the pilocarpine model of epilepsy'. *J. Neurophysiol.* 85, 1932–1940.

Morales, I., Guzmán-Martínez, L., Cerda-Troncoso, C., Farias, G. A., and Maccioni, R. B. (2014). Neuroinflammation in the pathogenesis of Alzheimer's disease. A rational framework for the search of novel therapeutic approaches. *Front. Cell Neurosci.* 8:112. doi: 10.3389/fncel.2014.00112

Moreira, P. I., Nunomura, A., Nakamura, M., Takeda, A., Shenk, J. C., Aliev, G., et al. (2008). Nucleic acid oxidation in Alzheimer disease. *Free Rad. Biol. Med.* 44, 1493–1505. doi: 10.1016/j.freeradbiomed.2008.01.002

Moriguchi, S., Marszalec, W., Zhao, X., Yeh, J. Z., and Narahashi, T. (2003). Potentiation of N-methyl-D-aspartate-induced currents by the nootropic drug nefiracetam in rat cortical neurons. *J. Pharmacol. Exp. Ther.* 307, 160–167. doi: 10.1124/jpet.103.050823

Multhaup, G., Schlicksupp, A., Hesse, L., Beher, D., Ruppert, T., Masters, C. L., et al. (1996). The amyloid precursor protein of Alzheimer's disease in the reduction of copper (II) to copper (I). *Science* 271, 1406–1409. doi: 10.1126/science.271.5254.1406

Muñoz, P., Zavala, G., Castillo, K., Aguirre, P., Hidalgo, C., and Núñez, M. (2006). Effect of iron on the activation of the MAPK/ERK pathway in PC12 neuroblastoma cells. *Biol. Res.* 39, 189–190.

Nakamura, M., Shishido, N., Nunomura, A., Smith, M. A., Perry, G., Hayashi, Y., et al. (2007). Three histidine residues of amyloid-beta peptide control the redox activity of copper and iron. *Biochemistry* 46, 12737–12743. doi: 10.1021/bi701079z

Nelson, P. T., Alafuzoff, I., Bigio, E. H., Bouras, C., Braak, H., Cairns, N. J., et al. (2012). Correlation of Alzheimer disease neuropathologic changes with cognitive status: a review of the literature. *J. Neuropathol. Exp. Neurol.* 71, 362–381. doi: 10.1097/NEN.0b013e31825018f7

Nicotra, A., Pierucci, F., Parvez, H., and Senatori, O. (2004). Monoamine oxidase expression during development and aging. *Neurotoxicology* 25, 155–165. doi: 10.1016/S0161-813X(03)00095-0

Nielsen, J. A., Mena, E. E., Williams, I. H., Nocerini, M. R., and Liston, D. (1989). Correlation of brain levels of 9-amino-1, 2, 3, 4-tetrahydroacridine (THA) with neurochemical and behavioral changes.' *Eur. J. Pharmacol.* 173, 53–64. doi: 10.1016/0014-2999(89)90008-3

Nochi, S., Asakawa, N., and Sato, T. (1995). Kinetic study on the inhibition of acetylcholinesterase by 1-benzyl-4-[(5,6-dimethoxy-1-indanon)-2-yl]methylpiperidine hydrochloride (E2020). *Biol. Pharm. Bull.* 18, 1145–1147. doi: 10.1248/bpb.18.1145

Nunomura, A., Perry, G., Pappolla, M. A., Friedland, R. P., Hirai, K., Chiba, S., et al. (2000). Neuronal oxidative stress precedes amyloid-beta deposition in Down syndrome. *J. Neuropathol. Exp. Neurol.* 59, 1011–1017. doi: 10.1093/jnen/59.11.1011

O'Carroll, A. M., Fowler, C. J., Phillips, J. P., Tobbia, I., and Tipton, K. F. (1983). The deamination of dopamine by human brain monoamine oxidase. Specificity for the two enzyme forms in seven brain regions. *Naunyn Schmiedebergs Arch. Pharmacol.* 322, 198–202.

O'Carroll, A. M., Tipton, K. F., Sullivan, J. P., Fowler, C. J., and Ross, S. B. (1987). Intra- and extrasynaptosomal deamination of dopamine and noradrenaline by the two forms of human brain monoamine oxidase. Implications for the neurotoxicity of N-methyl-4-phenyl-1, 2, 3, 6- tetrahydropyridine in man. *Biog. Amines* 4, 165–178.

Odetti, P., Angelini, G., Dapino, D., Zaccheo, D., Garibaldi, S., Dagna-Bricarelli, F., et al. (1998). Early glycoxidation damage in brains from Down's syndrome. *Biochem. Biophys. Res. Commun.* 132, 849–851. doi: 10.1006/bbrc.1998.8186

Ollis, D. L., Cheah, E., Cygler, M., Dijkstra, B., Frolow, F., Franken, S. M., et al. (1992). The α/β hydrolase fold. *Protein Eng.* 5, 197–211. doi: 10.1093/protein/5.3.197

Panayi, A. E., Spyrou, N. M., Iversen, B. S., and White, M. A. (2002). Determination of cadmium and zinc in Alzheimer's brain tissue using inductively coupled plasma mass spectrometry. *J. Neurol. Sci.* 195, 1–10. doi: 10.1016/S0022-510X(01)00672-4

Paoletti, P., Ascher, P., and Neyton, J. (1997). High-affinity zinc inhibition of NMDA NR1–NR2A receptors. *J. Neurosci.* 17, 5711–5725.

Park, I. H., Jung, M. W., Mori, H., and Mook-Jung, I. (2001). Zinc enhances synthesis of presenilin 1 in mouse primary cortical culture. *Biochem. Biophys. Res. Commun.* 285, 680–688. doi: 10.1006/bbrc.2001.5243

Parsons, C. G., Danysz, W., Bartmann, A., Spielmanns, P., Frankiewicz, T., Hesselink, M., et al. (1999). Amino-alkyl-cyclohexanes are novel uncompetitive NMDA receptor antagonists with strong voltage-dependency and fast blocking kinetics: *in vitro* and *in vivo* characterization. *Neuropharmacology* 38, 85–108. doi: 10.1016/S0028-3908(98)00161-0

Pei, J. J., An, W. L., Zhou, X. W., Nishimura, T., Norberg, J., Benedikz, E., et al. (2006). P70 S6 kinase mediates tau phosphorylation and synthesis. *FEBS Lett.* 580, 107–114. doi: 10.1016/j.febslet.2005.11.059

Percy, M., Moalem, S., Garcia, A., Somerville, M. J., Hicks, M., Andrews, D., et al. (2008). Involvement of ApoE E4 and H63D in sporadic Alzheimer's disease in a folate-supplemented Ontario population. *J. Alzheimers Dis.* 14, 69–84.

Pérez, V., and Unzeta, M. (2003). PF9601N, a new MAO B inhibitor, attenuates MPTP-induced depletion of striatal dopamine levels in C57/BL6 mice. *Nurochem. Int.* 42, 221–239. doi: 10.1016/S0197-0186(02)00091-8

Pérez, V., Marco, J. L., Fernández-Álvarez, E., and Unzeta, M. (1999). Relevance of benzyloxy group in 2-indolyl methylamines in the selective MAO-B inhibition. *Br. J. Pharmacol.* 12, 869–876. doi: 10.1038/sj.bjp.0702600

Pérez, V., Romera, M., Lizcano, J. M., Marco, J. L., and Unzeta, M. (2003). Protective effect of PF 9601N, a novel MAO B inhibitor, on dopamine lesioned PC12 cells. *J. Pharm. Pharmacol.* 55, 713–716. doi: 10.1211/002235703765344649

Perl, D. P. (2010). Neuropathology of Alzheimer's disease. *Mt Sinai J. Med.* 77, 32–42. doi: 10.1002/msj.20157

Perrone, L., Mothes, E., Vignes, M., Mockel, A., Figueroa, C., Miquel, M. C., et al. (2010). Copper transfer from Cu-Abeta to human serum albumin inhibits aggregation, radical production and reduces Abeta toxicity. *Chembiochem* 11, 110–118. doi: 10.1002/cbic.200900474

Perry, E. K., Perry, R. H., Blessed, G., and Tomlinson, B. E. (1978). Changes in brain cholinesterases in senile dementia of Alzheimer type. *Neuropathol. Appl. Neurobiol.* 4, 273–277. doi: 10.1111/j.1365-2990.1978.tb00545.x

Petersen, R. B., Nunomura, A., Lee, H. G., Casadesus, G., Perry, G., Smith, M. A., et al. (2007). Signal transduction cascades associated with oxidative stress in Alzheimer's disease. *J. Alzheimers Dis.* 11, 143–152.

Petousi, N., and Robbins, P. A. (2014). Human adaptation to the hypoxia of high altitude: the Tibetan paradigm from the pregenomic to the postgenomic era. *J. Appl. Physiol.* 116, 875–884. doi: 10.1152/japplphysiol.00605.2013

Praticò, 2008###Praticò, D. (2008). Evidence of oxidative stress in Alzheimer's disease brain and antioxidant therapy: lights and shadows. *Ann. N.Y. Acad. Sci.* 1147, 70–78. doi: 10.1196/annals.1427.010

Qian, J., and Noebels, J. L. (2005). Visualization of transmitter release with zinc fluorescence detection at the mouse hippocampal mossy fibre synapse. *J. Physiol.* 566, 747–758. doi: 10.1113/jphysiol.2005.089276

Qizilbash, N., Whitehead, A., Higgins, J., Wilcock, G., Schneider, L., and Farlow, M. (1998). Cholinesterase inhibition for Alzheimer's disease: a meta-analysis of the tacrine trials. *J. Am. Med. Assoc.* 280, 1777–1782. doi: 10.1001/jama.280. 20.1777

Ramadan, Z. B., Dostert, P., and Tipton, K. F. (1999). Some peculiar aspects of monoamine oxidase inhibition. *Neurobiology* 7, 159–174.

Ramadan, Z. B., and Tipton, K. F. (1998). Cyanide potentiates the inhibition of monoamine oxidase by hydrazine derivatives. *J. Neurochem.* 71, S36–S36.

Ramadan, Z. B., Wrang, M. L., and Tipton, K. F. (2007). Species differences in the selective inhibition of monoamine oxidase (1-methyl-2-phenylethyl) hydrazine and its potentiation by cyanide. *Neurochem. Res.* 32, 1783–1790. doi: 10.1007/s11064-007-9309-x

Reinikainen, K. J., Paljarvi, L., Huuskonen, M., Soininen, H., Laakso, M., and Riekkinen, P. J. (1988). A post-mortem study of noradrenergic, serotonergic and GABAergic neurons in Alzheimer's disease. *J. Neurol. Sci.* 84, 101–116. doi: 10.1016/0022-510X(88)90179-7

Religa, D., Strozyk, D., Cherny, R. A., Volitakis, I., Haroutunian, V., Winblad, B., et al. (2006). Elevated cortical zinc in Alzheimer disease. *Neurology* 67, 69–75. doi: 10.1212/01.wnl.0000223644.08653.b5

Rogers, J. T., Randall, J. D., Cahill, C. M., Eder, P. S., Huang, X., Gunshin, L., et al. (2002). An iron-responsive element type II in the 5-untranslated region of the Alzheimer's amyloid precursor protein transcript. *J. Biol. Chem.* 277, 45518–45528. doi: 10.1074/jbc.M207435200

Rogers, J., Webster, S., Lue, L. F., Brachova, L., Civin, W. H., Emmerling, M., et al. (1996). Inflammation and Alzheimer's disease pathogenesis. *Neurobiol. Aging* 17, 681–686. doi: 10.1016/0197-4580(96)00115-7

Rosini, M., Simoni, E., Milelli, A., Minarini, A., and Melchiorre, C. (2014). Oxidative stress in Alzheimer's disease: are we connecting the dots? *J. Med. Chem.* 57, 2821–2831. doi: 10.1021/jm400970m

Rottkamp, C. A., Raina, A. K., Zhu, X. W., Gaier, E., Bush, A. I., Atwood, C. S., et al. (2001). Redox-active iron mediates amyloid-b toxicity. *Free Rad. Biol. Med.* 30, 447–450. doi: 10.1016/S0891-5849(00)00494-9

Ruiz, A., Walker, M. C., Fabian-Fine, R., and Kullmann, D. M. (2004). Endogenous zinc inhibits GABA (A) receptors in a hippocampal pathway. *J. Neurophysiol.* 91, 1091–1096. doi: 10.1152/jn.00755.2003

Salkovic-Petrisic, M., Knezovic, A., Osmanovic-Barilar, J., Smailovic, U., Trkulja, V., Riederer, P., et al. (2015). Multi-target iron-chelators improve memory loss in a rat model of sporadic Alzheimer's disease. *Life Sci.* 136, 108–119. doi: 10.1016/j.lfs.2015.06.026

Samadi, A., Valderas, C., de los Ríos, C., Bastida, A., Chioua, M., González-Lafuente, L., et al. (2011). Cholinergic and neuroprotective drugs for the treatment of Alzheimer and neuronal vascular diseases. II. Synthesis, biological assessment, and molecular modelling of new tacrine analogues from highly substituted 2-aminopyridine-3-carbonitriles. *Bioorg. Med. Chem.* 19, 122–133. doi: 10.1016/j.bmc.2010.11.040

Samudralwar, D. L., Diprete, C. C., Ni, B. F., Ehmann, W. D., and Markesbery, W. (1995). Elemental imbalances in the olfactory pathway in Alzheimer's disease. *J. Neurol. Sci.* 130, 139–145. doi: 10.1016/0022-510X(95)00018-W

Sanz, E., Quintana, A., Hidalgo, J., Marco, J. L., and Unzeta, M. (2009). PF 9601N confers MAOB independent neuroprotection in ER-stress-induced cell death. *Mol. Cell. Neurosci.* 41, 19–31. doi: 10.1016/j.mcn.2009.01.005

Saura, J., Kettler, R., Da, P. M., and Richards, J. G. (1992). Quantitative enzyme radioautography with 3H-Ro 41-1049 and 3H-Ro 19-6327 *in vitro*: localization and abundance of MAO-A and MAO-B in rat CNS, peripheral organs, and human brain. *J. Neurosci.* 12, 1977–1999.

Sayre, L. M., Perry, G., Harris, P. L., Liu, Y., Schubert, K. A., and Smith, M. A. (2000). *In situ* oxidative catalysis by neurofibrillary tangles and senile plaques in Alzheimer's disease: a central role for bound transition metals. *J. Neurochem.* 74, 270–279. doi: 10.1046/j.1471-4159.2000.0740270.x

Schipper, H. M., Bennett, D. A., Liberman, A., Bienias, J. L., Schneider, J. A., Kelly, J., et al. (2006). Glial heme oxygenase-1 expression in Alzheimer disease and mild cognitive impairment. *Neurobiol. Aging* 27, 252–261. doi: 10.1016/j.neurobiolaging.2005.01.016

Schliebs, R. (2005). Basal forebrain cholinergic dysfunction in Alzheimer's disease–interrelationship with beta-amyloid, inflammation and neurotrophin signaling. *Neurochem. Res.* 30, 895–908. doi: 10.1007/s11064-005-6962-9

Schlief, M. L., Craig, A. M., and Gitlin, J. D. (2005). NMDA receptor activation mediates copper homeostasis in hippocampal neurons. *J. Neurosci.* 25, 239–246. doi: 10.1523/JNEUROSCI.3699-04.2005

Schlief, M. L., West, T., Craig, A. M., Holtzman, D. M., and Gitlin, J. D. (2006). Role of the Menkes copper-transporting ATPase in NMDA receptor-mediated neuronal toxicity. *Proc. Natl. Acad. Sci. U.S.A.* 103, 14919–14924. doi: 10.1073/pnas.0605390103

Schubert, D., Behl, C., Lesley, R., Brack, A., Dargusch, R., Sagara, Y., et al. (1995). Amyloid peptides are toxic via a common oxidative mechanism. *Proc. Natl. Acad. Sci. U.S.A.* 14, 1989–1993. doi: 10.1073/pnas.92.6.1989

Schubert, D., and Chevion, M. (1995). The role of iron in beta amyloid toxicity.' *Biochem. Biophys. Res. Commun.* 216, 702–707. doi: 10.1006/bbrc.1995.2678

Selkoe, D. J. (1994). Alzheimer's disease: a central role for amyloid. *J. Neuropathol. Exp. Neurol.* 53, 438–447. doi: 10.1097/00005072-199409000-00003

Serrano, M. P., Herrero-Labrador, R., Futch, H. S., Serrano, J., Romero, A., Fernandez, A. P., et al. (2016). The proof-of-concept of ASS234: Peripherally administered ASS234 enters the central nervous system and reduces pathology in a mouse model of Alzheimer's disease. *J. Psychiatry Neurosci.*

Serrano-Pozo, A., Qian, J., Monsell, S. E., Frosch, M. P., Betensky, R. A., and Hyman, B. (2013). Examination of the clinicopathologic continuum of Alzheimer disease in the autopsy cohort of the National Alzheimer Coordinating Center. *J. Neuropathol. Exp. Neurol.* 72, 1182–1192. doi: 10.1097/NEN.0000000000000016

Shan, W. J., Huang, L., Zhou, Q., Meng, F. C., and Li, X. S. (2011). Synthesis, biological evaluation of 9-N-substituted berberine derivatives as multi-functional agents of antioxidant, inhibitors of acetylcholinesterase, butyrylcholinesterase and amyloid-β aggregation. *Eur. J. Med. Chem.* 46, 5885–5893. doi: 10.1016/j.ejmech.2011.09.051

Shin, R. W., Iwaki, T., Kitamoto, T., Sato, Y., and Tateishi, J. (1992). Massive accumulation of modified tau and severe depletion of normal tau characterize the cerebral cortex and white matter of Alzheimer's disease: demonstration using the hydrated autoclaving method. *Am. J. Pathol.* 140, 937–945.

Shoffner, J. M. (1997). Oxidative phosphorylation defects and Alzheimer's disease. *Neurogenetics* 1, 13–19. doi: 10.1007/s100480050002

Silvestri, L., and Camaschella, C. (2008). A potential pathogenetic role of iron in Alzheimer's disease. *J. Cell Mol. Med.* 12, 1548–1550. doi: 10.1111/j.1582-4934.2008.00356.x

Smith, D. P., Smith, D. G., Curtain, C. C., Boas, J. F., Pilbrow, J. R., Ciccotosto, G. D., et al. (2006). Copper-mediated amyloid-beta toxicity is associated with an intermolecular histidine bridge. *J. Biol. Chem.* 281, 15145–15154. doi: 10.1074/jbc.M600417200

Smith, M. A., Hirai, K., Hsiao, K., Pappolla, M. A., Harris, P. L., Siedlak, S. L., et al. (1998). Amyloid-beta deposition in Alzheimer transgenic mice is associated with oxidative stress. *J. Neurochem.* 70, 2212–2215. doi: 10.1046/j.1471-4159.1998.70052212.x

Song, M. S., Rauw, G., Baker, G. B., and Kar, S. (2008). Memantine protects rat cortical cultured neurons against beta-amyloid-induced toxicity by attenuating tau phosphorylation. *Eur. J. Neurosci.* 28, 1989–2002. doi: 10.1111/j.1460-9568.2008.06498.x

Soreq, H., and Seidman, S. (2001). Acetylcholinesterase–new roles for an old actor. *Nat. Rev. Neurosci.* 2, 294–302. doi: 10.1038/35067589

Stasiak, A., Mussur, M., Unzeta, M., Samadi, A., Marco-Contelles, J. L., and Fogel, W. A. (2014). Effects of novel monoamine oxidases and cholinesterases targeting compounds on brain neurotransmitters and behavior in rat model of vascular dementia. *Curr. Pharm. Des.* 20, 161–171. doi: 10.2174/13816128113199990026

Stoltenberg, M., Bruhn, M., Sondergaard, C., Doering, P., West, M. J., Larsen, A., et al. (2005). Immersion autometallographic tracing of zinc ions in Alzheimer beta-amyloid plaques. *Histochem. Cell Biol.* 123, 605–611. doi: 10.1007/s00418-005-0787-0

Strolin-Benedetti, M., Dostert, P., and Tipton, K. F. (1992). Developmental aspects of the monoamine-degrading enzyme monoamine oxidase. *Dev. Pharmacol. Ther.* 18, 191–200.

Struble, R. G., Cork, L. C., Whitehouse, P. J., and Price, D. L. (1982). Cholinergic innervation in neuritic plaques. *Science* 216, 413–415. doi: 10.1126/science.6803359

Su, X. Y., Wu, W. H., Huang, Z. P., Hu, J., Lei, P., Yu, C. H., et al. (2007). Hydrogen peroxide can be generated by tau in the presence of Cu (II). *Biochem. Biophys. Res. Commun.* 358, 661–665. doi: 10.1016/j.bbrc.2007.04.191

Suh, S. W., Jensen, K. B., Jensen, M. S., Silva, D. S., Kesslak, P. J., Danscher, G., et al. (2000). Histochemically-reactive zinc in amyloid plaques, angiopathy, and degenerating neurons of Alzheimer's diseased brains. *Brain Res.* 852, 274–278. doi: 10.1016/S0006-8993(99)02096-X

Sultana, R., Mecocci, P., Mangialasche, F., Cecchetti, R., Baglioni, M., and Butterfield, D. A. (2011). Increased protein and lipid oxidative damage in mitochondria isolated from lymphocytes from patients with Alzheimer's disease: insights into the role of oxidative stress in Alzheimer's disease and initial investigations into a potential biomarker for this dementing disorder. *J. Alzheimers Dis.* 24, 77–84. doi: 10.3233/JAD-2011-101425

Sussman, J. L., Harel, M., Frolow, F., Oefner, C., Goldman, A., Toker, L., et al. (1991). Atomic structure of acetylcholinesterase from Torpedo californica: a prototypic acetylcholine-binding protein. *Science* 253, 872–879. doi: 10.1126/science.1678899

Syme, C. D., Nadal, R. C., Rigby, S. E. J., and Viles, J. H. (2004). Copper binding to the amyloid-beta (Abeta) peptide associated with Alzheimer's disease: folding, coordination geometry, pH dependence, stoichiometry, and affinity of Abeta-(1-28): insights from a range of complementary spectroscopic techniques. *J. Biol. Chem.* 279, 18169–18177. doi: 10.1074/jbc.M313572200

Terry, R. D., Gonatas, N. K., and Weiss, M. (1964). Ultrastructural studies in Alzheimer'spresenile dementia. *Ann. J. Pathol.* 44, 269–297.

Thies, W., and Bleiler, L. (2012). Alzheimer's association: Alzheimer's disease facts and figures. *Alzheimers Dement.* 8, 131–168.

Thies, W., and Bleiler, L. (2013). Alzheimer's disease: Facts and figures. *Alzheimer Dement.* 9, 208–215. doi: 10.1016/j.jalz.2013.02.003

Touchon, J., Bergman, H., Bullock, R., Rapatz, G., Nagel, J., and Lane, R. (2006). Response to rivastigmine or donepezil in Alzheimer's patients with symptoms suggestive of concomitant Lewy body pathology. *Curr. Med. Res. Opin.* 22, 49–59. doi: 10.1185/030079906X80279

Tougu, V., Karafin, A., and Palumaa, P. (2008). Binding of zinc (II) and copper (II) to the full-length Alzheimer's amyloid-beta peptide. *J. Neurochem.* 104, 1249–1259. doi: 10.1111/j.1471-4159.2007.05061.x

Traynelis, S. F., Burgess, M. F., Zheng, F., Lyuboslavsky, P., and Powers, J. L. (1998). Control of voltage-independent zinc inhibition of NMDA receptors by the NR1 subunit. *J. Neurosci.* 18, 6163–6175.

Tremblay, R., Chakravarthy, B., Hewitt, K., Tauskela, J., Morley, P., Atkinson, T., et al. (2000). Transient NMDA receptor inactivation provides long-term protection to cultured cortical neurons from a variety of death signals. *J. Neurosci.* 20, 7183–7192.

Tsang, D., Ho, K. P., and Wen, H. L. (1986). Ontogenesis of multiple forms of monoamine oxidase in rat brain regions and liver. *Dev. Neurosci.* 8, 243–250. doi: 10.1159/000112258

Uchida, Y., Takio, K., Titani, K., Ihara, Y., and Tomonaga, M. (1991). The growth inhibitory factor that is deficient in the Alzheimer's disease brain is a 68 amino acid metallothionein-like protein. *Neuron* 7, 337–347. doi: 10.1016/0896-6273(91)90272-2

Van Eersel, J., Bi, M., Ke, Y. D., Hodges, J. R., Xuereb, J. H., Gregory, G. C., et al. (2009). Phosphorylation of soluble tau differs in Pick's disease and Alzheimer's disease brains. *J. Neural Trans.* 116, 1243–1251. doi: 10.1007/s00702-009-0293-y

Vermeiren, Y., Van Dam, D., Aerts, T., Engelborghs, S., Martin, J. J., and De Deyn, P. P. (2015). The monoaminergic footprint of depression and psychosis in dementia with Lewy bodies compared to Alzheimer's disease. *Alzheimers Res Ther.* 7, 7. doi: 10.1186/s13195-014-0090-1

Vogels, O. J., Broere, C. A., ter Laak, H. J., ten Donkelaar, H. J., Nieuwenhuys, R., and Schulte, B. P. (1990). Cell loss and shrinkage in the nucleus basalis Meynert complex in Alzheimer's disease. *Neurobiol. Aging* 11, 3–13. doi: 10.1016/0197-4580(90)90056-6

Vogt, K., Mellor, J., Tong, G., and Nicoll, R. (2000). The actions of synaptically released zinc at hippocampal mossy fiber synapses. *Neuron* 26, 187–196. doi: 10.1016/S0896-6273(00)81149-6

Von Bernhardi, R., and Eugenín, J. (2012). Alzheimer's disease: redox dysregulation as a common denominator for diverse pathogenic mechanisms. *Antioxid. Redox Signal.* 16, 974–1031. doi: 10.1089/ars.2011.4082

Wang, C. Y., Wang, T., Zheng, W., Zhao, B. L., Danscher, G., Chen, Y. H., et al. (2010). Zinc overload enhances APP cleavage and Abeta deposition in the Alzheimer mouse brain. *PLoS ONE* 5:e15349. doi: 10.1371/journal.pone.0015349

Wang, L., Esteban, G., Ojima, M., Bautista-Aguilera, O. M., Inokuchi, T., Moraleda, I., et al. (2014). Donepezil+propargylamine+8-hydroxyquinoline hybrids as new multifunctional metal-chelators, ChE and MAO inhibitors for the potential treatment of Alzheimer's disease. *Eur. J. Med. Chem.* 80, 543–561. doi: 10.1016/j.ejmech.2014.04.078

Wang, X., Su, B., Zheng, L., Perry, G., Smith, M. A., and Zhu, X. (2009). The role of abnormal mitochondrial dynamics in the pathogenesis of Alzheimer's disease. *J. Neurochem.* 109, 153–159. doi: 10.1111/j.1471-4159.2009.05867.x

Westlund, K. N., Denney, R. M., Kochersperger, L. M., Rose, R. M., and Abell, C. W. (1988). Distinct monoamine oxidase A and B populations in primate brain. *Science* 230, 181–183. doi: 10.1126/science.3875898

White, A. R., Multhaup, G., Maher, F., Bellingham, S., Camakaris, J., Zheng, H., et al. (1999). The Alzheimer's disease amyloid precursor protein modulates copper-induced toxicity and oxidative stress in primary neuronal cultures. *J. Neurosci.* 19, 9170–9179.

Wilkinson, D., and Murray, J. (2001). Galantamine: a randomized, double-blind, dose comparison in patients with Alzheimer's disease. *Int. J. Geriatr. Psychiatry* 16, 852–857. doi: 10.1002/gps.409

Willard, L. B., Hauss-Wegrzyniak, B., Danysz, W., and Wenk, G. L. (2000). The cytotoxicity of chronic neuroinflammation upon basal forebrain cholinergic neurons of rats can be attenuated by glutamatergic antagonism or cyclooxygenase-2 inhibition. *Exp. Brain Res.* 134, 58–65. doi: 10.1007/s002210000446

Wright, C. I., Geula, C., and Mesulam, M. M. (1993). Neurological cholinesterases in the normal brain and in Alzheimer's disease: relationship to plaques, tangles, and patterns of selective vulnerability. *Ann. Neurol.* 34, 373–384. doi: 10.1002/ana.410340312

Wu, M. Y., Esteban, G., Brogi, S., Shionoya, M., Wang, L., Campiani, G., et al. (2015). Donepezil-like multifunctional agents: design, synthesis, molecular modelling and biological evaluation. *Eur. J. Med. Chem.* doi: 10.1016/j.ejmech.2015.10.001. [Epub ahead of print].

Wu, W., Lei, P., Liu, Q., Hu, J., Gunn, A. P., Chen, M., et al. (2008). Sequestration of copper from beta-amyloid promotes selective lysis by cyclen-hybrid cleavage agents. *J. Biol. Chem.* 283, 31657–31664. doi: 10.1074/jbc.M804722200

Xie, W., Stribley, J. A., Chatonnet, A., Wilder, P. J., Rizzino, A., McComb, R. D., et al. (2000). Postnatal developmental delay and supersensitivity to organophosphate in gene-targeted mice lacking acetylcholinesterase. *J. Pharmacol. Exp. Ther.* 293, 896–902.

Yamamoto, A., Shin, R. W., Hasegawa, K., Naiki, H., Sato, H., Kitamoto, T., et al. (2002). Iron (III) induces aggregation of hyperphosphorylated tau and its reduction to iron (II) reverses the aggregation: Implications in the formation of neurofibrillary tangles of Alzheimer's disease. *J. Neurochem.* 82, 1137–1147. doi: 10.1046/j.1471-4159.2002.t01-1-01061.x

You, H., Tsutsui, S., Hameed, S., Kannanayakal, T. J., Chen, L., Xia, P., et al. (2012). Ab neurotoxicity depends on interactions between copper ions, prion protein, and N-methyl-D-aspartate receptors. *Proc. Natl. Acad. Sci. U.S.A.* 109, 1737–1742. doi: 10.1073/pnas.1110789109

Youdim, M. B. H., Edmondson, D., and Tipton, K. F. (2006). The therapeutic potential of monoamine oxidase inhibitors. *Nat. Rev. Neurosci.* 7, 295–309. doi: 10.1038/nrn1883

Youdim, M. B. H., Maruyama, W., and Naoi, M. (2005). Neuropharmacological, neuroprotective and amyloid precursor processing properties of selective MAO-B inhibitor antiparkinsonian drug, rasagiline. *Drugs Today* 41, 369–391. doi: 10.1358/dot.2005.41.6.893613

Yu, W. H., Lukiw, W. J., Bergeron, C., Niznik, H. B., and Fraser, P. E. (2001). Metallothionein III is reduced in Alzheimer's disease. *Brain Res.* 894, 37–45. doi: 10.1016/S0006-8993(00)03196-6

Zheng, H., Gal, S., Weiner, L. M., Bar-Am, O., Warshawsky, A., Fridkin, M., et al. (2005). Novel multifunctional neuroprotective iron chelator-monoamine oxidase inhibitor drugs for neurodegenerative diseases: *in vitro* studies on antioxidant activity, prevention of lipid peroxide formation and monoamine oxidase inhibition. *J. Neurochem.* 95, 68–78. doi: 10.1111/j.1471-4159.2005.03340.x

Zhou, L. X., Du, J. T., Zeng, Z. Y., Wu, W. H., Zhao, Y. F., Kanazawa, K., et al. (2007). Copper (II) modulates *in vitro* aggregation of tau peptide. *Peptides* 28, 2229–2234. doi: 10.1016/j.peptides.2007.08.022

Zhu, X., Lee, H. G., Perry, G., and Smith, M. A. (2007). Alzheimer disease, the two-hit hypothesis: an update. *Biochim. Biophys. Acta* 1772, 494–502. doi: 10.1016/j.bbadis.2006.10.014

Zhukareva, V., Vogelsberg-Ragaglia, V., Van Deerlin, V. M., Bruce, J., Shuck, T., Grossman, M., et al. (2001). Loss of brain tau defines novel sporadic and familial tauopathies with frontotemporal dementia. *Ann. Neurol.* 49, 165–175.

Zigler, J. S. Jr., Jernigan, H. M. Jr., Garland, D., and Reddy, V. N. (2015). The effects of "oxygen radicals" generated in the medium on lenses in organ culture: inhibition of damage by chelated iron. *Arch. Biochem. Biophys.* 241, 163–172. doi: 10.1016/0003-9861(85)90372-8

Conflict of Interest Statement: The authors declare that the research was conducted in the absence of any commercial or financial relationships that could be construed as a potential conflict of interest.

Permissions

All chapters in this book were first published in SBDDDTND, by Frontiers Media SA; hereby published with permission under the Creative Commons Attribution License or equivalent. Every chapter published in this book has been scrutinized by our experts. Their significance has been extensively debated. The topics covered herein carry significant findings which will fuel the growth of the discipline. They may even be implemented as practical applications or may be referred to as a beginning point for another development.

The contributors of this book come from diverse backgrounds, making this book a truly international effort. This book will bring forth new frontiers with its revolutionizing research information and detailed analysis of the nascent developments around the world.

We would like to thank all the contributing authors for lending their expertise to make the book truly unique. They have played a crucial role in the development of this book. Without their invaluable contributions this book wouldn't have been possible. They have made vital efforts to compile up to date information on the varied aspects of this subject to make this book a valuable addition to the collection of many professionals and students.

This book was conceptualized with the vision of imparting up-to-date information and advanced data in this field. To ensure the same, a matchless editorial board was set up. Every individual on the board went through rigorous rounds of assessment to prove their worth. After which they invested a large part of their time researching and compiling the most relevant data for our readers.

The editorial board has been involved in producing this book since its inception. They have spent rigorous hours researching and exploring the diverse topics which have resulted in the successful publishing of this book. They have passed on their knowledge of decades through this book. To expedite this challenging task, the publisher supported the team at every step. A small team of assistant editors was also appointed to further simplify the editing procedure and attain best results for the readers.

Apart from the editorial board, the designing team has also invested a significant amount of their time in understanding the subject and creating the most relevant covers. They scrutinized every image to scout for the most suitable representation of the subject and create an appropriate cover for the book.

The publishing team has been an ardent support to the editorial, designing and production team. Their endless efforts to recruit the best for this project, has resulted in the accomplishment of this book. They are a veteran in the field of academics and their pool of knowledge is as vast as their experience in printing. Their expertise and guidance has proved useful at every step. Their uncompromising quality standards have made this book an exceptional effort. Their encouragement from time to time has been an inspiration for everyone.

The publisher and the editorial board hope that this book will prove to be a valuable piece of knowledge for researchers, students, practitioners and scholars across the globe.

List of Contributors

José Marco-Contelles
Laboratory of Medicinal Chemistry, Institute of General Organic Chemistry, Cajal Institute (CSIC), Madrid, Spain

Mercedes Unzeta, Irene Bolea and Gerard Esteban
Departament de Bioquímica i Biologia Molecular, Facultat de Medicina, Institut de Neurociències, Universitat Autònoma de Barcelona, Barcelona, Spain

Rona R. Ramsay
Biomedical Sciences Research Complex, University of St Andrews, St Andrews, UK

Alejandro Romero
Department of Toxicology and Pharmacology, Faculty of Veterinary Medicine, Complutense University of Madrid, Madrid, Spain

Ricard Martínez-Murillo
Neurovascular Research Group, Department of Molecular, Cellular and Developmental Neurobiology, Cajal Institute (CSIC), Madrid, Spain

M. Carmo Carreiras
Research Institute for Medicines and Pharmaceutical Sciences (iMed.ULisboa), Faculty of Pharmacy, University of Lisbon, Lisbon, Portugal

Lhassane Ismaili
Laboratoire de Chimie Organique et Thérapeutique, Neurosciences Intégratives et Cliniques EA 481, Université Franche-Comté, Université Bourgogne Franche-Comté, UFR SMP, Besançon, France

Rebecca E. Hughes and Rona R. Ramsay
School of Biology, BMS Building, University of St Andrews, St Andrews, UK

Katarina Nikolic
Department of Pharmaceutical Chemistry, Faculty of Pharmacy, University of Belgrade, Belgrade, Serbia

Dubravka Svob Strac and Nela Pivac
Division of Molecular Medicine, Rudjer Boskovic Institute, Zagreb, Croatia

Ilse J. Smolders
Department of Pharmaceutical Chemistry and Drug Analysis, Vrije Universiteit Brussel, Brussels, Belgium

Wieslawa A. Fogel
Department of Hormone Biochemistry, Medical University of Lodz, Lodz, Poland

Philippe De Deurwaerdere
Centre National de la Recherche Scientifique (Unité Mixte de Recherche 5293), Institut of Neurodegenerative Diseases, Bordeaux Cedex, France

Giuseppe Di Giovanni
Laboratory of Neurophysiology, Department of Physiology and Biochemistry, University of Malta, Msida, Malta

Dorotea Mück-Šeler and Matea Nikolac Perkovic
Division of Molecular Medicine, Rudjer Boskovic Institute, Zagreb, Croatia

Montse Sole
Departament de Bioquímica i Biologia Molecular, Facultat de Medicina, Institut de Neurociències, Universitat Autònoma de Barcelona, Barcelona, Spain

Keith F. Tipton
School of Biochemistry and Immunology, Trinity College Dublin, Dublin, Ireland

Laura Della Corte
Department of Neuroscience, University of Florence, Florence, Italy

Anna Stasiak
Department of Hormone Biochemistry, Medical University of Lodz, Lodz, Poland

Magdalena Majekova
Department of Biochemical Pharmacology, Institute of Experimental Pharmacology and Toxicology, Slovak Academy of Sciences, Bratislava, Slovakia

Milagros Medina
Departamento de Bioquímica y Biología Molecular y Celular, Facultad de Ciencias and BIFI, Universidad de Zaragoza, Zaragoza, Spain

Massimo Valoti
Dipartimento di Scienze della Vita, Università degli Studi di Siena, Siena, Italy

Mohammad A. Khanfar
Stark Lab, Institut fuer Pharmazeutische and Medizinische Chemie, Heinrich-Heine-Universitaet Duesseldorf, Duesseldorf, Germany
Faculty of Pharmacy, The University of Jordan, Amman, Jordan

Anna Affini, Kiril Lutsenko and Holger Stark
Stark Lab, Institut fuer Pharmazeutische and Medizinische Chemie, Heinrich-Heine-Universitaet Duesseldorf, Duesseldorf, Germany

Stefania Butini
Department of Biotechnology, Chemistry and Pharmacy, European Research Centre for Drug Discovery and Development, University of Siena, Siena, Italy

Jelica Vucicevic and Danica Agbaba
Department of Pharmaceutical Chemistry, Faculty of Pharmacy, University of Belgrade, Belgrade, Serbia

Lazaros Mavridis
School of Biological and Chemical Sciences, Queen Mary University of London, London, UK

Teodora Djikic and Kemal Yelekci
Department of Bioinformatics and Genetics, Faculty of Engineering and Natural Sciences, Kadir Has University, Istanbul, Turkey

John B. O. Mitchell
EaStCHEM School of Chemistry and Biomedical Sciences Research Complex, University of St Andrews, St Andrews, UK

Samuele Maramai, Sandra Gemma, Simone Brogi, Giuseppe Campiani and Margherita Brindisi
European Research Centre for Drug Discovery and Development and Department of Biotechnology, Chemistry and Pharmacy, University of Siena, Siena, Italy

Holger Stark
Institut fuer Pharmazeutische and Medizinische Chemie, Heinrich-Heine-Universitaet Duesseldorf, Duesseldorf, Germany

Robert Vianello
Computational Organic Chemistry and Biochemistry Group, Ruąer Boškovic´ Institute, Zagreb, Croatia

Carmen Domene
Department of Chemistry, King's College London, London, UK
Chemistry Research Laboratory, University of Oxford, Oxford, UK

Janez Mavri
Department of Computational Biochemistry and Drug Design, National Institute of Chemistry, Ljubljana, Slovenia

Gerard Esteban
School of Biochemistry and Immunology, Trinity Biomedical Sciences Institute, Trinity College Dublin, Dublin, Ireland

Moussa B. H. Youdim
Department of Pharmacology, Ruth and Bruce Rappaport Faculty of Medicine, Eve Topf and National Parkinson Foundation Center for Neurodegenerative Diseases Research, Haifa, Israel

José Marco-Contelles
Laboratory of Medicinal Chemistry, Institute of General Organic Chemistry, Spanish National Research Council, Madrid, Spain

Index

www.ingramcontent.com/pod-product-compliance
Lightning Source LLC
Chambersburg PA
CBHW050445200326
41458CB00014B/5076